MEDICAL RADIOLOGY

Diagnostic Imaging and Radiation Oncology

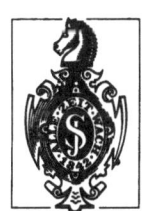

Innovations in Radiation Oncology

Contributors

K.K. Ang · R. Arriagada · H.T. Barkley, Jr. · M.M. Bortin · W.A. Brock
J.M. Brown · J.E. Byfield · G.T.Y. Chen · J.-M. Cosset · B.J. Cummings
L. Delclos · J.J. Diamond · T.J. Dougherty · G.H. Fletcher · F.A. Gibbs
G.P. Glasgow · E.S. Gragoudas · P.H. Gutin · G.E. Hanks · A.J. Hartz
R. Hawkins · R.M. Henkelman · R.T. Hoppe · J.-C. Horiot · R.L. Huckstep
T.J. Kinsella · S. Kramer · S.A. Leibel · R.R. Lichtman · R.D. Lindberg
M.H. Maor · P. McNulty · K.W. Mead · E.D. Montague · J.E. Munzenrider
J.R. Oleson · J. Papillon · L.J. Peters · M.E. Phelps · P.Y. Poon · T.A. Rich
W. Rider · J.M. Seddon · W.F. Sindelar · S. Strober · S.B. Sutcliffe · S.E. Taylor
J.E. Tepper · J.E. Till · Z. Tochner · M. Tubiana · M. Urie · C.C. Wang
T.E. Weisenburger · H.R. Withers · J.V. Wood · G.K. Zagars

Edited by

H. Rodney Withers and Lester J. Peters

Foreword by

Luther W. Brady and Hans-Peter Heilmann

With 111 Figures

Springer-Verlag
Berlin Heidelberg New York
London Paris Tokyo

H. Rodney Withers, M.D., D.Sc.
Director, Division of Experimental Radiation Oncology
Professor, Department of Radiation Oncology
University of California
Los Angeles, CA 90024
USA

Lester J. Peters, M.D.
Professor and Head, Division of Radiotherapy
The University of Texas M.D. Anderson Hospital and
Tumor Institute
Houston, TX 77030
USA

MEDICAL RADIOLOGY · Diagnostic Imaging and Radiation Oncology

Continuation of
Handbuch der medizinischen Radiologie
Encyclopedia of Medical Radiology

ISBN-13:978-3-642-83103-4   e-ISBN-13:978-3-642-83101-0
DOI: 10.1007/978-3-642-83101-0

Library of Congress Cataloging-in-Publication Data. Innovations in radiation oncology. (Medical radiology) Bibliography: P. Includes index. I. Cancer--Radiotherapy. I. Ang, K. K. (K.Kian) II. Withers, H. Rodney. III. Peters, Lester J., 1942-. IV. Series.
RC271.R3I44 1987   616.99'40642   87-19426
ISBN-13:978-3-642-83103-4 (U.S.)

2122/3130-543210

List of Contributors

K. KIAN ANG, M.D.
Associate Professor
Division of Radiotherapy
The University of Texas M.D. Anderson
Hospital and Tumor Institute
Houston, TX 77030
USA

RODRIGO ARRIAGADA, M.D.
Radiotherapy Department
Institute Gustave-Roussy
94800 Villejuif
France

H. THOMAS BARKLEY, Jr., M.D.
Associate Professor
Division of Radiotherapy
The University of Texas M.D. Anderson
Hospital and Tumor Institute
Houston, TX 77030
USA

MORTIMER M. BORTIN, M.D.
Scientific Director, International Bone
Marrow Transplant Registry
Professor, Department of Medicine
The Medical College of Wisconsin
Milwaukee, WI 53226
USA

WILLIAM A. BROCK, Ph.D.
Associate Professor
Department of Experimental
Radiotherapy
The University of Texas M.D. Anderson
Hospital and Tumor Institute
Houston, TX 77030
USA

J. MARTIN BROWN, D.Phil.
Professor
Division of Radiobiological Research
Department of Radiology
Stanford University Medical Center
Stanford, CA 94305
USA

JOHN E. BYFIELD, M.D., Ph.D.
Kern Regional Cancer Centre
Bakersfield, CA 933301
USA

GEORGE T.Y. CHEN, Ph.D.
Director, Division of Radiation Therapy
Physics
Professor, Department of Radiation
Oncology
University of Chicago
Chicago, IL 60637
USA

JEAN-MARC COSSET, M.D.
Radiotherapy Department
Institute Gustave-Roussy
Villejuif
France

BERNARD J. CUMMINGS, M.B., Ch.B.,
FRCPC
Professor, Department of Radiology
University of Toronto, Canada
Staff Radiation Oncologist
The Princess Margaret Hospital
500 Sherbourne Street
Toronto, Ontario M4X 1K9
Canada

LUIS DELCLOS, M.D.
Professor
Department of Clinical Radiotherapy
The University of Texas M.D. Anderson
Hospital and Tumor Institute
Houston, TX 77030
USA

JAMES J. DIAMOND, Ph.D.
Division of Research and Assessment
Services
American College of Radiology
Philadelphia, PA 19107
USA

THOMAS J. DOUGHERTY, Ph.D.
Head, Division of Radiation Biology
Department of Radiation Medicine
Roswell Park Memorial Institute
Buffalo, NY 14263
USA

GILBERT H. FLETCHER, M.D.
Professor
Department of Clinical Radiotherapy
The University of Texas M.D. Anderson
Hospital and Tumor Institute
Houston, TX 77030
USA

FREDERIC A. GIBBS, Jr., M.D.
Associate Professor
Division of Radiation Oncology
University of Utah Medical Center
Salt Lake City, UT 84132
USA

GLENN P. GLASGOW, Ph.D.
Professor
Head, Division of Therapeutic Physics
Department of Radiotherapy
Loyola University Medical Center
2160 South First Avenue
Maywood, IL 60153
USA

E.S. GRAGOUDAS, M.D.
Chief, Retina Service
Massachusetts Eye and Ear Infirmary
Associate Professor
Harvard Medical School
Boston, MA 02114
USA

PHILIP H. GUTIN, M.D.
Associate Professor
Departments of Neurological Surgery
and Radiation Oncology
Brain Tumor Research Center of the
Department of Neurological Surgery
University of California
San Francisco, CA 94143
USA

GERALD E. HANKS, M.D., F.A.C.R.
Director
Department of Radiation Oncology
Fox Chase Cancer Center
Philadelphia, PA 19111
USA

ARTHUR J. HARTZ, M.D., Ph.D.
Assistant Professor, Pennsylvania State
University School of Medicine
Director of Research, Milton S. Hershey
Medical Center
Hershey, P.A. 17033
USA

RANDALL HAWKINS, M.D., Ph.D.
Assistant Professor
Department of Radiological Sciences
University of California, Los Angeles
Los Angeles, CA 90024
USA

R. MARK HENKELMAN, Ph.D.
Professor and Associate Chairman
Department of Medical Biophysics
University of Toronto
Toronto, Ontario M4X 1K9
Canada

RICHARD T. HOPPE, M.D.
Associate Professor
Department of Therapeutic Radiology
Stanford University
Stanford, CA 94305
USA

JEAN-CLAUDE HORIOT, M.D.
Head, Department of Radiotherapy
Centre G.F. Leclerc
Professor of Radiotherapy
University of Dijon
21034 Dijon
France

RONALD L. HUCKSTEP, C.M.G., F.T.S.,
M.D., F.R.C.S., F.R.A.C.S
Professor and Chairman
Department of Traumatic and Ortho-
paedic Surgery and School of Surgery
The University of New South Wales
Kensington, Sydney
N.S.W., 2033 Australia

TIMOTHY J. KINSELLA, M.D.
Deputy Chief
Radiation Oncology Branch
National Cancer Institute
National Institutes of Health
Bethesda, MD 20892
USA

SIMON KRAMER, M.D., F.A.C.R
Distinguished Professor
Department of Radiation Therapy
& Nuclear Medicine
Thomas Jefferson University
Hospital
Philadelphia, PA 19107
USA

STEVEN A. LEIBEL, M.D.
Associate Professor
Department of Radiation Oncology
School of Medicine
University of California
San Francisco, CA 94143
USA

ROSEMARY R. LICHTMAN, Ph.D.
Assistant Research Psychologist
Department of Psychology
University of California
Los Angeles, CA 90024
USA

ROBERT D. LINDBERG, M.D.,
F.A.C.R.
Professor and Chairman
Department of Therapeutic
Radiology
Brown Cancer Center
Louisville, KY 40202
USA

MOSHE H. MAOR, M.D.
Associate Professor
Department of Radiotherapy
The University of Texas M.D. Anderson
Hospital and Tumor Institute
Houston, TX 77030
USA

P. MCNULTY, R.N.
Department of Radiation Medicine
Massachusetts General Hospital
Boston, MA 02114
USA

KEVIN W. MEAD, M.B.B.S, F.R.A.C.R,
F.R.C.R
Professor and Director
Institute of Oncology and Radiotherapy
Prince of Wales Hospital
Randwick, N.S.W. 2031
Australia

ELEANOR D. MONTAGUE, M.D.
Professor
Department of Clinical Radiotherapy
The University of Texas M.D. Anderson
Hospital and Tumor Institute
Houston, TX 77030
USA

JOHN E. MUNZENRIDER, M.D.
Associate Radiation Therapist
Department of Radiation Medicine
Massachusetts General Hospital
Associate Professor of Radiation Therapy
Harvard Medical School
Boston, MA 02114
USA

JAMES R. OLESON, M.D., Ph.D.
Associate Professor
Division of Radiation Oncology
Duke University Medical Center
Durham, NC 22710
USA

JEAN PAPILLON, M.D.
Professor of Radiotherapy
University of Lyon, and
Head, Radiotherapy Department
Centre Leon Berard
Lyon 69373
France

LESTER J. PETERS, M.D.
Professor and Head
Division of Radiotherapy
The University of Texas M.D. Anderson
Hospital and Tumor Institute
Houston, TX 77030
USA

MICHAEL E. PHELPS, Ph.D.
Professor, Chief, Division of Nuclear
Medicine and Biophysics
Chief, Laboratory of Nuclear Medicine
University of California
Los Angeles, CA 90024
USA

PETER Y. POON, M.B., F.R.C.P. (C)
Assistant Professor
Department of Diagnostic Radiology
University of Toronto
Toronto, Ontario M4X 1K9
Canada

TYVIN A. RICH, M.D.
Assistant Professor
Department of Radiotherapy
The University of Texas M.D. Anderson
Hospital and Tumor Institute
Houston, TX 77030
USA

WALTER RIDER, M.B., F.R.C.R.,
F.R.C.P.(C)
Professor Emeritus of Radiology
Otolaryngology and Medical Biophysics
P.O. Box 53, Niagara on the Lake
Ontario L0S 190
Canada

J.M. SEDDON, M.D.
Director, Epidemiology Unit
Massachusetts Eye and Ear Infirmary
Assistant Professor
Harvard Medical School
Boston, MA 02114
USA

WILLIAM F. SINDELAR, M.D., Ph.D.
Senior Investigator
Surgery Branch
National Cancer Institute
National Institutes of Health
Bethesda, MD 20892
USA

SAMUEL STROBER, M.D.
Professor
Division of Immunology
Department of Medicine
Stanford University
Stanford, CA 94305
USA

SIMON B. SUTCLIFFE, B.Sc., M.D.,
M.R.C.P., F.R.C.P.(C)
Associate Professor
Department of Radiology
University of Toronto
Toronto, Ontario M4X 1K9
Canada

SHELLEY E. TAYLOR, Ph.D.
Professor
Department of Psychology
University of California
Los Angeles, CA 90024
USA

JOEL E. TEPPER, M.D.
Associate Professor
Department of Radiation Medicine
Massachusetts General Hospital
Boston, MA 02114
USA

JAMES E. TILL, Ph.D.
Senior Scientist, Division of Biological
Research
Ontario Cancer Institute
Professor, Institute of Medical Science
School of Graduate Studies
University of Toronto
Toronto, Ontario M4X 1K9
Canada

ZELIG TOCHNER, M.D.
Visiting Physician
Radiation Oncology Branch
National Cancer Institute
National Institutes of Health
Bethesda, MD 20892
USA

MAURICE TUBIANA, M.D.
Professor of Radiotherapy
Director, Institut Gustave-Roussy
94800 Villejuif
France

M. URIE, Ph.D.
Assistant Radiation Biophysicist
Department of Radiation Medicine
Massachusetts General Hospital
Instructor in Radiation Therapy
(Radiation Biophysics)
Harvard Medical School
Boston, MA 02114
USA

C.C. WANG, M.D.
Head, Division of Clinical Services
Professor
Department of Radiation Medicine
Massachusetts General Hospital
Boston, MA 02114
USA

THOMAS H. WEISENBURGER, M.D.
Associate Clinical Professor
UCLA Department of Radiation
Oncology and
Director of Clinical Research
Cancer Foundation of Santa Barbara
Santa Barbara, CA 93105
USA

H. RODNEY WITHERS, M.D., D.Sc.
Director, Division of Experimental
Radiation Oncology
Professor
Department of Radiation Oncology
University of California
Los Angeles, CA 90024
USA

JOANNE V. WOOD, Ph.D.
Department of Psychology
University of California
Los Angeles, CA 90024
(currently Assistant Professor)
Department of Psychology
State University of New York at Stony
Brook, Stony Brook, NY 11794
USA

GUNAR K. ZAGARS, M.D.
Assistant Professor
Division of Radiotherapy
The University of Texas M.D. Anderson
Hospital and Tumor Institute
Houston, TX 77030
USA

Foreword

The series "Medical Radiology – Diagnostic Imaging and Radiation Oncology" is the successor to the well known "Encyclopedia of Medical Radiology/Handbuch der medizinischen Radiologie". This international handbook with its unique compilation of data in more than fifty volumes lags behind the fast developing knowledge in radiology today.

"Medical Radiology" brings the state of the art on special topics in a timely fashion. The first volume of the series was "Lung cancer", edited by Scarantino. This volume "Innovation in Radiation Oncology", edited by H.R. Withers and L.J. Peters, presents data on the development of new therapeutic strategies in different oncologic diseases. 57 authors wrote 32 chapters covering a broad range of topics. The innovations are at various levels of development, but were all chosen with the practicing radiation oncologist in mind. Perhaps not all of the innovations will survive the test of time, others have now become well established standard procedure in some centers. Also discussed is the assessment of the effectiveness of standard treatment and how it effects the quality of a patient's survival. The contributions have been grouped into 9 broad sections as outlined in the table of contents.

We think the second volume, as the whole series, will provide valuable reading for the general community of radiation oncologists.

LUTHER W. BRADY   HANS-PETER HEILMANN
Philadelphia   Hamburg

Preface

It is sometimes claimed that Radiation Oncology is a "mature" speciality with little change in practice year to year. That is not so. There is still much to be learnt and new approaches to be tried with the aim of reducing the problem of local recurrence, of normal tissue injury and hopefully also of metastasis. To achieve these aims requires cooperative efforts with other disciplines: general and specialized surgeons, medical oncologists, diagnostic radiologists, pathologists, physicists, nurses, to name some of the more common collaborators. Innovations in radiation oncology also require a better level of understanding between basic scientists and clinicians than is commonly the case: physicians need to appreciate the shortcomings and strengths of animal and in vitro research whilst basic scientists need to appreciate the accuracy required of radiobiology data if they are to be applied in the clinic, as well as appreciating both the problems and advantages of radiobiology data gathered from clinical experience.

In this volume we have gathered contributions from a great diversity of basic and clinical scientists. The contributors have written their chapters with the practicing radiation oncologist in mind. Their purpose was to present in sufficient, but not exhaustive, detail the current state of knowledge in topics that have emerged, for the most part, during the past 5 to 10 years. The first chapter sets the stage by reviewing the quality of radiation oncology as it is practiced in the majority of radiation oncology centers in the United States. The second chapter examines how we may better predict the possible causes of failure of conventional radiotherapy in order that the most appropriate of a variety of therapeutic options may eventually be offered to patients on an individual basis. The third chapter discussed how our therapeutic endeavors affect the quality of life, a problem created by our ability to be successful. Following these three introductory chapters there are 29 chapters by highly qualified specialists discussing the newest ideas in subjects of concern to the practicing radiation oncologist. Some chapters relate to the reader's own practice: others will discuss new techniques available only in certain referral centers. We hope that the work presented in this and subsequent volumes will convince the reader that radiation oncology has more "growing points" now than at any time in its history and that he or she must remain current in this innovative speciality.

H. RODNEY WITHERS
LESTER J. PETERS

Contents

1 General Aspects

1.1 Quality of Treatment: An Overview of the Patterns of Care Study in Clinical Radiation Therapy

Simon Kramer, Gerald E. Hanks, and James J. Diamond

CONTENTS

The increasing utilization of radiation therapy as a curative modality in cancer and the increasing contribution that full-time radiation oncologists have made to the practice has led to the "Patterns of Care Study" which has documented the level of care as well as the changes taking place in the management of patients across the whole spectrum of facilities in the United States. The study began in 1971 with the objectives to improve the quality and accessibility of radiation therapy in the United States. Supported by the National Cancer Institute and developed and performed under the aegis of the American College of Radiology (ACR), it took as its starting point a statement in *A Prospect for Radiation Therapy in the United States* (1968), the first "blue book" of the, then, Committee for Radiation Therapy Studies, which said "... cancer patients in the United States are being treated well in a few places, reasonably well in many others, and quite inadequately in a great many places."

Simon Kramer, M.D., Distinguished Professor
Thomas Jefferson University Hospital
Philadelphia, PA 19107, USA

Gerald E. Hanks, M.D., Director
Fox Chase Cancer Center
Philadelphia, PA 19111, USA

James J. Diamond, Ph.D.
American College of Radiology
Philadelphia, PA 19107, USA

Basic to our study was the concept that variability in care would lead to variability in outcome. Initially a feasibility study was funded by a grant from the National Cancer Institute to Thomas Jefferson University; one of us (S.K.) recruited a small working group of radiation therapists to assist in the planning.

The feasibility study established: 1) that the radiation therapy community would support and actively participate in a quality assessment effort; 2) that a general formalism could be developed for optimal radiation therapy; 3) that a method for assessing the present practice of radiation therapy could be developed in a format suitable for comparison with criteria of optimal radiation therapy care; 4) that a suitable organizational structure for the conduct of the study could be developed. At this time the decision was made to conduct the Patterns of Care Study (PCS) as part of the American College of Radiology's Commission on Radiation Therapy. The College is nationally based and represents both full-time and part-time radiation therapists. The past history and organizational structure of the ACR placed it in a unique position to promote this study.

Radiation oncology has several advantages which made the notion of a study of the Patterns of Care feasible. The relatively small number of treatment centers, physicians, and support staff, and the focus on management of cancer implied a commonality of interest and emphasis not necessarily inherent in other specialties and placed the discipline of radiation oncology in a favorable position for such a study.

The rationale of the Patterns of Care Study was defined as follows:
- differences exist across all types of practice
- these differences can be studied and documented
- these differences are important in the outcome of treatment
- these differences can be modified
- the effect of these modifications can be measured and documented

In addition, three assumptions were made regarding the study. The first was that the extent of the documentation of the pretreatment evaluation in patients' charts would reflect the quality of care delivered. The second was that "good processes" i.e. complete and appropriate pretreatment workup and treatment delivery are more likely to result in "good outcome." If a physician performs a careful and complete evaluation and treatment, then we may expect his patients to have a generally better outcome than if established procedures were not followed. The third was that quality of care could be improved by appropriate changes in the application and utilization of resources. It was assumed that once areas amenable to change had been defined by the study, the profession as a whole and the professional organizations responsible for scientific and educational programs would be receptive to well-documented recommendations for change.

Much of our work has been based upon the Donabedian model discussed in "Evaluating the Quality of Medical Care" (Donabedian 1966), leading to assessment of the areas of structure, process and outcome.

Structure encompasses the materials that are used to provide care. These include the qualification of the staff, their organization, physical facilities, and equipment. Process represents the techniques of information-gathering based upon history, physical examination and diagnostic tests and the subsequent delivery of appropriate therapy. Outcome assessment includes the changes in health status that can be related to the care delivered by the oncology team.

1 Facilities Master Lists

In assessing the processes of radiation therapy care, the PCS has compiled Facilities Master Lists (FML) for 1974, 1975, 1978 and 1980. Each list profiles radiation therapy practice for that year and identifies all physicians involved in the practice of radiation therapy, whether their practice was full-time or part-time, the type of facility in which they practice (university affiliated, community hospital or free-standing) and the number of new cancer patients treated.

The list provides a current inventory of the radiation oncology resources – both manpower and equipment – that are available and used in the care of cancer patients in the United States. A study of the information on the FML reveals

Table 1. Number of megavoltage facilities and number of nonrespondents for each FML survey

Survey	Date	Respondents	Non-respondents	Total
First	1974	1004	9	1013
Second	1975	1034	13	1047
Third	1978	1068	25	1093
Fourth	1980	1076	7	1083

Table 2. Number of newly accessioned radiation therapy patients and total resident population in the United States

Survey	Date	Newly accessioned Rx patients	U.S. resident population (000)	New Rx patients per 1,000 population
First	1973	304,020	208,680	1.46
Second	1974	312,548	210,191	1.49
Third	1977	350,028	215,080	1.63
Fourth	1979	377,837	218,777	1.73

changing patterns in the utilization of radiation therapy services.

While the FML provides a base for studying the demographics of radiation therapy, each list also denotes the population of eligible facilities from which a stratified random sample is taken for both PCS process and outcome studies.

In terms of emerging trends in radiation therapy, the FML surveys indicate a decline in the number of part-time radiation oncologists, changes in types of megavoltage equipment, and the increasingly dominant role that community hospitals are playing in radiation therapy treatment.

The number of facilities with megavoltage treatment machines identified in each FML survey conducted by the PCS is shown in Table 1. The total number of facilities increased by about 7% from the first to the fourth survey.

The total number of newly accessioned cancer patients reported by all responding facilities for each survey period is shown in Table 2. Also shown is the U.S. resident population for each survey period, as reported by the U.S. Bureau of the Census (Current Population Reports). Note that the ratio of new radiation therapy patients per 1,000 population (column 5) has increased by about 18% from the first to fourth survey.

The number of radiation therapists reported in each FML survey is shown in Table 3. Although there has been no significant change in the total

Table 3. Number of full-time and number of part-time therapists

Survey	Full-time[a]	Part-time	Not stated	Total
First	1080 (49%)	1114	6	2200
Second	1194 (55%)	955	5	2154
Third	1414 (65%)	763	4	2181
Fourth	1564 (72%)	600	–	2164

[a] At least 35 hours per week devoted to radiation therapy practice, research, or administration

Table 4. Number of facilities and new patients treated in facilities with solo therapists

		First FML survey	Fourth FML survey
Facilities	Full-time	199	261
	Part-time	65	60
	Total	264	321
Patient load	Full-time	54,178	69,013
	Part-time	7,205	7,022
	Total	61,383	76,835

Table 5. Number of megavoltage treatment units[a]

Survey	CO-60	ACC ≤10	ACC >10	Beta-tron	Total
Second	970	312	51	44	1377
Third	900	442	119	45	1506
Fourth	820	545	217	39	1621

[a] Data not obtained in first FML survey

number of therapists from the first to the fourth survey, the proportion who are practicing on a full-time basis has increased dramatically.

The number of facilities with a solo therapist reported in the first and fourth FML surveys is shown in Table 4 as is the number of new patients treated in these facilities. In 1980 30% of all facilities were staffed by solo practioners and 20% of new patients were treated in these facilities.

Overall, the number of treatment machines has increased by approximately 18% from the second to fourth survey (Table 5), while the total number of new patients treated per year (Table 2) has increased proportionately, leaving the ratio of new patients per treatment machine roughly stable at 233.

The FML surveys conducted by the PCS have documented a number of important characteristics of the practice of radiation therapy in the United States. The increasing use of radiation therapy nationally, the growth of solo practitioners and the shift away from part-time practice are certainly among the more important trends documented.

2 PCS Process Studies

In completing its national surveys, the PCS has determined a consensus of "best current management" for ten disease sites or types in which radiation therapy plays a major part in curative treatment. Table 6 shows the ten disease sites studied in 1973 and the number of patient records reviewed in each. Reaching a consensus on the best current management of a particular cancer consisted in organizing the decisions facing medical personnel in the pretreatment evaluation of the patient and the extent and nature of his tumor and displaying them graphically in "decision trees." The branches of these ten decision trees lead to appropriate treatment systems. Thus, the key decisions, or diagnostic tasks essential to the decisions for treatment and the actual management of the treatment comprised best current management. An example of a decision tree for carcinoma of the cervix is shown as Fig. 1.

Review committees were assembled to organize the literature and clinical experience of their members in each disease site. The consensus they developed was broadly based in that the committees were comprised of radiation therapists from several areas of the country and from different types of practice. Circumstances where the deliberative process failed to lead to a consensus naturally pointed out areas in which controlled clinical studies would have to be undertaken.

In its first Process Survey, the PCS compared the actual delivery of radiation therapy throughout the U.S., as of 1973, with the criteria for best

Table 6. Patterns of care study charts reviewed for 1973

Breast	1565	Bladder	1072
Testis	459	Prostate	901
Cervix	937	Larynx	1023
Hodgkin's	495	Ant. tongue	556
Corpus uteri	1018	Nasopharynx	308
Total cases			8334

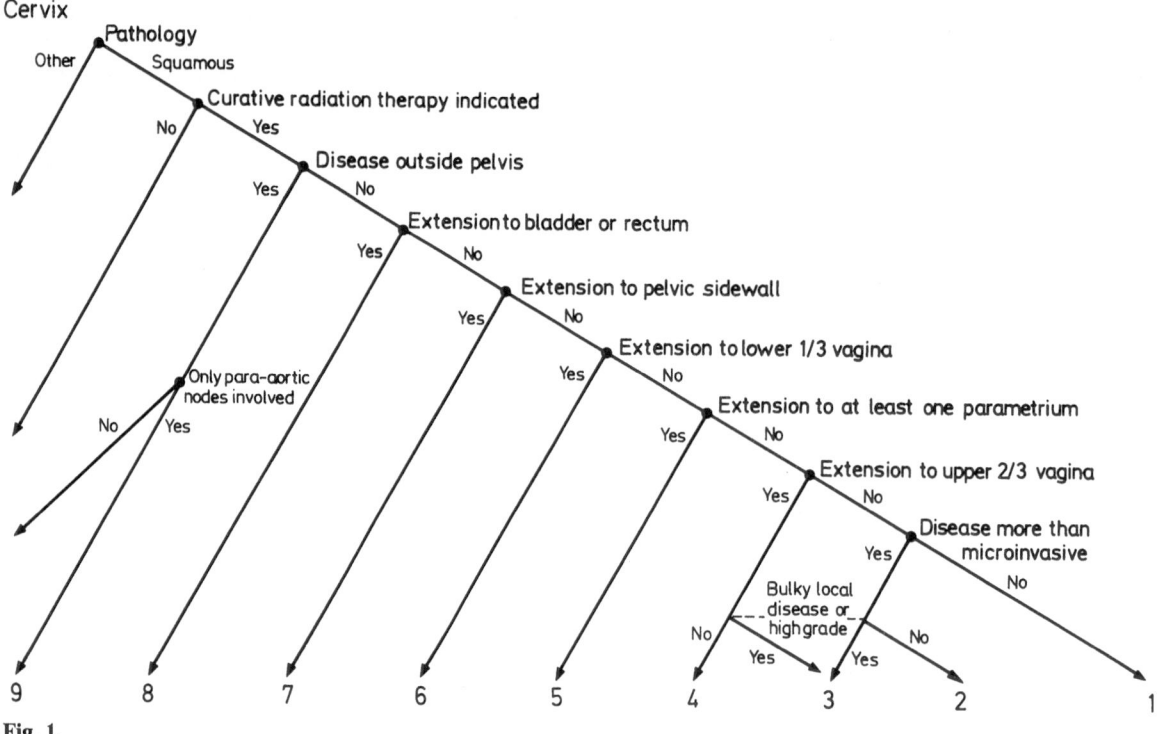

Fig. 1.

current management as discussed above. A stratified sample of radiation therapy facilities was selected to reflect the demographics of the U.S. The FML provided the population from which these facilities were sampled, and records of ten patients receiving definitive radiation therapy for each of the ten sites were reviewed.

Each facility selected to be included in a national PCS survey is invited by letter to participate. Upon agreement, they are sent a census form asking for a coded listing of all eligible patients for all disease sites in the survey. A simple random sample of eligible patients is selected from the census and a visit is scheduled. Information is taken from the radiation therapy and hospital records on-site by a team that consists of radiation therapist, medical physicist and nurse-data manager. Assessment of individual facilities is not done.

Information from the sampled records showed that, for each disease site, wide variation existed in the national practice in 1973 across all types of facilities. These variations were reported via newsletters and scientific papers to the professional community. The recognition of variations also pointed to the need to conduct Outcome studies.

This 1973 Process Survey revealed several findings:

– free standing, small institutions (less than 250 patients per year, part-time practitioners) were consistently below the national average for conformity with process criteria felt to be critical in patient management and treatment.
– large facilities (over 800 patients per year staffed by full-time radiotherapists with active residency training programs) were consistently above the national average in these critical processes.
– in all types of facilities, there are those that score well relative to a process-of-care composite and those that do not. This alerted PCS to the need for individual department profiles.
– lack of conformity and the identification of segments of practice that perform poorly offer an opportunity for educational efforts.

The wide variations found in the process studies led to measuring and documenting differences in outcome. For the first time, national, valid statistics could be cited to serve as a barometer as to how well radiation therapy performance in general compared to results reported by major national and international institutions.

3 PCS Outcome Studies – Six Sites

The Outcome Survey portion of the PCS program aims to correlate Process Survey Criteria with subsequent outcome data. Of course retrospective institutional studies have been done on treatment technique and outcome, along with prospective clinical studies, but an assessment of quality of care in terms of specific clinical hypotheses on a national basis has never been undertaken. Since individual institution retrospective studies are often based upon selected experiences, (selected patients, private patients, patients in clinical trial, etc.) they are frequently of limited statistical significance. By utilizing random samples of practices and patients, PCS can validly assess where patients are treated, special patient characteristics and treatment parameters, and even the frequency and accuracy of various staging systems. We reliably define inadequate practice operationally through the analysis of results as well as through consensus and validation by the practicing community.

The methods used in the Outcome Survey yield valid national estimates ("benchmarks") of survival complications and recurrence rates. Questionnaires were designed to document follow-up information on patients and their reactions to radiation therapy intervention with respect to these outcome variables. Furthermore, a detailed medical physics review was required to verify the accuracy of reported doses. The PCS developed precise anatomic dose points that were used by the physicist surveyors in calculating doses.

Of the original 314 institutions we visited in the Process Survey, 244 were visited in the Outcome Survey. The decrease in the number of institutions was based on the disproportionately small number of patient records available for survey in these facilities compared to the cost of obtaining them.

4 Cancer of the Cervix (Table 7)

The results of the national practice for treatment of cancer of the cervix with radiation therapy are extremely good in the early stages when compared with reported results from institutions from around the world (JAMPOLIS et al. 1975; MARCIAL 1977).

The results obtained in Stage III cervix cancer indicate an area for potential improvement. Complications are not stage related and the observed rate of 11% for Stage I cervix cancer is higher than anticipated (STROCKBINE et al. 1970).

Table 7. Patterns of care study-outcome surveys cancer of the cervix-national benchmarks[a]

Stage	No. of patients	Free of recurrence (%)	Major complications (%)	Survival (%)
I	275	89	11	88
II	210	72	11	82
III	81	29	14	44

[a] Actuarial analysis at 4 years

Table 8. Patterns of care study-outcome surveys Hodgkin's disease-national benchmarks[a]

Stage	No. of patients	Free of recurrence (%)	Major complications (%)	Survival (%)
IA	110	83	10	87
IIA	149	74	6	85
IIIA	74	59	7	77
IB, IIB, IIIB	66	50	13	68

[a] Actuarial analysis at 4 years

5 Hodgkin's Disease (Table 8)

Of the 399 Hodgkin's disease patients, 47 received planned chemotherapy and radiation therapy as their initial management. The four-year free of recurrence rates and survival by stage are excellent, and compare favorably with those reported from individual institutions exhibiting a special interest in Hodgkin's disease (KAPLAN 1968). Major complication rates of 4 to 12% were observed.

Four percent of the patients were treated with the involved field technique only, that is, with treatment fields limited to the areas showing clinical evidence of disease. They exhibited a high recurrence rate (46% at 4 yrs actuarial) outside the treated lymph node areas. The majority of the patients were treated with extended fields (58%) or total nodal irradiation (38%) and had a low recurrence rate.

6 Seminoma of the Testis (Table 9)

In the national results for seminoma of the testis, Stage I and Stage II patients exhibit the same (3%) low recurrence rates. Patients with Stage IC disease were defined as those without evaluation of their retroperitoneal nodes either by lymphangiog-

Table 9. Patterns of care study-outcome study seminoma of the testis-national benchmarks[a]

Stage	No. of patients	Free of recurrence (%)	Major complications (%)
IA	229	97	3
IC[b]	33	87	3
II	107	97	0
III	10	70	0

[a] Actuarial analysis of free of recurrence and major complications at 4 years.
[b] No evaluation of retroperitoneal nodes

Table 10. Patterns of care study-outcome surveys anterior tongue and floor of mouth-national benchmarks[a]

Stage	No. of patients	Free of recurrence (%)	Major complications (%)	Survival (%)
I	60	75	2	83
II	164	59	4	72
III	74	43	1	46
IV	107	21	4	30

[a] Actuarial analysis of free of recurrence and major complications at 2 years

raphy or intravenous pyelogram. This subgroup exhibits a significant increase in failure ($p < 0.01$), the first statistically valid demonstration of the necessity for evaluating the retroperitoneal nodes in seminoma in order to correctly stage the patient and determine the volume or areas to be irradiated.

Complications were infrequent (2%) and our data analysis has shown them to be in part related to excessive radiation doses.

7 Anterior Two-Thirds Tongue and Floor of Mouth (Table 10)

Outcome results for 405 patients treated for anterior two-thirds of tongue and floor of mouth show that the recurrence free rate in Stage I and II is lower than expected and is in part due to very poor control in the subgroup of patients who did not receive interstitial radiation as part of their treatment. The benchmark statistics for control of Stages III and IV cancer are affected by the poor outcome in a subgroup treated with radiation therapy alone rather than combined surgery and radiation. The low overall complication rates (1–4%)

Table 11. Patterns of care-outcome surveys carcinoma of the larynx-national benchmarks[a]

Stage	No. of patients	Free of recurrence (%)	Major complications (%)	Survival (%)
Glottic				
I	374	82	1	90
II	102	68	0	78
III	43	61	0	65
IV	8	37	0	23
Supraglottic				
I	24	78	13	78
II	37	45	3	68
III	38	49	5	54
IV	53	27	9	30

[a] Actuarial analysis of free of recurrence and major complications at 3 years

suggest that more aggressive therapy would have been appropriate, particularly in those patients treated with radiation therapy alone.

8 Cancer of the Larynx (Table 11)

A cancer free rate of 82% was observed in patients with early glottic cancer treated with radiation. A high recurrence rate was obtained in a subgroup of Stage III and IV patients partly due to not combining surgery with radiation. A similar phenomenon was seen in Stage III and IV anterior tongue and floor of mouth. Essentially no major complications were observed in glottic cancer, suggesting that a more aggressive radiation program might reduce recurrence rates. Benchmark statistics for supraglottic larynx cancer show the generally worse prognosis for this disease, as compared to glottic larynx.

9 Prostate (Table 12)

The favorable national averages for recurrence and complications in 617 patients with prostate cancer are quite comparable to those reported from individual institutions heavily involved in treating this disease. They illustrate why external radiation is assuming an increasingly important role in the management of prostate cancer. Complications were less frequent than had been previously observed (Ray et al. 1973).

Table 12. Patterns of care study-outcome surveys carcinoma of the prostate-national benchmarks[a]

Stage	No. of patients	Free of recurrence (%)	Major complications (%)	Survival (%)
A	56	85	9	91
B	293	77	2	88
C	268	59	6	76

[a] Actuarial analysis of free of recurrence and major complications at 3 years

We are in the process of completing the analysis of a ten year follow-up of men treated definitively in 1973 for adenocarcinoma of the prostate. Our preliminary findings show no difference in survival for treated stage A patients when compared with men of the same age without prostate cancer. In Stages B and C, however, the group with cancer have a poorer survival relative to the non-prostate-cancer cohort.

10 Future Plans

The national averages for cancer free survival and major complications of these six cancer sites commonly managed by radiation therapy are particularly good in patients with early disease. The PCS is currently involved in a continuing program of surveys that will monitor and record the changes in these benchmarks of care from 1973 to 1983, and at periodic intervals thereafter. These benchmarks will provide an important resource in cancer care.

The 1983 national survey will involve only *processes* of care in randomly-selected radiation therapy facilities. The disease sites to be surveyed will be cervix, Hodgkin's disease, prostate and breast. The survey will enable the PCS to track changes in the practice of radiation therapy and then to monitor trends evolving nationally and in different types of practice. Also included in this survey will be a study of palliative care in radiation therapy. For the first time, the PCS will collect national data on the treatment of metastatic disease including brain metastases, pain from bone metastases and obstructive symptoms. Over time, the patient outcome data will be collected for the patients receiving curative intent therapy for further study of process-outcome correlations.

The PCS intends this quality assessment survey to be the start of a quality assurance program for radiation therapy. Beginning in 1985, the ACR will conduct individual facility visits modelled after the PCS program in order to provide radiation therapists with feedback on their practice relative to regional or national norms established by the survey. This feedback loop completes the move toward the basic goal of the PCS – to improve the quality of care in radiation therapy in the United States.

References

Donabedian A (1966) Evaluating the quality of medical care. *Milbank Meml. Fund Quart.* 44:166–206

Jampolis S, Andras EJ, and Fletcher GH (1975) Analysis of sites and causes of failures of irradiation in invasive squamous cell carcinoma of the intact uterine cervix. *Radiology* 115:681

Kaplan HS (1968) Prognostic significance of the relapse free interval after radiotherapy in Hodgkin's disease. Cancer 22:1131–1136

Marcial VA (1977) Carcinoma of the cervix; present status and future. Cancer 39:945–958

Ray GR, Cassady JR, and Bagshaw MA (1973) Definitive radiation therapy of carcinoma of the prostate. *Radiology* 106:407–418

Strockbine MF, Hancock JE, and Fletcher GH (1970) Complications in 831 patients with squamous cell carcinoma of the uterine cervix treated with 3000 rads or more whole pelvic irradiation. *Am J Roentgenol* 108:293

U.S. Department of Commerce, Bureau of the Census, Current Population Reports

1.2 Predictive Assays

WILLIAM A. BROCK

CONTENTS

1 Introduction

The best method of predicting the radiocurability of individual human tumors is based upon tumor size, site, histologic type and grade, and host factors such as sex and age. Small tumors located such that normal tissues do not seriously limit total dose and those with "favorable" histology are more radiocurable than large tumors located over a critical normal tissue. The precision of prognosis based upon these features is relatively low; clini-

This investigation was supported by research grant CA-06294, awarded by the National Cancer Institute, grant HD-16843, awarded by the National Institute of Child Health and Human Development, and the Katharine Unsworth Memorial Fund.

WILLIAM A. BROCK, Ph.D., Associate Professor
The University of Texas M.D. Anderson Hospital and Tumor Institute
Houston, TX 77030, USA

cians have observed that the average response of different histological subtypes varies, and the range of sensitivities within each subtype varies almost as much. The need to predict radiocurability on an individual basis is now more important than ever because of the existence of different radiation modalities, the development of a broad range of chemotherapeutic drugs as an alternative treatment, and the possibility of combining drugs with radiation in addition to or as an alternative to surgery. Further, what is needed are assays precise enough to predict the results of treatment for a particular patient, not just to place him in a broad category of possibilities. This review outlines the need for developing better methods of predicting radiocurability, the present methods of prediction, and some prospects that are being developed for the future.

If a particular tumor is destined to receive radiotherapy as the only treatment, and if no alternative exists, then one might argue that a method for predicting radiocurability would not be useful; the tumor should simply be treated to an acceptable limit of tolerance for the relevant normal tissue. However, even in this simple case, knowledge that a tumor is more resistant than average might lead to the decision to risk a higher probability of normal tissue complications and give a larger total dose. But even more important, additional information about the radiocurability of the tumor allows other treatment modalities to be considered. If it is known before treatment that a tumor has a low probability for cure by conventional fractionated radiotherapy, then alternate therapy might be considered. For example, if a tumor is certain to fail radiotherapy because of poor oxygenation, then hypoxic cell sensitizers, hyperbaric oxygen, or neutron therapy could be considered. Although alternate modalities such as neutron therapy have not met with overwhelming success, it is likely that proper patient selection based on assays that would define the subset of patients best suited for neutrons would dramatically improve the results. If, for example, we could determine why carcinomas of the salivary gland respond well to neutron therapy, it would be possible to make measurements on individuals and select patients according to those features, not simply according to tumor type and location. Finally, treatment planning would benefit greatly by combining drug sensitivity testing with radiosensitivity testing. Development of tests for chemotherapy drug sensitivity has been ongoing for several years (HAMBURGER and SALMON 1977; VONHOFF 1983; and BAKER et al. 1986). These tests include clonogenic assays, xenograft testing, and biochemical assays, and in many cases sensitivity to particular drugs was demonstrated. If it becomes possible to develop tests for both drug and radiation sensitivity, then one might expect dramatic improvements in therapy. Therefore, assays for radiosensitivity, drug sensitivity, and the two in combination should be developed in parallel.

2 Predicting Radiocurability

In order to accurately predict radiocurability, ideally those factors that limit the cure of a tumor should be known. This is, of course, a difficult problem since curelimiting factors will differ from one individual to the next (PETERS et al., 1980). This leads to the conclusion that for each tumor, several features must be measured, analyzed, and weighed before an accurate prediction can be made. Any approach for developing a predictive assay should be an attempt to quantitate one or more curelimiting factors, not just any random measurable tumor parameter. These curelimiting factors can be classified as intrinsic to the tumor, related to tumor physiology, or related to host factors.

2.1 Intrinsic Factors

2.1.1 Tumor Size

As a tumor grows, the number of clonogenic cells in it increases, and since cell killing is an exponential function of radiation dose, increasing numbers of clonogenic cells in the tumor mean that a higher radiation dose is needed for cure. Although it is not yet possible to estimate the number of clonogenic cells in a tumor, it is generally agreed that larger tumors have more and, therefore, are harder to cure. Thus, an assessment of tumor size is a

necessary first measure for predicting and must be used in conjunction with any other measurement. The fraction of tumor cells that are clonogenic must vary considerably in different tumors, making a direct measure of tumor size only a rough approximation of clonogenic cell number. It is not known how many clonogenic cells are in any human tumor of any size. SUIT et al. (1965) estimated that animal tumors contain about 10^6 clonogenic cells per mm^3. However, assuming approximately equal radiosensitivities of mouse and human tumors, there is a large discrepancy in dose needed to cure mouse and human tumors; because of the relatively lower dose required to cure human tumors, they must have fewer clonogenic cells. It was estimated by TEPPER (1981) that human tumors might contain between 80 and 1200 clonogenic per mm^3. Human tumor cloning assays developed by SALMON et al. (1978) reveal an *in vitro* plating efficiency that is only a fraction of 1%, although recent techniques report a higher value, but these techniques are also only a rough estimate of clonogenic cell number. Until creative new techniques are developed that will estimate clonogenic cell number, tumor size remains an important parameter for predicting radiation response.

2.1.2 Cellular Radiosensitivity

Intrinsic cellular radiosensitivity is another feature that possibly limits cure, although this has not been proved. Cellular radiosensitivity refers to a combination of the level of damage sustained by a cell after a given dose of radiation and the ability of the cell to repair that damage. WEICHELSBAUM (1984) has recently reviewed his studies on early passage cultures of squamous cell carcinomas of the head and neck region. He suggested that, in general, the *in vitro* radiosensitivity of tumor cell lines has a rather narrow range, as measured by D_0. However, he reported significant differences in repair capacity, that is the ability to repair potentially lethal damage (PLD). One would argue that D_0 is not relevant in the clinical situation since clinical doses are generally on the shoulder of the survival curves, suggesting that the relevant factor of cellular radiosensitivity is the intrinsic ability of the cell to repair damage. This is further supported by recent publications by FERTIL and MALAISE (1981; 1985) and DEACON et al. (1984), who showed no correlation for the D_0 of over 50 human tumor cell lines with tumor radioresistance, but a strong correlation between *in vitro* survival at low doses and tumor radioresistance. If these observations are true, this parameter could have significant predictive value if it could be measured in individual cases.

Tumor cells change in intrinsic radiosensitivity as they progress through the cell cycle. The sensitivity to radiation cell killing can vary by as much as a factor of 5 as cells move through the cell cycle, and this has been shown to be true both *in vitro* (SINCLAIR and MORTON 1966; DEWEY and HUMPHREY 1962) and *in vivo* (GRDINA 1980). Dividing cells are usually more sensitive, while quiescent cells are more resistant, although this is not always true. Therefore, knowledge of the cell cycle distribution of the relevant cells in the tumor would be useful information for predictive assays.

2.1.3 Cell Heterogeneity

Another intrinsic factor is tumor cell heterogeneity, which exists in many tumors. This has been shown with chromosome markers, DNA distribution studies, and biochemical probes, all showing multiple tumor cell populations within tumors. The existence of tumor heterogeneity has considerable theoretical importance, since a small fraction of very resistant cells would be difficult to detect, but would be wholly responsible for treatment failure. Identifying the existence and sensitivity of tumor cell subpopulations would is very important for any predictive assay strategy, although such determinations may be extremely difficult with present technology.

2.2 Tumor Physiology

Features of tumor physiology include blood flow, pH, and oxygen tension, all of which can influence the level of radiation cell killing by their influence on initial radiation damage and on repair. Determining the oxygen concentration and the ability of a tumor to reoxygenate during fractionated radiotherapy could be crucial in predicting radiocurability. Tumor pH may reflect tumor hypoxia, since lower pH is due primarily to a build-up of lactic acid under anaerobic metabolism. The relevance of hypoxia in human tumors is still a controversy because direct measurements of human tumor cell hypoxia have not been made. In experimental systems, the effect of artificially induced hypoxia, hypoxic cell sensitizers, and hyperbaric oxygen have been measured and shown to be rele-

vant. However, human tumors, which usually grow slowly, may not be radiobiologically hypoxic though experimental tumors that outgrow their blood supply are. In addition, during fractionated radiotherapy, reoxygenation may occur to the extent that hypoxia becomes less relevant as a limiting factor in radiotherapy. However, because of the significant role oxygen plays in cellular radiosensitivity, hypoxia must be further explored and tested as a predictor of radiation response.

2.3 Host Factors

If a tumor is not sterilized by radiotherapy, it may be reduced to a volume and physiologic state such that the host immune system may be able to play a role in tumor cure. The role of the immune system has been demonstrated in many experimental systems and has been implicated by the response of patients with immune deficiencies and in the results of immunotherapy. An assessment of a patient's immune status and tumor immunogenicity could be useful for prediction.

3 Present Methods

As mentioned previously, tumor histologic type and size have been shown to be the most reliable predictors of tumor response. For example, breast carcinomas respond better than glioblastomas and, among a given set of breast carcinomas, smaller tumors will respond better. However, these indicators are not precise enough because of the clinical observation that tumors of identical histologic type and size have a wide range of responses.

3.1 Histology

Despite the shortcomings, histologic methods remain the most useful methods of predicting the prognosis of radiation therapy. Starting in 1939 (WARREN et al. 1939) and continuing to the present, reports of quantitating histological changes during fractionated radiotherapy have claimed an excellent correlation to prognosis. Measurements include the fraction of viable cells, the number of mitotic cells, the number of degenerating cells as assessed by nuclear morphology, and the state of differentiation before and after a test dose of radiation. The most complete study was carried out by GLUCKSMAN (1974) who, over a 30-year period, analyzed the histopathology of over 1400 patients. Histologic scores were grouped as favorable or unfavorable and compared to the 5-year survival rates of the patients. The accuracy of predicting favorable or unfavorable response was excellent. Other workers have obtained similar results (Dubranszky 1966; Walter et al. 1964; McGarrity and Garvan 1961), although Limburg et al. (1972) found no statistical correlation between histologic response and survival. In a review on this subject, Trott (1980) concludes that, at least in the case of carcinoma of the cervix, there is excellent prognostic value obtainable from the histologic response. One drawback to this method is that the histologic response is determined after the patient has received at least 10–15 Gy radiation. Thus, the number of surviving cells is less than 1% in all tumors, regardless of prognosis. This means that the method does not assess the actual survival or death of any clonogens, but only some general property of cellular degeneration or differentiation. In other words, success of this method would depend upon cells in resistant or sensitive tumors dying by different mechanisms, for example by entering a terminally differentiated state. Such measurements would have built-in inaccuracies because differences from tumor to tumor in the cell loss factor or dead tumor cell clearance would influence the histology score.

3.2 Labeling Techniques

Another histologic approach that takes into account survival uses autoradiography. In this assay, ^{3}H-dThd incorporation into DNA is measured at various times during radiotherapy, providing a dynamic estimate of the fraction of cells able to continue through S-phase after a test dose of radiation. Fettig et al. (1980) incubated biopsy samples taken from patients before and 10 days after a single dose of radiation in cultures containing ^{3}H-dThd. After the labeling index was determined, the response was classified as good if the index was reduced by at least 60% as a result of the radiation, and if there was a good correlation with the clinical outcome at 1 year. Tatra and Breitnicker (1980) found that labeling index had prognostic value in carcinoma of the uterine cervix, if it was derived after the first half of radiotherapy was administered. In this case they found that a positive labeling index was indicative of a bad prognosis. An assay utilizing labeling techniques has a sound rationale in that labeled cells must

be able to progress through the cell cycle and the assay is based upon cell survival. However, if the analysis is made too late in treatment, it may have no value for individualizing therapy. In addition, since the labeling index of all tumors will be much less than 1% after treatment, the method lacks sensitivity. Methods to assess the response must be performed early enough that differences in survival can be observed. Thus, if possible, it would be more logical to develop a technique to assess the response after 1 or 2 fractions, when the surviving fraction of tumor cells is relatively high. The added advantage of an early observation would be that different rates of cell clearance or turnover would influence the index to a lesser extent, making the measurement more accurate in terms of cell survival.

A technique has been developed recently that has the ability to detect S-phase cells in frozen tissue sections. This technique makes use of a monoclonal antibody against bromodeoxyuridine (BRDU), (Gratzner 1982) a nucleotide analogue, that is incorporated into DNA. Antibody binding to BRDU incorporated into S-phase cells is visualized by a fluorescence microscopy or, alternatively, the labeling index of single cell suspensions from tumors can be determined by flow cytometry. The advantage of frozen section analysis is an ability to perform differential cell counts. A definite advantage of BRDU is that it can be given to patients with little or no toxicity. Clinical studies using this technique have begun (Hoshino et al. 1985; 1986). So far results are preliminary, but this may be proven to be a method by which radiotherapy patients can be selected according to the growth fraction and/or growth rate of tumors.

4 Prospects for Predictive Assays

In general, any predictive assay would be useful as long as it could be used to some clinical advantage, that is, if it can identify that treatment modality with the highest probability of success. However, since validation of any method requires years for patient follow-up, random measurements of any available tumor parameter do not represent a practical approach. Attempts to develop a predictive assay must have as a basis some rational relationship to a known potential limiting feature for tumor cure. Since it stands to reason that treatment fails for different reasons in different situations, several parameters must be measured and the one predicting the worst outcome should be used to choose therapy. Therefore, methods should be developed to quantitate those factors that have proved to be important for tumor control in both experimental situations and in clinical observations. Hence, measurements of cellular sensitivity, the degree of tumor cell hypoxia, tumor cell kinetics, cytogenetics, and the capacity to repair radiation damage represent rational approaches to the problem. Discussed below is a review of some current approaches to measuring these parameters.

4.1 Intrinsic Cellular Radiosensitivity

Since PUCK and MARCUS (1956) described a method for determining cellular radiosensitivity, the sensitivity of a great number of different cell lines derived from human tumors has been determined. Recently, FERTIL and MALAISE (1981) compiled and analyzed published survival curve data from human lines with the aim of correlating *in vitro* sensitivity with the radiocurability of each tumor type. They found that a statistical correlation exists between the *in vitro* surviving fraction after 2.0 Gy of radiation and the 95% tumor control dose, which was estimated from clinical experience. They concluded that the relative radioresistance of melanomas, glioblastomas, and osteosarcomas is attributable in part to the intrinsic radioresistance of the tumor cells. DEACON et al. (1984) found a similar result showing a positive correlation between survival at 2.0 Gy and relative radiosensitivities of different tumor histology types. This agrees with the predictions of BARENDSEN (1980), who suggested that cellular radiosensitivity plays a role in tumor radiosensitivity, although he pointed out that such observations should be supplemented with other measurements, such as proliferation kinetics, to make prediction more accurate. However, these observations were made on established cell lines, which were long removed from the tumor.

4.1.1 Clonogenic Assays

The agar-suspension cloning technique (HAMBURGER and SALMON, 1977) has been used with some success in determining the sensitivity of primary human tumor cell cultures to chemotherapeutic agents. This approach to determining drug sensitivity has promise, but many technical details need to be evaluated and improved for each specific tumor type. The cell suspension technique and evaluation of the cell inoculum pose problems since cell type, number and viability, and the presence of cell clumps are critical factors. These problems have not been adequately solved. Nevertheless, radiation studies have been carried out on primary human tumor biopsy samples. Dose-response curves have been obtained from a variety of sites, especially melanomas, and survival values have fallen into the expected range of cell sensitivity, although significant differences were found between different biopsy specimens (GOOD et al. 1978; MEYSKENS 1980; COURTENAY et al. 1978). However, the main problem has been the unrealistically high radioresistance exhibited by many cultures. D_0 values for some melanomas have been greater than 100 Gy. The initial interpretation was that this represented true resistance, but from a radiobiological point of view, such high resistance is not possible. The reason for resistance is probably that most colonies from this assay developed from cell aggregates, not from single cells and it takes a much larger dose to kill an aggregate than a single cell (ROCKWELL 1985). Even though there are technical difficulties associated with this assay, it is important to pursue the development of the method because of theoretical value that individual survival curves might have. These methods need to be developed and tested as predictors of radiocurability.

BAKER et al. (1986) developed a method for primary culture of human tumor cells that makes use of a cell adhesive matrix, which promotes cell attachment, and a medium enriched in growth factors to promote cell growth. They reported a very high efficiency of tumor cell culture production (over 80%) and initial success with drug testing, including good clinical correlations, in a group of patients with all types of tumors. This method has been used by BROCK et al. (1985; 1985a) for radiosensitivity measurements in primary human tumor cell cultures. Cultures were irradiated after 24 hours of incubation and survival was quantitated by measuring the total number of growing cells 12 days later. Fig. 1 shows an irradiated stained culture plate and the survival curve derived from it. An analysis of the first 40 cultures taken from a variety of tumor types shows correlation with the radiosensitivities of different histology types and the expected wide variation of responses within each histology group. This method is sensitive at low radiation doses, which makes it ideal for calculating the potentially clinically relevant parameter survival at 2.0 Gy. The next step for

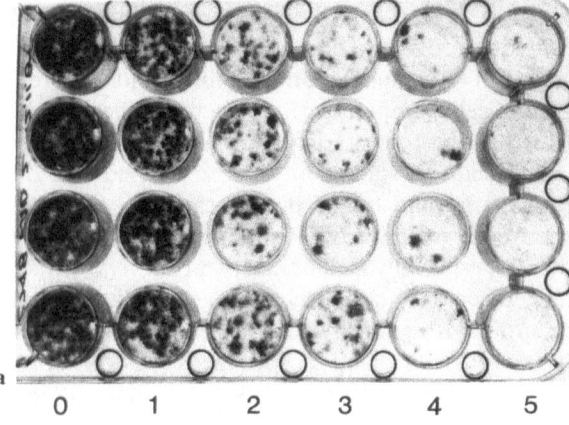

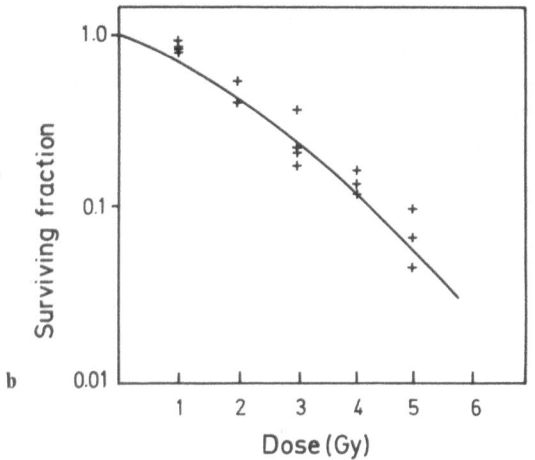

Fig. 1. a Photograph of a stained primary culture derived from a squamous cell carcinoma 13 days after inoculation after treatment. The radiation doses range from 0 to 5 Gy. **b** The "survival curve" derived from the culture shown in panel **a**. The crosses represent fraction of cell growth in each irradiated culture relative to controls. The solid line is a linear quadratic fit of the data. (Brock et al. 1985, with permission)

testing this culture technique is a retrospective clinical trial in which survival at 2.0 Gy will be determined for a group of radiotherapy patients and later compared to two-year local tumor control.

4.1.2 The Micronucleus Assay

Because of the technical difficulties associated with determining the radiosensitivity of human tumor cells in primary culture, alternative methods have been proposed. One of these is the micronucleus (MN) assay. The rationale for this assay is based upon the observation that the major mechanism

of reproductive cell death by radiation is through the production of chromosome aberrations (Carrano 1973; Bedford et al. 1978). The predominant aberration is the acentric fragment (Carrano and Heddle 1973), which, because it lacks a centromere, lags behind the segregating chromosomes during anaphase, and is, therefore, excluded from the nuclei in the daughter cells. These cytoplasmic acentric fragments form micronuclei, which are readily observable in cells after the first post-irradiation cell division. The presence of an MN in a cell is predictive of nonclonogenicity (Grote et al. 1981; Joshi et al. 1982a; 1982b). Midander and Revesz (1980) reported that the frequency of radiation-induced MN could be used to predict the D_0 of several cell lines. This assay has since been used to estimate cell killing, to determine the effects of dose-modifying agents such as misonidazole, hypoxia, and glutathione (Midander 1982a; 1982b; Brock et al. 1983), and to measure the relative biological effectiveness (RBE) of low and high linear energy transfer (LET) radiation (Bettega et al. 1980; Diehl-Marshall and Bianchi 1981). Fig. 2 shows the correlation between the cell survival curve determined by a conventional clonogenic method and one calculated from the MN frequency. It exemplifies the good correlation that exists between the MN assay and the clonogenic assay when the surviving fraction is 0.01 or greater. At lower survival levels, a significant fraction of irradiated cells is delayed or blocked from cell division, and, therefore, does not express MN

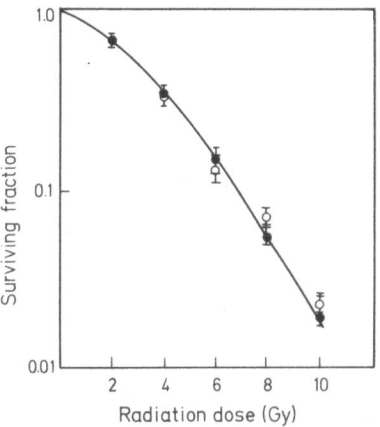

Fig. 2. Survival curve for Chinese hamster cells determined by standard colony formation assay (●) and as calculated from the radiation-induced MN frequency (○). MN were scored 24 hours after irradiation and surviving fraction calculated from the expression $SF = e^{-MN\ frequency/0.20}$

(BROCK and WILLIAMS 1985). The advantages of using the MN assay for determining the radiosensitivity in primary human cell cultures are that only one cell division is required after irradiation rather than the growth of colonies, and that high quality single-cell suspensions are not necessary.

In animal tumor systems, radiation-induced MN are expressed in a dose dependent fashion, but the relationship to tumor cure has not yet been tested. Because of the heterogeneous nature of tumors, however, interpreting of MN levels is difficult. For example, following a dose of radiation to a tumor or tumor cell suspension, the absolute number of MN expressed would depend upon several factors in addition to cellular radiosensitivity. Tumors contain a variable proportion of dividing cells and stationary cells, whether clonogenic or nonclonogenic, and stationary phase cells will not express MN. In addition, normal cells in the tumor would contribute to the cell count, but their radiosensitivity, even if they divide, is irrelevant. Because of these factors, it is not possible to derive an MN level that represents sensitivity or resistance. However, Streffer and coworkers (personal communication) suggested that MN in untreated tumors of the colon reflect tumor cell kinetics and cell loss. They found that a high level of spontaneous MN was associated with a better treatment outcome.

Another potential use of the MN assay does exist for determination of the RBEs of low and high LET irradiations, or of the effect of agents that modify radiation dose. Since MN levels do reflect cell killing, the MN levels induced by radiations of different qualities would be a measure of their relative abilities to kill cells. This has been demonstrated by PETERS et al. (1984) who used the MN assay to determine the RBE γ/n in two mouse tumors. Fig. 3 and 4 show their results, which were similar to the results of RBEs determined by conventional means. MIDANDER (1982a; 1982b) also showed the value of the MN assay to predict the effects of dose-modifying agents such as the effects of misonidazole in hypoxic cultured cells. He was also able to measure the relative sensitivity of cells derived from patients who were heterozygous or homozygous for a defect in glutathione synthesis. Finally, in mouse tumors, the radioprotective effect of the thiol agent WR-2721 has been measured by the relative MN levels and the protection factor obtained agreed with those determined by conventional assays (BROCK et al. 1983).

Since radiation-induced MN levels have a solid relationship to cell lethality, and since problems

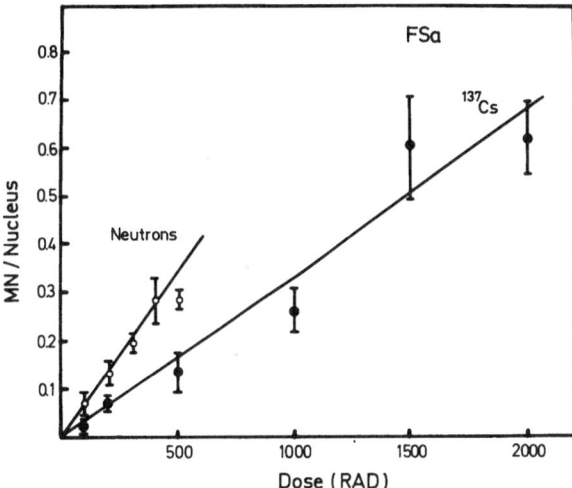

Fig. 3. MN induction in fibrosarcoma tumors (FSa) by photons (●) and 42 MeV neutrons (o). Animals were irradiated 24 hours before they were killed and MN was determined. The data points are means ± SE. (PETERS et al. 1985, with permission)

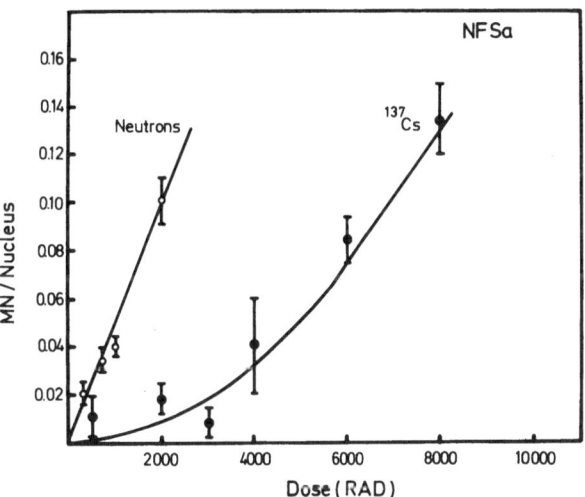

Fig. 4. MN induction in fibrosarcoma tumors (NFSa) by photons (●) and 42 MeV neutrons (o). Animals were irradiated 48 hours before they were killed and MN was determined. The data points are means ± SE. (PETERS et al. 1985, with permission)

of tumor heterogeneity with respect to normal or nondividing cells are not significant for RBE or dose modification determinations, the MN assay has potential as a predictive assay for human tumors. It may be possible to use this assay to select those patients most likely to benefit from neutron trials, or the assay could be included in protocols for testing the effectiveness of radiosensitizers.

4.1.3 Repair Capacity

Another intrinsic feature of cells is the ability to repair radiation damage. The potential importance of repair processes in tumor response to radiation have been discussed by WEICHELSBAUM (1984). The significance of the repair process is most dramatically demonstrated by the observation that as the number of fractions of radiation is increased, a larger total dose is needed for a similar biological effect. The importance of repair is also illustrated by patients suffering from the genetic disorder xeroderma pigmentosum, who are hypersensitive to ultraviolet light. *In vitro* studies with cells lines derived from the fibroblasts of these patients show a defect in repair capacity, showing that this defect is expressed in culture. In other words, variations in repair capacity influence radiation response. Thus, it is fair to assume that the shoulder on the survival curve is largely influenced by the repair capacity of the cells and a large shoulder on the curve reflects the response of a tissue requiring a much larger total dose of fractionated radiotherapy for an equal biological effect. Therefore, one strategy for a predictive assay would be to determine the ability of tumor cells to repair damage after low doses of radiation in primary cell cultures or explants from a tumor. Tumor cells with a large repair capacity might then best be treated by larger doses per fraction or by neutrons.

WEICHELSBAUM et al. (1982) studied the inherent ability of nine established human tumor cell lines to repair potentially lethal damage (PLD) in an attempt to correlate repair ability with the radiocurability of different tumor types. They found that tumors considered to be more nonradiocurable (osteosarcomas and melanomas) show greater PLD repair in culture than did more curable tumors (breast carcinomas and neuroblastomas). Other laboratories have also shown a variable ability in human tumor cells to repair PLD. The range of repair capacities was large, and some positive correlations with clinical outcome have been found.

In order to minimize the effect that long-term culturing might have on PLD repair, WEICHELSBAUM et al. (1985) studied 10 early passage tumor cell lines derived from the tumors of patients with head and neck squamous cell carcinomas. Some results were interesting. For example, the cell line that was the most radiosensitive (lowest D_0) and exhibited the highest ability to repair PLD, happened to have been derived from a patient for whom radiotherapy failed. The data are too few

for any firm conclusions, but they do suggest a potential use for this type of determination as a predictive assay.

A requirement for this type of approach would be development of a more practical methodology. For instance, since even early passage cell lines might deviate in repair capacity from the tumor cells of origin, the determination would best be made on primary cultures, or even on the tumor itself. By doing so, the assay could be done more quickly than currently possible due to the several weeks or months necessary to develop early passage lines and measure PLD repair, an approach that already suffers from the fact that cell lines are not easily derived from tumors. A new approach to measuring PLD repair in cells has been outlined by CORNFORTH and BEDFORD (1983). They have shown that radiation-induced chromosome breakage and repair can be examined in interphase cells by inducing premature chromosome condensation (PCC). This is a method of visualizing interphase chromosomes by fusing the irradiated cells with mitotic cells (JOHNSON and RAO 1970). HITTELMAN and RAO (1974) showed how this approach could be used to study radiation-induced chromosome breaks and repair. CORNFORTH and BEDFORD extended these studies to examine chromosome break repair and to correlate it with PLD repair. When the kinetics of PLD repair are measured by clonogenic assays and compared to the PCC method, they found that remaining damage mirrored the rate of repair, as shown in Fig. 5.

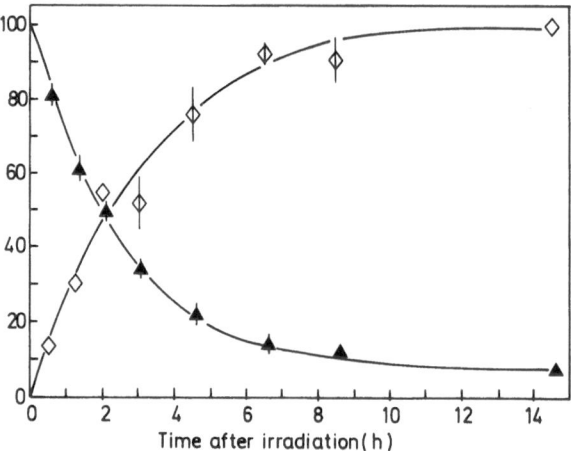

Fig. 5. The figure illustrates the relationship between repair of potentially lethal damage and the repair of broken chromosomes measured using the premature condensed chromosome technique. ▲ Percent PCC breaks remaining; ◇ Percent maximum PLD repair; AG 1522 Human fibroblasts plateau phase (600 rad). (COMFORTH and BEDFORD 1983, with permission)

On the surface this system seems to have excellent potential for estimating repair capacity in human biopsy specimens. Since it is possible to induce PCC in human tumor cells, this approach is technically feasible and should be tested. If PLD repair can be measured by this system, the results would be available only a couple of days after taking the biopsy specimen.

4.2 Measurements of Tumor Oxygenation

It is known from experimental work that hypoxic cells can be as much as three times more radioresistant than well-oxygenated cells. This has been documented not only *in vitro*, but also in animal tumors from radiobiologic data (GRDINA 1980) and in the selective binding of misonidazole to hypoxic cells (CHAPMAN et al. 1981). It has also been shown that hypoxia in mouse tumors can be responsible for resistance to radiocurability (SUIT et al. 1977). Hypoxia in human tumors has been inferred from tumor histology and from estimates of tumor tissue pO_2 (JAMIESON and VAN DEN BRENK 1965; MUELLER-KLIESER et al. 1981), although its importance in limiting cure in human tumors is not known. The problem has been difficult to study in humans without a direct method to assess its presence and to manipulate its degree. Clinical trials using neutrons, hyperbaric oxygen, and hypoxic cell sensitizers have been designed to overcome the potential hypoxic effect. However, the lack of clinical gain in the majority of patients in these studies suggests that hypoxia is not cure limiting in many human tumors. It is true that reoxygenation during treatment may minimize the consequences of hypoxia in human tumors, but it is commonly believed, although not yet proven, that in many human tumors radiotherapy fails because of a resistant subpopulation of hypoxic cells. Until proved false, hypoxia must be considered a candidate for producing tumor radioresistance because it does exist in human tumors and because oxygen is such an effective radiosensitizer.

4.2.1 Direct Measurements of Oxygen

It is now possible to make direct measurements of blood flow, oxygen extraction, and oxygen utilization in human tumors and normal tissues. The technique makes use of the positron emission tomograph (PET), which is an instrument that can obtain an image of *in vivo* positron-emitting nu-clides, such as oxygen-15. Oxygen-15 is produced by a cyclotron (half-life, 2 minutes), given to the patient by inhalation, and detected with a positron camera. Brain and breast tumors have been studied by this technique, and interesting results have been obtained. For example, blood flow in breast tumors was found to be higher in tumor than in normal tissues, except that it was low in necrotic tumor tissues. The oxygen-extraction ratio was lower in tumors, but the oxygen-consumption rate was higher, suggesting adequate oxygen supply to the tumors (BEANEY et al. 1984). In contrast, brain tumors have a lower oxygen consumption rate than normal brain tissue, in addition to having a low oxygen extraction rate (ITO et al. 1982). It has also been observed that ischemic normal tissues have the ability to increase their oxygen extraction ratio, which results in improved oxygen metabolism, but it appears that tumors do not have the same ability (BEANEY et al. 1984), probably due to differences in tumor microvasculature. Furthermore, since hypoxic tumor cells are likely to be at the limit of the oxygen diffusion distance, an increased demand could not be met by increased oxygen extraction anyway. At any rate, these results suggest that the cause of hypoxia in human tumors is due to a larger intercapillary distance than in normal tissues. Reoxygenation would be a result of cell killing and cell clearance. These conclusions are no different than what has been believed for years by the workers studying oxygen diffusion and tumor vasculature. However, oxygen-15 imaging can measure a patient's pretreatment oxygen status and so be used during therapy to monitor reoxygenation and possibly determine if pockets of hypoxia remain in the tumor.

4.2.2 Sensitizers and Other Probes of Hypoxia

Other potential methods for imaging hypoxia in tumors have been suggested. The hypoxic cell sensitizer misonidazole has been shown to bind selectively to intracellular sites in hypoxic cells. VARGHESE et al. (1980) and CHAPMAN et al. (1981) have shown that when radioactive misonidazole is given to multicellular spheroids or to mice bearing tumors, hypoxic areas can be identified by autoradiography. This work is very impressive in the mouse, but so far this approach has not been carried out in humans with positron imaging because of the lack of an active gamma- or positron-emitting nucleide of misonidazole. The search for a less toxic analogue that can be suitably labeled is under way. In the meantime, Chapman and co-workers have been carrying out studies using tritium-labeled sensitizer-adducts to hypoxic cells in humans. With this invasive technique, hypoxic cells have been identified in human tumor by autoradiography, proving the validity of this approach (CHAPMAN 1985).

Another potential metabolic approach for identifying hypoxic regions through imaging is to use labeled sugar analogs. The strategy would be to choose a nontoxic substrate that would be metabolized and preferentially concentrated in hypoxic tissues. An example proposed by PETERS et al. (1985), is to use radioactive pyruvate, labeled in the C1 position, so that its label is converted to radioactive CO_2 in aerobic tissues and removed, but in anerobic tissues where pyruvate is converted to lactic acid the label would remain. Preliminary studies were performed by PETERS et al. (1985) using $1\text{-}^{14}C$-pyruvate and a mouse fibrosarcoma that contains a high fraction of hypoxic cells. The hypoxic mouse tumors showed a preferential uptake of ^{14}C-pyruvate label to levels that would be imagable by PET as long as the C1 carbon is labeled with ^{11}C. This is a promising approach and should be expanded to include sugars and sugar analogs, which might give even better results. Examples would include glucose, 5-thio-D-glucose, 2-deoxy-D-glucose, or analogs of lactate and pyruvate, such as oxamate or oxalate.

4.2.3 Nuclear Magnetic Resonance

Nuclear magnetic resonance (NMR) is now being developed as a noninvasive method of measuring metabolism, including oxygenation and pH. These measurements can be determined spatially, thereby showing the "anatomy" of metabolic differences in a volume of tissue. Using NMR, the relative levels of inorganic phosphate, ATP, and phosphocreatine can be determined. The types of observations made so far include: a decrease in the phosphocreatine/ATP ratio and an increase in the Pi/ATP ratio as tumor volume increases, and a decrease in pH as the tumor volume increases (NG et al. 1982); all are suggestive of an increase in anaerobic metabolism with increasing tumor size. The relevance of these observations to tumor hypoxia or radioresponsiveness has not been determined. If the response of hypoxic regions within a tumor can be determined, NMR could be a valuable, noninvasive method for following tumor reoxygenation, possibly enabling accurate predic-

tion early in treatment. If patients with significant tumor cell hypoxia can be identified and even followed through the early stages of radiotherapy to determine the probability of treatment failure caused by hypoxia, then treatment could be altered to include hyperbaric oxygen, neutron therapy, or hypoxic cell sensitizers. At the very least, development of methods to measure tumor oxygenation before and during treatment will allow determination of the degree to which tumor hypoxia is responsible for tumor failure. If it turns out that this is a relatively small fraction of the patients, using this technique to select patients for an altered treatment should produce excellent results.

4.3 Cell Kinetics and Ploidy

In recent years, DNA levels and cell cycle distributions of tumor cell populations from the biopsies of individual patients biopsies have been determined by flow cytometry and have shown a great variation in both ploidy and in the cell cycle distribution. Further studies have searched for possible correlations between these features and their diagnosis and prognosis. For example, HOLM et al. (1980) showed that the DNA content (ploidy) of human squamous cell carcinomas correlates with histopathologic differentiation. Similar observations have been made for other tumors. In addition, higher levels of DNA are found more often in tumors in an advanced clinical stage. Therefore, it appears that this technique has potential as a diagnostic tool.

Correlations between cell kinetics, ploidy, or cell cycle phase distribution with the clinical outcome of radiotherapy have also been made. The most widely quoted publication is that of ATKIN and KAY (1979) who measured the cellular DNA content of over 1400 patient biopsy samples. They reported that in the case of uterine cervical carcinoma, a diploid or near diploid level of DNA predicts a worse local control rate and shorter survival time than does a triploid or greater DNA content. These results are subject to controversy because of inaccuracies of Feulgen DNA measurements and the minimal statistical significance of the data. In fact, JAKOBSON et al. (1984) found the opposite to be true for cervical carcinoma, the higher DNA content indicated a higher frequency of metastasis and lower survival time after radiotherapy. In their study, 171 patients were classified as having a G1 tumor cell DNA value of either less than or greater than 1.5 times the diploid

DNA level. A statistically significant higher local recurrence rate was found if the DNA level was 1.5 × diploid. However, JAKOBSEN and coworker's data clearly showed no correlation between DNA level and primary healing in these patients. HOLM (1982) reported a result for squamous cell carcinomas of the head and neck similar to those of JAKOBSEN et al. His results showed that a tumor cell DNA level greater than normal G_1 plus 2 standard deviations correlated with a more advanced clinical stage and poorer prognosis after radiotherapy. The favorable prognosis of near diploid levels appears to be true even for advanced clinical stages. This leaves open the question of whether or not high DNA levels are prognostic of tumor radiosensitivity. At present, there are several ongoing clinical studies for several tumor types and sites, all examining the value of the DNA index as a predictor of tumor cure by radiation.

Tumor cell proliferation during radiotherapy treatment is a potential reason for failure to cure, thereby making the overall treatment time an important factor (MACJEWSKI et al. 1983). An assessment of tumor cell kinetics prior to radiotherapy would make it possible to predict the optimum dose-fractionation schedule for an individual patient (THAMES et al. 1983; TROTT and KUMMERMEHR 1985). A new method has recently been developed for estimating tumor cell proliferation kinetics. This is a flow cytometric method for quantification of both cycling and noncycling S-phase cells and makes use of fluorescent labeled monoclonal antibodies against bromo-or iododeoxyuridine (GRATZNER 1982) that have been incorporated into DNA as a pulse label (DEAN et al. 1984). Estimates of the duration of S-phase and potential tumor doubling time are then calculated (BEGG et al. 1985). The validity and usefulness of this new methodology is now being tested in several laboratories.

5 Summary

It is clear from this discussion that the development of predictive assays has only begun and needs input from clinicians and researchers who are trying to identify those features of tumors that are responsible for radioresistance. The initial successes will be the development of methods which will group patients according to probable success after radiotherapy. However, ultimately a successful predictive assay, which may consist of a battery of tests, must not only be able to identify for an individual patient the possibility of failure after conventional radiotherapy, but also to identify the treatment modality with the greatest potential for success. Radiotherapy should be thought of as only one modality, to be used in combination with chemotherapy and surgery. Because of the unlimited possible combinations of radiation, drugs, surgery, hyperthermia, sensitizers, and so forth, predictive assays must be developed to aid in a rational choice of therapy for the individual patient. Therefore, one obvious necessity is collaboration between those who are testing for drug sensitivity and those testing for radiation sensitivity. Another area of research should include an examination of those factors that predict for the success of hyperthermia when used in combination with drugs or radiation, possibly in the area of tumor blood flow. Tumor cell heterogeneity with respect to radiation sensitivity is also an important problem. Small areas of heterogeneity due to hypoxia or to the presence of genetically radioresistant subpopulations are likely to be responsible for many failures, although identifying minor resistant subpopulations will be difficult. Possibly through the use of appropriate probes, flow cytometry will be able to identify the presence of rare but important resistant cells. Finally, the role of the host is of great importance. This factor may be the most difficult to assess. It will be necessary to assess the risk of radiation or combined therapy on late tissue damage and to oncogenesis. It will also be necessary to determine the role of the host immune system in influencing tumor cure and in the development of new cancers.

References

Atkin NB, Kay R (1979) Prognostic significance of modal DNA value and other factors in malignant tumors, based on 1465 cases. Br. J. Cancer 40:210–221

Baker F, Spitzer G, Ajani J, Brock W, Lukeman J, Pathek S, Tomasovic B, Thielvoldt D, Williams M, Vines C, Tofilon P (1986) Drug and radiation sensitivity measurements of successful primary monolayer cultureing of human tumor cells using cell-adhesive matrix and supplemented medium. Cancer Research 46:1263–1274

Barendsen GW (1980) Analysis of tumor responses by excision and *in vitro* assay of cellular clonogenic capacity. Br. J. Cancer 41, Suppl. IV:209–216

Beaney RP, Lammertsma AA, Jones T, McKenzie CG, Halnan KE (1984) Positron emission tomography for *in vivo* measurement of regional blood flow, oxygen utilisation, and blood volume in patients with breast carcinoma. Lancet 1:131–134

Bedford JS, Mitchell JB, Griggs HG, Bender MA (1978) Radiation-induced cellular reproductive death and chromosome aberrations. Radiat. Res. 76:573–586

Begg AC, McNally NJ, Shrieve DC, Karcher H (1985) A method to measure duration of DNA synthesis and the potential doubling time from a single sample. Cytometry 6:620–626

Bettega D, Bombana M, Pelucchi T, Poli A, Lombardi LT, Conti AMF (1980) Multinucleate cells and micronucleus formation in cultured human cells exposed to 12 MeV protons and -rays. Int. J. Radiat. Biol. 37:1–9

Brock WA, Williams M, Meistrich ML, Grdina DJ (1983) Micronucleus formation as a measure of surviving fraction in irradiated cell populations. In: Broerse JJ, Barendsen GW, eds., *Proceedings of the 7th International Congress of Radiation Research*. Amsterdam: Martinus Nijhoff, p B4–03.

Brock WA, Williams M (1985) Kinetics of micronucleus expression in synchronized irradiated Chinese hamster ovary cells. Cell Tissue Kinet. 18:247–254

Brock WA, Maor MH, Peters LJ (1985) Cellular radiosensitivity as a predictor of tumor radiocurability. Radiat. Res. 104:290–296

Brock WA, Williams M, Bhadkamkar VA, Spitzer G, Baker F (1985) Radiosensitivity testing of primary cultures derived from human tumors. In: Proceedings of the 3rd International Meeting on Progress in Radio-Oncology, Vienna, Austria, K.H. Karcher, ed.

Carrano AV (1973) Chromosome aberrations and radiation-induced cell death. I. Transmission and survival parameters of aberrations. Radiat. Res. 17:341–353

Carrano AV, Heddle JA (1973) The fate of chromosome aberrations. J. Theor. Biol. 38:289–304

Chapman JD (1985) Predictive assays for hypoxic cells in human tumors. *Abstracts for the Thirty-Third Annual Meeting of the Radiation Research Society*, Los Angeles, CA, p. 93

Chapman JD, Franko AJ, Sharplin JA (1981) A marker for hypoxic cells in tumors with potential clinical applicability. Br. J. Cancer 43:546–550

Cornforth MN, Bedford JS (1983) X-ray-induced breakage and rejoining of human interphase chromosomes. Science 222:1141–1143

Courtenay VD, Selby PJ, Smith IE, Mills J, Peckman MJ (1978) Growth of human tumour cell colonies from biopsies using two soft-agar techniques. Br. J. Cancer 38:77–81

Deacon J, Peckham MJ, Steel GG (1984) The radioresponsiveness of human tumors and the initial slope of the cell survival curve. Radiother. Oncol. 2:317–323

Dean PN, Dolbeare F, Gratzner H, Rice GC, Gray JW (1984) Cell cycle analysis using a monoclonal antibody to BrdUrd. Cell Tissue Kinet. 17:427–436

Dewey W, Humphrey R (1962) Relative radiosensitivity of different phases of the life cycle of L-P59 mouse fibroblasts and ascites and tumor cells. Radiat. Res. 16:503–530

Diehl-Marshall I, Bianchi M (1981) Induction of micronuclei by irradiation with neutrons produced from 600 MeV protons. Br. J. Radiol. 54:530–532

Dubranszky V (1966) Assessment of radiosensitivity of carcinoma of the cervix. J. Obstet. Gynecol. Br. Commonw. 73:41

Fertil B, Malaise E (1981) Inherent cellular radiosensitivity as a basic concept for human tumor radiosensitivity. Int. J. Radiat. Oncol. Biol. Phys. 7:621–629

Fertil B, Malaise EP (1985) Intrinsic radiosensitivity of human cell lines is correlated with radioresponsiveness of

human tumors: analysis of 101 published survival curves. Int. J. Radiat. Oncol. Biol. Phys. 11:1699–1707

Fettig O, Kaltenbach FB, Kloke WD (1980) Der „³H-thymidine-test" zur Beurteilung der Strahlensensibilität des collum carcinomas. Arch. Gynak. 213:283

Glucksman A (1974) Histological features in the local radiocurability of carcinomas. In: Friedman M, ed. *The Biological and Clinical Basis of Radiosensitivity*. Springfield: Thomas, p. 203–218

Good M, Lavin M, Chen P, Kidson C (1978) Dependence of cloning method on survival of human melanoma cells after ultraviolet and ionizing radiation. Cancer Res. 38:4671–4675

Grdina DJ (1980) Variations in radiation response of tumor subpopulations. In: Myen RE, Withers HR *Radiation Biology in Cancer Research*. New York: Raven Press, p. 353–363

Grote SJ, Joshi GP, Revell SH, Shaw CA (1981) Observations of radiation-induced chromosome fragment loss in live mammalian cells in culture, and its effect on colony-forming ability. Int. J. Radiat. Biol. 39:395–408

Hamburger AW, Salmon SE (1977) Primary bioassay of human tumor stem cells. Science 197:461–463

Hittelman WN, Rao PN (1974) Premature chromosome condensation. I. Visualization of -ray induced chromosome damage in interphase cells. Mutat. Res. 23:251–258

Holm L-E (1982) Cellular DNA amounts of squamous cell carcinomas of the head and neck region in relation to prognosis. Laryngoscope 92:1064–1069

Holm L-E, Jakobsson P, Killander D (1980) DNA and its synthesis in individual tumor cells from human upper respiratory tract squamous cell carcinomas. Laryngoscope 90:1209–1224

Hoshino T, Nagashima T, Murovic J, Levin EM, Levin VA, Rupp SM (1985) Cell kinetic studies of in situ human brian tumours with bromodeoxyuridine. Cytometry 6:627–632

Hoshino T, Nagashima T, Murovic JA, Wilson CB, Edwards MSB, Gutin PB, Davis RL, DeArmond SJ (1986) In situ cell kinetic studies on human neuroectodermal tumours with bromodeoxyuridine labelling. J Neurosurg 64:453–459

Jakobsen A (1984) Prognostic impact of ploidy level in carcinoma of the cervix. Am. J. Clin. Oncol., in press

Jamieson D, van den Brenk HAS (1965) Oxygen tension in human malignant disease under hyperbaric conditions. Br. J. Cancer 19:139–150

Johnson RT, Rao PN (1970) Mammalian cell fusion: Induction of premature chromosome condensation in interphase nuclei. Nature 226:717–722

Joshi GP, Nelson WJ, Revell SH, Shaw CA (1982a) X-ray-induced chromosome damage in live mammalian cells, and improved measurements of its effects on their colony-forming ability. Int. J. Radiat. Biol. 41:161–181

Joshi GP, Nelson WJ, Revell SH, Shaw CA (1982b) Discrimination of slow growth from non-survival among small colonies of diploid Syrian hamster cells after chromosome damage induced by a range of X-ray doses. Int. J. Radiat. Biol. 42:283–296

Limburg H, Napp JH, Willbrand V (1972) Die prognostische Beurteilung des Kollumkarzinoms nach Strahlenbehandlung durch Probeentnahme und Scheidenabstrich. Geburtshilfe und Frauenheilkunde 12:723

Maciejewski B, Preass-Bayer G, Trott KR (1983) The influence of the number of fractions and of overall treatment time on local control and late complication rate in squamous cell carcinoma of the larynx. Int. J. Radiat. Oncol. Biol. Phys. 9:321–328

McGarrity KA, Garvan JM (1961) Results of assessment of irradiation response in the treatment of carcinoma of the uterine cervix by evaluation of serial biopsies. In: Ilberg, P.L.T., ed. *Radiobiology, Proceedings of the 3rd Australasian Conference.* London: Butterworth, p. 206

Meyskens, F.L. (1980) Human melanoma colony formation in soft agar. In Salmon, S.E., ed. *Cloning of Human Tumor Stem Cells.* New York: Alan R. Liss, p. 85–99

Midander J (1982a) Oxygen enhancement ratios for glutathione-deficient human fibroblasts determined from the frequency of radiation induced micronuclei. Int. J. Radiat. Biol. 42:195–198

Midander J (1982b) Radiation-dose dependence of the formation of micronuclei in misonidazole treated cell cultures. Acta Radiol. Oncol. 21:133–137

Midander J, Revesz L (1980) The frequency of micronuclei as a measure of cell survival in irradiated cell populations. Int. J. Radiat. Biol. 38:237–242

Mueller-Klieser W, Vaupel P, Manz R, Schmidseder R (1981) Intracapillary oxygen hemoglobin saturation of malignant tumors in humans. Int. J. Radiat. Oncol. Biol. Phys. 7:1397–1404

Ng TC, Evanochko WT, Hiramoto RN, Ghanta VK, Lilly MB, Lawson AJ, Corbett TH, Durant JR, Glicoson JD (1982) ^{31}P NMR spectroscopy of *in vivo* tumors. J. Magnetic Resonance 49:271–286

Peters LJ, Withers HR, Thames HD, Fletcher GH (1980) The problem: Tumor radioresistance in clinical radiotherapy. In: Fletcher GH, Nervi C, Withers HR, eds. *Biological Basis and Clinical Implications of Tumor Radioresistance* New York: Masson Publishing, p. 1–11

Peters LJ, Hopwood LE, Withers HR, Suit HD (1984) Predictive assays of tumor radiocurability. Cancer Treat. Symp. 1:67–74

Peters LJ, Brock W, Johnson T (1985) Predicting radiocurability. Cancer 55:2118–2122

Puck TT, Marcus PI (1956) Action of X-rays on mammalian cells. J. Exp. Med. 103:653–666

Rockwell S (1985) Effects of clumps and clusters on survival measurements with clonogenic assays. Can. Res. 45:1601–1607

Sinclair WK, Morton RA (1966) X-ray sensitivity during the cell generation cycle of cultured Chinese hamster cells. Radiat. Res. 29:450

Suit HD, Howes AE, Hunter N (1977) Dependence of response of a C_3H mammary carcinoma to fractionated irradiation. Radiat. Res. 72:440–454

Tatra C, Breitnicker G (1980) Der klinische Wert histoautoradiographischer Untersuchungen während der Strahlentherapie des Zervixkarzinoms. Strahlentherapie 150:487

Trott KR (1980) Can tumour response be assessed from a biopsy? Br. J. Cancer 41, Suppl. IV: 163–170

Trott KR, Kummermehr J (1985) What is known about tumour proliferation rates to choose between accelerated fractionation or hyperfractionation? Radiother. & Oncol. 3:1–9

Varghese AJ, Whitmore GF (1980) Binding to cellular macromolecules as a possible mechanism for the cytotoxicity of misonidazole. Cancer Res. 40:2165–2169

VonHoff DD, Clark GM, Stogdill BJ (1983) Prospective clinical trial of a human tumor cloning system. Cancer Res. 43:1926–1931

Walter LH, Harrison CV, Glucksman A, Cherry CP (1964) Assessment of response of cervical cancers to irradiation by routine histological methods. Br. J. Medicine 1:1673

Warren S, Meigs JV, Severance AP, Jaffe HL (1939) The significance of the radiation reaction in carcinoma of the cervix uterine. Surg. Gynecol. Obstet. 69:645

Weichelsbaum RR, Schmit A, Little JB (1982) Cellular factors influencing radiocurability of human malignant tumors. Br. J. Cancer 45:10–16

Weichelsbaum RR (1984) The role of DNA repair processes in the response of human tumors to fractionated radiotherapy. Int. J. Radiat. Oncol. Biol. Phys. 10:1127–1134

Weichelsbaum RR, Dahlberg W, Little JB, Ervin TJ, Miller D, Hellman S, Reinwald JG (1985) Cellular X-ray repair parameters of early passage squamous cell carcinoma lines derived from patients with known responses to radiotherapy. Br. J. Cancer, in press

1.3 Quality of Survival

James E. Till

CONTENTS

1 Introduction

A new and fertile field of cancer research has begun to take shape over the past decade. It is based on an increasing awareness of the need for ways to measure aspects of the quality of life, with particular emphasis on those related to health. This development can be attributed to several factors, some arising from within oncology, and others external to it. One example of an internal factor is a sensitivity to the limits of current therapies, in that treatments that may prolong survival also may involve significant treatment-related effects on quality of survival. Another example is general acceptance of the principle that even when we cannot cure, care should still be the best possible. The success or failure of that care can only be evaluated by measuring any improvement in the quality as well as the quantity of life (TILL et al. 1984). Alleviation of symptoms and distress and, where possible, the preservation of function remain worthwhile objectives for treatment. Factors external to oncology include the rise of consumerism and its emphasis on the perspective of the patient,

together with an increasing interest in health maintenance and the prevention of disability as well as disease treatment (LALONDE 1974; MCKEOWN 1979). These concepts are illustrated by the World Health Organization's (1958) definition of health: "Health is a state of complete physical, mental and social well-being and not merely the absence of disease or infirmity".

In oncology, where increasing numbers of alternative therapies are becoming available, and where patient preferences among these alternatives are becoming increasingly important, reliable and valid information about quality of survival is seldom available. One important role of the newly-developing field is to make up for this deficiency. This area of research should be of particular interest to radiation oncologists, in that the unique potential of radiation therapy to preserve organ function as well as organ structure might be expected to yield improved quality of survival in comparison with the surgical alternatives.

There has always, of course, been interest in any morbidity associated with cancer and the patient's treatment, and many efforts have been made to assess and report such morbidity. For example, the Karnofsky Scale of Performance Status (KARNOFSKY and BURCHENAL 1949) has been used for more than 3 decades (see Section 3.1). It is based on the perspective of the physician rather than the patient, and thus addresses only one of the two most important aspects of an assessment of quality of survival. These two aspects may be viewed as: i) an assessment of engagement in life tasks, and ii) an assessment of the *satisfaction* derived from engagement in life tasks (MCCULLOUGH 1984). The former aspect can be assessed using objective criteria, by health professionals such as the physician or nurse, based on a shared perspective and widely-held value systems. The latter aspect cannot; it requires the inclusion of subjective information, based on the patient's own perspective and unique personal value system. It is a major theme of this Chapter that for some, if not all, uses of assessments of quality of survival,

Supported by a research grant from the National Cancer Institute of Canada and by career investigator support from the Ontario Cancer Treatment and Research Foundation.

James E. Till, Ph. D
Ontario Cancer Institute
Toronto, Ontario M4X 1K9, Canada

this subjective aspect based on the patient's perspective cannot and should not be ignored; it is an essential component of any comprehensive evaluation of quality of survival.

An illustration of the importance of the patient's subjective perspective is provided by a study of SUGARBAKER et al. (1982), designed to link treatment consequences to quality of life for patients with soft-tissue sarcoma. The major finding was that the initial hypothesis, that limb-sparing surgery plus irradiation would provide improved quality of life when compared to amputation, could not be substantiated. Instead, some evidence was obtained that, in terms of sexual relations, the amputated patients might even have adjusted better. However, two different methods for elicitation of data about sexual functioning yielded different results; a significant reduction in sexual functioning was detected for patients who received the limb-sparing treatment regimen, compared with the amputees, when patients were interviewed, but *not* when they provided self-reports of sexual functioning. Less sexual dysfunction was reported when some of the amputees were interviewed than in their self-report assessments, while a similar degree of sexual dysfunction was reported by the limb-spared group for both types of assessments. These results serve to emphasize a second major theme: that measurements of the patient's perspective may be very sensitive to the methods used to collect data.

The long-term goal of studies of quality of survival should always be to find ways to improve the care of patients. The existence of data such as those of SUGARBAKER et al. should serve as a stimulus to seek ways to ensure that function as well as structure is preserved, so that the quality of survival is enhanced.

2 Methodological Criteria

As illustrated by the work of SUGARBAKER et al. (1982), collection of data on quality of survival from the patient's perspective is limited at present mainly by methodological problems. As stressed at a recent conference on methodology in behavioral and social cancer research, the development and refinement of appropriate research methodology merits a very high priority (MILDER 1984). It is essential that the questionnaires (usually referred to as "instruments" in the jargon of the field) used to measure aspects of quality of survival

Table 1. Summary of Methodological Criteria

1. Conceptual scope
2. Feasibility
3. Psychometric properties
   Reliability
   Validity
   Availability of norms
   Sensitivity to change
4. Method of data collection

should be demonstrated, by systematic and rigorous testing, to have the properties required of any other meaningful measurement tool. Criteria which may be applied to assess the properties of instruments for the measurement of quality of survival have been discussed elsewhere (see, for example, NUNNALLY 1967; TUGWELL and BOMBARDIER 1982; FAYERS and JONES 1983; CIAMPI et al. 1983; TILL et al. 1984). Some of these criteria will be summarized briefly below (see also Table 1).

2.1 Conceptual Scope

Quality of survival is a broadly-defined concept involving many dimensions. Even when other factors such as housing, employment, finances, etc. (WARE 1984) are omitted, and attention is restricted to health status (an aspect of quality of life that is usually identified as important; see, for example, CAMPBELL 1981), one is still dealing with a multidimensional concept. Thus, the first issue to be faced in any assessment of quality of survival is the conceptual scope of the measures to be used. This choice is in turn largely determined by the purposes of the investigation. For the objective of evaluation of a particular treatment modality for patients with a particular disease, the choice of variables can be restricted to those which the disease affects, with particular attention to those likely to be influenced by treatment. Usually, a tradeoff must be made between the breadth of scope of the assessment and the depth of the examination of any particular aspect. Preliminary work must be done to ensure that the conceptual scope of the measurement is not too narrow, so that some important aspects are not unintentionally omitted. Conversely, the conceptual scope should also not be so broad that unnecessary information is collected, thus imposing an inappropriate burden on the patient.

2.2 Feasibility

The instrument must be capable of being used successfully to obtain results that are free of mistakes or missing data. To ensure feasibility, a method of assessment should be relatively simple, easy to understand, and should not make excessive time demands on the patient, or on those responsible for data collection.

2.3 Psychometric Properties

These properties include reliability, validity, availability of appropriate norms, and sensitivity to change (CIAMPI et al. 1983). They are usually termed "psychometric properties" (NUNNALLY 1967), because of pioneering work in this area on the measurement of subjective emotional states (BAROFSKY 1984).

Reliability may be defined as the degree to which results are free of random error. Major approaches to the assessment of reliability include internal consistency, test-retest stability, and inter-observer reliability. Internal consistency can be checked when several items in the instrument are likely to be measuring the same underlying phenomenon; such inter-related items should correlate with each other in a reliable instrument. Test-retest stability (reproducibility) is examined by analysis of the correlation obtained when the instrument is applied more than once to the same individuals, on the assumption that no changes have occurred during the time between tests. Inter-observer reliability involves an assessment of the extent to which different observers obtain the same measurement scores when the instrument is applied to the same individuals; it cannot be assessed for instruments based on patients' self-reports.

Validity may be defined as the degree to which an instrument measures what it is supposed to measure. If some "gold standard" exists, then the *criterion* validity of the instrument can be tested by comparison of the results obtained using the instrument to those obtained using the gold standard. However, in studies of quality of survival, a suitable gold standard is seldom, if ever, available. Validity must be established by testing the extent to which the results obtained with the instrument are compatible with other relevant evidence. Gradually, a body of indirect evidence is accumulated to support the validity of the measure

(MORROW 1984). There are usually at least three types of validity: First, the instrument should demonstrate *content* and *face* validity, in that it is both comprehensive and credible (TUGWELL and BOMBARDIER 1982). Second, it should show various aspects of *construct* validity, in that the results of the method make sense, that is, match with the hypothesized expectations of the investigator when compared with other indirect assessments. There are two main types of construct validity (TUGWELL and BOMBARDIER 1982): *convergent* construct validity, which involves an assessment of how well the results of the instrument agree with those obtained from other accepted methods, and *divergent* construct validity, which involves an assessment of how well the method under consideration demonstrates differences in groups of patients which would be expected to show differences. For example, a valid measure of physical function should generally reflect poorer physical health according to stage of disease, that is, show the expected gradient effect with stage of disease. A third form of validity, *predictive* validity, is demonstrated when an instrument is shown to be able to predict the value of some other (dependent) variable of interest. Evidence of validity provided by a combination of approaches is the most convincing; techniques of testing for the different types of validity are available (for an example, see MORROW 1984). The importance of avoiding errors of validity has been emphasized by TUKEY (as quoted in CAMPBELL 1978): "It is often much worse to have a good measurement of the wrong thing than to have a poor measurement of the right thing – especially when, as is so often the case, the wrong thing will in fact be used as an indicator of the right thing."

Availability of norms, that is, availability of results for reference populations, is often vital in interpreting results, and particularly for judging the extent to which an instrument is applicable to various populations, such as patients in different age groups or different diagnostic categories.

Sensitivity to change is very important in a clinical context, especially when the purpose is to assess the effect of a treatment. It should be demonstrated that the instrument can detect the smallest clinically significant change of interest to the investigator. An instrument may be reliable, but of little use in detecting subtle but important changes induced by a treatment, simply because it excludes certain items.

2.4 Methods of Data Collection

The method of data collection used (such as an interview, self-report, provision of information by family member, etc.) can have a major influence on the results obtained, as illustrated by the results of SUGARBAKER et al. (1982) summarized above.

3 Examples of Instruments for Use in Oncology

It is beyond the scope of this Chapter to attempt any comprehensive critical review of all the instruments currently used to assess the multiple components of quality of survival. Examples of measures of physical functioning, measures of psychosocial functioning, and some measures of health status of broader scope have been summarized by CIAMPI et al. (1983). The proceedings of the workshop conference on methodology sponsored by the American Cancer Society in April, 1983, also contains many examples of instruments designed to assess a variety of variables relevant to oncology (see, for example, SINGER 1984). Only two selected examples will be discussed below, to illustrate approaches that have been taken to the development and characterization of instruments. These are the Karnofsky Performance Status Scale (KPS) and Linear Analogue Self-Assessment (LASA).

3.1 The Karnofsky Performance Status Scale (KPS)

The 11-category KPS is the best-known instrument used in oncology; it has been in use since the 1940's (KARNOFSKY and BURCHENAL 1949). A 5-category abbreviated version is also widely used (ZUBROD et al. 1960). The categories of the KPS range from normal functioning ("normal, no complaints, no evidence of disease", score 100) to dead (score 0). The purpose of the KPS is to rate the patient's performance during various stages of illness. It has been used for research purposes as a stratifying variable and as an eligibility criterion in randomized trials, and as an outcome measure to evaluate response to treatment and to assess the impact of treatment on quality of survival (AISNER and HANSEN 1981; IRWIN et al. 1982; IRWIN and GOTTLIEB 1982). It has also been used by clinicians in treatment decisions for individual patients.

The conceptual scope of the KPS is somewhat limited. Emphasis is placed on a physician's assessment of the patient's physical capabilities. Information about psychosocial functioning from the perspective of the patient is not sought. Nor are the scores assigned to the various categories of the scale based on any formal method of measuring preferences, such as those used by TORRANCE et al. (1976) and LLEWELLYN-THOMAS et al. (1982).

The feasibility of the KPS is very well-established, as illustrated by its popularity. However, in spite of its wide use both in clinical research and in treatment decisions, very little attention has been paid to the psychometric properties of the instrument. Only recently have some attempts been made to assess its reliability and validity (HUTCHINSON et al. 1979; YATES et al. 1980; MOR et al. 1984; SCHAG et al. 1984). Taken together, they provide a useful case study of the issues to be dealt with in assessing the psychometric properties of an instrument. HUTCHINSON et al. (1979) were the first to point out deficiencies in the reliability and validity of the KPS. SCHAG et al. (1984) have confirmed these deficiencies, and made some very useful suggestions about approaches that could be used to improve the reliability and validity of the KPS. For example, they suggested ways in which more detailed information about the four main elements of the KPS (work, self-care, daily activity and evidence of disease) could be obtained from a routine clinical interview and used to make a more accurate assessment of the KPS.

3.2 Linear Analogue Self-Assessment (LASA)

Linear analogue self-assessment, using visual analogue scales, is a well-established method of obtaining subjective information, based on the patient's perspective, in an efficient way (BOND and LADER 1974; PRIESTMAN and BAUM 1976; HUSKISSON 1982; OBERST 1984). The approach is simple; the subject is presented with a 10-cm line, "anchored" at each end with statements that define the extremes of the scale (for an example, designed to assess an aspect of voice quality in laryngeal cancer, see Fig. 1). The subject marks the position on the line that corresponds to his/her own assessment. A measurement of the location of the mark relative to the total length of the scale provides a quantitative score for that scale. PRIESTMAN and BAUM (1976) used LASA scales to assess the quality of survival of patients with breast cancer, and similar approaches are being explored by others

(PRESANT et al. 1981; COATES et al. 1983; SELBY et al. 1984). For example, SELBY and colleagues (1984) have recently reported the results of a careful study of the properties of a series of LASA scales developed for the investigation of patients with breast cancer. The approach used is worthy of note; it is based on the concept of "modules" of LASA scales, which could, if necessary, be combined in different ways. For example, in their study, an 18-item module was designed to assess general health problems, based on the dimensions used in a well-known behaviorally-based measure of health status, the Sickness Impact Profile (BERGNER et al. 1981), which has itself been used by others (JOHNSON et al. 1983) to assess the quality of life of radiation therapy patients. This module based on the Sickness Impact Profile was combined with a 13-item module designed to assess major problems associated with breast cancer. Each item of the instrument was evaluated for feasibility, reliability and validity. It appeared easy to use, acceptable and reliable in these assessments. Most items appeared to be valid when compared to alternative measurement methods including the Sickness Impact Profile, and clinical evaluation by a physician. The correlations between items were analysed by factor analysis and seemed to fit with the clinical features of breast cancer. The method distinguished between clinically distinct groups of patients and detected changes with time.

A module of LASA scales has also been developed for assessment of voice quality for patients with laryngeal cancer following radiation therapy (LLEWELLYN-THOMAS et al. 1984a; SUTHERLAND et al. 1984; LLEWELLYN-THOMAS et al. 1984b). Voice quality is an aspect of quality of survival that is of particular concern for patients with laryngeal cancer (HARWOOD and RAWLINSON 1983). It can be influenced significantly by choice of treatment, in that radiation therapy can preserve the larynx and surgery may not. Survival without relapse for patients with localized disease is high (greater than 80%) after treatment with either radiation therapy or surgery (KAPLAN et al. 1984), so that differences in quality of survival can have a significant impact on treatment decisions. The voice is also an aspect of quality of survival that is uniquely amenable to study. It can be recorded, and thus can be preserved, stored, and made available for assessment at different times, in a variety of ways. It provides a very useful model for study of an aspect of quality of life that involves a limited number of variables.

a Effort required to speak

Able to speak without any effort	————————	Able to speak only with great effort

b Ability to use the telephone

Able to use telephone as usual	————————	Completely unable to use telephone

Fig. 1 a, b. Examples of LASA scales used to obtain self-assessments of voice quality. **a** Example of a scale designed to assess a symptom. **b** Example of a scale designed to assess a functional area. One such scale was prepared for each of the 16 voice quality dimensions. Patients are asked to place a vertical mark on each scale at a position that best described their own state over the past week (LLEWELLYN-THOMAS et al. 1984a)

Previous work concerned with the assessment of voice following therapy for laryngeal cancer has been focussed on objective physiological measures such as phonation range, air flow rate, or electrical activity of the laryngeal musculature (see, for example, ORR et al. 1972). This kind of approach does not provide information about aspects of voice quality which may be of particular concern from the patient's viewpoint, such as the ability of patients to work, to use the telephone, or to converse with their families. LASA scales have the advantage that they permit such information to be collected quickly and easily, while incorporating the patient's own point of view about his/her own voice-related abilities. An example of LASA scales used to obtain self-assessment of voice quality is shown in Fig. 1.

Work designed to provide an initial test of the reliability and validity of the use of LASA scales to assess voice quality has been reported (LLEWELLYN-THOMAS et al. 1984a; SUTHERLAND et al. 1984). The aspect of reliability that was examined was test-retest stability. This aspect (see Section 2.3) refers to the extent to which an instrument produces results that are consistent when applied repeatedly to patients whose clinical state is not expected to change between assessments. A total of 16 attributes of voice quality and function were selected; a separate LASA scale of the kind shown in Fig. 1 was used for self-assessment of each attribute. Taken together, the results for all 16 attributes indicated that LASA scores were generally reliable, sensitive to clinical change, yet stable when clinical status is unaltered (LLEWELLYN-THOMAS et al. 1984a). The validity of the LASA scores now needs to be investigated further (SUTH-ERLAND et al. 1984).

LASA scales are simple, convenient, versatile and reliable, but can pose difficulties in coding and analysis of data (FAYERS and JONES 1983).

4 Conclusions and Future Directions

The examples summarized above represent only two of many approaches that have been taken to the development of measures of aspects of the quality of survival for patients with malignant disease. Other examples of recent systematic work on the development of instruments especially designed for studies in oncology have been reported by SPITZER et al. (1981), SCHIPPER et al. (1984), and MORROW (1984). These examples serve to illustrate the importance of properties of the instruments. As in every other area of scientific investigation, the usefulness of the data obtained is critically dependent on the properties of the methods of measurement that are used. This is particularly true in the case of data based on patients' self-assessments. It is only recently that oncologists have begun to appreciate that reliable and valid data can be collected in this way; however, such reliability and validity cannot be taken for granted. It must be demonstrated using the kinds of approaches outlined above. No shortcuts are possible; time-consuming tests of reliability and validity must be carried out prior to the use of any such methodology in clinical trials or as a source of information to patients regarding the impact of proposed treatments on the quality of survival. These methodological issues demand immediate attention, in view of the rapidly developing interest in the application of quality of life measures in cancer clinical trials (FAYERS and JONES 1983; VAN DAM et al. 1984; TILL et al. 1984).

Since the impact of changes in a patient's quality of life may be expected to be dependent on that patient's value system, the problem of measuring quality of survival is inextricably linked to the problem of measuring values. Future research needs to emphasize the centrality of value differences among patients (BARD 1984). A remarkable example has been provided by MOUNT and SCOTT (1983) of a young patient who in dying commented that his last year had been the best year of his life, even though the final months had been characterized by physical deterioration and considerable suffering. Clearly, this patient did not give physical functioning a very high importance or value in his overall assessment of the quality of his survival over those months. As MOUNT and SCOTT (1983) point out, scales oriented toward the health care professional's view of quality of survival, such as the Karnofsky KPS or the QL Index of SPITZER et al. (1981), are unlikely to deal adequately with the issue of individual value differences.

Values are equally important in decisions. When treatments differ in their consequences, individuals with different value systems will rank them differently in terms of desirability, and for this reason will make different choices. An example of the significance of value judgments for clinical decision-making is provided by the work of McNEIL et al. (1981), who found that 20% of volunteers stated that, for laryngeal cancer, they would choose radiation therapy with preservation of laryngeal function over surgery with loss of laryngeal function, even under hypothetical circumstances where surgery was assumed to yield a 60% 3-year survival rate but irradiation was assumed to yield a lower survival rate of 40%. It is clear that these particular subjects suggested that they would be willing to trade off 20% differences in 3-year survival in order to preserve laryngeal function. These findings illustrate the importance of value differences among patients.

Other directions for future work (TILL et al. 1984) include further research on the difficult problem of how to aggregate the multiple components of quality of life, so that, if necessary, it might be possible to use a single index to summarize the quality of survival. Another important area is the development of techniques to help patients to understand the implications of alternative therapies, and then to assist them to choose among these alternatives in ways that are consistent with their attitudes toward the multiple components of quality of survival, and toward any tradeoffs between quality and quantity of survival. Much remains to be done, but the essential first step is the realization by oncologists that ways of approaching these difficult issues are indeed available, and that, by application of the kinds of criteria summarized in Section 2, such methods can be subjected to rigorous tests of their ability to provide meaningful data.

References

Aisner J, Hansen HH (1981) Commentary: Current status of chemotherapy for non-small cell lung cancer. Cancer Treat Rep 65:979–986

Bard M (1984) Summary of the informal discussion of function states: Quality of life. Cancer 53 (Supplement): 2327

Barofsky I (1984) Response. Cancer 53 (Supplement): 2299–2302

Bergner M, Bobbitt RA, Carter WB, Gilson BS (1981) The Sickness Impact Profile: Development and final revision of a health status measure. Med Care 19:787–805

Bond A, Lader MH (1974) The use of analogue scales in rating subjective feelings. Br J Med Psychol 47:211–218

Campbell A (1981) The Sense of Well-Being in America: Recent Patterns and Trends. McGraw-Hill, New York, p 15

Campbell A (1978) Poor measurement of the right thing. In: Goldfield ED (ed) Proceedings of the American Statistical Association, Social Statistics Section: 1977 Part I. American Statistical Association, Washington, p 120

Ciampi A, Silberfeld M, Till JE (1983) Health status indices: Some approaches and their limitations in oncology. Ontario Psychologist 15:4–14

Coates A, Dillenbeck CF, McNeil DR, Kaye SB, Sims K, Fox RM, Woods RL, Milton GW, Solomon J, Tattersall MHN (1983) On the receiving end – II. Linear analogue self-assessment (LASA) in evaluation of aspects of the quality of life of cancer patients receiving therapy. Eur J Clin Oncol 19:1633–1637

Fayers PM, Jones DR (1983) Measuring and analysing quality of life in cancer clinical trials: A review. Statistics in Medicine 2:429–446

Harwood AR, Rawlinson E (1983) The quality of life of patients following treatment for laryngeal cancer. Int J Rad Oncol Biol Phys 9:335–338

Huskisson EC (1982) Measurement of pain. J Rheumatol 9:768–769

Hutchinson TA, Boyd NF, Feinstein A (1979) Scientific problems in clinical scales, as demonstrated in the Karnofsky Index of Performance Status. J Chron Dis 32:661–666

Irwin PH, Gottlieb A, Kramer S, Danoff B (1982) Quality of life after radiation therapy: a study of 309 cancer survivors. Social Indicators Research 10:187–210

Irwin PH, Gottlieb A (1982) The quality of life after radiation therapy: health status. Social Indicators Research 11:105–108

Johnson JE, King KB, Murray RA (1983) Measuring the impact of sickness on usual functions of radiation therapy patients. Oncology Nursing Forum 10:36–39

Kaplan MJ, Johns ME, Clark DA, Cantrell RW (1984) Glottic carcinoma. The roles of surgery and irradiation. Cancer 52:2641–2648

Karnofsky DA, Burchenal JH (1949) The clinical evaluation of chemotherapeutic agents in cancer. In: Macleod CM (ed) Evaluation of Chemotherapeutic Agents. Columbia University Press, New York, 191–205

Lalonde M (1974) A New Perspective on the Health of Canadians. A Working Document, Queen's Printer, Ottawa

Llewellyn-Thomas H, Sutherland HJ, Tibshirani R, Ciampi A, Till JE, Boyd NF (1982) The measurement of patients' values in medicine. Med Decis Making 2:449–462

Llewellyn-Thomas HA, Sutherland HJ, Hogg SA, Ciampi A, Harwood A, Keane T, Till JE, Boyd NF (1984a) Linear analogue self-assessment of voice quality in laryngeal cancer. J Chron Dis 37:917–924

Llewellyn-Thomas HA, Sutherland HJ, Ciampi A, Etezadi-Amoli J, Boyd NF, Till JE (1984b) The assessment of values in laryngeal cancer: Reliability of measurement methods. J Chron Dis 37:283–291

McCullough L (1984) The bioethicist's view of quality of life. Presented at the Fifth Annual Meeting of the Society for Clinical Trials, Miami

McKeown T (1979) The Role of Medicine. Dream, Mirage or Nemesis? Princeton University Press, Princeton

McNeil BJ, Weichselbaum R, Pauker S (1981) Speech and survival: Tradeoffs between quality and quantity of life in laryngeal cancer. N Engl J Med 305:982–987

Milder JW (1984) Introduction. Cancer 53 (Supplement): 2217

Mor V, Laliberte L, Morris JN, Wiemann M (1984) The Karnofsky Performance Status Scale: An examination of its reliability and validity in a research setting. Cancer 53:2002–2007

Morrow GR (1984) The assessment of nausea and vomiting: Past problems, current issues, and suggestions for future research. Cancer 53 (Supplement):2267–2278

Mount BM, Scott JF (1983) Whither hospice evaluation. J Chron Dis 36:731–736

Nunnally JC (1967) Psychometric Theory. McGraw-Hill, New York

Oberst MT (1984) Patients' perceptions of care: Measurement of quality and satisfaction. Cancer 53 (Supplement):2366–2373

Orr NM, Hamilton MD, Glennie JM (1972) Variations in voice quality with laryngeal tumors and radiotherapy of larynx. Br J Disord Communic 7:135–140

Presant CA, Klahr C, Hogan L (1981) Evaluating quality-of-life in oncology patients: Pilot observations. Oncology Nursing Forum 8:26–30

Priestman TJ, Baum M (1976) Evaluation of the quality of life in patients receiving treatment for advanced breast cancer. Lancet 1:899–901

Schag CC, Heinrich RL, Ganz PA (1984) Karnofsky Performance Status revisited: reliability, validity and guidelines. J Clin Oncol 2:187–193

Schipper H, Clinch J, McMurray A, Levitt M (1984) Measuring the quality of life of cancer patients: The Functional Living Index – Cancer: Development and validation. J Clin Oncol 2:472–483

Selby PJ, Chapman JAW, Etezadi-Amoli J, Dalley D, Boyd NF (1984) The development of a method for assessing the quality of life of cancer patients. Br J Cancer 50:13–22

Singer JE (1984) Some issues in the study of coping. Cancer 53 (Supplement):2303–2313

Spitzer WO, Dobson AJ, Hall J, Chesterman E, Levi J, Shepherd R, Catchlove BR (1981) Measuring the quality of life of cancer patients: A concise QL-index for use by physicians. J Chron Dis 34:585–598

Sugarbaker PH, Barofsky I, Rosenberg SA, Gianola FJ (1982) Quality of life assessment of patients in extremity sarcoma clinical trials. Surgery 91:17–23

Sutherland HJ, Llewellyn-Thomas H, Hogg SA, Keane TJ, Harwood AR, Till JE, Boyd NF (1984) Do patients and physicians agree on the assessment of voice quality in laryngeal cancer? J Otolaryngol 13:325–330

Till JE, McNeil BJ, Bush RS (1984) Measurement of multiple components of quality of life. Cancer Treatment Symposia 1:177–181

Torrance GW (1976) Social preferences for health states: An empirical evaluation of three measurement techniques. Socioecon Plann Sci 10:129–136

Tugwell P, Bombardier C (1982) A methodologic framework for developing and selecting endpoints in clinical trials. J Rheumatol 9:758–762

Van Dam FSAM, Linssen CAG, Couzijn AL (1984) Evaluating 'quality of life' in cancer clinical trials. In: Cancer Clinical Trials: Methods and Practice. Buyse ME, Staquet MJ, Sylvester RJ (eds), Oxford University Press, Oxford, p 26

Ware JE jr (1984) Conceptualizing disease impact and treatment outcomes. Cancer 53 (Supplement):2316–2323

World Health Organization (1958) Constitution of the World Health Organization. In: The First Ten Years of the World Health Organization. World Health Organization, Geneva p 459

Yates JW, Chalmer B, McKegney FP (1980) Evaluation of patients with advanced cancer using the Karnofsky Performance Status. Cancer 45:2220–2224

Zubrod CG, Schneiderman M, Frei E, Brindley C, Gold LG, Shnider B, Oviedo R, Gorman J, Jones R, Jonsson U, Colsky J, Chalmers T, Ferguson B, Dederick M, Holland J, Selawry O, Regelson W, Lasagna L, Owens AH (1960) Appraisal of methods for the study of chemotherapy of cancer in man: Comparative therapeutic trial of nitrogen mustard and triethylene thiophosphoramide. J Chron Dis 11:7–33

2 Conservation Therapy

2.1 Head and Neck

2.1.1 Functional Surgery and Radiotherapy in Head and Neck Cancer

GILBERT H. FLETCHER

CONTENTS

1 Introduction

The management of cancers of the head and neck should be as conservative as is consistent with tumor eradication because of appearance and the vital functions of the upper respiratory and digestive tract. Examples are preservation of an important functional organ such as the larynx or, in cancers of the oral cavity and oropharynx, minimizing the difficulty in swallowing and impairment of speech by limiting the amount of tissues removed. Although shoulder motion is a less important function, it can be preserved by saving the spinal accessory nerve. Conservatism applies when surgery alone or radiation therapy alone is used and in the combination of surgery and irradiation.

This investigation was supported in part by grants CA06294 and CA16672 awarded by the National Cancer Institute, U.S. Department of Health and Human Services.

GILBERT H. FLETCHER, M.D., Professor of Radiotherapy
The University of Texas M.D. Anderson Hospital
and Tumor Hospital
Houston, TX 77030, USA

Preservation of life has priority and therefore a more conservative treatment is only acceptable if the control rates are equal.

Because of the multiple combinations of radiation alone, surgery alone, and the combined treatment, individualization of treatment is required to minimize damage to cosmesis and function.

General principles will be discussed first, and some treatment schemes for the various anatomical sites of the head and neck area will be reviewed.

2 General Principles

2.1 The Sigmoid Dose Response Curve

There is not an "all or none" cancerocidal dose. Because of the randomness of cell killing, the probability of controlling a tumor can be plotted on a curve, a portion of which is very steep if the tumor population is homogeneous (Fig. 1). With

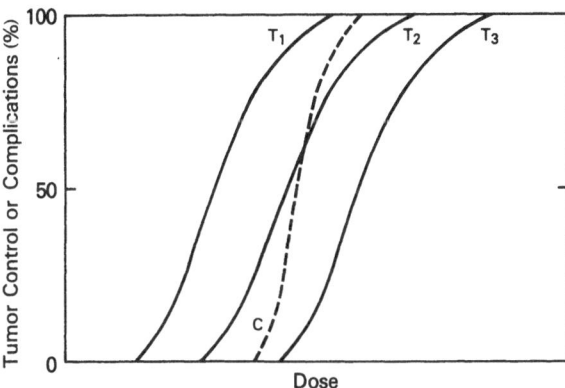

Fig. 1. The therapeutic ratio relates the probability of tumor control to that of a treatment complication for a given dose of radiation. If curve C represents the dose response relationship for an unacceptable normal tissue injury, and curves T_1, T_2 and T_3 represent tumor control probabilities for say 3 increasing stages of the same tumor, then the therapeutic ratio would be strongly positive for T_1 with a high percentage of uncomplicated cures possible; marginally positive for T_2 with a maximum for 20–25% of uncomplicated cures possible; and negative for T_3 for which curative treatment by radiotherapy would be contraindicated. (From PETERS 1985, in press)

Table 1. Incidence of recurrence at the primary site in 946 primary determinate cases treated for the most part by surgery alone[a]. (From FARR and ARTHUR 1972)

Primary Site	Recurrence (%)
Hard palate	73
Base of tongue	61
Tonsil	53
Soft palate	52
Pharyngeal wall	48
Gingiva	46
Buccal mucosa	41
Floor of mouth	39
Anterior tongue	38
Supraglottic larynx	23
Lip	14

[a] 90% of the patients were treated by surgery alone

Table 2. Recurrence at the primary site following multimodality treatment for stages III or IV squamous cell carcinoma of the head and neck. (From VIKRAM et al. 1984a)

Surgery only 1960–1970		Surgery + postop. irradiation 1975–1980	
Satisfactory margins	Unsatisfactory margins	Satisfactory margins	Unsatisfactory margins
39%	73%	2%	10.5%

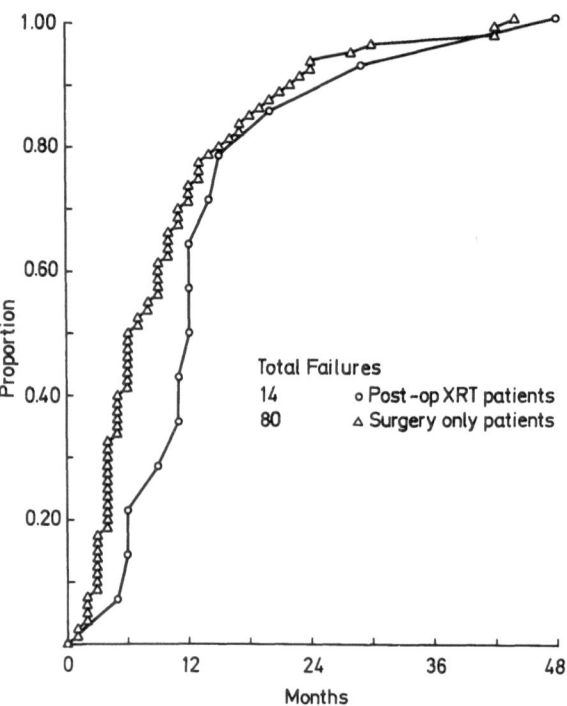

Fig. 2. Cumulative rate of failures above the clavicles in pyriform sinus tumors. Almost half of the failures in the surgery only group have appeared by 6 months. (From FLETCHER GH 1983)

a relatively small increment of dose, the probability of control can be increased from 25% to 75%, whereas to increase the probability of control from 80% to 95%, the dose must be increased considerably more because the curve flattens out. There is also a sigmoid response curve for complications (Fig. 1), and there is an interplay between radiocurability and tolerance. One would like to cure all patients, but this goal cannot be achieved, and it is unwise to attempt to increase control rates beyond a certain point because of the excessive complications all patients would experience. This concept is even more important if cosmesis and preservation of function are goals, and if salvage surgery for radiation failures is an available "back-up" option.

2.2 Treatment Strategy in the Combination of Surgery and Irradiation

Surgery alone for the primary lesion and metastases in lymph nodes in the neck results in a high incidence of failures (Tables 1 and 2). This has prompted the increasing use of the combination of surgery and irradiation in the last two decades.

Optimally, the surgical procedures should be limited to the removal of the gross masses for the following reasons:

1. Faster healing reduces the interval between the surgical procedure and the initiation of irradiation. Malignant clonogens can repopulate rapidly after a surgical procedure as shown by the rate of appearance of clinically manifest recurrences above the clavicles in patients with a tumor of the pyriform sinus (Fig. 2). In a series of patients with squamous cell carcinoma of the head and neck, an increased failure rate was related to the delay between the surgical procedure and the initiation of postoperative irradiation (Table 3). Because of the diminished cell loss in an accelerated repopulation there is a higher proportion of malignant clonogens than in a nonchallenged tumor cell population.

2. It must be well understood that when postoperative irradiation is planned there is no benefit to be derived from trying to remove all microscopic disease, which cannot be done in all patients

Table 3. Recurrences in the head and neck of patients electively irradiated postoperatively for stages III and IV epidermoid carcinoma of the head and neck. (From VIKRAM et al. 1980)

Nodal status at surgery	Radio-therapy ≤ 6 wks postop.		Radio-therapy > 6 wks postop.[a]	
	No.	%	No.	%
Negative	0/5	0	0/3	0
Positive at one level	0/18	0	3/11	27
Positive at multiple levels	2/25	8	12/32	37.5
Total	2/48	4	15/46	32.5

[a] In the patients with a delay over 6 weeks there was no palpable disease at the time of the initiation of irradiation

Table 4. Comparison of failure rate at the primary site between patients treated by surgery only and patients treated by surgery and postoperative irradiation. (From FELDMAN and FLETCHER, 1982)

	Oral cavity	Oropharynx
Memorial Sloan-Kettering Cancer Center (NYC)[a]		
All stages in determinate patients[b] 1960 to Dec. 1964	38%–73%[c]	48%–61%[c]
UT M. D. Anderson Hospital		
T3 or T4 lesions[d] Primary or primary neck 1955 to Aug. 1976	22% (11/48)	32% (14/44)

[a] 90% of the patients were treated by surgery alone (FARR HW, ARTHUR K, 1972)
[b] Excludes patients lost to follow-up or dead of intercurrent disease
[c] Range of percentages of recurrences for various anatomical sites
[d] Evaluable patients treated by surgery and postoperative irradiation

anyway. The increase in radicalism of the surgical procedure might be counterproductive by increasing the delay before the start of irradiation.

3. There is less scar tissue and, therefore, less possibility of hypoxia of the tumor cells left behind, which increases the effectiveness of postoperative irradiation.

4. Complications, e.g., pharyngeal strictures, are less frequent and less severe if, for instance in pyriform sinus tumors, only gross cancer is removed with a limited partial pharyngectomy.

5. Diminished surgical manipulation provides less opportunity for disseminating tumor cells into the blood stream.

The radiation doses administered with limited surgery, provided all gross disease has been removed, need not be more, and perhaps may be less, than with a more radical procedure, since there is less scarring and delay before the initiation of irradiation.

3 Oral Cavity and Oropharynx

Impairment of speech and difficulty in swallowing make a patient an oral cripple. The disability increases with the extent of the resection and how much of the remaining tongue is bound down. In squamous cell carcinoma of the oral cavity and oropharynx, surgery alone is not often successful (Tables 1 and 2). Commando-type operations allow wider margins of resection, but are cosmetically unsatisfactory and can be very disabling, especially when the primary tumor is in the oropharynx. Combined treatment permits a less mutilating surgical procedure, and data shows that

postoperative irradiation increases the control rates (Table 4).

Early tumors of the faucial arch can be easily controlled by radiation therapy and with present techniques using mixed photon and electron beams there is little dryness of the mouth. In the main, tumors of the base of the tongue, tonsillar fossa, and pharyngeal walls are best treated by irradiation.

4 Larynx and Hypopharynx

Tumor limited to one vocal cord can be equally well controlled by partial laryngectomy or irradiation. With a partial laryngectomy the voice is always raspy, and with irradiation it is usually normal. When the tumor extends outside the true cords or to the anterior commissure, surgical procedures, even if less than a total laryngectomy, produce severe voice deficit and the voice is better if the patient is treated with irradiation. However, if most of the muscle has been destroyed by cancer, the voice may not be quite perfect, although still quite acceptable. Table 5 shows that with primary irradiation for T_1 lesions the control rate is 90% and for T_2 lesions 75%. With salvage surgery for failures, the control rate is close to 100% for T_1 lesions and 90% for T_2 lesions. At least 30% of the failures appear after 3 years and these are probably new lesions developing usually in pa-

Table 5. Squamous cell carcinoma of the vocal cords failures at anytime during follow-up. (From FLETCHER and GOEPFERT, 1984b)

Stage	No. of patients	No. of failures	No. of patients salvaged	Ultimate failures (%)
1948 thru 1973 (analysis 1976)				
T_1	332	37 (11%)	31	1.8
T_2	175	46 (26%)	36	5.7
1974 thru 1977 (analysis 1982)				
T_1	99	7 (7%)	6	1
T_2	27	7 (26%)	4	11

Table 6. Preservation of normal laryngeal function in patients treated by radiation therapy for primary tumors of supraglottic larynx. 1964 through 1972 (analysis December 1976). (From FLETCHER and GOEPFERT, 1984a)

Stage	No. of patients	Failures	Severe edema[a]	Percent laryngeal voice preserved
T_1[b]	18	1	0	94.5% (17/18)
T_2	37	4	4	78.5% (29/37)
T_3	23	4	2	74.0% (17/23)
T_4	13	6	1[c]	54.0% (7/13)

[a] Necessitating either temporary or permanent tracheostomy
[b] Of 16 patients irradiated between January 1973 and December 1979, one experienced a failure that was surgically salvaged and another had a laryngectomy for focal necrosis (analysis March 1982)
[c] Tracheostomy for severe edema at 10 months and laryngectomy for recurrence at 33 months

Table 7. Local-regional failures by histologic types after resection and postoperative irradiation. (From MCNANEY et al., 1983)

Histology	No. of patients	Failures		
		Primary site[a]	Neck	Primary site and neck
Malignant mixed	13	1	0	0
Adenocarcinoma	17	2	2	1
Mucoepidermoid (low grade)	9	0	0	0
Mucoepidermoid (high grade)	15	1	2	0
Acinic cell	5	0	0	0
Adenoid cystic	15	1	0	0
Unclassified	1	0	0	0
Other	2	0	0	0
Total	77	5	4	1

[a] Including the facial nerve into the base of the skull

Table 8. Local-regional failures by extent of facial nerve resection. (From MCNANEY et al. 1983)

Extent of resection of facial nerve	No. of patients	Failures		
		Primary site	Neck	Primary site and neck
Total	21	3	2	0
Partial	21	1	1	0
No resection	35	1	1	1
Total	77	5	4	1

Table 9. Squamous cell carcinoma of the head and neck. (From FLETCHER 1984)

Various anatomical sites Irradiation of whole neck in initially N_0 neck (primary controlled) 1970–1973 (analysis July 1976)	Supraglottic larynx Irradiation of subdigastric and midjuglar nodes in initially N_0 neck (primary controlled) 1948–1978 (analysis 1980)
1/60[a]	0/108[a]

[a] Number of failures/number of patients treated

tients who continue to smoke. Giving higher doses in an attempt to improve these control rates would, at best, yield a minimal increase but the incidence of severe edema, which was less than 1% in the series reported in Table 5, would increase and in many patients the quality of the voice would be compromised.

In tumors of the supraglottic larynx, a normal voice is preserved in a high percentage of T_1 and T_2 lesions (Table 6). More extensive tumors of the supraglottic larynx can be treated with a partial laryngectomy and postoperative irradiation, preserving the glottis (FLETCHER and GOEPFERT 1984b). The larynx can also be preserved in selected patients with tumors of the pyriform sinus and hypopharynx by treatment using primary irradiation, or conservation surgery followed by postoperative irradiation.

5 Parotid Tumors

Sacrifice of the facial nerve is a very disfiguring procedure. After removal of gross parotid cancer, microscopic residual disease can be controlled by

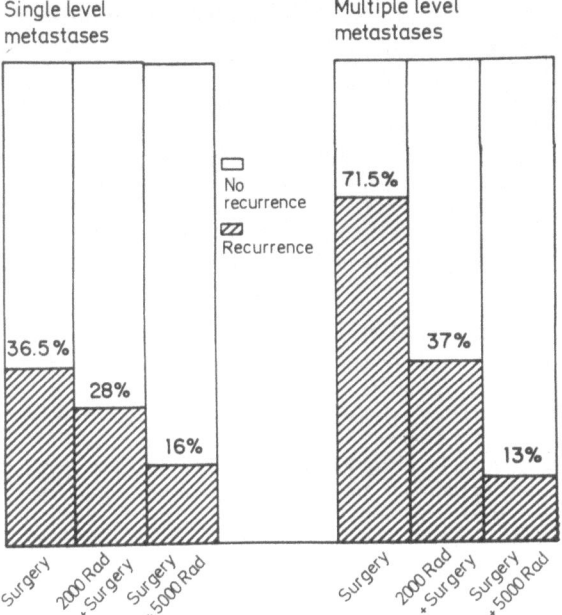

Single level metastases / Multiple level metastases

No recurrence

Recurrence

Single level metastases:
36.5% Surgery
28% 2000 Rad + Surgery
16% Surgery + 5000 Rad

Multiple level metastases:
71.5% Surgery
37% 2000 Rad + Surgery
13% Surgery + 5000 Rad

Fig. 3. Comparison of the rates of recurrences in the neck among patients treated by surgery alone or surgery with 20 Gy given preoperatively (historically derived from Strong E, 1969) and patients treated by surgery and 50–60 Gy given postoperatively. Almost all the recurrences were in patients with a delay of more than 6 weeks before the start of irradiation. (From VIKRAM et al. 1984b)

postoperative irradiation irrespective of the histology (Table 7). Table 8 shows that the control rates are not decreased by preserving the facial nerve. The facial nerve, or part of it, should only be sacrificed if a segment is grossly involved by tumor.

6 Management of Neck Disease

6.1 Elective Irradiation of the Lymphatics

Even if neck lymph nodes are clinically negative, there is a possibility of occult infestation becoming

Fig. 4a, b. Patient seen on May 1, 1968, with an ulcerated lesion on the laryngeal surface of the epiglottis extending to the left false and true cords. In the right midjugular chain, there was a node 3 cm in diameter and in the left one 4- to 5-cm. Biopsy: Grade IV squamous cell carcinoma. On May 7, 1968, a laryngectomy and a bilateral neck dissection were done. There were positive nodes in both sides of the neck. The irradiation was delayed for 2 months because of slow wound healing. **a** A midline dose of 60 Gy was given to the upper neck; after 45 Gy, the posterior margin of the parallel opposing portals was moved forward to exclude the spinal cord and an additional 15 Gy were given with a 9-MeV electron beam. **b** The lower neck received 50 Gy given dose in 5 weeks with an anterior portal, the stoma being shielded. The patient had a recurrence in the left neck 11 months after irradiation. (From FLETCHER et al. 1970)

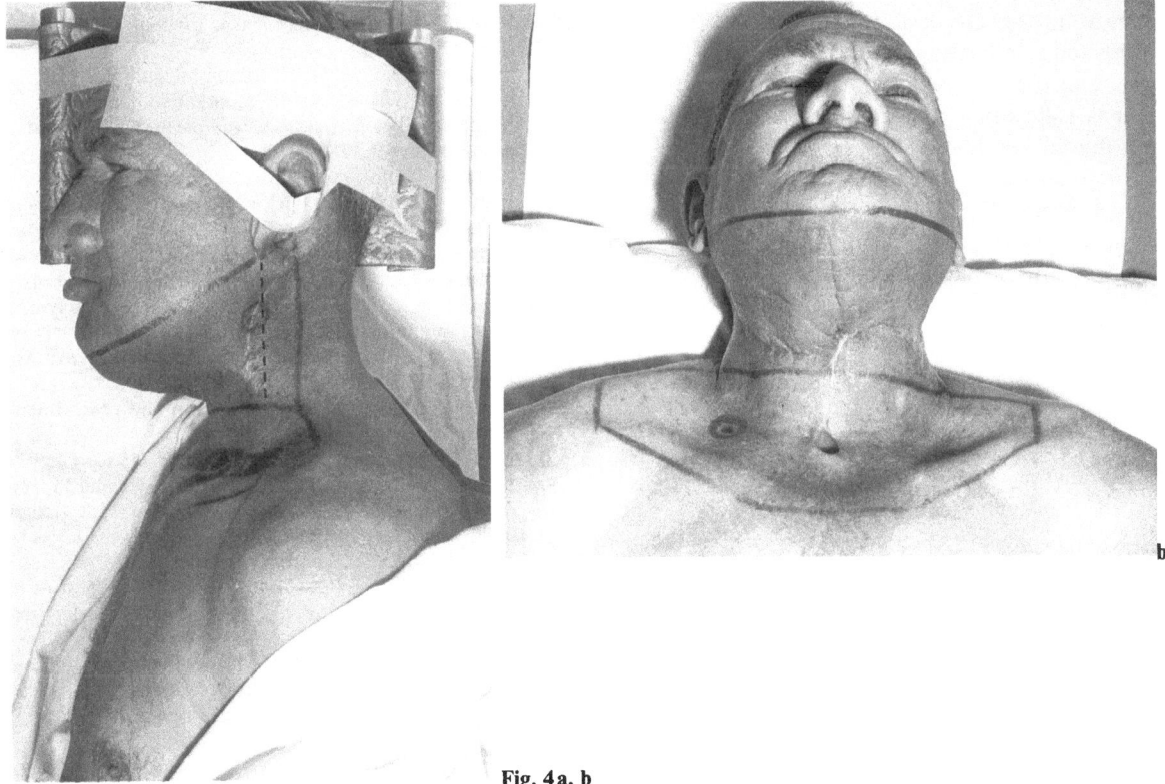

Fig. 4a, b

clinically manifest later. The frequency of this infestation varies with the anatomical location of the primary tumor, being highest for the base of the tongue, tonsillar fossa, pyriform sinus, and nasopharynx tumors (FLETCHER et al. 1980). Elective irradiation with 45–50 Gy ensures almost all patients freedom from developing clinical disease at a later date (Table 9). These moderate doses are not accompanied by significant late sequelae.

An elective neck dissection is an alternative method of treating subclinical metastases in cervical lymph nodes, but it affects cosmesis. If one does a classic radical neck dissection, which includes the removal of the sternocleidomastoid muscle, jugular vein, and the spinal accessory nerve, impairment of shoulder function is added to the cosmetic deficit.

6.2 Management of Clinically Positive Neck Metastases

Radical neck dissection alone is not very effective in controlling metastatic lymph node disease and postoperative irradiation has to be given (Fig. 3). Irradiation alone is very effective for nodes that are no more than 3 cm in diameter (SCHNEIDER et al. 1975). Using the shrinking field technique, high doses can be given to small volumes without compromising cosmesis and function. There are some data indicating that if surgery consists of less than the conventional radical neck dissection and is followed by irradiation, control rates are not diminished (JESSE et al. 1978).

Figure 4 shows an example of the edema of the face and upper neck after a conventional bilateral radical neck dissection removing the sternocleidomastoid muscle and the jugular vein on both sides. In this patient there was delay in healing and therefore irradiation postoperatively was delayed and the disease recurred in the neck.

7 Summary

When the management of head and neck cancers is approached with a view to preserving function, not only is the quality of life improved but in many clinical situations control rates are also improved. Because of the biology and radiobiology of cancer the effectiveness of the combination of surgery and irradiation can be increased by using a diminished surgical procedure.

References

Farr HW, Arthur K (1972) Epidermoid carcinoma of the mouth and pharynx. J Laryngol Otol 86:243–253

Feldman M, Fletcher GH (1982) Analysis of the parameters relating to failures above the clavicles in patients treated by postoperative irradiation or squamous cell carcinomas of the oral cavity or oropharynx. Int J Radiat Oncol Biol Phys 8:27–30

Fletcher GH (1983) The scientific basis of the present and future practice of clinical radiotherapy. Int J Radiat Oncol Biol Phys 9:1073–1082

Fletcher GH (1984) Lucy Wortham James Lecture. Subclinical disease. Cancer 53:1274–1284

Fletcher GH, Lindberg RD, Jesse RH Jr (1970) The combination of radiation and surgery in oropharynx and laryngopharynx squamous cell carcinomas. In: Saegesser F and Pettavel J (eds) Surgical oncology. Hans Huber Publishers, Bern, Switzerland, pp. 347–366

Fletcher GH, Jesse RH Jr, Lindberg RD, Westbrook KC (1980) Neck nodes In: Fletcher GH (ed) Textbook of radiotherapy, 3rd edn. Lea & Febiger, Philadelphia, pp. 249–271

Fletcher GH, Goepfert H (1984a) Irradiation in management of squamous cell carcinoma of the larynx. In: English GM (ed) Otolaryngology. J.B. Lippincott Co., Philadelphia, pp. 1–53

Fletcher GH, Goepfert H (1984b) Role of irradiation in the treatment of laryngeal cancr. In Ferlito A (ed) Cancer of the larynx, Vol. III, CRC Press, Boca Raton, 69–114, 1985

Jesse RH, Ballantyne AJ, Larson D (1978) Radical or modified neck dissection: a therapeutic dilemma. Am J Surg 136:516–519

McNaney D, McNeese MD, Guillamondegui OM, Fletcher GH, Oswald MJ (1983) Postoperative irradiation in malignant epithelial tumors of the parotid. Int J Radiat Oncol Biol Phys 9:1289–1295

Peters LJ (1987) Biology of radiation therapy. In Thawley SE and Panje WR (eds): Comprehensive Management of Head and Neck Tumors, W.B. Saunders Co, Philadelphia, pp 13

Schneider JJ, Fletcher GH, Barkley HT Jr (1975) Control by irradiation alone of nonfixed clinically positive lymph nodes from squamous cell carcinoma of the oral cavity, oropharynx, supraglottic larynx, and hypopharynx. Am J Roentgenol 123:42–48

Strong EW (1969) Preoperative radiation and radical neck dissection. Surg Clin North Am 49:271

Vikram B, Strong EW, Shah J, Spiro RH (1980) Elective postoperative irradiation therapy in stage III and IV epidermoid carcinoma of the head and neck. Am J Surg 140:580–584

Vikram B, Strong EW, Shah JP, Spiro R (1984a) Failure at the primary site following multimodality treatment in advanced head and neck cancer. Head Neck Surg 6:720–723

Vikram B, Strong EW, Shah JP, Spiro R (1984b) Failure in neck following multimodality treatment in advanced head and neck cancer. Head Neck Surg 6:724–729, 1984

2.1.2 Uveal Melanoma: Conservative Treatment with Radiation Therapy

JOHN E. MUNZENRIDER, EVANGELOS S. GRAGOUDAS,
PATRICIA MCNULTY, JOHANNA M. SEDDON,
MACIA URIE

CONTENTS

Supported in part by NIH Grant CA 21239.

JOHN E. MUNZENRIDER, M.D.
EVANGELOS S. GRAGOUDAS, M.D.
MACIA URIE, Ph. D.
JOHANNA M. SEDDON, M.D.
Harvard Medical School
Boston, MA 02114, USA

PATRICIA MCNULTY, R.N.
Massachusetts General Hospital
Boston, MA 02114, USA

1 Introduction

Uveal melanomas are relatively rare, with approximately 1,500 cases being diagnosed annually in the U.S. They are equally common in males and females, have an age-adjusted incidence which approximates 12% of the rate of cutaneous melanoma, and infrequently occur in blacks. Albert has recently reviewed intraocular melanomas, discussing etiology, histogenesis, histopathology, diagnostic criteria and various treatment modalities (ALBERT 1982). The overwhelming majority occur in adults in the middle years; only 101 of 6,358 cases in the Registry of Ophthalmic Pathology at the Armed Forces Institute of Pathology (AFIP) was less than 20 years old (BARR et al. 1981). Approximately 75% of the patients experience visual symptoms which prompt medical consultation and diagnosis of the tumor; approximately half the patients with symptoms complain of decreased vision (GRAGOUDAS et al. 1985b).

Traditional treatment has been enucleation after clinical diagnosis since biopsy was not generally feasible. Diagnostic criteria have been less than perfect in the general ophthalmological community with false positive rates approximating 20% reported in eyes submitted to the AFIP for review prior to 1964 (FERRY 1964) and between 1964 and 1974 (SHIELDS and ZIMMERMAN 1973). However, diagnostic accuracy in the general ophthalmological community has significantly improved, with only 48 non-melanomas being found in 744 eyes (6.4%) enucleated with a clinical diagnosis of ciliochoroidal melanoma (CHANG et al. 1984). False positive rates in patients evaluated at major referral and teaching centers have been extremely low, ranging from 2.7–8% (CHANG et al. 1984). Utilizing indirect ophthalmoscopy, fundus photography, fluorescein angiography and ultrasound, diagnostic accuracy is quite high and treatment decisions can be based on clinical evaluation only.

2 Relationship of Metastasis to Enucleation

Because of a peak in mortality of about 8% during the second year after enucleation it has been postulated that surgery contributed to most deaths from metastatic disease by disseminating tumor cells or by lowering the host's immunological defense mechanisms (ZIMMERMAN, MCLEAN, and FOSTER 1978; ZIMMERMAN, MCLEAN 1979). However, others have concluded that death within two years after enucleation could be due only exceptionally to tumor dissemination at surgery because the growth rates of uveal melanoma were generally far too low (MANSCHOT and VAN PEPERZEEL 1980). Nevertheless, they suggested that preoperative irradiation with two daily doses of 4 Gy each be given to prevent artificially induced distant metastases, and, if there was extra-scleral extension, postoperative radiation to doses in the range of 50 to 60 Gy be added.

In discussions advocating early enucleation to prevent metastatic dissemination, no recognition is generally given to the possibility that radiation therapy alone might permanently sterilize the tumor, with the added advantage of preserving the eye with some potential for useful vision.

3 Prognostic Factors in Uveal Melanoma Outcome

Prognostic factors have been evaluated after enucleation in 267 patients, 230 (86%) of whom had surgery at the Massachusetts Eye and Ear Infirmary between 1953 and 1973 prior to the introduction of proton therapy; the other patients were pathology referrals to that institution after enucleation elsewhere (SEDDON et al. 1983). Median follow-up was 17 years (8–28 years). Multivariate analysis identified five leading prognostic factors: number of epithelioid cells per high power field, largest tumor dimension, location of anterior tumor margin, invasion to line of transection, and pigmentation of tumor.

4 Conservative Treatment Techniques

The controversy over whether enucleation is beneficial or harmful in terms of survival has continued (ALBERT 1979; BONIUK 1979; JACOBIEC 1979; MAUMENEE 1979; SHIELDS and AUGSBURGER 1980), but there is no argument that patients undergoing enucleation immediately lose the sight of that eye.

Local excision (FOULDS 1977, PAYMAN and RAICHAND 1979) and photocoagulation (MEYER-SCHWICKERATH and VOGEL 1977; SHIELDS and AUGSBURGER 1980) can achieve tumor control and preservation of vision in some patients, but have limited applicability.

Over half a century ago interstitial irradiation using radon seeds was reported to have produced persisting regression of a uveal melanoma until death of the patient from intercurrent disease three years later (MOORE 1930). STALLARD (1966) described a patient dying of renal carcinoma 17.5 years after application of radon seeds for treatment of bilateral choroidal melanomas. Over the past two decades significant experience has been reported with plaque therapy using Cobalt-60 or Ruthenium-106/Rhenium-106, and more recently with Iodine-125. Vision has been preserved in significant numbers of patients treated with these techniques; initial survival experience is no worse than after enucleation.

During the past decade, external beam therapy using protons or helium ions has been shown to provide a high probability of local control of uveal melanoma, with good visual preservation rates and cosmesis equal to or better than that achieved with any other form of therapy.

The remainder of this chapter will discuss conservative radiotherapy techniques, with major emphasis on the use of external proton and helium ion beams.

5 Brachytherapy with Surface Applicators

In a classic paper STALLARD (1966) presented results in 105 patients treated by Cobalt-60 scleral plaques and 2 treated with radon seeds. Doses to the tumor base and summit were 18,000 to 36,000 r, and 7,000–14,000 r respectively in 79 patients receiving a single application, with higher doses given to 26 patients receiving more than one application. Treatment resulted in tumor recession to a flat pigmented scar in 31 of 35 (89%) eyes with tumors less than 7.5 mm diameter, and 52 of 72 (72%) patients with larger tumors. Metastases developed in none of the former and in 10 of the latter, with median follow-up times of 4–5 years. In a later report, 78 of the 107 (73%) patients were alive, with 11% of the patients dying a melanoma-related death. Fifty-one treated eyes had been retained, representing 65% of the survivors and 48% of the original 107 patients (MAC-

FAUL 1977). Complications included perimacular exudates, punctate retinal hemorrhages, vitreous hemorrhage, neovascular glaucoma, partial scleral sloughing and superficial punctate keratitis. Cataract was observed in ten patients (9%) between two and seven years after treatment.

Extensive additional experience has been gained using plaques of Cobalt-60 (ROTMAN et al. 1977; BRADY et al. 1984), Ruthenium-106/Rhenium-106 (LOMMATZSCH 1983; BUSSE et al. 1985), Iodine-125 (SEALY et al. 1976, 1980; ROTMAN et al. 1984; ROBERTSON et al. 1983), Radon-222 (STALLARD 1966; EHLERS 1975; DAVIDORF 1976), Tantalum-182 and Gold-198 (CHENERY et al. 1978), and Iridium-198 (JAPP et al. 1982).

Most patients have been treated with Cobalt-60 and with Ru-106/Rh-106; it has been suggested that Iodine-125 may be preferable, and clinical experience with that isotope is increasing. The choice of isotope should probably depend upon the height of the tumor treated: Ru-106/Rh-106 and I-125 for relatively low tumors, I-125 and Ir-192 for medium tumors, and Co-60 for highly elevated tumors.

Although the majority of tumors treated with plaques have regressed and the affected eye has been retained, complication rates have been fairly high, especially when tumors were located near the optic nerve and macula.

6 Radiotherapy: External Beams Using Charged Particles

Accelerated charged particles can treat small targets within the eye with minimal scatter and no radiation beyond the end of the particle range. Extensive experience has been developed at the Harvard Cyclotron Laboratory in proton beam therapy of uveal melanomas, involving a collaborative effort between that laboratory, the Radiation Medicine Department of Massachusetts General Hospital, and the Retina Service of the Massachusetts Eye and Ear Infirmary. A similar effort has developed at Berkeley, involving collaboration between the Lawrence Berkeley Laboratory and the Ocular Oncology Unit of the University of California-San Francisco. Proton therapy of uveal melanomas has been ongoing for several years in the U.S.S.R. (CHUVILO et al. 1984), was begun at the Swiss Institute for Nuclear Research (SIN) in Viligen, Switzerland, in 1984, and will commence at Upsala, Sweden, in 1988.

6.1 Protons: Preclinical Studies

In preclinical studies using monkeys, normal eyes and simulated ocular tumors were treated with single proton doses of 50–100 Gy using a 7 or 10 mm diameter beam. Opaque areas of edematous retina and choroid developed within 20 hours in each eye, while immediately outside the visible lesion, the retina and choroid appeared entirely normal (CONSTABLE and KOEHLER 1974; CONSTABLE et al. 1975). At longer intervals (42–51 months) there were chorioretinal changes within the irradiated area, but normal retinal architecture was preserved immediately outside the discrete retinal proton scar (GRAGOUDAS et al. 1979).

6.2 Protons: Clinical Studies

The technique was then adapted to the treatment of human intraocular melanoma, with encouraging results (GRAGOUDAS et al. 1985a and b, 1984, 1982, 1980, 1977).

6.2.1 Technique

Tantalum rings measuring 2.5 mm in diameter are sutured to the sclera around the perimeter of the tumor as defined by transillumination or by indirect ophthalmoscopy at surgery in the majority of patients. Some anterior ciliary body lesions and/ or peripheral choroid lesions which can be adequately seen by transillumination have been treated with a light field set-up only. The computerized treatment planning program employed at Harvard has been described (GOITEIN and MILLER 1983). Patients are treated in a seated position immobilized with an individually molded face mask and bite block, with voluntary fixation on an external light source positioning the eye during treatment after initial radiographic or light-field set up. Mean movement during treatment of 0.5 mm ± 0.3 mm was observed in 41 treatments of 11 patients, with maximum movement of 1.2 mm (VERHEY et al. 1982). A margin of 1.5 mm is allowed around the visible base of the tumor to allow for motion during treatment, set-up error and microscopic extension. A wide-angle fundus photograph of a patient with a posterior melanoma is shown in Fig. 1a, while in Fig. 1c the aperture designed from the treatment planning program is shown, encompassing the tumor outlined by scleral clips. Relationship of the radiation field to other ocular

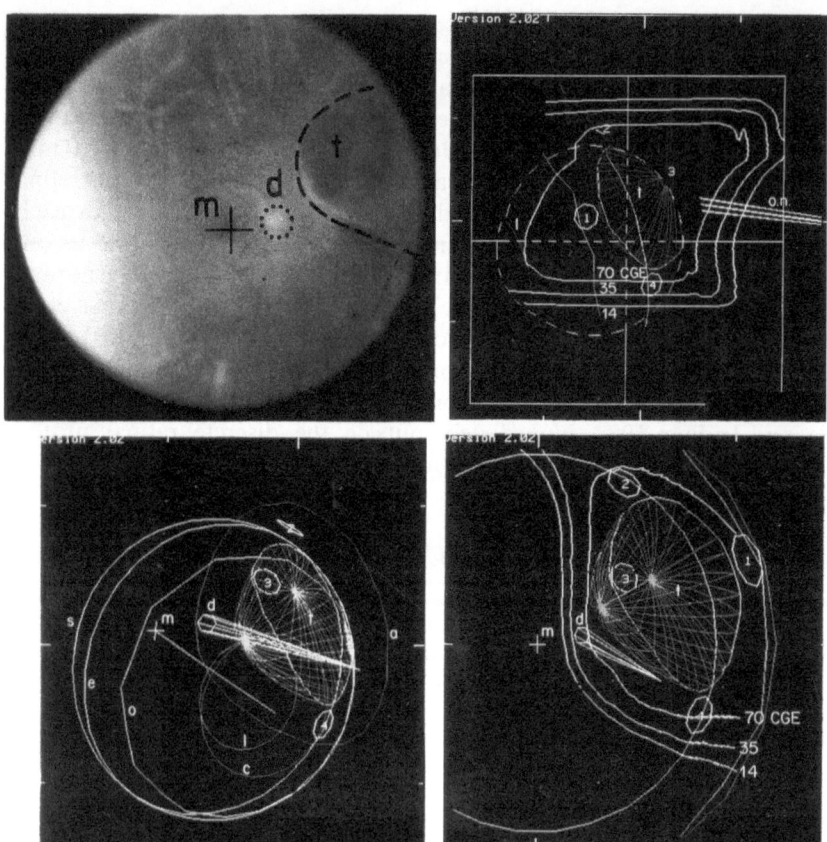

Fig. 1. **a** Wide angle fundus photograph of uveal melanoma (*t*) showing its relationship to the optic disc (*d*), and the macula (*m*). **b** Lateral dose distribution around tumor, showing clips (*1, 2, 3, 4*), optic nerve (*o.n.*), and 14, 35, and 70 CGE isodose lines. **c** Aperture (*a*) to treat tumor (shown in **a**) with relationship of aperture projection to tumor base, disc, and macula. *1, 2, 3,* and *4* are clips, *l* lens, *c* cornea, *o* ora serrata, *e* equator and *s* sclera. **d** "AP" dose distribution on fundus showing disc receiving less than 70 CGE, and macula receiving less than 14 CGE

structures is also seen. Fig. 1b and 1d show the lateral and "AP" dose distribution, with the disc lying immediately outside the high dose volume, and the macula receiving a negligible dose.

6.2.2 Clinical Material

Between July 1975 and August 1984, 526 melanomas were treated in 524 patients. The 268 female and 266 male patients ranged in age from 14 to 84 years, with two-thirds being in the sixth or seventh decade. Tumors were divided into small, medium, large, and extra-large categories, depending on maximum tumor diameter and height. Distribution of patients by size of lesion is given in Table 1. Sixty percent of the patients had tumors with maximum diameter larger than 15 mm and/or height larger than 5 mm. Virtually all patients received five treatments with 94% receiving a total dose of 70 Cobalt Gy equivalents (CGE, proton Gy times RBE 1.1); approximately 90% were treated in seven or eight days. Two-thirds of the patients presented with secondary serous retinal detachment; resolution of that detachment was the

Table 1. Uveal melanoma. Tumors by stage 7/75–6/84

Stage	Diameter (mm)	Height (mm)	Number	%
Small	≤ 10	≤ 2	25	5
Medium	10.1–15	2.1–5	183[a]	35
Large	15.1–20	5.1–10	258[a]	49
Extra-large	> 20	> 10.1	60	11
Total			526[a]	

[a] Two patients had two tumors each, one medium and one large; 526 eyes treated in 524 patients

Table 2. Uveal melanoma metastases

Stage	Total patients	Metastases	
		Number	7%
Small	25	0	0
Medium	181	4	0
Large	258	19	7.4
Extra-large	60	10	1.7
Total	524	33	6.3%

earliest sign of tumor regression, appearing as early as one week and as late as two years after treatment. On a few occasions, the detachment increased after radiation.

6.2.3 Regression

Tumor regression was seen as early as one or as late as 48 months after treatment, but generally was observed between 4 and 21 months. Total disappearance of the tumor, or formation of a flat scar at the tumor site does occur in some cases. In a detailed analysis of tumor size after treatment relative to initial tumor dimensions, 89% of 372 tumors decreased in size after treatment, based on clinical, photographic, and/or ultrasonic evaluation. Slight increases in size (0.5–1.5 mm) were noted in 9 tumors observed early after treatment; based on earlier observation such enlargement did not represent tumor growth, since on further followup regression did occur. Definite growth did occur in 4 patients in this series, while in 27 no change in size could be demonstrated. It must be emphasized that early slight increase in size or failure to regress is not an indication for enucleation or additional treatment, which should be carried out only after documented increase in tumor size. Mean decrease in tumor height was greater in large and extra-large (3 and 2.8 mm decrease, respectively) tumors than in small and medium (1.3 and 1.6 mm mean height decrease, respectively) tumors (GRAGOUDAS et al. 1985b).

6.2.4 Regrowth

Definite tumor growth in the treated area was observed in only 8 of 484 eyes (1.7%) observed between six and 108 months after treatment (median and mean followup of 18 and 24 months respec-

tively). In two patients, one of whom had a "ring melanoma", new tumors appeared well outside the treated area.

6.2.5 Metastasis and Survival

Metastasis and survival have been analyzed in 510 patients treated through June 30, 1984 (GRAGOUDAS et al. 1985c). Twenty-five percent of the patients had been treated at least 30 months prior to that date, with mean and median followup for the group being 18 and 23 months, respectively. Thirty-three patients (6.5%) developed metastasis, with nineteen dying from that cause and 14 still alive receiving chemotherapy at the time of the analysis. Metastasis was documented between 3 and 51 months after therapy (median 23 months); 25% and 75% were diagnosed by 12.5 and 31.3 months respectively. Twenty-eight had metastatic liver involvement, while skin and lung were involved in 3 and 2 patients, respectively.

Multivariate analysis with Cox's proportional hazards model was carried out in a group of 491 patients, 28 of whom developed metastasis. Patients with extrascleral extension (12) and with anterior tumors who were treated with a light field set-up only (12) were excluded from this analysis. Three independent variables associated with a greater likelihood of metastasis were identified: largest tumor diameter, more anterior tumor location, and age at treatment older than 59 years. Patients with tumor diameter greater than 15 mm had a 22.3 times higher metastatic rate than patients with tumors less than 10 mm in diameter ($p < 0.007$). Actuarial curves for time to metastasis by tumor diameter are shown in Fig. 2.

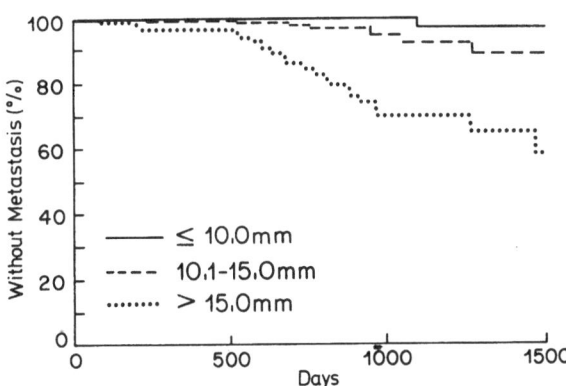

Fig. 2. Kaplan-Meier actuarial curve for time to metastasis by largest tumor diameter (GRAGOUDAS et al. 1985c)

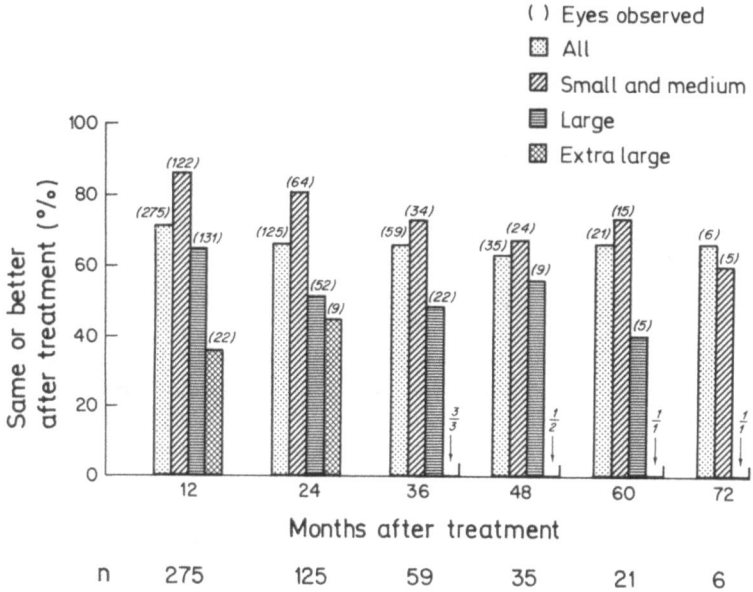

Fig. 3. Uveal melanomas. Relative visual acuity initially and after proton treatment

6.2.6 Complications and Vision After Treatment

Surgical complications were few with transient diplopia observed in patients requiring disinsertion of the inferior oblique muscle to adequately place the tantalum marker rings in posterior tumors. Moist eyelid desquamation with permanent epilation occurs in patients whose eyelids cannot be completely retracted from the irradiation field. Punctal occlusion has also been seen, requiring insertion of a Jones tube for control of tearing in one patient. Epithelial keratopathy in a few cases generally responded to use of artificial tears, although one patient required a soft contact lens. Cataracts were successfully extracted in 15 of 80 patients developing lens changes, being predominantly in patients with large choroidal or ciliary body tumors in whom a large portion of the lens was irradiated. Rubeosis iridis with neo-vascular glaucoma was observed in 16 patients and vitreous hemorrhage in 12. Radiation retinopathy involving the fovea was seen in 35 eyes, while radiation papillopathy developed in 7, and progressed to optic atrophy in two cases. The development of these complications is related to the location of the tumor.

Twenty-five eyes were enucleated, 12 for neovascular glaucoma, 3 for tumor growth (two within and one outside the irradiated volume), and 10 for other complications. Histological changes in eyes removed after treatment have been described (Seddon JM et al. 1983; Zinn KM et al. 1981).

Initial visual acuity was 20/100 (6/30) or better in 82% of treated eyes, with approximately two-thirds remaining at that level after treatment. Functional outcome in terms of relative visual acuity after treatment is shown in Fig. 3. Overall, approximately two-thirds of treated eyes had vision the same or better than that present initially. The lesser degrees of visual preservation occurred in eyes with larger and with more posteriorly placed tumors.

Visual acuity after treatment has been studied in a subgroup of 60 eyes thought to be at increased risk for visual loss because the tumor was located within 3 mm of the macula (Gragoudas et al. 1984). Even in this high-risk group, visual acuity remained the same in 47%, was better in 20%, and worse in 33%, with 58% having vision of 20/100 or better at the last observation; 72% had that level of vision before treatment. Vasculopathy with decreased vision did develop in 22% of these 60 patients. However, even when doses to the macula were in the 60–70 CGE range, visual function was preserved in the majority of eyes for 6–82 (mean 18) months.

6.2.7 Proton Energy Required

The frequency distribution of required proton beam penetration for 94 patients treated at the Harvard Cyclotron was determined. One patient required a depth of penetration of 33 mm and two a depth of 30 mm; 90% of the tumors required beam penetration of 27 mm or less. A beam energy of 60 MeV was judged probably adequate to treat all 94 patients; one accelerating protons to 50 MeV would have been adequate for slightly more than half the lesions treated (GOITEIN et al. 1983).

6.3 Helium Ions

Helium ions, like protons, exhibit excellent dose localization properties. They have an average RBE of 1.3, compared to 1.1 used clinically for the Harvard proton beam. Clinical results of treating choroidal melanomas with helium ions (CHAR and CASTRO 1982; SAUNDERS et al. 1985) appear to be as promising as for protons, with clinical indications being similar. Seventy-five patients were treated between January 1, 1978 and December 31, 1982. Diagnostic criteria and treatment-planning techniques were similar to those employed at the Harvard Cyclotron Laboratory. Three patients had small tumors, 24 medium tumors, and 48 large tumors, with small tumors being less than 10 mm in diameter and 3 mm thick, and large being greater than 15 mm in diameter and/or 5 mm thick. Twenty patients received 70 Gy equivalents (53.8 helium Gy × RBE 1.3) while the remaining 55 patients received 80 Gy equivalents.

6.3.1 Regression, Local Control, and Metastasis

Regression was observed 1–24 months after treatment, beginning generally six to eight months after treatment. Forty-nine of 54 lesions (91%) followed for at least one year after treatment decreased by 15–100% (mean 45%) of the original height as measured by A-mode ultrasound. With a mean follow-up of 22 months (3–60 months), four of 20 patients (20%) receiving the lower dose and one of 55 (2%) at the higher dose have recurred locally. Two of the early low-dose failures were attributed to inadequate tumor coverage; a third was in a patient with a "ring" melanoma involving the entire ciliary body, with regrowth occurring in a non-irradiated site initially thought to be uninvolved. The two other failures, one at each dose level, were attributed to inherent tumor radio-sensitivity. All five were free of evident disease, four after enucleation, and one after re-irradiation. No

distant metastases have developed following treatment, although two patients were thought to have lung metastases at the time of treatment: one died three months after therapy and the other was alive 28 months following treatment.

6.3.2 Complications and Vision After Treatment

Post treatment complications included neovascular glaucoma in 10 patients (13%); one received two courses of 70 Gy equivalents, and the other nine received 80 Gy equivalents. Radiation vasculopathy involving the macula or disc was observed in 11 patients. Six eyes developed cataracts, associated with decreased visual acuity in three. Acute eyelid reaction and lash epilation developed in patients in whom the lids could not be totally retracted; two patients had "dry eyes" and four required treatment for tear duct stenosis. Six eyes were enucleated, four for tumor recurrence, one because of neovascular glaucoma and visual loss, and one because of pain and uncertainty regarding tumor status because of lens opacification. Histopathologic findings in these enucleated eyes have been published (CHAR DM et al. 1983; GRIZZARD WS et al. 1984).

Approximately two-thirds of the patients (35/54) retained vision of 20/100 or better in the treated eye, with the most common cause of poor vision after treatment being radiation vasculopathy in eyes bearing tumors close to the macula or optic disc.

6.4 Indications for Heavy Charged Particles

From this experience, heavy charged particle therapy is the preferred treatment for uveal melanomas located at all sites within the eye, with the possible exception of very large tumors whose treatment would necessitate including 40 to 50% of the eye within the high dose volume. Even in those patients, treatment of a functional eye would be justified when vision was poor or absent in the fellow eye. However, expectation for visual preservation in such cases is low, with a definite risk that enucleation would be necessary at some time in the future. Further followup of particle-treated patients will be needed to determine ultimate impact of such therapy on survival and visual outcome. However, available evidence indicates that survival clearly is not compromised (SEDDON et al.

1985), local control is being observed in almost all treated eyes, and useful vision is preserved in the majority of patients.

7 Survival in Surgically-Treated Patients

Survival in 267 patients treated surgically with follow up of 8–28 years has been evaluated (SEDDON et al. 1983). Eighty-nine patients (33%) were alive at the time of the study, four with melanoma metastases. Forty-three percent had died of metastatic melanoma, 8.6% from metastases from another primary, and 16% from other causes. Metastatic disease was seen at intervals after enucleation ranging from one month to 27 years, with 25%, 50% and 75% occurring within 18, 42, and 96 months respectively. The liver was involved in 61% of the metastatic cases. Five, ten, and 15 year survival rates based on melanoma related deaths were 74%, 63%, and 55% respectively.

7.1 Survival in Conservatively Treated and in Enucleated Patients

Survival experience for three groups of uveal melanoma patients was compared in a non-randomized study of 120 patients treated by proton beam irradiation between 1975 and 1981, 235 patients treated by enucleation between 1953 and 1973, and 161 patients treated by enucleation between 1975 and 1981 (SEDDON et al. 1985). One proton patient with gross extra-scleral extension seen at clip placement for proton planning was excluded from analysis, as were 31 patients with histological extra-scleral extension in the earlier enucleation and 20 in the later enucleation group. Patients enucleated during the earlier (1953–1973) period were 6.32 times as likely to die of melanoma as were the proton treated patients (95% confidence interval 1.7–23.51); patients undergoing enucleation during the later period (1975–1981) were 3.06 times as likely to die of melanoma as proton treated patients (95% confidence interval 0.81–11.54). Tumor size and more anterior location of anterior tumor margin were significant prognostic factors in all three groups. Enucleation patients in the later period had a longer interval from presentation to treatment and generally larger tumors than those enucleated in the earlier period. Two of the five leading prognostic factors determined in the previous study (SEDDON et al. 1983) could be ascertained in the three groups:

proton-treated patients were at higher risk than those in either surgery group in that they had larger tumors and a greater percentage of more anteriorly located tumors. Since the median follow-up for the proton group was only 2.3 years, the comparisons are valid only for the early post-treatment period.

Tumor related mortality has also been assessed in Cobalt-60 plaque treated patients (BRADY LW et al. 1984), with no survival disadvantage being found in irradiated patients compared to enucleated patients in the early follow-up period.

8 Summary

Conclusive demonstration that successful treatment of uveal melanoma can be accomplished without removal of the involved eye constitutes one of the major oncologic triumphs of the latter part of the 20th century. Available data indicate that very high rates of local control can be achieved with either heavy charged particle external beam radiotherapy or radio isotope episcleral plaque brachytherapy. Not only is local tumor control being achieved with globe preservation in the vast majority of patients, but most treated patients are retaining a globe with vision at least as good as it was before therapy.

These gains have not been achieved at a cost of increased mortality, since irradiated patients have survival rates at least as good as those observed after enucleation. Further observation will be required to see if these initial dramatic and encouraging results will be maintained. Additional study is needed to clarify indications for the two types of radiotherapy.

Acknowledgements. Sincere and grateful appreciation is expressed to ANNE LESLIE MACAULAY and BARBARA GRYZBEK for their assistance in preparation of this manuscript, and to PATRICIA MCNULTY and KATHLEEN EGAN for providing data on uveal melanoma patients.

References

Albert DM (1982) Intraocular melanoma. In: DeVita VT Jr, Hellman S, Rosenberg SA (eds) Cancer: Principles and Practice of Oncology. J.B. Lippincott, Philadelphia, pp 1171–1180

Albert D (1979) Toward resolving the ocular melanoma controversy, Arch Ophthalmol 97:451–452

Barr CC, McLean IW, Zimmerman LE (1981) Uveal melanoma in children and adolescents, Arch Ophthalmol 99:2133–2136

Bedford MA (1973) The use and abuse of cobalt plaques

in the treatment of choroidal malignant melanomata, Trans Ophthalmol Soc UK 93:139–143

Boniuk M (1979) A crisis in the management of patients with choroidal melanoma, Am J Ophthalmol 87:840–842

Brady LW, Shields JA, Augsburger JJ, Day JL, Saunders WM, Castro JR, Munzenrider JE, Gragoudas E (1984) Posterior uveal melanomas. In: Phillips TL, Pistenmaa DA (eds) Radiation Oncology Annual 1983. Raven Press, New York, pp 233–245

Brady LW, Shields SA, Augsburger JJ, Day JL (1982) Malignant intraocular tumors, Cancer 49:578–585

Busse H, Muller R-P, Kroll P (1983) Results of ^{106}Ru/Rh-radiation of choroidal melanomas, Ann Ophthalmol 15:1146–1149

Chan B, Rotman M, Randall GR (1972) Computerized dosimetry of ^{60}Co ophthalmic applicators, Radiol 103:705–707

Chang M, Zimmerman LE, McLean I (1984) The persisting pseudomelanoma problem, Arch Ophthalmol 102:726–727

Char DH (1984) Therapeutic options in uveal melanoma, Am J Ophthalmol 98:796–799

Char DH, Castro JR (1982) Helium ion therapy for choroidal melanoma, Arch Ophthalmol 100:935–938

Char DH, Crawford JB, Castro JR, Woodruff KH (1983) Failure of choroidal melanoma to respond to helium ion therapy, Arch Ophthalmol 101:236–241

Char DH, Lonn LI, Margolis LW (1977) Complications of cobalt plaque therapy of choroidal melanomas, Am J Ophthalmol 84:536–541

Char DH, Phillips TL (1982) The potential for adjuvant radiotherapy in choroidal melanoma, Arch Ophthalmol 100:247–248

Chenery SG, Fitzpatrick PJ, Japp B, Galbraith DM, Leung PMK (1978) Treatment of choroidal melanoma with radio-isotopes, Int J Radiat Oncol Biol Phys (Suppl 2):123

Chenery SG, Galbraith DM, Leung PMK (1977) Application of small ^{60}Co beams in the treatment of malignant melanoma at the optic disc, Int J Radiat Oncol Biol Phys 2:1021–1026

Chenery SG, Japp B, Fitzpatrick PJ (1983) Dosimetry of radioactive gold grains for the treatment of choroidal melanoma, Brit J Radiol 56:415–420

Chuvilo IV, Goldin LL, Rhoroshkov VS, Blokhin SE, Brehev VM, Vorontsov IA, Ermolayev VV, Kleinbock YaL, Lomakin MI, Lomanov MF, Medvec VYa, Miliokhin NA, Narinsky VM, Pavlonsky LM, Shimchuck GG, Ruderman AI, Monzul GD, Shuvalov EL, Kiseliova VN, Marova EI, Kirpatovskaya LE, Minakova EI, Krymsky VA, Brovkina AF, Zarubeo GD, Reshetkinova IM, Kaplina AV (1984) ITEP synchrotron proton beam in radiotherapy, Int J Radiat Oncol Biol Phys 10:185–195

Constable IJ, Koehler AM (1974) Experimental ocular irradiation with accelerated protons, Investig Ophthalmol 13:280–287

Constable IJ, Koehler AM, Schmidt RA (1975) Proton irradiation of simulated ocular tumors, Investig Ophthalmol 14:547–555

Davidorf FM, Makley TA, Lang JR (1976) Radiotherapy of malignant melanoma of the choroid, Trans Am Acad Ophthal and Otol 81:849–861

Ehlers G, Batley F, Kartha M (1975) Radiotherapeutic management of malignant melanoma of the eye, Amer J Roentgenol Rad Ther Nuc Med 123:486–491

Ferry AP (1964) Lesions mistaken for malignant melanoma of the posterior uvea, Arch Ophthalmol 72:463–469

Foulds WS (1977) Experience of local excision of uveal melanomas, Trans Ophthalmol Soc UK 97:412–415

Freundlich HF (1949) A new beta-ray applicator using fission products, Nature 164:308–310

Goitein M, Gentry R, Koehler AM (1983) Energy of proton accelerator necessary for treatment of choroidal melanomas, Int J Radiat Oncol Biol Phys 9:259–260

Goitein M, Miller T (1983) Planning proton therapy of the eye, Med Phys 10:275–283

Gragoudas ES, Seddon J, Goitein M, Verhey L, Munzenrider JE, Urie M, Suit HD, Blitzer P, Koehler A (1985a) Current results of proton beam irradiation of uveal melanomas, Ophthal 92:284–291

Gragoudas ES, Seddon J, Goitein M, Verhey L, Munzenrider J, Urie M, Polivogianis L, Egan K, Suit HD, Austin-Seymour M, Koehler A (1985b) Proton beam irradiation of uveal melanomas. Presented at the 89th annual meeting of the Amer. Acad. of Ophthalmology, Atlanta, GA, November, 1984

Gragoudas ES, Seddon J, Egan KM, Polivogianis L, Goitein M, Verhey L, Munzenrider JE, Austin-Seymour M, Urie M, Koehler A (1985c) Prognostic factors for metastasis following proton beam irradiation, Ophtalmol 93:675–680, 1986

Gragoudas ES, Goitein M, Seddon J, Verhey L, Munzenrider J, Urie M, Suit HD, Blitzer P, Johnson KN, Koehler A (1984) Preliminary results of proton beam irradiation of macular and paramacular melanomas, Brit J Ophthalmol 68:479–485

Gragoudas ES, Goitein M, Verhey L, Munzenrider J, Urie M, Suit H, Koehler A (1982) Proton beam irradiation of uveal melanomas: results of 5 1/2 year study, Arch Ophthalmol 100:928–934

Gragoudas ES, Goitein M, Verhey L, Munzenrider J, Suit HD, Koehler (1980) Proton beam irradiation: an alternative to enucleation for intraocular melanomas, Ophthalmol 87:571–581

Gragoudas ES, Zakov NZ, Albert DM, Constable IJ (1979) Long-term observations of proton-irradiated monkey eyes, Arch Ophthalmol 97:2184–2191

Gragoudas ES, Goitein M, Koehler AM, Verhey LJ, Tepper JE, Suit HD, Brockhurst R, Constable I (1977) Proton irradiation of small choroid malignant melanomas. Am J Ophthalmol 83:665–673

Grizzard WS, Torczynski E, Char DH (1984) Helium ion charged-particle therapy for choroidal melanoma, Arch Ophthalmol 102:576–578

Jakobiec FA (1979) A moratorium on enucleation for choroidal melanoma? Am J Ophthalmol 87:842–846

Japp B, Payne D, Gallie B (1982) Individualized Ir-192 wire moulds for the treatment of large accessible malignant melanomas of the choroid, Int J Radiat Oncol Biol Phys 8:113

Kiehl H, Kirsch I, Lommatzsch P (1984) Das Überleben nach Behandlung des malignen Melanoms der Aderhaut: Vergleich von konservativer Therapie (^{106}Ru/^{106}Rh Applikator) und Enukleation ohne und mit postoperativer Orbitabestrahlung, 1960 bis 1979, Klin Mbl Augenheilk 184:2–14

Lavin PT, Albert DM, Seddon JM (1984) A deficit survival analysis to assess the natural history of uveal melanoma, J Chron Dis 37:481–487

Lommatzsch PJ (1983) B-irradiation of choroidal melanoma with ^{106}Ru/^{106}Rh applicators, Arch Ophthalmol 101:713–717

Lommatzsch PJ (1974) Treatment of choroidal melanoma

with ^{106}Ru/^{106}Rh applicators, Survey Ophthalmol 19:85–100

Long RS, Galin MA, Rotman M (1971) Conservative treatment of intraocular melanomas, Trans Acad Ophth and Otol 75:84–93

MacFaul PA (1977) Local radiotherapy in the treatment of malignant melanoma of the choroid, Trans Ophthalmol Soc UK 97:421–427

Manschot WA, van Peperzeel HA (1980) Choroidal melanoma: enucleation or observation? A new approach, Arch Ophthalmol 98:71–77

Maumenee AE (1979) An evaluation of enucleation in the management of uveal melanomas, Am J Ophthalmol 87:846–847

Meyer-Schwickerath G, Vogel M (1977) Treatment of malignant melanomas of the choroid by photocoagulation, Trans Ophthalmol Soc UK 97:416–420

Moore RF (1930) Choroidal sarcoma treated by the intraocular insertion of radon seeds, Brit J Ophthalmol 14:145–152

Packer S, Rotman M (1980) Radiotherapy of choroidal melanoma with Iodine-125, Ophthalmol 87:582–590

Packer S, Rotman M, Fairchild RG, Albert DM, Atkins HL, Chan B (1980) Irradiation of choroidal melanoma with Iodine-125 ophthalmic plaque, Arch Ophthalmol 98:1453–1457

Payman GA, Raichand M (1979) Full thickness eye wall resection of choroidal neoplasms, Ophthalmol 86: 1024–1036

Robertson DM, Earle J, Anderson JA (1983) Preliminary observations regarding the use of Iodine-125 in the management of choroidal melanoma, Trans Ophthalmol Soc UK 103:155–160

Rotman M, Packer S, Bosworth J, Chiu-Tsao ST (1984) I-125 ophthalmic applicators in the treatment of choroidal melanoma, Int J Radiat Oncol Biol Phys 10 (Suppl 2):107–108

Rotman M, Long RS, Packer S, Moroson H, Galin MA, Chan B (1977) Radiation therapy of uveal melanomas, Trans Ophthalmol Soc UK 97:431–435

Saunders WM, Char DH, Quivey JM, Castro JR, Chen GTY, Collier JM, Cartigny A, Blakely EA, Lyman JT, Woodruff KH, Tobias CA (1985) Precision, high dose radiotherapy: helium ion treatment of uveal melanoma, Int J Radiat Oncol Biol Phys 11:227–233

Sealy R, Buret E, Cleminshaw H, Stannard C, Hering E, Shackleton D, Korrubel J, LeRoux PLM, Sevel D, van Oldenborgh M, van Selm J (1980) Progress in the use of iodine therapy for tumors of the eye, Brit J Radiol 53:1052–1060

Sealy R, LeRoux PLM, Rapley F, Hering E, Shackleton D, Sevel D (1976) The treatment of ophthalmic tumors with low-energy sources, Brit J Radiol 49:551–554

Seddon JM, Gragoudas ES, Albert DM, Polivogianis L, Hsieh CC, Friedenberg GR (1985) Survival after treatment of uveal melanoma: a comparison between proton irradiation and enucleation, Am J Ophthalmol 99: 282–290

Seddon JM, Gragoudas ES, Albert DM (1983) Ciliary body and choroidal melanomas treated by proton beam irradiation, Arch Ophthalmol 101:1402–1408

Seddon JM, Albert DM, Lavin PT, Robinson N (1983) A prognostic factor study of disease-free interval and survival following enucleation for uveal melanoma, Arch Ophthalmol 101:1894–1899

Shields JA, Zimmerman LE (1973) Lesions simulating malignant melanoma of the posterior uvea, Arch Ophthalmol 89:466–471

Shields JA, Augsburger JJ, Brady LW, Day JL (1982) Cobalt plaque therapy of posterior uveal melanomas, Ophthalmol 89:1201–1207

Shields JJ, Augsburger JJ (1980) On the melanoma controversy, Am J Ophthalmol 90:266–268

Stallard HB (1966) Malignant melanoblastoma of the choroid, Mod Probl Ophthal 7:16–38

Verhey LJ, Goitein M, McNulty P, Munzenrider JE, Suit HD (1982) Precise positioning of patients for radiation therapy, Int J Radiat Oncol Biol Phys 8:289–294

Zimmerman LE, McLean IW, Foster WD (1978) Does enucleation of the eye containing a malignant melanoma prevent or accelerate the dissemination of tumor cells? Brit J Ophthalmol 62:420–425

Zimmerman LE, McLean IW (1979) An evaluation of enucleation in the management of uveal melanomas, Am J Ophthalmol 87:741–760

Zinn KM, Stein/Pokorny K, Jakobiec FA, Friedman AH, Gragoudas ES, Ritch R (1981) Proton beam irradiated epithelial cell melanoma of the ciliary body, Ophthalmol 88:1315–1321

2.2 Breast

2.2.1 Conservative Therapy for Breast Cancer

Eleanor D. Montague and Luis Delclos

CONTENTS

1 Introduction

Recent reports have indicated that clinically favorable breast cancer can be successfully treated by excision of the gross tumor in the breast and axilla followed by radiation therapy of moderate dose. Proper emphasis has been given to creating a field of treatment in which only subclinical disease exists, so that 45–50 Gy tumor dose delivered to the breast and regional lymphatics can be expected to control 90% of the treated areas (Fletcher et al. 1980).

This investigation was supported in part by grants CA06294 and CA16672 awarded by the National Cancer Institute, U.S. Department of Health and Human Services.

Eleanor D. Montague, M.D., Professor
Luis Delclos, M.D., Professor
The University of Texas M.D. Anderson
Hospital and Tumor Institute
Houston, TX 77030, USA

Table 1. Contraindications to conservation surgery and radiation

Primary tumor
>4 cm
Multiple (clinical or radiologic)
Grave signs
Subareolar location or Paget's disease
Nodes
N_2
N_3
Breast
Too small for excision of tumor
Prosthetic implants that may encapsulate giving poor cosmetic results

2 Selection of Patients

Patients are clinically suitable for conservation surgery and irradiation if the primary tumor-bearing area is equal to or less than 4 cm in a breast ample enough for a good cosmetic result after excision of the tumor; Table 1 lists tumor and patient contraindications for breast-saving procedures. It is important for a team consisting of a diagnostic radiologist, surgeon, radiotherapist, medical oncologist and pathologist to engage in the selection, treatment, and follow-up of such patients.

3 Technique

3.1 Surgery

A number of terms are used for breast conservation surgery: wedge excision, segmental mastectomy, partial mastectomy, and tylectomy are all more or less synonymous and imply resection of the tumor with a generous margin consisting of a segment or wedge of the breast.

At the University of Texas M. D. Anderson Hospital and Tumor Institute at Houston, prior to 1974, the primary cancer was removed by excisional biopsy. More recently, a segmental mastectomy has been performed; an elliptical incision conforming to the contour of the breast is used for tumors in the upper half of the breast and a radial incision for lower quadrant tumors. The aim of surgery is to remove all of the gross disease with a tumor-free margin. If a biopsy is performed prior to referral, a reexcision of the site of tumor and scar is performed whenever possible since recurrent tumor after irradiation occurred in 9% of patients without reexcision and 2% with reexcision (MONTAGUE and SCHELL 1983).

Whether it is necessary to perform a complete axillary dissection or a dissection of the lateral axilla is still being debated; there is a higher incidence of retrograde breast and arm edema with full axillary lymph node dissection. Our preference at the U.T.M.D. Anderson Hospital is to perform a dissection lateral to the pectoralis minor muscle through a separate incision. The incision is placed near the anterior axillary line immediately behind the fold created by the lateral margin of the pectoralis major muscle and is directed inferiorly toward the lower aspect of the axilla allowing creation of an axillary skin flap, which adequately exposes the lateral axillary contents. The axillary adipose tissue and contained lymph nodes medial to the thoracodorsal bundle, inferior to the axillary vein and lateral to the edge of the pectoralis minor muscle are removed en bloc. The long thoracic nerve is visualized but not disturbed. Hemostatis is secured, the wound irrigated, and a single cathether placed in the apex of the wound prior to closure of subcutaneous tissue and fat. This incision and approach to the axilla results in a scar that is barely visible when the arms are at the sides or on abduction to 90 degrees.

Two incisions, one for the primary tumor and the other for the axillary dissection, are preferred even when the primary tumor is in the upper quadrant. This manuever prevents retraction of the breast toward the axilla and poor orientation of the nipple and areola and separates the incision of the primary, which may require a boost, from the axillary incision, which does not.

3.2 Radiation

3.2.1 Fields

From 1955 to 1975, all patients treated with conservation surgery had only the primary tumor removed, followed by irradiation to the breast, ax-

Table 2. Areas irradiated[a] following excision of a carcinoma and dissection of the lateral axilla. (From MONTAGUE et al. 1979)

Histology of nodes	Radiotherapy fields	
	Outer quadrants primary	Central or inner quadrants primary
–	Breast	Breast
		Internal mammary chain nodes
+	Breast	Breast
	Internal mammary chain	Internal mammary chain
	Supraclavicular and axillary apex	Supraclavicular and axillary apex

[a] Without axillary dissection irradiation is delivered to the breast, axilla, internal mammary chain, and supraclavicular nodes. With axillary dissection the low and central axilla is treated only with N_2 nodes or extra-nodal tumor extension.

illa, internal mammary lymph node chain, and supraclavicular lymph nodes regardless of the clinical status of the axilla. The supraclavicular and axillary lymph nodes received 50 Gy tumor dose/5 weeks through an anterior supraclavicular-axillary field and a posterior axillary field opposing the low and central axilla. Since 1974, a dissection of the lateral axilla has been done and the radiation fields are tailored according to the histology of the axilla and the site of the primary tumor in the breast (Table 2). The posterior axillary field is not used unless extranodal disease or lymph nodes greater than 3 cm are described in the specimen. With negative or small positive lymph nodes, only the axillary apex is treated with supraclavicular and internal mammary lymph nodes (Fig. 1) and the axillary field is omitted for noninvasive or small invasive tumors in the outer quadrants with histologically negative lymph nodes.

Through medial and lateral tangential fields, the breast is irradiated with ^{60}Co without bolus for 45–50 Gy tumor dose/5 weeks (25 fractions) calculated in the area of the tumor. In the early years, only open fields were used, but in the last 8 years this has been changed to a combination of parallel-opposed open and wedge filtered fields, unless the tumor is circumareolar. In this location, open fields deliver a built-in boost because of the heterogeneity of dose. With computed tomography (CT) scan treatment planning, a cold region may appear when a separate internal mammary-tangential junction line overlies a full breast; however, divergence and penumbra of beams are not shown in the scan and, in fact, there have been no recurrences at the junction or lateral to it. Recently, CT scan treatment planning has been performed in every patient; patients with an unusual tumor position, unusual breast shape, or both, have multiple cuts with superimposed isodose curves. The CT scan identifies whether the entire breast is within the tangential fields with a separate internal mammary chain field or whether the internal mammary lymph node chain should be incorporated within the tangential fields (Fig. 2).

To avoid upper lung fibrosis, all but very heavy set patients receive to the supraclavicular-axillary apex portal 40 Gy given dose/4 weeks (20 fractions) with ^{60}Co and additional 5 Gy (stage I) or 10 Gy given dose (stage II) with electrons. Since the first internal mammary lymph node space is in the supra clavicular-axillary apex portal and would receive little or no irradiation from 7–10 Mev, the internal mammary portal, irradiated with 13–15 Mev, is raised to include the first interspace to bring the total dose 45 Gy tumor dose (Fig. 1).

The majority of patients treated with conservation surgery and irradiation have a straight-on internal mammary chain field with ^{60}Co for 45 Gy tumor dose/5 weeks at 3–4 cm depth: However, in recent years, to reduce paramediastinal fibrosis and to avoid irradiating the heart, expecially when doxorubicin (Adramycin) is included in an elective chemotherapy program, ^{60}Co is used to deliver only 20 Gy followed for the remainder of the treatment by electrons of appropriate energy. Electrons only can be used if the electron beam has enough skin sparing to avoid excessive skin reaction, both acute and late.

The lateral position and depth of the internal mammary lymph nodes are evaluated in each patient: lymphoscintigraphy allows measurements of the distance of the lymph nodes from the midline at each interspace, and ultrasound or CT scan gives the depth of the pleural reflection, i.e., the depth of the lymph nodes. Lymph nodes shown by lymphoscintigraphy have always been included in the usual straight-on internal mammary portal; therefore, if a straight-on internal mammary portal with ^{60}Co or 4 Mev is used, lymphscintigraphy for location of lymph nodes appears unnecessary. Whenever the internal mammary nodes are irradiated within the tangential fields, or with electrons, lymphoscintigraphy is necessary to assure adequate coverage. Fig. 2 is a treatment planning scan on a patient whose breast would be incompletely irradiated if a separate internal mammary field

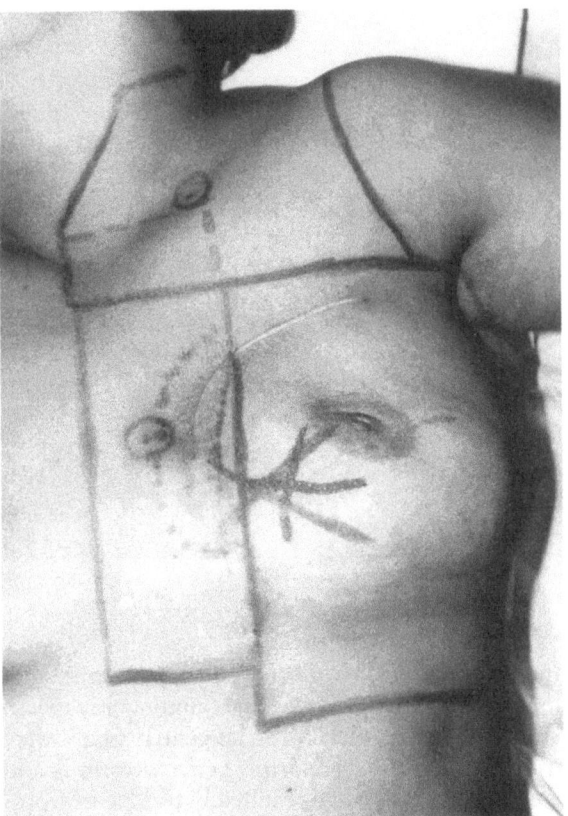

Fig. 1. Patient was 44 years old and presented in 1980 with a 3.5-cm upper inner quadrant carcinoma, which was excised; a dissection of the lateral axilla revealed 18 histologically negative lymph nodes. Because the low and central axilla had been dissected and did not require irradiation, the superior border of the tangential field was raised. The posterior axillary field was not used. With ^{60}Co, the breast received 50 Gy tumor dose/5 weeks (25 fractions) with a combination of open: wedged fields. The tumor bed was then boosted with 7 Mev electrons for 10 Gy/5 days. The internal mammary portal received 20 Gy given dose with ^{60}Co and an additional 30 Gy given dose with 13 Mev electrons. The supraclavicular-axillary apex portal received 40 Gy given dose/4 weeks with ^{60}Co, and an additional 10 Gy given dose with 9 Mev electrons. The internal mammary portal was raised to include the first internal mammary space and medial supraclavicular area, and with 13 Mev, the entire chain received 45 Gy tumor dose. Patient remains well in 1986. From MONTAGUE, ROMSDAHL et al. (1983)

were used; consequently the technique was changed to include the internal mammary lymph nodes (solid dot) within the tangential fields.

3.2.2 Junctions

Because the technique used for advanced local and regional cancer was initially carried over to the patients with early and clinically favorable disease,

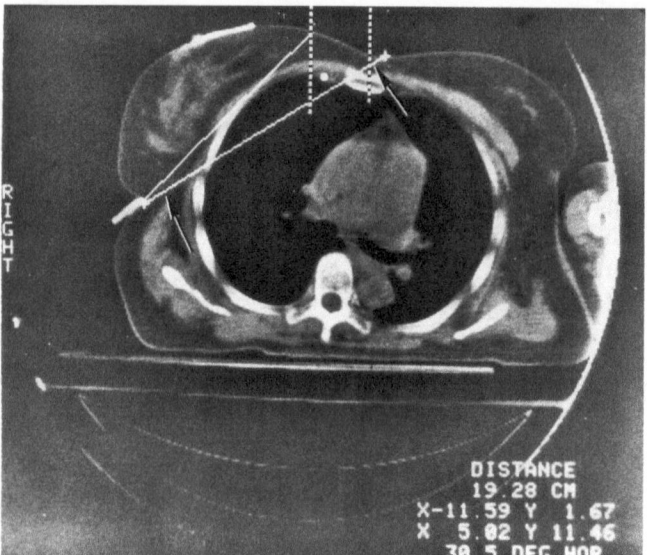

Fig. 2. Planning CT scan following segmental mastectomy. The scar is outlined with a lead strip in a patient with an excised upper inner quadrant primary tumor. The internal mammary lymph nodes were 3.5-cm from the midline of the sternum in the second and third interspaces on lymphoscintigraphy (*solid dot*). With a separate internal mammary chain field (*dotted lines*), the base of the breast was not being irradiated. Consequently the medial tangential field was moved 1.5-cm to the opposite side of the midline to cover the entire breast and internal mammary lymph nodes (*arrows* show the tangential portals used). (From Montague, Romsdahl et al. 1983)

the junction lines both between the tangential and internal mammary chain fields and supraclavicular-axillary apex field with tangential fields were irradiated with each portal, i.e., twice, to avoid a cold area. This often resulted in a ridge of fibrosis of the junction lines. A hot spot at the junctions can be avoided by irradiating the line with one portal only and careful blocking the line from the other portal. When a separate internal mammary chain field is used, it abuts the tangential fields in the middle of the field and no overlap of fields is permitted. Another approach to avoid junctional hot spots developed at the Joint Center for Radiation Therapy is to use a half beam block with the supraclavicular field, and an angulated tangential beam block to match the vertical edge (Svensson, Chin et al. 1983).

3.2.3 Boost

No boost is delivered with noninvasive carcinoma or with a unifocal well-differentiated tumor completely removed or with a negative re-excision of a primary site. An electron boost of appropriate voltage (6 to 20 Mev available) of 10 Gy/5 days is delivered to the depth measured with a CT planning scan (Fig. 3a). In the supine position, the breast flattens to a degree that 7–12 Mev are usually adequate. Surgical clips outlining the margins of excision are also helpful. Boost doses greater than 10 Gy (15–20 Gy) for positive or unknown margins of excision may be delivered by interstitial

implantation (^{192}Ir) if the tumor is appropriately located. An implant is not recommended with a tumor adjacent to the chest wall or in the subareolar position, in which instance the boost is delivered through medial and lateral reduced portals with compression with a bridge or postural compression (Fig. 3b, c).

3.2.4 Implant Techniques

Formerly we implanted the ^{192}Ir wire in Teflon tubing spacing the wires 1 cm apart with linear intensities around 0.6 mc/cm (radium equivalent) for single planes and 0.3 mc/cm (radium equivalent) for double planes and often crossed the ends, but we have now substituted stainless steel needles (modified from Henschke) with Teflon balls tailoring the needle spacing to the thickness of tissue to irradiate; spacing varies between 1 and 2 cm with preference for single planes. This type of implant causes less trauma and leaves no "exit scars" on the breast. When possible, the needles enter into the breast tissue from the least visible side (outer quadrant or below the breast) and do not show up in the inner upper area of the breast, something that many women appreciate, since it allows them to wear low-cut dresses and swim suits.

If needles must be passed under the nipple, they are implanted deeply keeping the hot areas around the needles away from the nipple (Fig. 4a–c) (Fig. 5a–c).

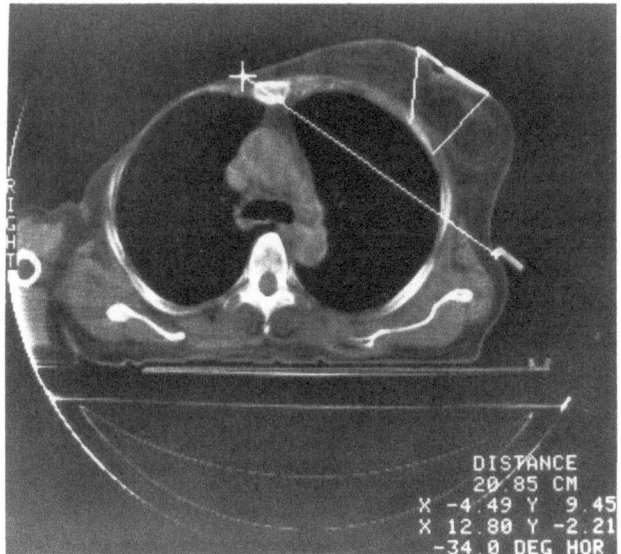

a

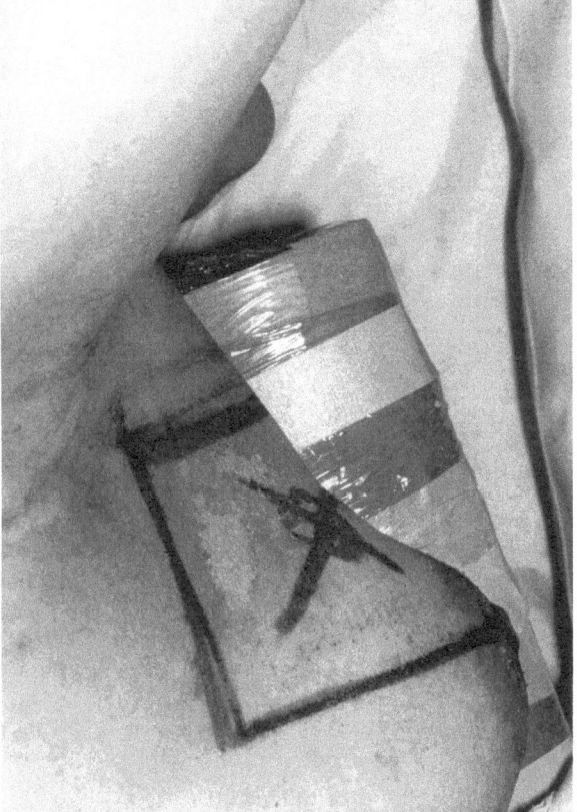

b

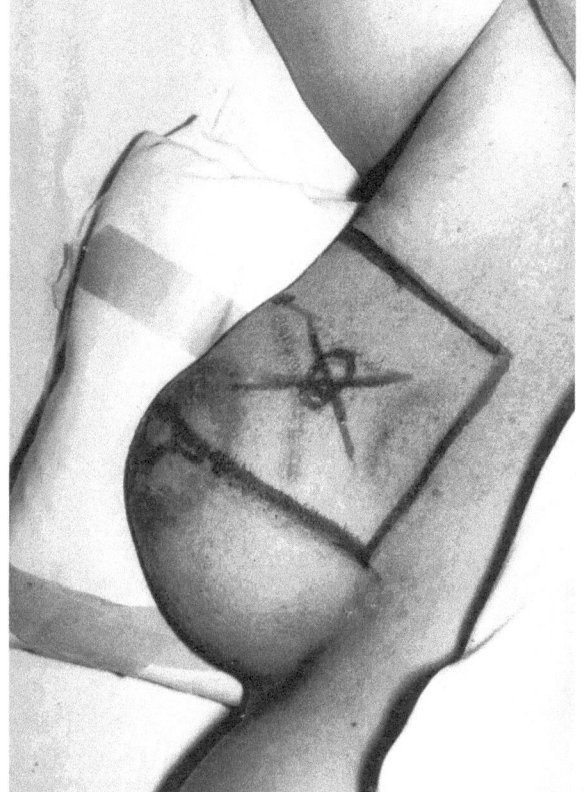

c

Fig. 3a–c. Modified boost technique. Patient presented in 1981 with a 3.5-cm carcinoma in the upper and central portions of the breast adjacent to the chest wall; it was excised with a close margin at the base; 18 axillary lymph nodes were histologically negative.

Since a boost of 15 Gy tumor dose at 4.5-cm depth necessitated a high skin dose with electrons and since the upper half of the areola had to be included for adequate margin at the tumor site, electrons were not indicated. Because the tumor was adjacent to the chest wall, an interstitial implant would not be effective. Therefore, after 50 Gy tumor dose to the breast, internal mammary chain, and supraclavicular-axillary apex portals, a boost of 15 Gy tumor dose was delivered in 7 days by turning the patient alternately into an anterior and posterior oblique position compressing the breast by its own weight on a rolled pad. **a** CT planning showing the scar outlined by a lead strip and the direct measurements from both ends of the scar to the chest wall. The medial end of the scar is 4.5-cm from the chest wall and the lateral end of the scar exceeds 5-cm. **b** The medial boost portal. **c** The lateral boost portal. (From MONTAGUE, ROMSDAHL et al. 1983)

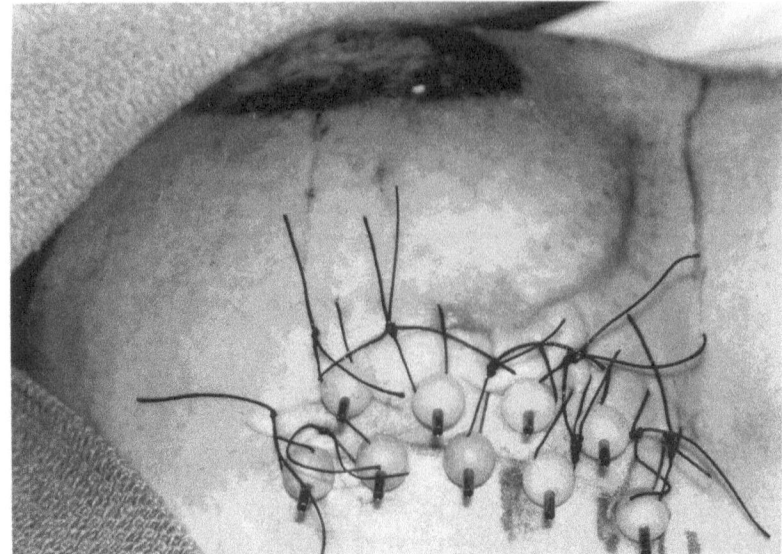

Fig. 4a–c. Example of a new technique of breast implantation.
a Staggered double-plane implant for the left upper outer quadrant.
b Radiographs of the implant.
c Isodose of the implant. The patient can wear a lowcut dress without showing unsightly exit scars

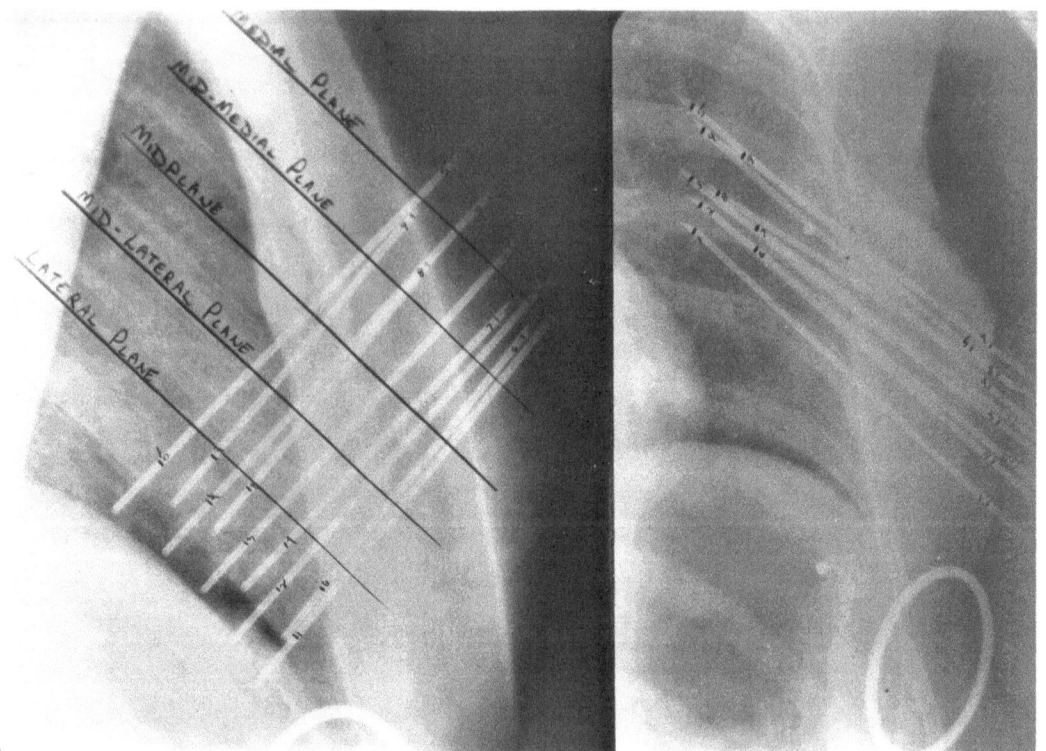

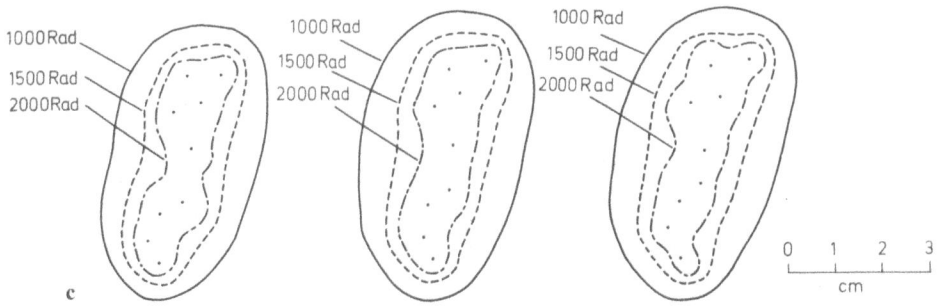

Fig. 5a–c. Single-plane implant with stainless steel needle guides for iridium (wires). **a** The needles are inserted from the lateral half of the breast and deep under the nipple. **b** Entrance points are in the lateral half of the right breast. **c** No exit points are visible on the medial half of the right breast. Compare with the normal left breast

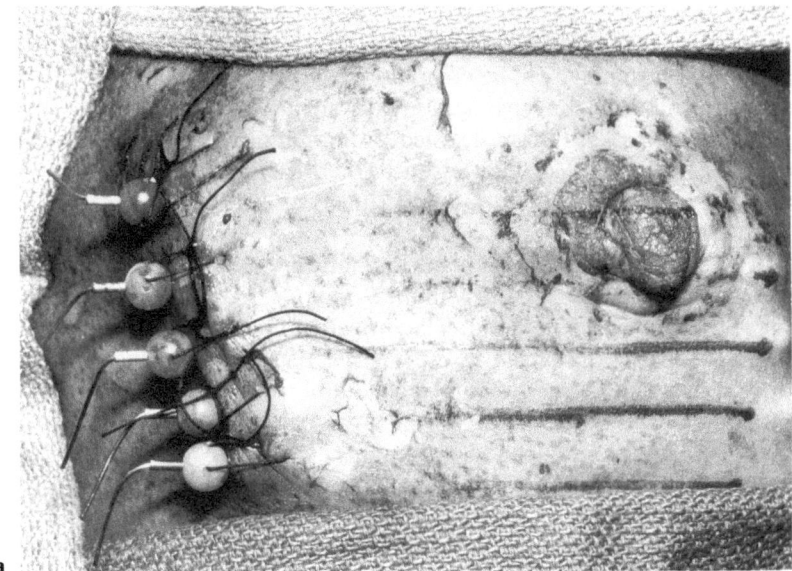

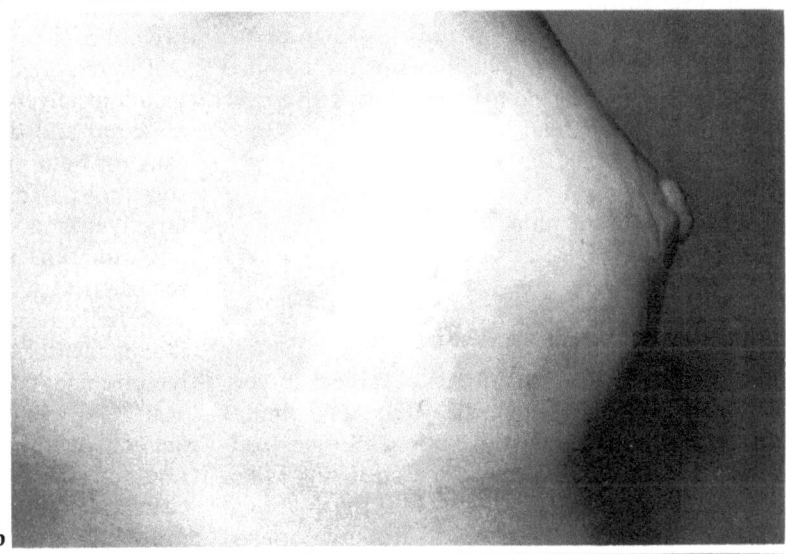

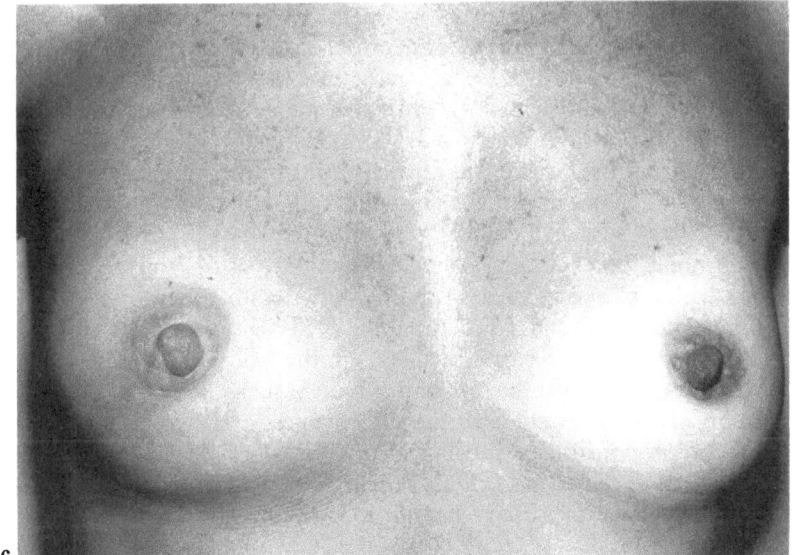

3.2.5 Dosimetry

Now that dosimetry can be computerized, calculations for all implants have been greatly simplified. The concepts used were learned from Quimby (Glasser et al. 1961), Patterson-Parker (Meredith 1967), and Pierquin-Dutreix (Pierquin and Dutreix 1967).

For small volumes single-plane implants are recommended and for larger volumes, a staggered double-plane system is used. The implant follows the contour of the breast in every case. In some locations it is necessary to combine a double-plane implant with a single-plane, in which case the single-plane needles are loaded with higher linear intensity iridium.

Neither with the single plane nor with the staggered double plane do we attempt to give a uniform dose through the target volume, since the dose required at the periphery is less than at the center. Typically, as in this implant, the nominal implant dose is specified to correspond with a dose rate of 40–60 cGy/hour.

4 Results of Conservation Surgery and Radiation

4.1 Clinical Trials

Major progress in the reduction of radical surgery for breast cancer was achieved with several clinical trials, two conducted by the National Surgical Adjuvant Breast Project and the second by the Milan Tumor Institute. From 1969–1975, the National Surgical Adjuvant Breast Project trial randomized patients with a clinically negative axilla to 1 of 3 treatment: radical mastectomy, total mastectomy followed by local-regional irradiation, or total mastectomy alone without any treatment of the axilla; 40% of the patients having radical mastectomy had histologically positive lymph nodes, but only 14.2% of the patients receiving total mastectomy only have had clinical growth of axillary lymph nodes necessitating axillary dissection. Patients with a clinically negative axilla treated with total mastectomy and irradiation have had no greater incidence of recurrence (2.0%) in the axillary lymph nodes than having had a radical mastectomy, (1.8%) attesting to the effectiveness of 45–50 Gy in controlling subclinical disease, since it would be expected that these patients also had a 40% incidence of axillary lymph node involvement (Table 3).

Table 3. NSABP B-04 Protocol. Randomized patients with clinically negative axilla. (From Fisher et al. 1980)

Radical mastectomy Positive axillary histology	Total mastectomy + irradiation Axillary recurrence[a]	Total mastectomy alone Subsequent axillary node growth
40%	1.8%	14.2%

[a] Following 5 Gy tumor dose/5 weeks (25 fractions).
NSABP (National Surgical Adjuvant Breast Project)

In 1973, Veronesi began a trial at the Milan Tumor Institute for patients with Stage I disease randomizing radical mastectomy or quadrantectomy, axillary dissection, and radiotherapy to the breast; in the third year of the trial, 12 cycles of cyclophosphamide, methotrexate, and 5-fluorouracil were added to the treatment of patients with histologically positive lymph nodes. In 1983 the actuarial and disease-free survival rates were the same in both groups (Fig. 6a, b). Of interest, the subset of patients with histologically positive axillary lymph nodes treated with quadrantectomy and radiation had a statistically significant higher relapse-free survival than those patients treated with radical mastectomy. One must ask whether the incidental irradiation of internal mammary lymph nodes caused an improvement.

In 1972, at the Institute Gustave-Roussy, a similar trial was begun with $T_1 N_0 N_1$ stages with randomization to either mastectomy or local excision of the primary and low axillary dissection followed by breast irradiation; if lymph nodes were involved, complete axillary dissection was done. Fig. 7a and 7b shows that the patients treated with conservation surgery and irradiation have fared as well as those treated with mastectomy. At 5 years, 6% of the patients treated with conservation surgery have had local recurrence compared with 10% following mastectomy.

In 1976, the National Surgical Adjuvant Breast Project (Fisher et al. 1985) began a trial for patients with tumors up to 4 cm in size. After axillary dissection in every patient, breast treatment was randomized to segmental mastectomy alone, segmental mastectomy and 50 Gy/25 fractions in 5 weeks to the breast (no boost) or total mastectomy. Recurrence in the breast occurred in 28% of women treated with segmental mastectomy alone and in 8% if the breast was irradiated after segmental mastectomy. Life table estimates based

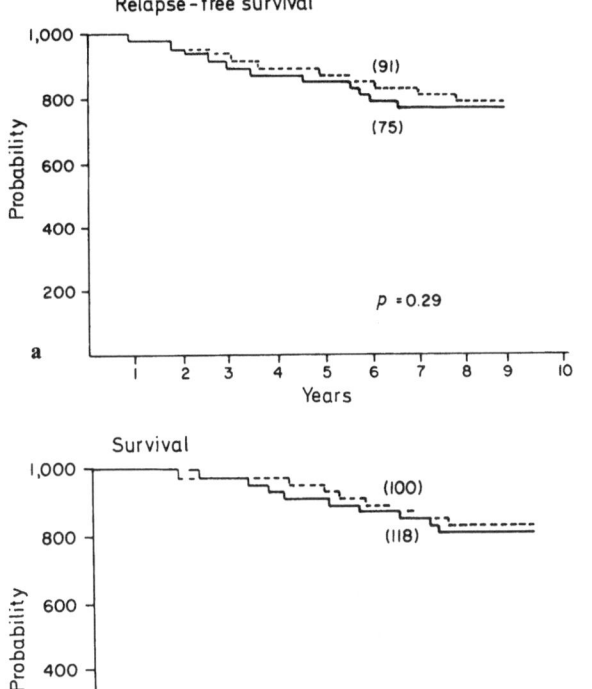

Fig. 6. a Acturial overall survival for 349 patients treated by Halsted mastectomy (——) and 352 patients treated by quadrantectomy (---), axillary dissection, and radiotherapy for breast cancers of small size up to 2-cm. **b** Actuarial diseasefree survival for 349 patients treated with Halsted mastectomy and 352 patients treated by quadrantectomy, axillary dissection, and radiotherapy for breast cancers of small size up to 2-cm. (From VERONESI 1983)

on data from 1843 women result in the same 5 years survival and disease-free survival rates (Fig. 8).

4.2 Retrospective Reports

This retrospective analysis was made of 1,073 patients with TIS T_1 T_2 N_0 N_1 M_0 breast cancer treated at U.T.M.D. Anderson Hospital between 1955 and 1980; 728 patients were treated with radical or modified radical mastectomy alone, while 345 were treated with conservation surgery and irradiation. All patients were treated by the same group of physicians and had biopsy-proved breast cancer. Radical surgery consisted of the standard or modified radical mastectomy.

Table 4 shows similar local-regional recurrence rates in patients treated with conservation surgery and irradiation or radical mastectomy. Although the total number of patients with recurrent disease was the same in both groups (4.9% versus 5.6%), those patients treated with radical mastectomy alone had a higher incidence of regional nodal recurrence than patients treated with conservation surgery and irradiation. The 5- and 10-year disease survival rates are shown in Table 5 and Fig. 9.

Of the patients developing breast or chest wall recurrences, 71% of patients treated with conservation surgery and irradiation and 66% of patients treated with radical mastectomy relapsed before the fifth year of follow-up. The 4 recurrences developing in an intact breast after the sixth follow-up year were in quadrants other than the original quadrants.

Although results obtained in nonrandomized studies are difficult to compare with each other, there has been remarkable agreement in the results

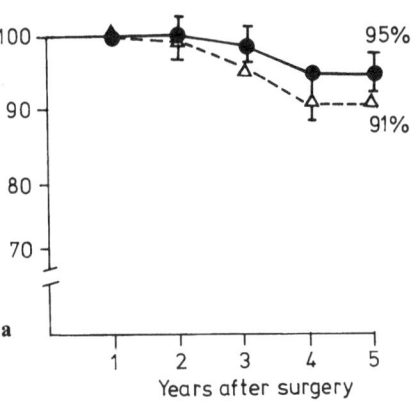

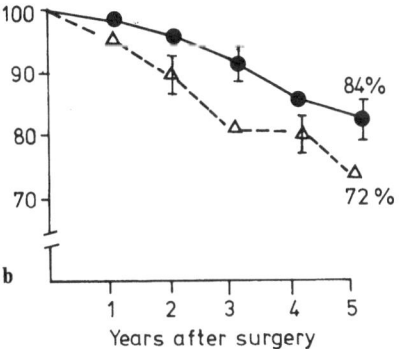

Fig. 7. a Survival curves according to surgical treatment: tumorectomy – 88 patients, 8 deaths; mastectomy – 91 patients, 6 deaths. **b** Relapse-free survival according to surgical treatment: tumorectomy 88 patients, 11 relapses or deaths; mastectomy – 91 patients, 19 relapse or deaths. ●——● Tumorectomy; △---△ Mastectomy. (From SARRAZIN, LE et al. 1983)

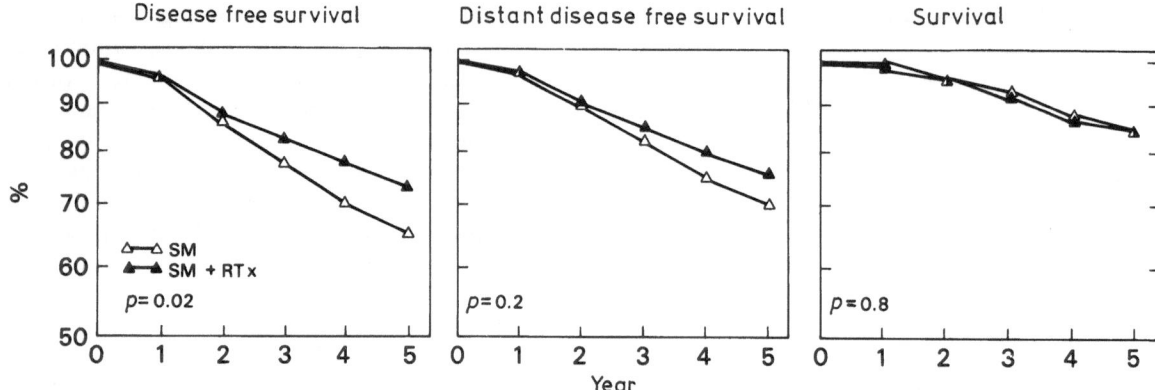

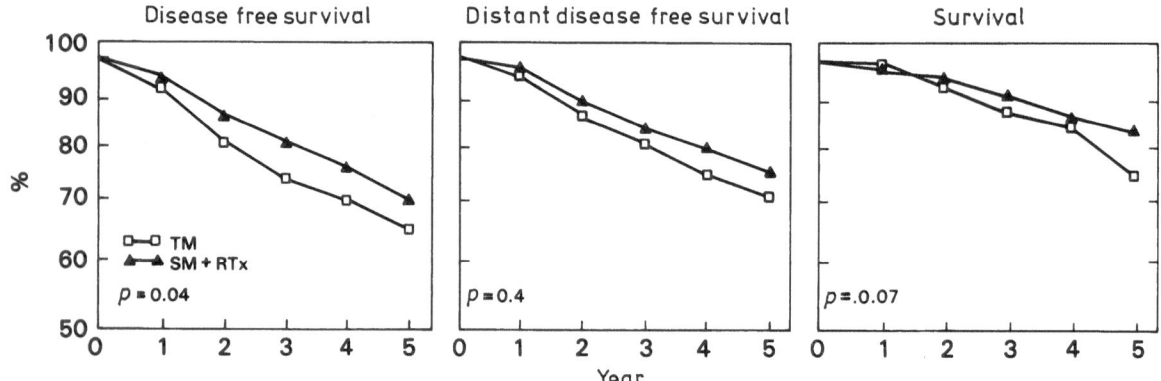

Fig. 8. a Life-table analysis showing disease-free survival, distant-disease-free survival, and overall survival of patients treated by segmental mastectomy (SM) or by segmental mastectomy with radiation (SM + RTx) who had specimen margins free of tumor. **b** Life-table analysis showing disease-free survival, distant-disease-free survival, and overall survival of patients treated by total mastectomy (TM) or by Segmental Mastectomy plus Radiation (SM-RTx). (From FISHER, BAUER et al. 1985)

Table 4. Sites of local-regional recurrences[a] 1955–1980. Analysis, March 1983. (From MONTAGUE, 1984)

	Conservation surgery + irradiation			Radical or modified radical Mastectomy		
	(No.)	Breast	Nodes	(No.)	Chest wall	Nodes
Minimal breast cancer[b]	(54)		1[c]	(134)		1
Stage I[d] (T₁ N₀)	(134)	8	1	(225)	6	6
Stage II[d] (T₁ N₀)	(157)	8	1	(370)	19	14
No. of patients with recurrence	17/345 = 4.9%			41/728 = 5.6%		

[a] A patient may have more than one site of recurrence.

[b] Includes 20 patients with microinvasion (≤ 5 mm) and 34 with noninvasive intraductal carcinoma.

[c] Regional lymphatics untreated.

[d] Prior to 1974 patients treated with conservation surgery had only clinical evaluation of axillary nodes

Table 5. 5- and 10-Year disease-free survival rates 1955–1980. Analysis, March 1983. (From MONTAGUE 1984)

	No. of patients	Conservation surgery + irradiation		No. of patients	Radical or modified radical mastectomy alone	
		5 yr. (%)	10 yr. (%)		5 yr. (%)	10 yr. (%)
Minimal breast cancer	54	97	92	134	97	95
Stage I: $T_1 N_0$	134	85	78	224	88	80
Stage II: $T_1 N_1$; $T_2 N_0 N_1$	157	78	73	370	77	65

No statistical significant between any group

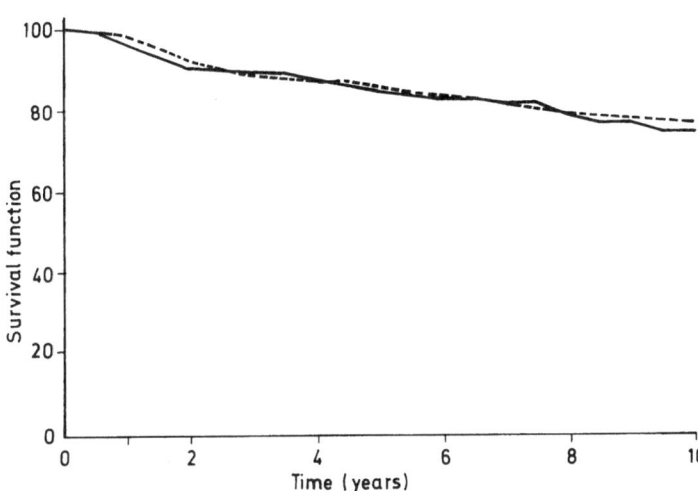

Fig. 9. Disease-free survival rates of patients treated with conservation surgery and irradiation or with radical or modified radical mastectomy. — — Conservation surgery and irradiation; --- radical or modified radical mastectomy alone. (From MONTAGUE 1984)

of conservation surgery and irradiation (HARRIS and HELLMAN 1984; CALLE et al. 1984; PIERQUIN et al. 1980; AMALRIC et al. 1983; PROSNITZ 1983; CLARK 1982).

There is general agreement that inadequate excision and increasing primary size play major roles in increasing the risk of tumor recurrence in the breast (HELLMAN et al. 1980; HARRIS and HELLMAN 1984; CLARK et al. 1982; AMALRIC et al. 1983). An attempt is being made to evaluate the pathologic predictors of increased risk of recurrence; SCHNITT et al. (1984) estimated 39% recurrence in a group of patients with extensive intraductal carcinoma, high nuclear grade, and high mitotic index. VILCOQ et al. (1981) reported increased breast recurrences in young patients.

There is no suggestion in the nonrandomized or randomized studies that radiation therapy interferes with the ability to give chemotherapy or adversely influences the survival of patients with positive lymph nodes receiving chemotherapy.

Various reports have been complied supporting the conclusion that a recurrence in the intact breast

is not as prejudicial to patient survival as chest wall recurrence following a radical or modified radical mastectomy (AMALRIC et al. 1982; CALLE et al. 1979; DELOUCHE and BACHELOT 1980; KURTZ et al. 1983a; KURTZ et al. 1983b; PAPILLON 1975; PROSNITZ et al. 1980; PROSNITZ et al. 1983). As has already been reported, the survival rate of patients with recurrence in the lymph nodes can be expected to be lower than the survival rate of patients with recurrent tumor only in the breast (CLARK 1982).

4.3 Cosmetic Results

Although cosmetic results vary depending on both the surgical and the radiation technique, they are good to excellent in 75% of patients. The radiotherapist must avoid junction overlaps by carefully setting up fields and by reducing the volume to be irradiated. For example, if a lateral axillary dissection is done and the lymph nodes are positive but smaller than 2 cm in size, only the axillary apex should be irradiated.

4.4 Complications of Treatment

A previous report from the U.T.M.D. Anderson Hospital described the longterm complications of protracted irradiation of 70 Gy for far-advanced cancer of the breast. This report showed that long-term follow-up is necessary since 18% of severe complications developed after 10 years (SPANOS et al. 1980). However, if patients treated with 50 Gy in 5 weeks (25 fractions) have a good cosmetic result at 5 years, complications are likely to remain minimal, whereas if there is early fibrosis of the breast and soft tissues, there can be severe complications in 10–15 years. At U.T.M.D. Anderson Hospital, it is our impression that the addition of polychemotherapy before or after radiation may add to the fibrosis but much less so than concomitant chemotherapy and radiation.

The incidence of symptomatic radiation pneumonitis has been reduced significantly (19% to 2%) with the mixture of photons and electrons for supraclavicular and internal mammary fields. Two instances of tender nodules within the irradiated fields were biopsied with the diagnosis of fat necrosis; both occurred in heavy-set women. Patients with collagen vascular diseases do not tolerate radiation; our only instance of necrosis of soft tissue occurred in a patient with generalized scleroderma.

In 1974, when it was decided that histologic evaluation of the axilla was necessary, the first 9 patients at U.T.M.D. Anderson Hospital had a complete axillary dissection. Six of these patients developed significant arm edema, as well as severe retrograde breast edema. Following the dissection, breast edema can occur prior to be radiation and has clinical manifestations similar to inflammatory carcinoma with skin changes of erythema, peau d'orange, and wheals. Radiation therapy does not appear to make the edema worse, but the skin thickening on follow-up xeromammograms can be confused with recurrent disease, so that all clinicians should be made aware of the problem. Following the high incidence of complications with a complete axillary dissection, it was decided to perform only a dissection lateral to the pectoralis minor muscle with only an occasional patient experiencing transient upper arm edema and mild breast edema since the reduction in surgery.

4.5 Incidence of Other Cancer

Table 6 is an analysis of all patients with stages I and II breast cancer treated at U.T.M.D. Anderson Hospital, 6% of whom have developed a can-

Table 6. Bilateral breast cancer: consecutive presentation: Stage I and II (T_1 N_0 N_1): analysis May, 1983 incidence of contralateral breast cancer correlated with the treatment of the first breast 1948–1980. (From MONTAGUE 1984)

Treatment	No. of patients developing second breast primary (%)[a]
Surgery only	30/576 (5.2%)
Peripheral lymphatic XRT	27/553 (4.9%)
Peripheral lymphatic + electron beam to chest wall	7/321 (2.2%)
Irradiation of chest wall with tangential portals after simple mastectomy	5/228 (2.2%)
Preop XRT and radical mastectomy	18/473 (3.8%)
Wedge excision or segmental mastectomy	6/316 (1.9%)

63/1891 (3.3%)

[a] Denominator excludes patients with simultaneous bilateral breast cancer (0–6 months within diagnosis of one breast cancer) and patients treated in unknown fashion for one breast cancer prior to referral.
$p = 0.038$

Table 7. Incidence of multiple primary cancers excluding breast in patients with breast cancer treated with surgery alone or surgery and irradiation[a] 1948–1978. Analysis, November 1980. (From MONTAGUE and SPANOS et al. 1983a)

	Surgery alone	Surgery and irradiation
Total number of patients	700	3,713
Number of patients developing second primary tumors after treatment to breast	9(1.3%)[a]	75(2.0%)[a]

[a] $P = 0.19$

cer in the remaining breast. When the incidence of second breast malignancy is studied as function of the treatment to the first breast, it is seen that patients who were treated with combined surgery and radiation therapy for the first breast cancer have no greater incidence of a second breast cancer (3.3%) than patients whose first breast cancer was treated with surgery alone (5.2%). These data were accumulated from patients treated between 1948 and 1980. There is no evidence, at least in these patients, that the radiation therapy used in the treatment of the first breast cancer is conducive to the development of a second breast cancer; the same findings have been reported by MCCREDIE et al. (1975) and HANKEY et al. (1983).

Table 7 shows the incidence of other primary tumors in patients with breast cancer treated from 1948 through 1978 at U.T.M.D. Anderson Hospital. There is no statistical difference between the patients treated with surgery alone and those treated with combined surgery and irradiation. The most common second primary malignancies, excluding skin cancer, in both groups were gynecological and colorectal cancers, and in the last 4 years under review, an increasing incidence of lung cancer.

5 Summary

An important step in the development of a scientific basis for combined surgery and irradiation for solid tumors, in general, was the concept of subclinical disease derived from elective irradiation of clinically negative areas undisturbed by any surgical procedure. These data showed that 45–50 Gy tumor dose in 5 weeks (5 fractions/week) eliminated most of the expected occult deposits. The basic concept has to be adjusted for 3 parameters: the density of infestation, hypoxia due to scar tissue and edema, and regrowth of residual cancer if the interval between surgery and radiation therapy is prolonged.

The concept of electively irradiating subclinical disease with modest doses was a radical departure from the previous tenet of radiation that there is a cancerocidal radiation dose linked with the histology and not the volume of cancer. The successful combination of conservation surgery for gross disease and irradiation for subclinical tumor in the treatment of early breast cancer is but one example of the clinical application of the concept and should not be thought of as a unique and unexpected event.

References

Amalric R, Santamaria F et al. (1982) Radiation therapy with or without primary limited surgery for operable breast cancer: A 20 year experience at the Marseilles Cancer Institute. Cancer 49:30–34

Amalric R, Santamaria F et al. (1983) Conservation therapy of operable breast cancer: Results at five, ten and fifteen years in 2,216 consecutive cases. In: Harris JR, Hellman S, and Silen W (eds) Conservative Management of Breast Cancer: New Surgical and Radiotherapeutic Techniques. J.B. Lippincott Co., Philadelphia, pp. 15–21

Calle R, Pilleron JP et al. (1979) Conservation management of operable breast cancer: Ten years experience at the Foundation Curie. Cancer 42:2045–2053

Calle R, Pilleron JP et al. (1984) Breast Carcinoma: Experience of the Curie Institute. In: Ames F., Blumenschein G, and Montague E (eds) Current Controversies in Breast Cancer. University of Texas Press, Austin, pp. 121–128

Clark RM, Vilkinson RH et al. (1982) Breast Cancer: A 21 year experience with conservative surgery and radiation. Int J Radiat Oncol Biol Phys 8:967–975

Delouche G, and Bachelot F (1980) Tumorectomie et radiotherapie pour les petits cancers du sein operables d'emblee. Resultats at 5 et 10 ans. J Eur Radiother 1:133

Fisher B, Montague E et al. (1980) Findings from NSABP Protocol No. B-04 comparison of radical mastectomy with alternative treatments for primary breast cancer. I. Radiation compliance and its relation to treatment outcome. Cancer 46:1–13

Fisher B, Bauer M et al. (1985) Five-year results of a randomized clinical trial comparing total mastectomy and segmental mastectomy with or without radiation in the treatment of breast. New Eng J Med 11:665–673

Fletcher GH, Montague ED et al. (1980) Radiotherapy in the management of nondisseminated breast cancer. In: Fletcher GH, Textbook of Radiotherapy, 3rd edn. Lea & Febiger, Philadelphia, pp. 527–579

Glasser O, Quimby EH, Taylor LS, Weatherwax JK, Morgan RH (1961) Physical Foundations of Radiology, 3rd edn. Harper and Row, New York

Hankey BF, Curtis RE et al. (1983) A retrospective cohort analysis of second breast cancer risk for primary breast cancer patients with an assessment of the effect of radiation therapy. JNCI 70:797–804

Harris JR, Hellman S (1984) The treatment philosophy, technique, and results of primary radiation for early breast cancer at the Joint Center for Radiation Therapy. In: Ames FC, Blumenschein GR, and Montague ED (eds) Current Controversies in Breast Cancer. University of Texas Press, Austin, pp. 111–119

Hellman S, Harris JR et al. (1980) Radiation therapy of early carcinoma of the breast without mastectomy. Cancer 46:988–994

Kurtz JM, Spitalier JM et al. (1983a) Results of salvage surgery for local failure following conservation therapy of operable breast cancer. In: Vaeth JM (ed) Frontiers of Radiation Therapy and Oncology. S Karger, Basel, pp. 84–90

Kurtz JM, Spitalier JM et al. (1983b) Late breast recurrence after lumpectomy and irradiation. Int J Radiat Oncol Biol Phys, in press

McCredie JA, Inch WR et al. (1975) Consecutive primary carcinoma of the breast. Cancer 35:1472–1477

Meredith WJ (1967) Radium Dosage: The Manchester System, 2nd edn, E & S Livingston, London

Montague ED (1984) Conservation treatment of early breast cancer. Cancer 53:700–704

Montague ED, Gutierrez AE et al. (1979) Conservation surgery and irradiation for the treatment of favorable breast cancer. Cancer 43:1048–1061

Montague ED, Romsdahl MM et al. (1983) The University of Texas M. D. Anderson Hospital technique for treatment of early breast cancer with conservation surgery and irradiation. In: Harris JR, Hellman S, and Silen W (eds) Conservation Management of Breast Cancer: New Surgical and Radiotherapeutic Techniques. J. B. Lippincott Co., Philadelphia, pp. 225–238

Montague ED, Schell SR et al. (1983) Conservation surgery and irradiation in the treatment of breast cancer. In: Vaeth JM (ed) Frontiers of Radiation Therapy and Oncology. S. Karger, Basel, pp. 76–83

Montague ED, Spanos Jr. WJ et al. (1983a) Conservative treatment and non-invasive or small-volume breast cancer. In: Feig S (ed) Breast Carcinoma: Current Diagnosis and Treatment. Masson Publishing, New York, pp. 429–432

Papillon J (1975) Conservative treatments of early breast cancer by tumorectomy and irradiation. In: Castro (ed) Current Concepts in Breast Cancer and Tumor Immunology. Bernie Huber, 117

Pierquin B, Dutreix A (1967) Towards a new system in curietherapy (endocurietherapy and plesiocurietherapy with non-radioactive preparation). Br J Radiol 40:184–186

Pierquin B, Woen R et al. (1980) Radical radiation therapy in breast cancer. Int J Radiat Oncol Biol Phys 6:17–24

Prosnitz LR, Golderberg IS et al. (1980) Primary radiotherapy for stage I and II breast cancer: A follow-up report from four east coast university hospitals. Int J Radiat Oncol Biol Phys 6:1339–1340

Prosnitz LR, Goldenberg IS et al. (1983) Radiotherapy for carcinoma of the breast instead of mastectomy. An update. In: Vaeth JM (ed) Frontiers of Radiation Therapy and Oncology, Karger S, Basel, pp. 69–75

Sarrazin D, Le GM et al. (1983) Conservative treatment versus mastectomy in T1 or small T2 breast cancer-A randomized clinical trial. In: Harris JR, Hellman S, and Silen W (eds) Conservative Management of Breast Cancer: New Surgical and Radiotherapeutic Techniques. J. B. Lippincott Co., Philadelphia, pp. 101–111

Schnitt SJ, Connolly JL et al. (1984) Pathologic predictors of early local recurrence in stage I and II breast cancer treated by primary radiation therapy. Cancer 53:1049–1057

Spanos WJ Jr., Montague ED et al. (1980) Late complication of radiation only for advanced breast cancer. Int J Radiat Oncol Biol Phys 6:1473–1476

Svensson GK, Chin LM et al. (1983) Breast treatment techniques at the Joint Center for Radiation Therapy. In: Harris JR, Hellman S, and Silen W (eds) Conservative Management of Breast Cancer: New Surgical and Radiotherapeutic Techniques. J. B. Lippincott Co., Philadelphia, pp. 239–255

Veronesi U (1983) Conservative treatment in breast cancer of limited size. In: Feig S (ed) Breast Carcinoma: Current Diagnosis and Treatment Publishing, New York, pp. 429–432

Vilcoq JR, Calle R et al. (1981) The outcome of treatment by tumorectomy and radiotherapy of patients with operable breast cancer. Int J Radiat Oncol Biol Phys 7:1327–1332

2.2.2 Responses to Treatment and Quality of Life After Radiation Therapy for Breast Cancer

Rosemary R. Lichtman, Shelley E. Taylor, and Joanne V. Wood

CONTENTS

Although breast cancer remains the foremost site of cancer deaths in American women today, the five-year survival rate for early, localized breast cancer has risen to 87% (American Cancer Society, 1982). Primary treatment for Stage I and Stage II breast cancers often involves radiation therapy, in the form of external beam radiation and/or iridium needle implants (Bluming 1982; Calle et al. 1978; Check 1981; Fisher et al. 1985; Harris et al. 1983; Mustakallio 1972). Consequently, an ever-increasing percentage of women being treated for breast cancer receive some form of radiation therapy.

Given the increase in the use of radiation therapy as a primary treatment in early breast cancer and the corresponding improved survival rates, it becomes important to consider the degree of compliance with treatment, short-term responses to treatment, and long-term quality of life after radiation therapy. Although there has been little research to date addressing these issues directly, there are indications that psychological factors

Rosemary R. Lichtman, Ph.D., Shelley E. Taylor, Ph.D., Joanne V. Wood, Ph.D.
University of California
Los Angeles, CA 90024, USA

may affect patient decision-making concerning compliance with radiation therapy used to treat other types of cancer (McNeil et al. 1982) and patient reactions to such treatment (Andersen et al.; Peck and Boland 1977; Rotman et al. 1977).

More specifically, past studies have found that patients may experience heightened anxiety (Andersen et al.; Peck and Boland 1977) and/or depressed mood (Mitchell and Glicksman 1977; Peck and Bolland 1977) during radiation therapy. Patients are often fearful of radiotherapy. Frequently indicated are fears of "being burned" (Peck 1972), of pain, scarring, and death (Peck and Boland 1977), of the inability to continue normal sexual functioning Rotman et al. 1977) and fear of the loss of social acceptance due to "contamination from the radioactivity" (Rotman et al. 1977). The research described here focused on the question of reactions to radiation therapy and quality of life for breast cancer patients after radiation treatment.

As part of a study investigating psychological adjustment in a group of 78 breast cancer patients, recruited from a three-physician private oncology practice in the Los Angeles area, reactions to radiation therapy were ascertained. Information was gathered through: a patient interview, the patient's responses to questionnaire materials including standardized adjustment measures, an interview with a person close to the patient, patient charts, and interviewer and physician ratings of patient adjustment to illness. The demographic attributes of the patients in the sample are presented in Table 1.

1 Responses to Radiation Therapy

For the 43 patients receiving radiation therapy, compliance was 100%. This rate is identical to that found in another study of cancer patients' reactions to radiation therapy (Peck and Boland 1977). It appears that, whatever difficulties pa-

Table 1. Characteristics of breast cancer patients in sample

Age		
Range: 29–78 years	(Median = 53)	
Marital Status		
Married	$n = 55$	(71%)
Single, divorced, separated	$n = 15$	(19%)
Widowed	$n = 8$	(10%)
Employment Status		
Unemployed	$n = 40$	(51%)
Employed	$n = 38$	(49%)
Full-time	$n = 20$	(26%)
Part-time	$n = 18$	(23%)
Education		
Range: 7th grade to M. A.	(Median = 1 year college)	
Time since surgery		
Range: 2–60 months	(Median = 25.5 months)	
Type of treatment		
Nonsurgical only	$n = 3$	(4%)
Surgical	$n = 75$	(96%)
Lumpectomy	$n = 26$	(34%)
Mastectomy	$n = 2$	(3%)
Simple	$n = 29$	(37%)
Modified radical	$n = 9$	(12%)
Halsted radical	$n = 9$	(12%)
Additional therapy after surgery	$n = 68$	(92%)
Radiation	$n = 43$	(58%)
Radiation therapy only	$n = 16$	(22%)
Radiation and chemotherapy	$n = 21$	(28%)
Multiple regimens	$n = 6$	(8%)
Other		
Chemotherapy only	$n = 23$	(31%)
Immunotherapy only	$n = 2$	(3%)
No therapy after surgery	$n = 6$	(8%)
No information	$n = 14$	
Stage at diagnosis		
Stage I	$n = 24$	(31%)
Stage II	$n = 43$	(55%)
Metastatic	$n = 11$	(14%)

tients have in response to radiation therapy, they are not great enough to cause them to discontinue therapy.

Those in our sample who received radiation therapy reported that they generally found it to be tolerable. Specifically, the women were asked to rate the unpleasantness of radiation therapy on a five-point scale. Twenty-five percent of the women rated it "1", "not at all unpleasant" 22% rated it "2", 16% rated it "3", 19% rated it "4", and 19% rated it "5", "extremely unpleasant". The mean rating was 2.8, suggesting that the women generally found the radiation therapy to be only moderately unpleasant. Interestingly, those women receiving the more extensive doses of radiotherapy did not rate it significantly more unpleasant.

For those women who found the therapy unpleasant, typical complaints about the external beam radiation concerned: (1) the physical side effects of the treatment, both systemic and local, i.e., nausea, fatigue, a skin reaction similar to sunburn and, for some, temporary difficulty in swallowing; (2) the logistics of getting to the therapy sessions (since the full course of external beam radiation treatment required daily outpatient visits for four to six weeks); and (3) the smell in the radiation therapists' office.

No other studies have yet reported the reactions of women receiving iridium needle implants as therapy for their breast cancer. Women in the present study receiving iridium implants complained about (1) a second hospitalization, with its unpleasant reminder of the earlier one, (2) fears due to a lack of information about the procedure itself, and (3) the isolation in the hospital due to the requirements of the procedure. One women noted that she felt like a leper.

2 Reasons for Compliance

Despite these various fears and side effects, all of the women to whom radiation therapy was recommended completed the prescribed treatment plan. The 100% compliance rate for radiation therapy may be compared to compliance with chemotherapy among this sample, which was 92%. Since radiation therapy generally has less toxic and noxious side effects and generally is prescribed for shorter periods of time than chemotherapy, it is not surprising that patients were somewhat more likely to adhere to the radiation treatments.

As in compliance with chemotherapy (See TAYLOR et al. 1984), several other reasons may be offered to explain the high rate. First, physicians generally advise radiation patients that it is not an optional treatment but a potentially life-saving treatment. Consequently, patients are likely to comply with the scheduled treatments even though they are bothered by the side effects. Second, radiation therapy fits the norms of treatments that show high rates of adherence generally (DIMATTEO and DINICOLA 1982). That is, it is administered in a hospital or office setting by trained professionals using advanced technical equipment. Third, since the radiation therapy is actively monitored by a physician, non-compliance is easily detected and may be immediately followed up. Thus, not complying is made very difficult. Fourth, primary radiation therapy employed in conjunction with lumpectomy is preferred to mastectomy by most patients, even with the attendant side effects. Therefore, patients may be highly motivated to follow through. Fifth, medications appear to relieve some of the physical complaints generated by the treatments. Finally, patients may have been better able to adhere to the radiation therapy because of their spontaneous use of coping techniques to deal with the unpleasant side effects. We now turn to this issue.

3 Coping with Radiation Therapy

Patients were asked if they did anything to counteract the side effects of the external beam radiation therapy; all but four of the 24 women who indicated that they felt at least some unpleasantness had done something to try to alleviate the situation. Eight of the women took medication to treat a particular complaint of nausea, fatigue, or "sunburn", five slept more than usual to counteract the fatigue, one made a change in her diet to alleviate the nausea.

In addition, six women used psychological techniques to counteract the side effects. Although the number of people using such techniques was actually small, the likelihood is that, increasingly, cancer patients will be adopting these techniques in the future to control the side effects of therapy such as radiation. Therefore, we will discuss them in some detail.

Several women used self-guided imagery (i.e., controlled vivid imagination of a pleasing scene or experience) as a method of controlling side effects (SHEIKH 1985). Typically, a patient would imagine either a peaceful scene to induce a calm state of mind during the therapy, or she would imagine a scene in which the radiotherapy took on the status on an ally doing battle with the foe, cancer.

Distraction (i.e., systematically choosing to ignore the side effects and think of something else instead) was also used as a means of coping with the radiation therapy. For example, one woman used distraction (thinking of her daughter's upcoming wedding) during the treatment to relieve her fear and anxiety.

Other patients used techniques of relaxation training, including deep breathing and muscle relaxation (JACOBSON 1938; WOLPE 1958). These techniques involve taking slow, deep breaths and progressively relaxing all of the muscles of the body, in order to induce a state of full relaxation. Some of the women had previously learned these techniques in another setting, such as natural childbirth or stress management, and found them effective in coping with the side effects of radiation therapy as well.

Most women reported that their actions helped in counteracting the side effects of radiation therapy. They were asked to indicate on a five-point scale how much the techniques they used had helped them. Seven of the women who had used coping techniques indicated that they had helped "very much", a rating of "5", two women rated their effect a "4", four rated the effect a "3", four rated it a "2", and two said that their efforts had helped "not at all." The mean rating was 3.4, suggesting that the women generally found their coping techniques to be moderately successful at alleviating the side effects which they experienced.

Because psychological coping techniques for dealing with physical problems have sometimes been associated with non-traditional treatments for cancer, the question may be legitimately posed: Does use of these techniques undermine compliance with traditional therapies? Patients were asked if using such psychological coping techniques made them more or less inclined to follow through with their prescribed, traditional therapies. Twenty-three percent reported that these psychological coping techniques made them more inclined to follow through with the therapy recommended by their physician. No patients felt less inclined to follow through, and 77% said it was irrelevant to their decisions about compliance with the treatment recommendations.

4 Adjustment and Quality of Life After Treatment for Cancer

Because increasing numbers of patients are surviving cancer after undergoing such treatments as radiotherapy, it is important to assess overall adjustment to the cancer experience. Studies of patients still close to their treatments have suggested that some may have difficulty in adjusting to the diagnosis of cancer and treatment for it. In one study of patients receiving radiation therapy, over one-half of the sample indicated that they were "having serious problems in living concerning internal thoughts and/or interpersonal relations" (MITCHELL and GLICKSMAN 1977). However, another study found that although emotional reactions generally occurred in patients who had had radiotherapy, they were always mild or moderate, never severe (PECK and BOLAND 1977).

Few studies have looked at these quality of life issues once therapies have been completed. Our own research addressed this issue. Because there is no generally agreed-upon measure of adjustment, composite measures are desirable. In particular, we employed measures of the patient's adjustment from several different individuals, including the patient herself (both in her verbal and in later written appraisals), a psychological interviewer, and her oncologist. We included measures developed for our particular study as well as standardized measures which have been used successfully with other populations of chronically-ill individuals. The eventual score of psychological adjustment was determined by a factor analysis of all these individual measures. The statistical approach draws upon the shared variance among measures in coming up with a single composite measure. The final measure included:

1. the woman's self-rating of adjustment. During the interview, the patient made a verbal assessment of her current overall adjustment on a scale going from 1 (very bad) to 5 (very good).

2. the women's report of psychological distress. During the interview, the patient was asked to indicate her present level of anxiety, fear, anger, and depression, each on a scale of 1 (not at all) to 4 (very much). These ratings were then summed to provide the indication of current psychological distress.

3. the total score on the Profile Of Mood States. The Profile of Mood States, or POMS (McNAIR and LORR 1964) was completed as part of a questionnaire left with the patient. It measured the woman's current emotional adjustment, asking her to specifically consider how she had been feeling during the past week. Its subscales measure tension, confusion, vigor, depression, and anxiety.

4. The Index of Well-Being Score. This was also included in the questionnaire. The Index of Well-Being Score (CAMPBELL et al. 1976) is derived from of a combination of ratings on a ten-item scale concerning the patient's current affect and a rating of present satisfaction.

5. the interviewer's rating of the patient on the Global Adjustment to Illness Scale. The Global Adjustment to Illness Scale (GAIS) (DEREGOTIS 1975) has been used successfully to differentiate patient adjustment to serious illness. The GAIS is a 100-point scale, broken down into ten deciles, ranging from "severely impaired adjustment" (1–10) to "excellent adjustment" (91–100). For each category, specific guidelines are provided regarding the psychological and behavioral symptomatology that would be required in order to rate the patient in that range. Once a decile is selected for a patient, the rating is further specified by the placement within that range. Interviewers rated patient adjustment at the time of the interview.

6. the oncologist's GAIS rating. This rating was made by the oncologist caring for the patient and was based on the most recent office visit.

The results from our study indicate that having had some form of radiation therapy did not negatively affect patient psychological adjustment after cancer. For women with good physical prognoses who had had radiation therapy, psychological adjustment after breast cancer was generally high, and long-term quality of life was generally reported to remain the same or even be improved over the pre-illness level. Patients who had had primary radiation therapy generally had had lumpectomies rather than mastectomies for their surgical treatment. We found that these lumpectomy-radiotherapy patients were significantly better adjusted after their treatments than were the mastectomy patients ($r=0.35$, $p<0.002$), with the Halsted radical patients the least well adjusted of that latter group. Two factors appeared to be mediators in the effect the type of surgical treatment had on adjustment (TAYLOR et al. 1983). First, the concern with breast loss and body disfigurement was greater among the mastectomy patients; when its effects were partialled out, the correlation between surgical treatment and adjustment dropped ($r=0.24$, $p<0.03$). Second, the mastectomy patients reported greater deterioration in affectional and sexual functioning than did the lumpectomy-radiotherapy patients. When these variables were individually partialled out, the original treatment-adjustment relationship declined (partial correlation controlling for changes in frequency of marital affection: $r=0.22$, $p<0.09$; partial correlation controlling for changes in frequency of sexual intercourse: $r=0.28$, $p<0.05$).

Generally, patients in this sample appeared to adjust well to the cancer experience. The mean sample rating on the oncologists' GAIS ratings of the patients can provide a more comparative measure of adjustment since it has been used to rate adjustment to other illness as well. The mean physicians' rating for the patients in this sample was 82: "Very good adjustment. Minimal psychological symptomatology associated with the illness. Good functioning in most life activities. Involved in a broad spectrum of interests. Socially active with high life investment. Worries occasionally about problems associated with illness, but maintains good control. Adjustment to illness and relations with treatment staff are very good. "This level of adjustment is comparable to that found in other studies of cancer patients (DEROGATIS et al. 1979).

How can one account for the generally high levels of adjustment that are found after treatment for cancer? It can be argued that part of the explanation stems from the patient's own need to evaluate herself as coping well, rather than perceiving herself as a victim of adversity (TAYLOR et al. 1983). One way of achieving this positive self-evaluation is through a process known as downward social comparison. That is, cancer patients may compare their adjustment, their physical status, or other aspects of their current situation, with cancer patients who are less advantaged by comparison. By selecting a comparison woman who has coped very poorly, is very ill, or is unfortunate in other ways, a cancer patient may selectively focus on attributes of her particular situation in which she has an advantage, and consequently feel better about herself. For example, a woman who has had a lumpectomy may focus on her minimal surgery as compared to a patient who has had a mastectomy. A woman has had a mastectomy but with no nodal involvement may focus on the fact that she does not require chemotherapy as others did.

In some cases, in order to cast their current condition in a more positive light, women even create hypothetical others who are coping more poorly than they are.

"You read about a few who handle it (the diagnosis and treatment of cancer) well, but it seems like the majority really feel sorry for themselves, and I don't think they cope with it very well. I don't understand it, because it doesn't bother me at all."

Overall, then, by making her own level of adjustment appear good by comparison, a cancer patient increases her good feelings about herself.

So far, we have emphasized the fact that most breast cancer patients seem to cope fairly well. Generally, they adjust satisfactorily to the diagnosis, prognosis, and therapies. What is perhaps more notable is the fact that some patients report beneficial effects that the experience has had on their lives. In particular, the cancer experience appears to prompt at least a proportion of cancer patients to search for meaning in their lives. The search for meaning involves the need to understand why the crisis occurred and what its impact has been. Slightly over half of the cancer patients we interviewed reported that the cancer experience had caused them to reappraise their lives. For example, a 61-year old woman remarked:

"You can take a picture of what someone has done, but when you frame it, it becomes significant. I feel as if I were, for the first time, really conscious. My life is framed in a certain amount of time. I always knew it, but now I can see it, and my life is made better by the knowledge."

Another said:

"I have much more enjoyment of each day, each moment. I am not so worried about what is or isn't, or what I wish I had. All those things you get entangled with just don't seem to be part of my life right now."

For others, the meaning gained from the experience was self-knowledge:

"The ability to understand myself more fully is one of the greatest changes I have experienced. I have faced what I went through. It's a bit like holding up a mirror to one's face when one can't turn around. I think that is a very essential thing."

Typically, individuals reordered their priorities, giving low priority to such mundane concerns as housework, petty quarrels, and involvement in other people's problems and high priority to relationships with spouse, children, and friends, personal projects, or just plain enjoyment of life (Lichtman, 1982):

"You take a long look at your life and realize that many things that you thought were important before are totally insignificant. You find out that things like relationships are really the most important things you have – the people you know and your family – everything else is of minor importance. It's very strange that it takes something so serious to make you realize that."

Not every cancer patient construes positive meaning from the cancer experience, and it would be misleading to suggest that all can. However, when positive meaning can be construed, it produces significantly better psychological adjustment. The cancer threat, then, is perceived by many to have been the catalytic agent for restructuring their lives along more meaningful lines, with an overall beneficial effect.

5 Conclusions

Both the results of the present study and previous research indicate that cancer patients respond well to radiation therapy and often achieve a high quality of life following their experience with cancer and its treatments. In the present study, compliance with radiation therapy was 100%, and women undergoing radiation therapy reported only moderate side effects as a consequence of the treatment. These figures are comparable to other studies of radiotherapy patients. Part of the reason for the high level of compliance and relatively low levels of reported discomfort was the spontaneous effort these women made to counteract the side effects they experienced. These efforts included medications and rest as well as psychological coping techniques such as imaging, distraction and relaxation. These latter techniques may be used increasingly in the future to help alleviate the adverse consequences of treatment.

Long-term quality of life after radiation therapy for breast cancer appears to be high. Most of the women in the present study were well adjusted following the cancer experience. They had occasional worries, but otherwise led full and active lives. Indeed, some women reported that the cancer experience had actually enriched their lives, enabling them to reorder priorities and find meaning in their activities. While it would be foolish to suggest that, overall, cancer is a psychologically beneficial experience, it would be equally unwise to portray it as a psychologically devastating one. Rather, like all chronic diseases, cancer creates substantial problems for its victims which can threaten, challenge, and in some cases, ennoble its victims.

References

American Cancer Society (1982) Cancer facts and figures, 1983. American Cancer Society, New York

Andersen BL, Karlsson JA, Anderson B, Tewfik HH (in press) Anxiety and cancer treatment: Response to stressful radiotherapy. Health Psych

Bluming AZ (1982) Treatment of primary breast cancer without mastectomy: Review of the literature. Amer J Med 72:820–828

Calle R, Pilleron JP, Schlienger P, Vilcog JR (1978) Conservative management of breast cancer. Cancer 42:2045–2053

Campbell A, Converse PE, Rodgers WL (1976) The quality of American life: Perceptions, evaluations, and satisfactions. Russell Sage Foundation, New York

Check WA (1981) Breast-saving surgery, radiation for early cancer gaining advocates. JAMA 245:661–664

Derogatis LR (1975) The global adjustment to illness scale (GAIS). Clinical Psychometric Research, Baltimore

Derogatis LR, Abeloff MD, Melasaratos N (1979) Psychological coping mechanisms and survival time in metastatic breast cancer. JAMA 242:1504–1508

DiMatteo MR, DiNicola DD (1982) Achieving patient compliance: The psychology of the medical practitioner's role. Pergamon Press, New York

Fisher B, Baver M, Margolese R (1985) Five-year results of a randomized clinical trial comparing total mastectomy and simple mastectomy with or without radiation in the treatment of breast cancer. N Engl J Med 312:665–675

Harris J, Hellman S, Silen W (eds) Conservative management of breast cancer. Lippincott, Philadelphia

Jacobson E (1938) Progressive relaxation. University of Chicago Press, Chicago

Lichtman RR (1982) Close relationships after breast cancer. Doctoral dissertation, University of California, Los Angeles

McNair DM, Lorr M (1964) An analysis of mood in neurotics. J Abnorm Psych 69:620–627

McNeil BJ, Pauker SG, Sox HC, Tversky A (1982) On the elicitation of preferences for alternative therapies. N Engl J Med 306:1259–1262

Mitchell GW, Glicksman AS (1977) Cancer patients: Knowledge and attitudes. Cancer 40:61–66

Mustakallio S (1972) Conservative treatment of breast cancer – review of 25 years follow-up. Clin Radiol 23:110–116

Peck A (1972) Emotional reactions to having cancer. Amer J Roent Rad Ther Nuc Med 114:591–599

Peck A, Boland J (1977) Emotional reactions to radiation treatment. Cancer 40:180–184

Rotman M, Rogow LR, DeLeon G, Heskel N (1977) Supportive therapy in radiation oncology. Cancer 39:744–750

Sheikh AA (ed) (1985) Imagery: Current theory, research and application. John Wiley, New York

Taylor SE, Lichtman RR, Wood JV (1984) Compliance with chemotherapy among breast cancer patients. Health Psych 6:533–562

Taylor SE, Lichtman RR, Wood JV, Bluming AZ, Dosik GM, Leibowitz RL (1985) Illness-related and treatment-related factors in psychological adjustment to breast cancer. Cancer 55:2506–2513

Taylor SE, Wood JV, Lichtman RR (1983) It could be worse: Selective evaluation as a response to victimization. J Soc Issues 39:19–40

Wolpe J (1958) Psychotherapy by reciprocal inhibition. Stanford University Press, Stanford

2.3 Soft Tissue Sarcoma

2.3.1 UCLA Combined Modality Limb Salvage Protocols for Soft Tissue Sarcomas

Thomas H. Weisenburger

CONTENTS

1 Background

Innovations in any field are usually based on a substantial foundation of previous efforts of workers in that field. The UCLA Limb-Salvage protocol is no exception. It combines preoperative chemotherapy and radiation with a surgical resection that allows a functioning limb. The combination of preoperative chemotherapy and radiation was chosen to treat subclinical deposits of malignant cells which may not be resected with the grossly evident disease when limb sparing surgery is done. This multi-modality approach has been built upon previous experiences with the combination of radiation and surgery, and the discovery of active chemotherapy agents.

The concept of adding radiation to surgery, though mentioned early in the history of radiation therapy, even for soft tissue sarcomas (Pusey 1902,

Thomas H. Weisenburger, M.D.,
Associate Clinical Professor
UCLA Department of Radiation Oncology and
Director of Clinical Research
Cancer Foundation of Santa Barbara
Santa Barbara, CA 93105, USA

Leucutia 1935), was systematically applied to cancers of the head and neck and soft-tissue sarcomas in the 1960's, with the publication of the results of the first significant clinical trials in the early 1970's. These studies demonstrate that radiation given to undisturbed lymphatics at high risk for recurrence (Fletcher 1972a, Fletcher 1972b) or after removal of clinically evident tumor (Suit et al. 1973, Lindberg 1972, Lindberg et al. 1975) can control subclinical disease (both microscopic and macroscopic, clinically non-appreciable, extension) which might surround the gross tumor. The M.D. Anderson experience with the use of radiation in the primary management of patients with soft tissue sarcomas clearly demonstrated that combined modality treatment could result in local control of approximately 80% of extremity sarcomas with very acceptable function in the majority of patients (Lindberg et al. 1977). For the larger and more proximal tumors of the thigh, the failure rate approached 30%. Similar series utilizing surgical excision without radiation resulted in > 80% local recurrence rates (Martin et al. 1965), indicating that radiation can control subclinical deposits of soft tissue sarcoma in patients who have had the gross tumor excised.

In the late 1960's and early 1970's there was much interest in combining chemotherapy agents, recently found to be active, with surgery alone and surgery and radiation (DiPietro et al. 1970, O'Bryan et al. 1973, Haskell et al. 1974). In a pilot study at UCLA, 44 patients with sarcomas, both soft tissue and skeletal, were treated with multimodality therapy (Morton et al. 1976). Eight received preoperative intra-arterial doxorubicin, 5 had surgery followed by postoperative radiation, 14 received preoperative intra-arterial doxorubicin and radiation followed by resection, and 17 had resection alone. The conclusions were that combined therapy yielded superior results compared to resection alone and that limb sparing surgical procedures were possible more often in the group that received pre-operative intra-arterial doxorubicin and radiation than in the group that received preoperative chemotherapy alone. It was also the impression of the surgeons that the resections performed after preoperative chemotherapy and radiation therapy could not have always been accomplished without the preoperative combined treatment.

2 UCLA Limb Salvage Protocols for Soft Tissue Sarcomas

2.1 Chemotherapy

The intra-arterial infusion of doxorubicin delivers 30 mg per day for three days, for a total of 90 mg. The arterial catheter must be placed in a high flow vessel. Flourescein is injected and the skin in the region being infused is examined with ultraviolet light to insure that there is not a high concentration of doxorubicin reaching the cutaneous tissues (which can result in significant skin reactions). This procedure is repeated daily during the infusion of the doxorubicin and, if necessary, the catheter is repositioned.

2.2 Radiotherapy

Radiation is given with large fractions over a short time following the infusion of intra-arterial doxorubicin to exploit a relatively high concentration of the drug in the tumor. The radiation is not given concurrently, since the patients are at bed rest during the infusion to insure that the catheter does not become dislodged. Initially, ten fractions of 350 cGy were given over 12 to 14 days with the radiation beginning within three days of the completion of the intra-arterial infusion (WEISENBURGER et al. 1981). This dose regimen, given over two weeks was thought to be approximately equivalent to 50 Gy, given in 25 fractions over 5 weeks. The NSD Formula (ELLIS 1971) was used to make the approximation. It was postulated that this preoperative regimen of chemotherapy and radiation would effectively control subclinical deposits of tumor cells at the periphery of the clinically apparent tumor and therefore allow wide excision to replace amputation in most patients. The total dose of radiation has been modified in subsequent versions of the protocols (vide infra).

Because soft tissue sarcomas tend to spread along fascial planes (CANTIN et al. 1968), the radiation fields are defined to include all tissue planes at risk from the origin to the insertion of involved muscle groups. Anterior and posterior parallel op-posed fields are employed in the majority of cases, sparing as much tissue as possible either medially or laterally to minimize long term side effects. This requires large fields in most instances, but they seem justified by data (LINDBERG et al. 1977) indicating that approximately 30% (10 of 31) of local recurrences were marginal or geographic when 5 cm margins were used. Because of the large field sizes, patients are often treated using extended SSDs or TSDs of 125 to 150 cm. Most of the patients have been treated with 6 or 10 mev photon beams, although ^{60}Co was used occasionally. A computer program for dose calculation involving irregular fields (CUNNINGHAM et al. 1970) was used to evaluate the uniformity of the dose delivered. Because of the extended treatment distances used in most instances, there is an acceptable variation of within $+/-10\%$ of the prescribed dose using this technique.

2.3 Surgery

Surgery consists of wide excision 7–14 days after the completion of the irradiation. The exact procedure varies with the location of the tumor, but the intent is to be as conservative as possible consistent with complete excision (EILBER et al. 1980).

3 Results

Seventy-seven patients with non-metastatic soft tissue tumors were treated according to this protocol between 1975 and March 1981. The median follow-up for this group is 60 months. The majority had grade III tumors (78%) with some grade II (19%) and a few grade I (3%). Histological analysis of the surgical specimen revealed that an average of approximately 80% of the tumor was necrotic. The survival of the group is 67% at 5 years. Comparison with the data from the American Joint Committee study (RUSSELL et al. 1977) indicates that, at the least, the survival of these patients is not jeopardized by this limb salvage approach. Only 3 of 77 (4%) have developed local recurrence. Life table analysis yields a local control rate of 95% at 60 months which compares favorably with previously published reports (SUIT et al. 1973, LINDBERG 1972, LINDBERG et al. 1975, LINDBERG et al. 1977). However, 19 (25%) of these patients had complications requiring reoperation, and in 17 the complications were considered to be major. Eight developed wound necrosis, which healed but required hospitalization and grafting in some cases. Six developed lymphoedema. Five patients sustained femoral fractures (four of these 5 had had periosteal stripping performed to provide tumor clearance: all healed after fixation with intramedullary rods). Three patients required amputations because of complications and three for local recurrence for an overall limb salvage rate of 71/77 (92%).

4 Modifications of the Protocol

A local recurrence rate of <5% is quite acceptable, and difficult to improve upon. The next step, therefore, was to maintain the excellent local control rate while decreasing the incidence of complications. It was elected in March 1981 to maintain the existing chemotherapy and to reduce the dose of radiation to 350 cGy × 5.

One hundred and seven patients have been treated with this regimen. With a median follow-up of only 20 months, several interesting observations can be made. The amount of necrosis in the surgical specimen decreased from 80% to approximately 20%, indicating a clear dose response effect. In addition, the complication rate has been lower, with 15% of the patients requiring reoperation because of complications. Four patients have had amputations, two primarily because of major vessel involvement and two because of recurrence. The most important result is, however, that despite the shorter follow-up, 9 patients developed local recurrence. At 36 months after treatment, by which time essentially all local recurrences will have become evident, life table analysis yields a local control rate of 86%, compared with a value of 95% in the earlier series of 77 patients.

Since the complications can be treated, the protocol has again been modified to improve the probability of local control of the tumor by increasing the radiation dose to 8 fractions of 350 cGy over 10 days. Also, because intraarterial administration of doxorubicin is technically demanding, its efficacy is being compared in a randomized fashion with intravenous administration. Thirty patients have been treated, but, since the protocol was begun only in March 1985, no useful analysis is yet possible.

5 Discussion

It is clear from the data presented that this combination of preoperative chemotherapy and radiation followed by limb-sparing surgery provides an

Table 1. Local control and complications for the various series

Series-dose	No. patients	Local control[a]	Complications[b]
I-35 Gy	77	95% 60 mo	25%
II-17.5 Gy	120	86% 36 mo	15%
III-28 Gy	30	N/A[c]	N/A[c]

[a] Life table analysis
[b] Requiring reoperation
[c] Not assessed

excellent local control rate for soft tissue sarcomas while preserving function. What is not a clear is the reason for the success of this protocol. It may be due in part to the fact that these patients often undergo two surgical procedures, an excisional biopsy for diagnosis and the re-excision following the preoperative therapy. It has been shown that 49 of 98 patients (50%) of patients who have had an excisional biopsy will have gross disease evident at the time of re-excision (GIULIANO, personal communication, 1985). The presence of gross disease following the initial excision of the primary probably decreases the local control rate if a second, definitive, excision is not performed. The use of large fractions may also have contributed to the excellent results obtained in this series of patients. If the shoulder of the survival curve is large there may be an advantage in using large individual fractions, since each fraction would exceed the range of the shoulder and fall on the straight line or logarithmic portion of the survival curve (SHANK and CHU, 1984). The delivery of the radiation shortly after giving the doxorubicin may have increased the therapeutic ratio, since the concentration of the drug would be increased, but this is conjectural, since such enhancement has not been established.

The difference between the local recurrence rate in those who received the higher and lower doses of radiation (Table 1) clearly indicates a dose response effect, and demonstrates the significant contribution of radiation to the local control rate. A clear definition of the relative benefits of the surgery, chemotherapy and radiation in this protocol may, however, never be possible.

References

Cantin J, McNeer GP, Chu FC, Booker RJ (1968) The problem of local recurrence after treatment of soft tissue sarcoma. Ann. Surg. 168:47–53
Cunningham JS, Shrivastava PN, Wilkinson JM (1970)

Computer calculation of dose within an irregularly shaped field. Proceedings of the American association of Physicists in Medicine Hodgkin's Disease Workshop. Chicago, Illinois

DiPietro S, dePalo GM, Molinari R, Gennari L (1970) Clinical trials with Adriamycin by prolonged arterial infusion. Tumori 56:233–244

Eilber FR, Mirra J, Grant TT, Weisenburger TH, Morton DL (1980) Is amputation necessary for sarcomas? A seven year experience with limb salvage. Annals of Surgery 192:431–437

Ellis F (1971) Nominal standard dose and the ret. Br. J. Radiol. 44:101–108

Fletcher GH (1972a) Local results of irradiation in the primary management of localized breast cancer. Cancer 29:545–551

Fletcher GH (1972b) Elective irradiation of subclinical disease in cancers of the head and neck. Cancer 29:1450–1454

Giuliano A (1985) Personal communication

Haskell CM, Silverstein MJ, Rangel DM, Hunt JS, Sparks FC, Morton DL (1974) Multimodality cancer therapy in man: a pilot study of Adriamycin by arterial infusion. Cancer 33:1485–1490

Leucutia T (1935) Radiotherapy of sarcoma of soft parts. Radiology 25:403–415

Lindberg RD (1972) The role of radiation therapy in the treatment of soft-tissue sarcome in adults. In: Proceedings of Seventh National Cancer Conference. Philadelphia, Pennsylvania, J.B. Lippincott Co., pp 883–888

Lindberg RD, Fletcher GH, Martin G (1975) The management of soft tissue sarcomas in adults: surgery and postoperative radiotherapy. Journal de Radiologie et d'Electrologie 56:761–767

Lindberg RD, Martin RG, Romsdahl MM, McMurtrey MJ (1977) Management of Primary Bone and Soft Tissue Tumors. Year Book Medical Publishers, Chicago, pp 289–298

Martin RG, Butler JJ, Albores-Saavedra J (1965) Soft-tissue tumors: surgical treatment and results. In: Tumors of Bone and Soft Tissue. Year Book Medical Publishers, Inc., Chicago, pp 333–347

Morton DL, Eilber FR, Townsend CM, Grant TT, Mirra JJ, Weisenburger TH (1976) Limb salvage from a Multidisciplinary treatment approach for skeletal and soft tissue sarcomas of the extremity. Annals of Surgery 184:268–278

O'Bryan RM, Luce JK, Talley RW, Gottlieb JA, Baker LH, Bonadonna G (1973) Phase II evaluation of Adriamycin in human neoplasia. Cancer 32:1–8

Pusey WA (1902) Cases of sarcoma and Hodgkin's disease treated by exposure to x-rays: a preliminary report. JAMA 38:166–169

Russell WO, Cohen J, Enziger F, Hajdu SI, Heise H, Martin RG, Meissner W, Miller WT, Schmitz RL, Suit HD (1977) A clinical and pathological staging system for soft tissue sarcomas. Cancer 40:1562–1573

Shank B, Chu F (1984) Fractionation in radiation therapy: Theoretical basis, experimental, and clinical studies, Cancer Investigation 2:165–176

Suit HD, Russel WO, Martin RG (1973) Management of patients with sarcomas of soft tissue in an extremity. Cancer 31:1247–1255

Weisenburger TH, Eilber FR, Grant TT, Morton DL, Mirra JJ, Steinberg M, Rickles D (1981) Multidisciplinary "Limb Salvage" treatment of soft tissue and skeletal sarcomas. Int J Radiat Oncol Biol Phys 7:1495–1499

2.3.2 M.D. Anderson Hospital Experience

H. Thomas Barkley, Jr., Robert D. Lindberg, and Gunar K. Zagars

CONTENTS

1 Introduction

Sarcomas arising from extra skeletal sites have excited medical interest out of proportion to their incidence for many years. Despite their comparative rarity much has been, and continues to be, written about their histology, patterns of growth, and especially their treatment. In the past, it was common for the tumor to be massive at time of presentation, a characteristic of many being that they caused no discomfort or decrease in function until they reached enormous size. The patient with such disease was lulled into a sense of complacency due to the deliberate growth pattern of many of the histologic varieties and the lack of symptoms. Others were simply overwhelmed by the rapidity of growth and lost the opportunity for early diagnosis and treatment. For such manifestations of disease, surgery was the only available treatment of worth. Since many of the lesions had the deceptive appearance of complete encapsulation, enuc-

H. Thomas Barkley, Jr., M.D., Associate Professor
Gunar K. Zagars, M.D.
The University of Texas M.D. Anderson Hospital
and Tumor Institute
Houston, TX 77030, USA

Robert D. Lindberg, M.D.
Brown Cancer Center
Louisville, KY 40202, USA

leation was attempted with an almost universal consequence that the sarcoma recurred locally. The recommended treatment for lesions appearing in the extremities became amputation or disarticulation. Unfortunately disease appearing in the head and neck, thorax, retroperiteum, etc. could not be handled in this way and enucleation, debulking or no treatment was the fate of these unfortunate victims. Radiation therapy was attempted for many of those who could not be operated upon but equipment restrictions of depth dose characteristics and acute reactions prevented the application of suitable tumor doses and gained for these tumors the reputation of being "radioresistant".

As the medical profession and the general population became more aware of the serious nature of the soft tissue sarcoma, earlier manifestations of the stages of the disease presented for treatment. Over the past 35 years, certain principles by which soft tissue sarcomas should be treated have been acknowledged, but there is a considerable controversy ongoing concerning the manner in which these principles are to be accomplished. In case of extremity lesions, the preservation of function is paramount. The major schools of thought, with respect to local control, have been reduced to two: (1) soft part resection and (2) limited excision and postoperative radiation therapy with or without the addition of chemotherapy. There are numerous variations on these themes as exemplified by the use of combinations of interstitial irradiation, intra-arterial chemotherapy, pre- and postoperative radiation etc. When the lesion is large and infiltrative, or adjacent to bone or joints, or in the head and neck, thorax or retroperitoneum, soft part resection with secure margins is not feasible, and other means must be employed for control of disease. Generally, the only universal approach for any anatomic site is a combination of limited resection and irradiation.

There is a considerable literature available concerning the importance of proper initial approach to soft tissue sarcomas. Despite this fact, a large number of patients arrive at referral centers after incisional biopsy, piecemeal excision or enucleation without margin, frequently done in the anticipation of a benign tumor. It is obvious that in contrast to the intense interest within the cancer centers, soft tissue sarcoma is not the diagnosis most frequently entertained by the medical practitioner when faced with a tumor of trunk or extremities. The initial approach has definite consequences in the planning of subsequent treatment and may indeed have deleterious prognostic significance.

2 Material and Methods

From 1963 to date, more than 1000 patients with soft tissue sarcoma have been treated at UT M.D. Anderson Hospital. Through 1982, 959 of these have been placed in a data base, showing the following treatment categories: surgery 334, radiotherapy 67, perfusion 34, surgery and postoperative irradiation 458 and preoperative irradiation and surgery, 66. By July 1983, 313 patients had been treated by some form of limited surgical procedure and postoperative irradiation 5 years or more prior to the analysis. (These patients form the basis of the report to follow.)

If, on admission, there was suspicion of minimal residual disease either by palpation or a review of the pathology report, re-excision was performed at MDAH prior to the course of irradiation. Table 1 shows that this assessment was correct approximately two thirds of the time.

Radiation treatment parameters have varied little over this period. The majority of patients were treated by ^{60}Co until 1977, since which time 6 MeV photons have been utilized. Since 1971, the total dose for low grade lesions has been 60 Gy, 65–66 Gy for high grade lesions. Prior to this time the respective doses were 65 and 70 Gy. Since the change, normal tissue sequelae have lessened with the reduced doses and no change in local control has been noted. Initially, extremity treatment fields are parallel opposed, equally loaded open and 45° wedge pair extending cephalad and caudad 7 or 5 cm beyond the scar of excision if possible for high grade and low grade lesions respectively. After a dose of 50 Gy, the fields are reduced symmetrically and again at 60 Gy for those who are to receive 65–66 Gy. When the surgical scar is adjacent to elbow, wrist, knee or ankle, the additional radiation is given by means of an appropriate electron beam energy using an appositional field.

Table 1. Treatment of soft tissue sarcomas by limited resection and radiation therapy. Results of re-excision prior to irradiation

Reason for re-excision	Specimen positive	Specimen negative
Gross residual	3	2
Questionable margins	21	12

For the remainder of the patients, depending on site and assessment of risk, the reduced fields may be treated either with appositional electrons, continued photon irradiation, or a combination of both.

In other regions treatment is individualized for the anatomic site with compensating filters, anterior posterior weighting, and other appropriate maneuvers. When indicated, the entire dose may be given by electron beam, or by high energy photon beams for deeply seated abdominal or pelvic disease. The prescribed total dose is reduced for retroperitoneal tumors to about 55 Gy and the overall time is extended by reducing the fractional dose size to 1.7–1.8 Gy, depending on the volume required or the habitus of the patient.

3 Results

Analysis of results in the past (Suit et al. 1975) has led to emphasis on certain aspects of disease presentation. Those features of the disease which appear to have the greatest impact on prognosis both for local control and survival are 1) size of the primary lesion, 2) histologic grade, 3) and anatomic site.

The relationship of primary control and recurrence to size of primary is seen in Table 2. There is a clear but not statistically significant increase in local recurrence as the size of the primary tumor increases. The oft repeated warning that these lesions are prone to extend widely along fascial planes seems somewhat exaggerated in view of the low incidence of recurrence outside the treatment field in spite of the conservative nature of the surgery and the modest margins of the radiation portals. The average number of recurrences outside these portals is 5% and is not greater with increasing size of the primary lesion.

In the time frame covered by this series of patients, all specimens were graded histologically either by the original pathologist or, at our request, Dr. R. Ayala who kindly acted as referee. All but

Table 2. Treatment of soft tissue sarcomas by limited resection and radiation therapy. Size of primary related to control surgery + radiation therapy (1963–1978) analysis 1983

Size	Total treated	Permanently controlled	Recurrence in field	Recurrence outside field
≤ 5 cm	126	103(82)[a]	18(14)	5(5)
5 to ≤ 8 cm	72	55(76)	13(18)	4(7)
> 8 cm	115	81(70)	28(24)	6(7)
Total	313	239(76)[a]	59(19)	15(5)

[a] Per cent of total treated

Table 3. Treatment of soft tissue sarcomas by limited resection and radiation therapy. Histologic grade related to control surgery + radiation therapy (1963–1978) analysis 1983

Grade	Total treated	Permanently controlled[a]	Recurrence in field	Recurrence outside field
1	71	62(87)[b]	7(10)	2(3)
2	150	109(73)	33(22)	8(5)
3	90	67(74)	18(20)	5(6)
Total	311	238	58	15

[a] Two patients not graded, 1 controlled, 1 failed in field
[b] Number in parentheses are percentages

Table 4. Soft tissue sarcoma MDAH grading system (1981). (Fibrosarcoma will be graded I–III)

Grade I	Desmoidal fibromatosis Well-differentiated liposarcoma Dermatofibrosarcoma protuberans Hemangiopericytoma Epithelioid hemangioendothelioma
Grade II	Myxoid liposarcoma (not cellular) Myxoid malignant fibrohistiocytoma Chondrosarcoma — mesenchymal — extra skeletal
Grade III	Rhabdomysarcoma Synovial sarcoma Malignant fibrohistiocytoma Leiomyosarcoma Pleomorphic liposarcoma Epithelioid and clear cell sarcoma

Table 5. Treatment of soft tissue sarcomas by limited resection and radiation therapy. Histologic grading assigned by diagnosis related to control. Surgery + radiation therapy (1963–1978) analysis (1983)

Assigned grade	Total treated	Permanently controlled	Recurred in field	Recurred outside field
1	47	43(92)[a]	2(4)	2(4)
2	77	55(71)	71(22)	5(7)
3	189	141(75)	40(21)	8(4)
Total	313	239	59	15

[a] per cent of total treated

Table 6. Treatment of soft tissue sarcomas by limited resection and radiation therapy

	Stage grouping
Stage IA	G1, T1, N0, M0 well-differentiated tumor 5 cm or less in diameter; no regional lymph nodal or distant metastases
Stage IB	G1, T2, N0, M0 well-differentiated tumor more than 5 cm in diameter; no regional lymph nodal or distant metastases
Stage IIA	G2, T1, N0, M0 moderately differentiated tumor 5 cm or less in diameter; no regional nodal or distant metastases
Stage IIB	G2, T2, N0, M0 5 cm in diameter; no regional lymph nodal or distant metastases
Stage IIIA	G3, T1, N0, M0 poorly differentiated tumor 5 cm or less in diameter; no regional lymph nodal or distant metastases
Stage IIIB	G3, T2, N0, M0 poorly differentiated tumor more than 5 cm in diameter; no regional lymph nodal or distant metastases
Stage IIIC	Any G, T1, T2; N1, M0 tumor of any differentiation, any size; regional lymph nodal metastases but no distant metastases
Stage IVA	Any G, T3, any N, M0 tumor of any differentiation of malignancy demonstrating clear radiographic evidence of destruction of cortical bone (with invasion) and histopathologic confirmation of invasion major artery or nerve, with or without regional lymph nodal metastases but without distant metastases
Stage IVB	Any G, any T, any N, M1 tumor with distant metastases

two of the cases were graded in this manner, these two having insufficient tissue submitted following excision elsewhere to make the decision. Table 3 shows that the incidence of recurrence in-field for grades 2 and 3 is essentially the same and approximately twice as great as that for grade 1. When the in-field and out-of-field recurrences are

Table 7. Treatment of soft tissue sarcomas by limited resection and radiation therapy. Status by stage at 5 or more years after treatment

Stage	Total treated	NED	Primary	Cause of failure				ID 2nd P
				P+DM	P+N+DM	N+DM	DM	
IA	34	31	—	—	—	—	2	1
IB	28	23	—	1	—	—	2	2
IIA	54	44	—	—	—	1	8	1
IIB	82	42	3	5	—	3	26	3
IIIA	24	16	2	—	—	—	6	—
IIIB	56	21	3	5	2	1	20	4
IIIC	6	4	—	—	—	1	1	—
IVA	29	16	4	1	—	—	7	1
Total	313	197	12	12	2	6	72	12

P+DM,   primary+distant metastasis
P+N+DM, primary+nodal+distant metastasis
N+DM,   nodal+distant metastasis
DM,   distant metastasis
ID,   intercurrent disease
2nd P,   second primary

summed for grades 2 and 3 and compared to grade 1, the difference reaches a level of significance at $X^2 = 6.018$, p = 0.025, 1 df. Again the local aggressiveness does not manifest itself by extensive out-of-field recurrence.

Since 1978, rather than grade the lesions individually, a grade has been assigned by diagnosis (Table 4). This approach is felt to be justified by: 1) the lack of specific universally acceptable criteria for grading and 2) the constantly evolving diagnostic criteria as more is learned about the origins of these lesions. This has made a change in the distribution by grade, more than doubling those assigned to grade 3. However, Table 5 shows that in comparison with Table 3, the incidence of control and recurrence remain the same by grade, except for an improvement in the results of grade 1.

Information concerning size and grade is used in staging the patients according to the staging system suggested by the American Joint Committee on Cancer (1983) (Table 6). Table 7 shows the ultimate disease free survival at 5 years by stage.

Several features of interest may be extracted from Table 6. The ultimate failure rate in the primary site with or without distant metastases is seen to be 26 patients or 8%. As seen in Tables 1, 2 and 3, 74 primary recurrences in or beyond the limits of the radiation fields were noted. Forty-eight recurrences, or 65% of these were salvaged by further surgery although 15 patients went on

to succumb to 1) distant metastases (13) or 2) intercurrent disease (2) after the salvage procedure.

In general, the extent of the salvage surgery was dictated by the location of the primary lesion and the procedure did not exceed what would have been required by an attempt at surgical cure originally.

Distant metastases remain the most ominous prognostic factor in patients with soft tissue sarcomas. Although a few patients with metastases to the lung only which were resectable have been salvaged surgically, this approach is not feasible for the majority. Reference to Table 7 shows that distant metastases alone were the ultimate cause of failure in 23% of the patients (72/313). Complete (100%) primary control without concomitant control of distant metastases will only improve long term survival by 4%. Eighty-two percent of the distant metastases occur by 2 years after treatment. Only 1.6% have occurred at intervals greater than 60 months after treatment.

Although a previous randomized experience with adjuvant chemotherapy in our institution (LINDBERG et al. 1977) was not positive, numerous other attempts have been and are being made to control the appearance of distant metastases. Excellent reviews of the subject by Edmonson (1984) and Rosenberg (1984) have recently appeared. Obviously, the development of an effective, relatively non-toxic chemotherapeutic regimen would be of great benefit.

4 Conclusions

1. Local control of soft tissue sarcomas, particularly of the extremities, can be reliably achieved by limited surgical excision followed by radiotherapy in the event of local recurrence, disease free status is frequently achieved by further (salvage) surgery.
2. Functional competence is preserved in the vast majority of patients without increased risk of serious complication.
3. Ultimate disease control is a function of the incidence of distant metastases which, either alone or in conjunction with primary recurrence, account for 88% of disease related failure.

References

Beahrs OH, Myers MH (eds), Manual for Staging of Cancer (1983) Second Edition, American Joint Committee on Cancer JB Lippincott Company, Philadelphia

Suit HD, Russell WO, Martin RG (1975) Sarcoma of soft tissue: Clinical and histopathologic parameters and response to treatment. Cancer 35:1478–1483

Lindberg RD, Murphy WK, Benjamin RS et al. (1977) Adjuvant chemotherapy in the treatment of primary soft tissue sarcomas: a preliminary report. In: Management of Bone and Soft Tissue Tumors, Yearbook Medical Publishers, Inc. Chicago, p 343–352

Edmonson JH (1984) Role of adjuvant chemotherapy in the management of patients with soft tissue sarcomas. Cancer Treatment Reports 68(9):1063

Rosenberg SA (1984) Prospective randomized trials demonstrating the efficacy of adjuvant chemotherapy in adult patients with soft tissue sarcomas. Cancer Treatment reports 68(9):1067

2.4 Rectum and Anal Canal

2.4.1 Conservative Management of Cancer of the Rectum

JEAN PAPILLON

CONTENTS

1 Introduction

The purpose of conservative treatment is the control of rectal carcinoma without bowel resection. Conservative treatment by irradiation has long been a subject of controversy, because it contradicts two generally held notions: first, that adenocarcinoma of the rectum is only slightly radiosensitive; second, that rectal cancer can only be cured by radical surgery, i.e., en bloc resection of the bowel segment bearing the tumor and the lymphatic drainage areas.

These traditional views may now be challenged. During the past 15 years substantial progress has been made in the earlier detection of rectal cancer, in knowledge of the natural history of the disease, and in the practice of radiotherapy. It is now accepted that radical surgery is not the only means of treating rectal cancer and that conservative treatment by local surgery or by intracavitary irradiation may be alternatives to major surgery in certain cases.

Irrespective of the method used, conservative treatment has a purely local effect. It involves only the primary tumor and a limited margin of surrounding tissues but does not concern the lymphatic chains. Accordingly, such a treatment is only applicable to tumors, which are thought to have no lymphatic spread. Before the decision for conservative treatment is taken, two conditions must be met: (1) strict selection of the tumors with regard to the probability of lymphatic involvement, and (2) regular follow-up, accepted by the patient, after treatment.

2 Selection

Most patients treated conservatively are elderly, poor surgical risks, with tumor of the lower half of the rectum, which would require radical surgery with permanent colostomy.

With respect to the probability of lymph node involvement, three criteria based on histologic and clinical data should be considered.

2.1 Histologic Grading

Multiple biopsies of the rectal tumor should be performed to assess the histologic type of the tumor with a satisfactory degree of accuracy. Poorly differentiated and colloid carcinomas must be excluded because of their high rate of lymphatic dissemination. Well or moderately well-differentiated adenocarcinomas may be accepted for local therapy.

JEAN PAPILLON, M.D., Professor
28, rue Laennec
F-69008 Lyon

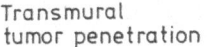
Transmural
tumor penetration

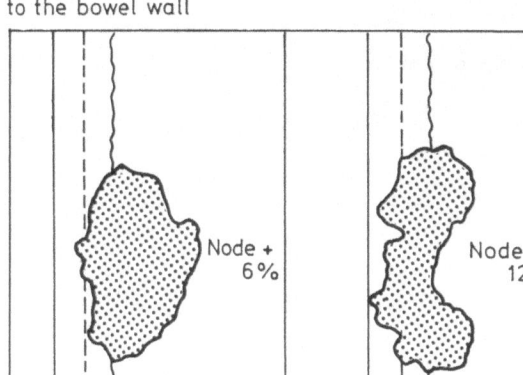
Tumor confined
to the bowel wall

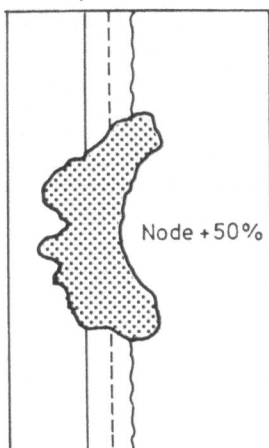

Fig. 1. The probability of lymphatic spread is related to the local spread of a rectal cancer. Tumors which have spread beyond the rectal wall have a high rate of lymph node involvement (50%), whereas well-differentiated adenocarcinomas confined to the rectal wall have a much lower lymphatic risk: 6% in cases of polypoid tumor, 12% in cases of ulcerative tumor. (From Papillon 1982)

2.2 Local Spread

It has been shown (Morson 1966; Hermanek 1982) that there is a close relationship between local spread and lymphatic spread of rectal cancer. Tumor confined to the bowel wall have a low probability of lymph node metastasis (6–12%), whereas tumors with extrarectal spread have a much higher chance of lymphatic spread (up to 50%). Only tumors confined to the rectal wall may be treated conservatively. York Mason (1976) and Nicholls et al. (1982) have demonstrated that the assessment of configuration, size, consistency and mobility of the tumor enables the clinician to evaluate the degree of infiltration of the tumor in the rectal wall rather well. They showed that tumors confined to the bowel wall are correctly identified in 80% of cases. In case of doubt, the radiotherapist has an additional means of evaluation of local spread at his disposal. The shrinkage of the tumor between the 1st day and the 21st day after two applications of contact x-ray therapy may help to select tumors which have no transmural penetration and are suitable for conservative irradiation (Fig. 1).

Limited well differentiated adenocarcinomas, not more than 4.5 cm in length and 3 cm in width,

can be accepted for intracavitary irradiation. Polypoid lesions well accessible up to 12 cm above the anal verge are the most suitable; ulcerative carcinomas up to 9 cm from the anal verge can also be treated with good chance of success as long as the tumors are freely mobile and certainly confined to the bowel wall (Fig. 2).

Indications

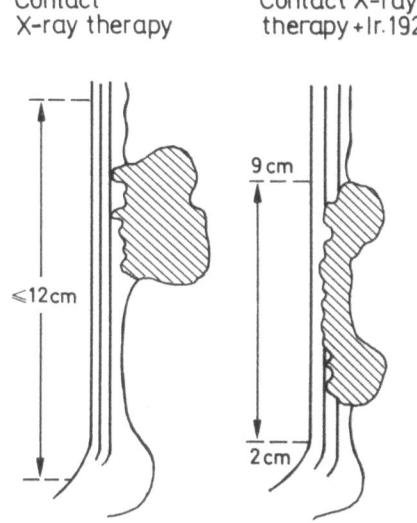

Size ≤ 4.5 cm x 3 cm

Fig. 2. Well-differentiated adenocarcinomas confined to the bowel wall (3rd week test) and smaller than 4.5 × 3 cm may be treated by intracavitary irradiation. Polypoid tumors up to 12 cm from the anal verge are suitable for contact x-ray therapy. Ulcerative carcinomas of the lower half of the rectum are suitable for contact x-ray therapy combined with Iridium 192 implant. (From Papillon 1982)

All deeply infiltrating or circumferential tumors and those which are not completely mobile are contraindications of the method.

2.3 Absence of Palpable Metastatic Nodes in the Mesorectum

GABRIEL et al. (1935), TURNBULL (1974), and NICHOLLS et al. (1982) have demonstrated that the first lymph nodes to harbor metastases are usually those situated in the perirectal tissues immediately or a few centimeters above the primary tumor and that discontinuous spread is very uncommon. Enlarged metastatic nodes are always indurated and easy to distinguish from inflammatory lymph nodes (TURNBULL 1974). If the tumor is situated low in the rectum, it is possible to search for and to detect such metastatic lymph nodes by a careful digital examination as long as this investigation is properly performed, preferably with the patient in the knee-chest position. In the series of the Centre Léon Bérard, a hard nodule was discovered above the primary tumor in 23 cases, all of which proved to be metastatic at the time of surgery.

Obviously, beside these specific investigations, general clinical work-up is mandatory, requiring chest x-ray, double contrast barium enema or colonoscopy, liver ultrasound, and CEA level.

3 Follow-Up

After treatment of the rectal tumor, patients must be followed up regularly and carefully in order to detect local or regional failures as early as possible. Many recurrences can be treated effectively by major surgery and a number of patients will be cured.

Follow-up consists essentially of digital and endoscopic examination in the search for any changes in the treated area or any hard nodule in the perirectal area. Cytologic examination of scrape smears taken in the irradiated area may be helpful in evaluating the nature of some residual ulcers during the first weeks following completion of irradiation.

Local and general examination should be performed four times a year during the first two years, three times a year up to the 5th year and once a year after the 5th year. In addition, a double contrast enema or a colonoscopy must be carried out every two or three years.

Clinical follow-up is a demanding task. It should be performed by the radiation oncologist, who was in charge of the treatment, because he will remember all the details of the features of the tumor and will be in a better position to observe any changes in the treated area.

4 Methods of Irradiation

In the control of limited rectal cancers, external beam irradiation is much less efficient than intracavitary irradiation consisting of contact x-ray therapy supplemented, when necessary, by interstitial curietherapy.

4.1 Contact X-Ray Therapy

The basic method of intracavitary irradiation uses the Philips RT 50 machine, well adapted to intrarectal applications. The characteristics of the tube are as follows: low voltage (50 kV), short focal distance (4 cm), high dose-rate (20 Gy per min in air with a filter of 0.5 mm Al) and substantial absorption of x-ray beam (90%) in the first 2 cm. The field of irradiation is circular and is 3 cm in diameter. Two overlapping fields can be used, one upper and one lower, for tumors larger than 3 cm. The x-ray tube is light and easily held in one hand of the operator (Fig. 3). During the treatment the patient is in the knee-chest position. The tip of the x-ray tube is inserted in a special proctoscope held by the other hand of the operator (Fig. 3). The treatment consists of 4 applications given over a period of 6 weeks. It is carried out in the outpatient department and is compatible with normal active life. It is well tolerated and easily applicable to elderly, frail or handicapped patients.

The high exposure dose given at every application (25 to 40 Gy) produces rapid shrinkage of the exophytic part of the lesion. Hence at the second (8th day) and third application (21st day) the tumor has a greatly reduced size and the degree of shrinkage is an indicator of the degree of infiltration of the rectal wall by the tumor. The total exposure dose is 100 to 140 Gy. The fourth application is given on day 42, when all of the exophytic part of the lesion has been destroyed.

4.2 Iridium Implant

Curietherapy is used only as a supplementary method to give a booster dose of radiation to the bed of the tumor when the cancer is ulcerative

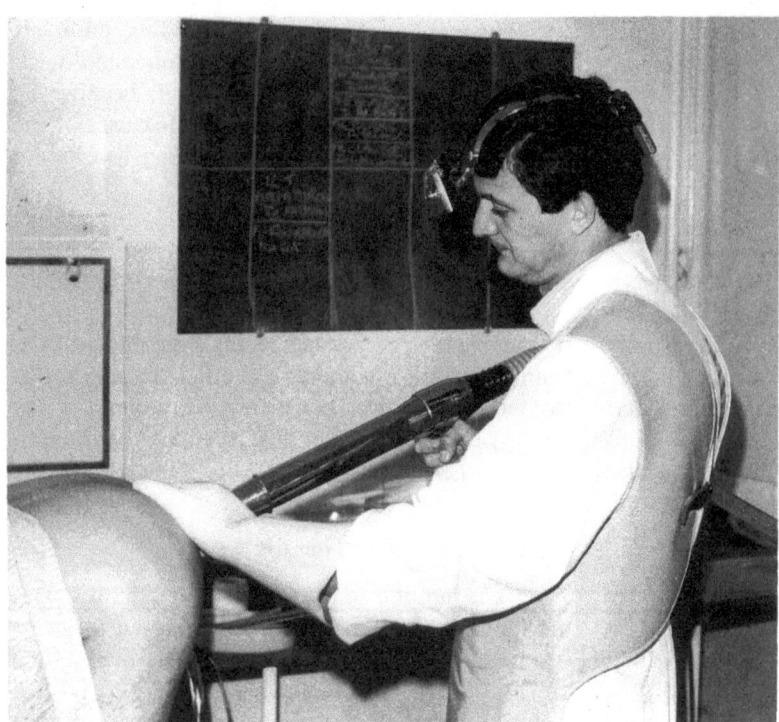

Fig. 3. During the treatment, the operator has a forehead lamp and wears a leaded rubber apron and a leaded rubber left glove. The x-ray tube held by his right hand is fitted in the treatment applicator, which is firmly held by his left hand. (From PAPILLON 1982)

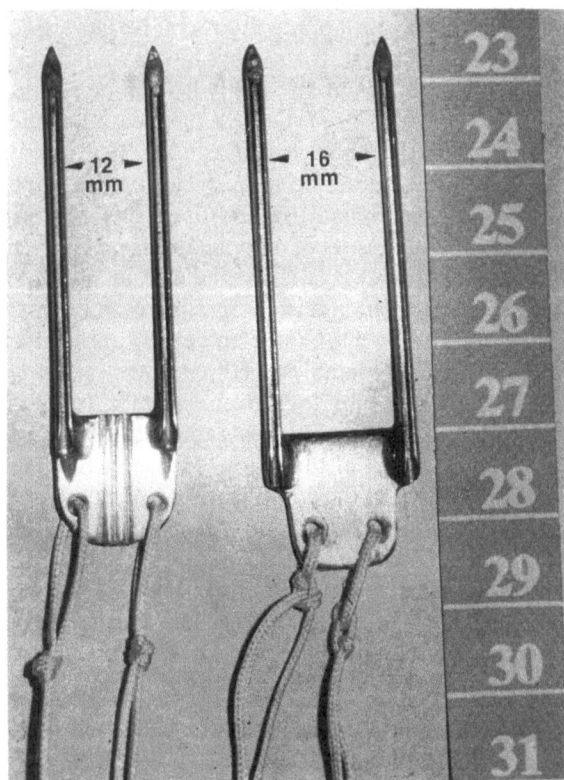

Fig. 4. Steel forks used for Iridium 192 implant. They have two prongs 16 mm or 12 mm apart. Each prong is preloaded with an Iridium wire 4 cm long. (From PAPILLON 1982)

or slightly infiltrating. The material used is a rigid steel fork with two straight hollow prongs preloaded with two Iridium wires 4 cm long (Fig. 4). The insertion of the fork requires only local anesthesia. It is performed with the patient in the knee-chest position. The dose delivered is 20 to 40 Gy within 24 to 36 hours. This treatment takes place one month after the last application of contact x-ray therapy. It increases the chance of local control of the cancer and is used in 50% of the cases.

5 Results

The three most important studies of intracavitary irradiation have been conducted at the Centre Léon Bérard, Lyon, France by J. PAPILLON (1982), at the Highland Hospital, Rochester, New York, by SISCHY (1982; 1984), and at the Cleveland Clinic by JELDEN et al. (1984).

At the Centre Léon Bérard, 245 patients have been treated and followed more than 5 years. All patients accepted had true invasive well differentiated or moderately well differentiated adenocarcinomas. In situ carcinomas, cancers in polyps and degenerated villous tumors were excluded from this series. The results at 5 and 10 years are reported in Tables 1 and 2. At 5 years, 187 (76%)

Table 1. Rectal cancer. Results of intracavitary irradiation experience at the centre Léon Bérard, Lyon

	No. of cases	Alive and well (%)	Dead of interc. disease (%)	Dead of cancer (%)	Dead postop. (%)
At 5 yrs	245	76.3	13.2	8.9	1.6
At 10 yrs	186[a]	55.4	33.3	9.1	2.2

[a] No patients lost to follow-up

Table 2. Rectal cancer. Treatment failures after intracavitary irradiation. Experience at the centre Léon Bérard based on 245 cases followed more than 5 years

	No. of cases	Alive + well	Death of cancer	Postop. death
Local failures	13 (5.3%)	3[a]	9[c]	1
Nodal failures	12 (4.9%)	3[b]	8	1

[a] 2 after AP resection, 1 after low anterior resection
[b] 1 after AP resection, 2 after lymphadenectomy without colostomy (only one node involved)
[c] Out of nine patients, four were inoperable because of extent of disease or general condition

Table 3. Rectal cancer. Results of intracavitary irradiation. Experience at the highland hospital, Rochester N.Y (SISCHY 1984)

No. of cases followed from 18 mths to ten years	Control	Treatment failures
121	95%	5%

Table 4. Rectal cancer. Superiority of intracavitary irradiation on local excision and electrocoagulation with regard to the rate of local failures

Methods	References	Rate of local failures (%)
Intracavitary irradiation	(PAPILLON 1982, SISCHY 1984)	5
Local excision	(MORSON 1966, HERMANEK 1982)	10–20
Electrocoagulation	(MADDEN 1971, CRILE 1972, CULP 1976)	13–25

patients were alive and well. Among them, 181 had normal ano-rectal function, six had permanent colostomy after abdomino-perineal resection: for local failure (three), for nodal failure (one), or for presumed local failure in whom the operative specimen was tumor-free (two). The rate of death of cancer is 8.9%. At 10 years, of 186 patients 55.4% were alive and well. The rate of death of cancer is 9.1% (Table 1). Among the 245 patients followed more than 5 years, 5.3% developed local recurrences and 4.9% had nodal failures (Table 2).

The series of SISCHY (1984) is reported in Table 3. It shows a tumor control rate in the same range as that in the Lyon series.

In comparing intracavitary irradiation with local excision or electrocoagulation, stress may be placed on the fact that contact x-ray therapy is a true ambulatory treatment. Iridium 192 implant requires hospital admission for 2 or 3 days, but no general anesthesia. Tolerance of the procedure is excellent. There is no risk of perforation or rectovaginal fistula when the treatment is properly applied. The only reaction, noted in 50% of the patients, is a short period of mild proctitis which does not last more than 2 weeks. The scar after irradiation remains supple without any retraction; it is easy to appreciate the consistency of the treated area and of the adjacent rectal wall during

the follow-up period. The rate of local failure is low (Table 4).

In medical practice there are few situations comparable to the patient with limited cancer of the low rectum. We may now propose with the same probability of success two therapeutic modalities as different as abdominoperineal resection and intracavitary irradiation. Abdominoperineal resection means major surgery and a correspondingly long hospitalization and convalescence with a mortality rate which is not negligible in the elderly, with important genitourinary morbidity and a permanent colostomy. Contact x-ray therapy involves a simple ambulatory treatment. Interestingly, it was the influence of eminent surgeons that led to the introduction of contact x-ray in America. They have transferred to their radiotherapist a treatment which they considered to be safer and more effective than electrocoagulation or local excision for limited rectal cancers.

6 New Approaches

6.1 Elective Lymphadenectomy

One of the main objections made to conservative treatment is the lack of knowledge of the absence or presence of metastatic lymph nodes. The problem of positive regional lymphatic spread and its management should be considered in relation to the morbidity of extra treatment and the life expectation of the patient. Although most patients treated conservatively are elderly and a poor surgical risk, conservative treatment may be applied to middle aged, robust, even young patients. In the latter case, after control of the rectal tumor has been achieved, uncertainty remains concerning the possibility of lymphatic dissemination. To remove this uncertainty, an elective inferior mesenteric and perirectal lymphadenectomy should be considered and carried out 2 to 3 months after completion of the intracavitary irradiation. The technique of the operation is as follows:

Through a midline incision the liver is examined and the paraaortic and common external iliac nodes are palpated to check that the tumor has not spread throughout the abdomen. Then the sigmoid colon is freed from its congenital adhesions to the peritoneum in the left iliac fossa. Left and right ureters are identified at the level of the iliac arteries. The posterior parietal peritoneum is incised above and below the origin of the inferior mesenteric artery. The incision follows the right side of the rectum and crosses in front of the rectum, entering the pouch of Douglas before continuing along the left side of the rectum up to the origins of the sigmoid arteries. Inferior mesenteric nodes are resected after the artery has been isolated at its origin. The dissection is extended along the artery up to the trunk of the sigmoid arteries. Sigmoid nodes are excised, and if there is any suspicion about their nature they are sent for frozen section examination.

The dissection of the mesorectum is then undertaken. The operator enters the retrorectal space with his right hand. The posterior surface of the rectum is freed from the sacrum down to the levator ani muscles. Then the inferior mesenteric lymphadenectomy is performed with excision of all tissues bearing lymph nodes surrounding the artery. The lateral ligaments of the rectum are stretched and the superior hemorhoidal pedicle is isolated at its origin and held in a ligature. With his left hand, the operator pulls this pedicle above and to the left, while the assistant, with his right hand, pushes the rectosigmoid colon anteriorly and to the left. A good exposure of the mesorectum is thus obtained. The bifurcation of the superior hemorrhoidal artery is identified and the principal nodes are excised and sent for frozen section. The dissection is continued succesively along the right, and then the left branch of the superior he-

morrhoidal artery up to their entry into the muscular layer of the rectal wall, and any lymphatic tissue is excised. This dissection which exposes the posterior and lateral sides of the rectum with minimal blood loss, permits excision of the anorectal lymph nodes. Ligation of one of the branches of the superior hemorrhoidal artery may be necessary if its termination is surrounded by fibrotic tissue. Sometimes the nodes may be adherent to the rectal wall, which is repaired with silk thread. Then the middle hemorrhoidal pedicles are sectioned near their points of origin and tissues bearing lymph nodes are excised up to the rectal wall. The next stage of the operation is the excision of the posterior obturator lymph nodes situated at the bifurcation of the primitive iliac artery. A succion drain is put into the posterior rectal space and brought out through the left or right iliac fossa. The pelvic and parietal peritoneum is sutured and the abdomen is closed.

Recovery after surgery is rapid, and in a series of 30 patients at the Centre Léon Bérard no complications have been recorded (Mayer et al. 1982).

If one or several nodes are found involved at frozen section, radical surgery should be carried out immediately. If pathologic study of the specimen does not show any metastatic nodes, the patient is followed as usual. In the series of 30 surgical procedures performed in Lyon, a metastatic node was found in one patient who is alive and well 10 years after abdominoperineal resection. In all the other cases, no involved node was found and no regional recurrences have occurred so far.

This surgery performed in patients not older than 55 or 60 years has proved to be reliable and in some respects may be compared to the neck dissection for carcinoma of the tongue or to the pelvic lymphadenectomy for carcinoma of the uterine cervix. It is conceived as a joint effort of the radiation oncologist and the surgeon and has contributed to make conservative treatment safer.

6.2 Extension of the Field of Conservative Treatment by Combination of External Beam and Intracavitary Irradiation

Goligher (1977) emphasizes that for elderly patients in poor social conditions or living alone, a colostomy may become a major problem. Patients feel isolated, depressed and lose all interest in feeding and looking after themselves. The situation may produce profound psychological upset.

Special effort should be made to spare such patients a permanent colostomy.

Conventional conservative procedures, either surgical or radiotherapeutic, are only applicable to a small proportion of patients with rectal cancer (5–10% of cases); the great majority of patients have to undergo extensive surgery and one in two will have a permanent colostomy. In poor surgical risk patients it would be rational to try to extend the field of conservation without jeopardizing the chance of control of the disease. For this purpose external beam irradiation can be used as a first approach.

Preoperative external beam irradiation has proved to be more effective than expected. Beside the reduction of the rate of local treatment failures, two points, not commonly stressed, must be emphasized:

1. In several series (STEVENS et al. 1977; KLIGER-MAN 1977; BRENNER et al. 1979; ROE et al. 1982) the occurrence of Dukes'A tumors is significantly greater after preoperative irradiation (27–45%) than after surgery (15–25%). This indicates that some tumors that had involved the perirectal fat to some extent, may have shrunk in such a manner that they became confined to the rectal wall.

2. Some tumors may be controlled by external beam irradiation alone. WILLIAMS and HORWITZ (1956), WANG and SCHULTZ (1962), STEVENS et al. (1977), BUGAT et al. (1981), ROE et al. (1982), BOU-LIS-WASSIF (1982), and SISCHY (1982) reported that, after preoperative irradiation, when the operation does not take place in the first 2 weeks, some operative specimens are free of tumor cells, the lesion being totally sterilized. In such cases, extensive surgery could have been theoretically avoided.

These examples indicate that external beam irradiation may convert tumors suitable for abdominoperineal resection into lesions amenable to conservative treatment. Such an approach would be

Fig. 5. Isodose distribution of external beam irradiation using Cobalt 60 for cancer of the rectum. The patient is in the prone position. Radiation is delivered through a 9 × 12 cm sacral field using Cobalt 60 arc therapy, 120 degrees. The axis of rotation is 10 cm depth. A dose of 30 Gy is delivered in 10 fractions within 12 days. The tumor area receives a higher dose, up to 39 Gy. The 70% isodose encompasses the perirectal area and most sites of regional lymphatic spread with satisfactory protection of the urinary bladder. According to the site and spread of the tumor, the target-volume may be displaced laterally to the right or left side

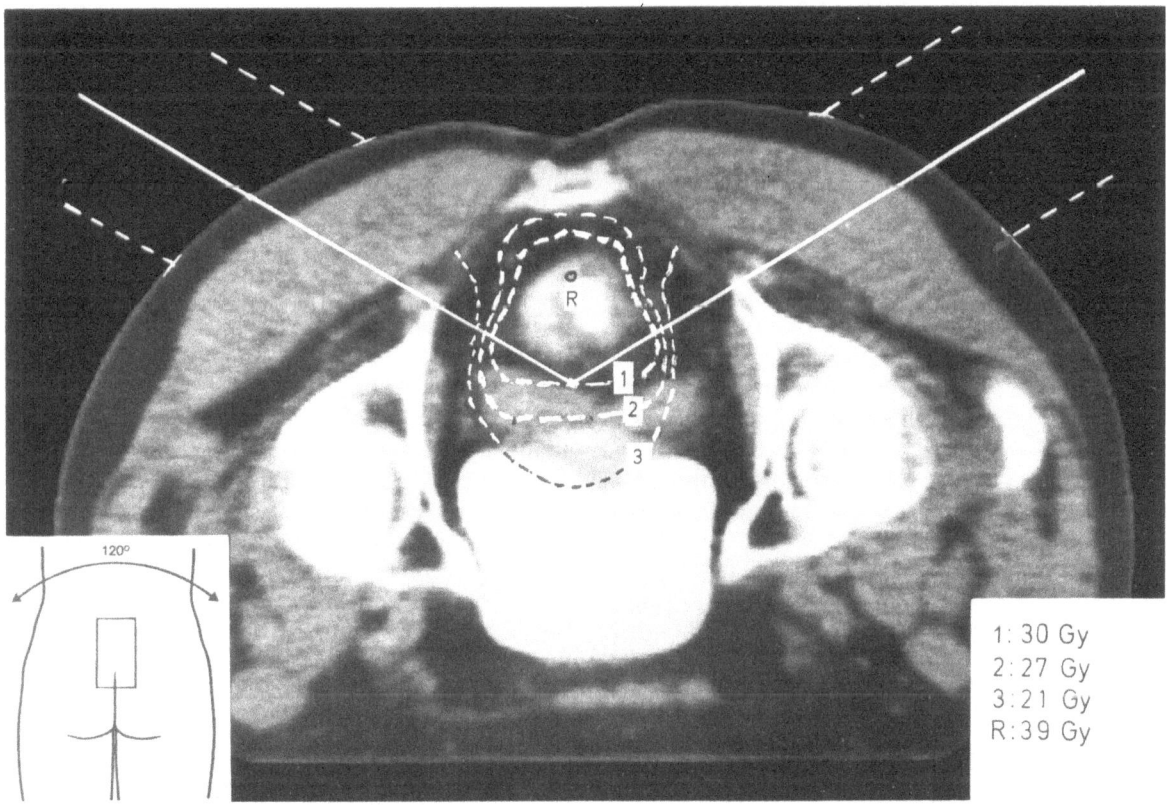

1: 30 Gy
2: 27 Gy
3: 21 Gy
R: 39 Gy

especially useful in elderly and frail patients with tumors of the lower half of the rectum, 4 to 6 cm in diameter, mobile, too large and too thick to be suitable for intracavitary irradiation but whose clinical examination indicates that they are still confined to the bowel wall or have slight extra-rectal spread.

Many techniques of preoperative external beam irradiation of rectal cancer have been reported in the literature. The method used at the Centre Léon Bérard, Lyon, is quite different from most of them. It consists of delivering a tumor-dose of 30 Gy calculated at 10 cm depth, in 10 fractions within 12 days by Cobalt 60, arc therapy, 120 degree, through a posterior field measuring 9×14 cm. The patient is in the prone position. The isodose distribution shows that the target-volume is well adapted to the peri-rectal and posterior pelvic area. The center of the irradiated area receives 39 Gy in 10 fractions (Fig. 5).

The main characteristics of this method are as follows:

1. Limited target-volume, which encompasses the most important sites of regional spread of rectal cancer.
2. Satisfactory protection of the small bowel and urinary bladder.
3. Non-homogeneous dose with a hot spot centered on the tumor area.
4. Short overall treatment time (12 days). Treatment starts on Monday and ends on Friday of the following week. It includes only one week-end.

The tolerance is good: proctitis usually, does not last more than 3 weeks and is easily relieved by steroid enemas.

Since 1977, this technique has been applied to 155 patients and has proved to be very effective. All these patients had rectal tumors not suitable for contact x-ray therapy. Some had very large, infiltrating tumors with impaired mobility. Others had tumors moderately infiltrating but whose size (larger than 4 cm) or site (very close to the anus) make them unsuitable for conventional conservative procedures.

The results of treatment were evaluated two months after completion of irradiation at which time two groups of patients were identified (Table 5).

The first group consisted of 82 patients either in good general condition or with substantial residual disease. They underwent radical surgery with curative intent, either abdominoperineal re-

Table 5. Rectal cancer. Role of external beam irradiation (3000 rad in 12 days). Experience at the Centre Léon Bérard, Lyon (J. PAPILLON)

No. of cases		No. of cases
155 ←2 Month rest→	Radical surgery	82
	Tentative conversion into conservation	73

Median age 75 yrs.

section (65) or low anterior resection (17) (Fig. 6). In 14 cases (17%) the operative specimen was tumor-free. Histologic findings are presented in Table 6. Patients with liver metastasis and treated with palliative intent are excluded from this analysis. The effectiveness of the external beam irradiation by Cobalt 60, 30 Gy in 12 days, is shown by the high rates of Dukes'A and tumor-free specimens.

The second group consists of 73 elderly patients with a median age of 75 years (poor surgical risks) with moderately infiltrating, mobile T2 tumors of the low rectum. The purpose of external beam irradiated was attempted conversion of the tumor into a lesion amenable to conservation therapy. When the residual disease was limited, an Iridium implant often combined with contact x-ray therapy was carried out 60–70 days after completion of Cobalt therapy. Forty-six patients have been followed more than 3 years.

In this group of 46 elderly patients, 7 died of cancer, 1 died postoperatively after treatment failure, 23 have been controlled by first intention, 2 after subsequent radical surgery, and 13 died of intercurrent disease locally controlled. The rate of death of cancer or postoperatively is 17.3% (Table 7).

This experience supports a plea in favor of external irradiation prior to intracavitary therapy for more advanced lesions. The efficacy of the technique described, assessed 8 weeks later, is greater than usually thought. Extending the eligibility criteria for conservative therapy in poor risk patients allows a larger number of such patients to avoid both major surgery and permanent colostomy, without sacrificing ultimate control of the disease.

7 Conclusion

Intracavitary irradiation has gained an established place in the conservative treatment of rectal cancer. The purpose of external beam irradiation as

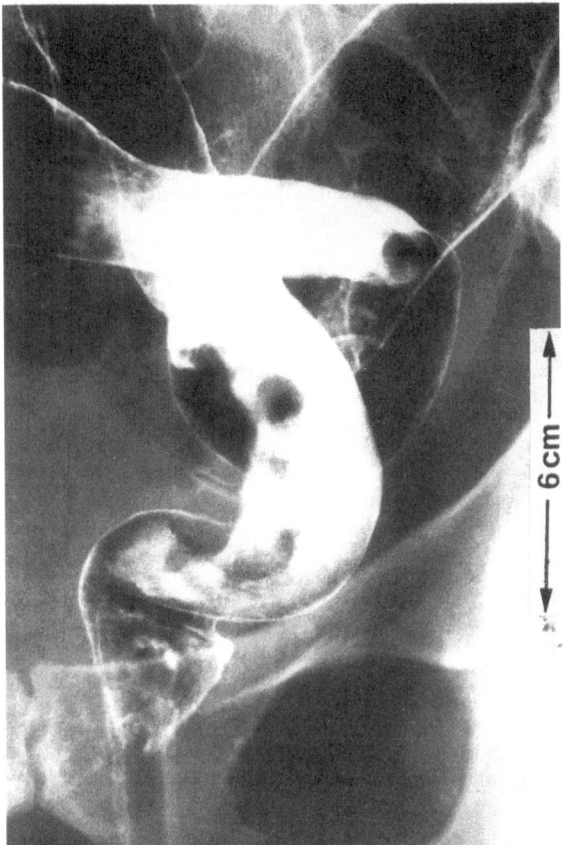

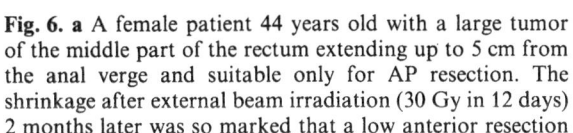

a

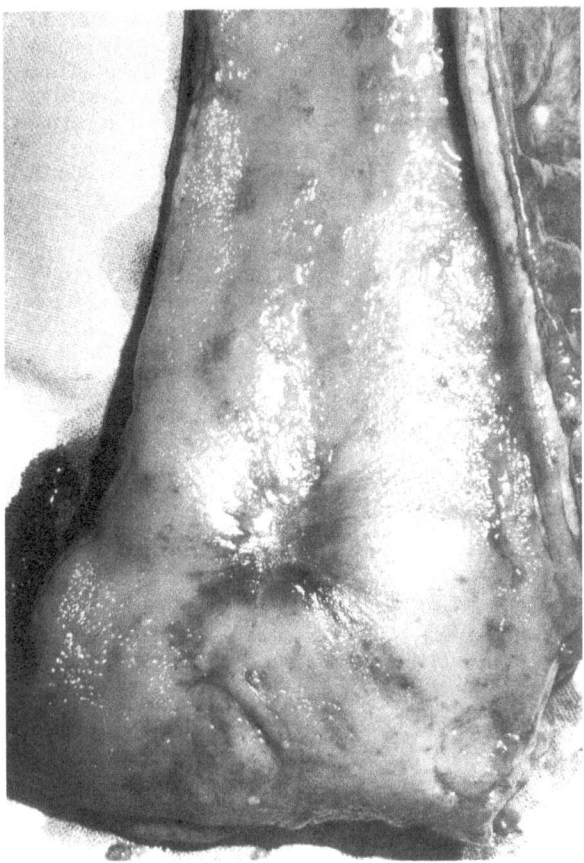

b

Fig. 6. a A female patient 44 years old with a large tumor of the middle part of the rectum extending up to 5 cm from the anal verge and suitable only for AP resection. The shrinkage after external beam irradiation (30 Gy in 12 days) 2 months later was so marked that a low anterior resection could be performed. b Tumor-free operative specimen of low anterior resection with colo-anal anastomosis. The patient is alive and well with normal anal function more than 4 years after surgery

Table 6. Rectal cancer. Histologic study of operative specimen after preoperative irradiation (3000 rad in 12 days). Experience at the Centre Léon Bérard, Lyon (82 cases)

Tumor-free op. specimen	Dukes'A	Dukes'B	Dukes'C
17%	32.9%	23.1%	26.8%

Table 7. Tentative conversion of moderately advanced tumors (T_2) from radical into conservative treatment minimum follow-up: 3 yrs, median age: 75 yrs

No. of cases	Alive + well	Death of int. disease	Death of cancer	Post-operative death
46	25[a]	13	7	1

[a] 23 with normal anal function, 2 with permanent colostomy

a first approach is not only to make radical surgery safer but also to try to enlarge the framework of conservative methods. This new policy may only be developed in a climate of mutual understanding between surgeons and radiotherapists. Both share a common responsibility and should choose the most appropriate protocol in order to give each patient the best chance of cure and a satisfactory quality of life following treatment.

References

Boulis Wassif S (1982) The role of preoperative adjuvant therapy in the management of borderline operability rectal cancer. Clin Radiol 33:353–358

Brenner J, Seligman BR, Lanter B (1979) Adjuvant radiotherapy and chemotherapy in the treatment of operable adenocarcinoma of the rectum. In 2d Intern Conf on Adjuv Therap Cancer 1979. Tucson, New York: Grune and Stratton

Bugat R, Nguyen TD, El Safadi N, Naja A, Combes PF (1981) L'irradiation ré-opératoire des cancers du rectum. A propos d'une série de 96 cas. Bull Cancer (Paris) 68:363

Crile G, Turnbull RB (1972) The role of electrocoagulation in the treatment of carcinoma of the rectum. Surg Gynecol Obstet 135:391–396

Culp CE (1976) Conservative management of certain selected cancers of the lower rectum. In: Controversy in surgery. Philadelphia: WB Saunders 404–414

Gabriel WB, Dukes CE, Bussey HJR (1935) Lymphatic spread in cancer of the rectum. Br J Surg 23:395

Goligher JC (1977) Surgery of the anus, rectum and colon, 3rd ed., Charles C Thomas, Springfield IL

Hermanek P (1982) Aufgaben des Pathologen bei Diagnose und Therapie. In: Gall EP, Hermanek P, Schweiger M, eds. Das Rektumkarzinom. Erlangen, Germany: Perimed Fachbuch Verlaggesellschaft, 40–48

Jelden G, Lavery I, Antunez AR, Fazio Y, Jagelman D, Weakley F (1984) Definitive treatment of rectal carcinoma with intracavitary radiation therapy. Third Annual Meeting of the European Society for Therapeutic Radiology and Oncology. Jerusalem. Abstracts 125

Kligerman MM (1977) Radiotherapy of rectal cancer. Cancer 39:896–900

Madden JL, Kandalaft S (1971) Clinical evolution of electrocoagulation in the treatment of cancer of the rectum. Am J Surg 122:347

Mayer M, Papillon J, Bobin JY, Ardiet JM (1982) La lymphadénectomie mésentérique inférieure et périrectale dans le traitement conservateur des cancers de la partie inférieure de l'ampoule rectale. Chirurgie 108:479–483

Morson BC (1966) Factors influencing the prognosis of early cancer of the rectum. Proc R Soc Med 59:607–608

Nicholls RJ, Mason AY, Morson BC, Dixon AK, Kelsey FRY I (1982) The clinical staging of rectal cancer. Br J Surg 69:404–409

Papillon J (1982) Rectal and anal cancers. Conservative treatment by irradiation. An alternative to radical surgery. New York, Springer Verlag

Roe JP, Kodner IJ, Walz B, Fry RD (1982) Preoperative radiation therapy for rectal carcinoma. Dis Colon Rectum 25:471–473

Sischy B (1982) The place of radiotherapy in the management of rectal adenocarcinoma. Cancer 50:2631–2637

Sischy B (1984) Ten years experience with endocavitary irradiation of rectal cancer. Third Annual Meeting of the European Society of Therapeutic Radiology and Oncology. Jerusalem. Abstract 124

Stevens KRJ, Fletcher WS, Allen CV (1977) Value of preoperative irradiation for adenocarcinoma of the rectosigmoid. (Abstr) Digestion 16:278

Turnbull RBJ (1974) Carcinoma of the rectum. Nonresective treatment. Dis Colon Rectum 17:588–590

Wang CC, Schulz MD (1962) The role of radiation therapy in the management of carcinoma of the sigmoid, rectosigmoid and rectum. Radiology 79:1–5

Williams IG, Horwitz H (1956) The primary treatment of adenocarcinoma of the rectum by high voltage roentgenrays (1000 kV). Am J Roentgenol 76:919–928

York Mason A (1976) Rectal cancer: the spectrum of selective surgery. Proc R Soc Med 69:237–244

2.4.2 Treatment of Cancer of the Anal Canal

Bernard J. Cummings and John E. Byfield

CONTENTS

The combination of radiation and chemotherapy has many theoretical attractions, but a clear demonstration of improvements in tumor control rates without coincidental increases in toxicity has generally proven elusive. The changing patterns of management of anal cancer provide an opportunity to compare the results of various combinations of radiation, chemotherapy and surgery with traditional methods of treatment. In North America, radical resection by abdominoperineal resection had become the established treatment. In Europe, and in France especially, a tradition of treatment by radical radiation therapy had been maintained. While there is as yet no conclusive proof that the combination of chemotherapy, radiation and surgery improves survival, the greatly increased numbers of patients who retain anal function and avoid a colostomy, and the acceptable levels of acute toxicity, suggest that the combination has genuine advantages.

Primary carcinomas of the anal canal are uncommon, occurring at a rate of only 0.5 to 1 per 100,000 people. Most arise from the squamous or

Bernard J. Cummings, M.B.
500 Sherbourne Street
Toronto, Ontario M4X 1K9, Canada

John E. Byfield, M.D.
Kern Regional Cancer Centre
Bakersfield, CA 933301
USA

transitional epithelium. About 75% are classified as squamous carcinomas and 20% as basaloid carcinomas (synonyms, cloacogenic or transitional cell carcinoma). Since the results of treatment of these two major histological subtypes by surgery or by radiation are similar, and depend more on the extent of the carcinoma than on the histological type, they may, in general, be treated similarly. These carcinomas present in a predominantly locoregional distribution, well suited to management by radiation therapy. At presentation, about 33% have inguinal and/or pelvic node metastases (Boman et al. 1984; Golden and Horsley 1976), and 10% have more distant metastases. Local pelvic recurrence and regional node failure are also more common than systemic metastases if relapse occurs after apparently successful initial treatment of the primary anal cancer (Boman et al. 1984; Cummings 1982).

The three major treatment alternatives are radical surgical resection, radical radiation therapy, and combined radiation and chemotherapy used either alone or as an adjuvant to limited or radical surgical resection. However, any comparison of reported series is partly confounded by the differences in the histopathological and clinical staging systems used, in case selection, and in the ways in which results have been reported. The relatively small numbers of patients with anal carcinoma also make the conduct of conventionally designed clinical trials difficult.

1 The Primary Tumor

Local excision, with preservation of anal function, has been recommended for patients with superficial squamous cell cancers up to 2 cm diameter which have not infiltrated the sphincter muscles, since the risk of lymph node metastases from these tumors was less than 3% (Boman et al. 1984). However, since 35% of basaloid carcinomas less than 2 cm diameter had involved regional lymph nodes local excision was not considered appropriate for that histological type. Only one of 13 patients with small superficial squamous cell carcinomas treated by local excision suffered local recurrence in the Mayo Clinic series, but these patients represented only 7.5% of all patients with anal canal cancer seen over a 25 year period (Boman et al. 1984). Other centers, perhaps less selective, recorded higher local recurrence rates after local excision (Golden and Horsley 1976).

Following the much more commonly used abdominoperineal resection, five year survival rates in the absence of adjuvant therapy of from 33% to 69% have been described (Boman et al. 1984; Golden and Horsley 1976). The main disadvantages of abdominoperineal resection are the small, but appreciable, risk of up to 5% postoperative mortality, the need for colostomy, and the sexual dysfunction which may result from damage to the presacral plexus. Tumor recurrence in the pelvis or in the pelvic or inguinal lymph nodes occurred in about 30% (Boman et al. 1984; Cummings 1982).

Radical radiation therapy has also been used effectively, with five year survival rates ranging from 31% to 70%, rates numerically similar to those reported by centers which have favored surgical resection (Cummings 1982). Following radiation therapy, about 75% of patients did not need a colostomy (Cummings 1982; Papillon 1982). Residual carcinoma, or local recurrence, was found in about 30% of those treated by radical radiation. Serious local radionecrosis or anal stricture requiring surgical management was reported in up to 20% in several series (Cummings 1982), but Papillon (1982) demonstrated that the risks of serious complications could be reduced to about 5% by careful attention to radiation technique and dose.

In 1974, Nigro and his colleagues reported complete clinical or histological regression of primary anal carcinomas in three patients who had been treated by a protocol of preoperative radiation therapy (3000 cGy/3 weeks) combined with a concurrent five day intravenous infusion of 5-Fluorouracil (5-FU) and a bolus injection of Mitomycin C (MTC), followed about six weeks later by abdominoperineal resection. Michaelson et al. (1983) subsequently reported a 59% response rate (complete plus partial responses) with 5-FU and MTC without radiation in patients with advanced measurable anal canal carcinoma. The original protocol described by Nigro has been modified by many investigators (Fig. 1). Combined chemo- and radiotherapy is no longer considered solely an adjuvant to abdominoperineal resection, but has also been evaluated as definitive treatment.

In the early years of treatment with combined chemotherapy and radiation therapy, complete clinical regression of the anal carcinoma was frequently noted by the time abdominoperineal resection was performed some weeks later. The clinical findings were mirrored by the absence of residual histologically identifiable tumor in most patients. Following the commonly used dose of 3000 cGy in three weeks, complete clinical regression occurred most frequently when the primary carcinoma was less than 5 cm in diameter (Nigro et al. 1983). Several investigators (Flam et al. 1983; Michaelson et al. 1983; Nigro et al. 1983; Sischy et al. 1982) eventually elected to biopsy the area of the original carcinoma approximately four weeks after the end of the radiation therapy, and to perform abdominoperineal resection only in those who still had histologically identifiable carcinoma. In order to reduce the risk of delayed healing, it was recommended that biopsies should be narrow and deep, rather than being an attempt at wide local excision of the residual scar (Nigro et al. 1983). There was good correlation between complete regression as measured by clinical examination and by histology, and very few patients later developed pelvic recurrence after the primary cancer had regressed completely. Random biopsies, as opposed to biopsy of clinically suspicious areas, may therefore be unnecessary, since they may just as easily miss areas of residual carcinoma and they do not remove the need for careful followup.

There is very little information on the results of preoperative radiation alone (and none at all of preoperative chemotherapy alone) with which to compare preoperative chemotherapy and radiotherapy. Preoperative radiation was usually given only to patients with locally advanced disease, and at doses greater than 3000 cGy in 3 weeks. For example, Frost et al. (1984) reported that, following 4000 to 4600 cGy in 4 to 5 weeks, 11 of 26 patients with locally advanced tumors had no demonstrable tumor in the surgical specimen. Some further information on the response to medium dose radiation alone can be deduced from the split course radiation protocols of Papillon who estimated that about one third of his patients had no clinically detectable residual tumor eight weeks after a minimum tumor dose of 3000 cGy in three weeks by a direct perineal Cobalt-60 beam (maximum dose 4200 cGy) (Papillon – personal communication).

5-Fluorouracil and MTC were combined with radical external beam radiation therapy by CUMMINGS et al. (1980, 1984) and by SISCHY et al. (1982). Both groups eventually adopted split course therapy because of unacceptable acute toxicity from concurrent combined chemotherapy and high dose radiation. Both reported local control rates better than 90%, with very few patients needing colostomy. Fifteen of the 30 patients in CUMMINGS' series (1984) had tumors larger than 5 cm diameter. The anal canal was not biopsied after treatment unless there were clinical grounds for suspecting residual or recurrent cancer. Serious late complications which required surgical intervention were no more common after combined radical radiation and chemotherapy than after radiation alone, during the period of 24 to 78 months over which the patients were followed (CUMMINGS et al. 1984). There have been no reports of significant toxicity after major resections following medium dose preoperative chemotherapy and radiation, but further experience will be needed before the safety of surgical resection for residual cancer or for complications after high dose radiation and chemotherapy can be compared with that following radical radiation alone.

None of these series of preoperative or definitive radiation and chemotherapy has yet matured to a point where observed five year survival and complication rates are available for substantial numbers of patients. Actuarial survival rates are similar to those for surgical resection or radiation therapy alone, but the difficulties of comparing different series have been commented on previously. The most easily identifiable benefit seems likely to be a reduction in the number of patients who require a colostomy (CUMMINGS et al. 1984; NIGRO et al. 1983).

While there has been widespread enthusiasm as a result of the high primary tumor control rates following radiation and chemotherapy, several authors have demonstrated that very good results can be achieved with radical radiation therapy alone, especially with small primary carcinomas. Thus, CANTRIL et al. (1983) reported local control of 18 of 22 (82%) tumors up to 5 cm diameter with external beam treatment of 6500 cGy in 6 $^1/_2$ weeks. PAPILLON (1982) controlled primary carcinomas up to 4 cm diameter in 86% of 88 patients treated by either one stage or two stage radium needle interstitial therapy, and in 90% of 39 patients treated with split course Cobalt-60 irradiation and interstitial iridium-192. Even when the tumors were larger than 4 cm, the control rate was

76% (44 of 58). PAPILLON (1982) suggested that chemotherapy be added to pelvic radiation only for those patients with fixed, unresectable carcinomas, or with deeply infiltrating tumors which involve more than two thirds of the circumference of the anal canal, or the vaginal mucosa, or in whom pelvic metastatic nodes are detectable at presentation. However, in North America at least, many centers appear to have adopted a policy of using combined chemotherapy and radiation therapy for all patients.

2 The Lymph Nodes

In the review of the surgical literature by GOLDEN and HORSLEY (1976), about 33% of patients who underwent abdominoperineal resection were found to have perirectal and superior hemorrhoidal lymph node metastases. These lymph nodes are not irradiated by interstitial radiation techniques but can be treated by external beam therapy. The importance of including the presacral area in the radiation volume to cover the local lymph nodes has been stressed (PAPILLON 1982), and the upper border of the pelvic radiation volume has usually been at the midsacrum in both the radical and preoperative radiation and chemotherapy protocols (CUMMINGS et al. 1984; NIGRO et al. 1983). This restriction of the superior extent of the radiation field reduces the risk of late radiation enteritis. The adequacy of this treatment volume, which does not include all the lymph nodes up to the origin of the superior hemorrhoidal artery, which are usually removed at abdominoperineal resection, can be inferred from the absence of histologically involved nodes in those treated by preoperative chemotherapy and radiation and radical resection, and from the continued low rates of pelvic recurrence or distant metastases in patients who did not undergo laparotomy and resection.

Inguinal lymph node metastases were found at some time in the course of disease in 30% of the patients surveyed by GOLDEN and HORSLEY (1976). Only 20% of those who had inguinal metastases at the time of presentation were salvaged by inguinal dissection. However, provided the primary area remained controlled, the five year survival rate was 60% following node dissection when the inguinal metastases did not appear until three months or more after the primary tumor was treated. Radiation alone has generally been used only for unresectable or extensive inguinal node metastases, and although local control was

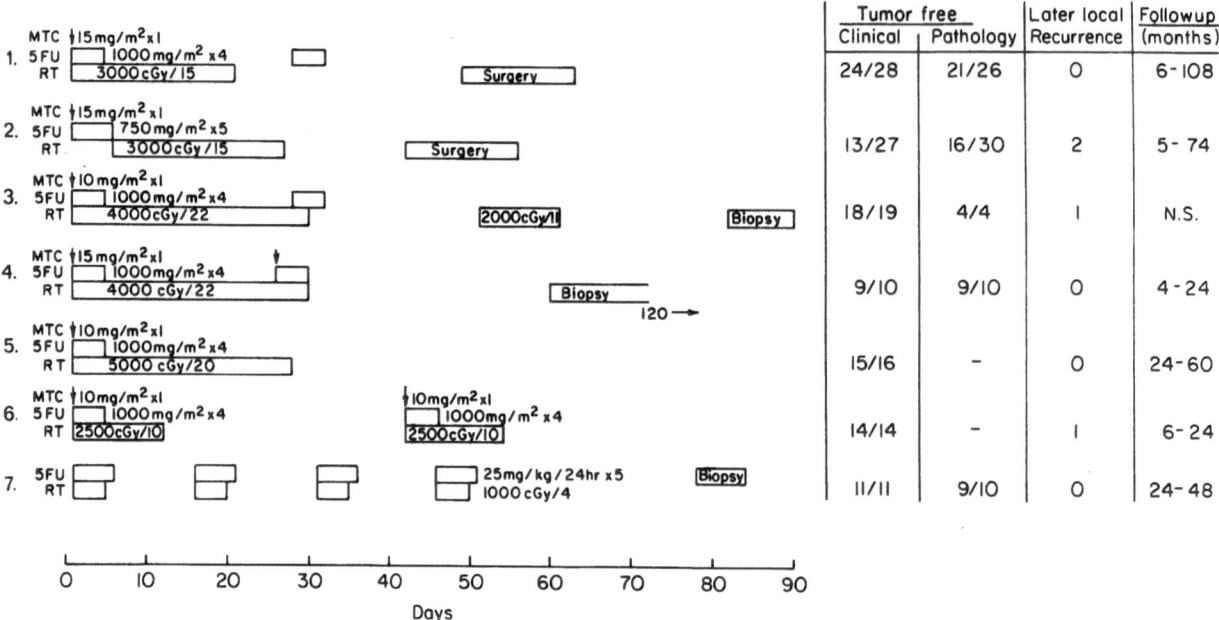

Fig. 1. Schedules used for the treatment of anal cancer. The original references should be consulted for full details. *MTC* Mitomycin C; *5-FU* 5-Fluorouracil; *RT* radiation therapy; *N.S.* not stated. 1. NIGRO et al. (1983); 2. MICHAELSON et al. (1983); 3. SISCHY et al. (1982); 4. FLAM et al. (1983); 5.+6. CUMMINGS et al. (1984); 7. BYFIELD et al. (1983)

achieved in about 20% (CUMMINGS 1982; PAPILLON 1982), some combination of radiation and inguinal node resection has usually been preferred (PAPILLON 1982). Several of the series shown in Fig. 1 included small numbers of patients with inguinal node metastases which were managed similarly to the primary carcinoma. The response of these lymph nodes paralleled that of the primary tumor, and, following radiation and chemotherapy, surgical resection can be reserved for those patients in whom a residual mass or induration raises doubts as to local control.

Prophylactic irradiation of the inguinal lymph nodes is worthwhile in order to reduce the usually reported 10% to 20% rate of late node relapse (PAPILLON 1982; STEARNS et al. 1980). Elective node dissection is not recommended because of the small numbers of positive nodes found, and because of the side effects of bilateral groin dissection (STEARNS et al. 1980). However, the radiation dose required to sterilize subclinical disease in the inguinal lymph nodes may be quite low when radiation is combined with chemotherapy, with correspondingly low morbidity. ROUSSEAU et al. (1973) used radiation alone and reported late node failure in only 1 of 61 patients after elective irradiation of the inguinofemoral nodes with 6000 cGy in 6 weeks. With either a single course of chemotherapy or with two courses during split course treatment, there has not been a single inguinal node relapse in the Princess Margaret Hospital series of 40 patients who received as little as 2400 cGy in 2 $^{1}/_{2}$ weeks (median followup 24 months, range 6 to 78 months). When prophylactic inguinal irradiation is given, it is advisable to use techniques which reduce irradiation of the femoral head and neck as much as possible.

3 Advanced Disease

The development of programs of combined radiation and chemotherapy has led to more aggressive treatment of patients who have had incomplete primary surgical resections, or who later develop pelvic recurrence or regional metastases after resection (QUAN et al. 1978; WANEBO et al. 1981). Although significant tumor regression is often seen, it is not yet possible to determine if salvage rates will be higher than the 20% obtained previously by surgery or by radiation therapy alone (CUMMINGS 1982).

The role of maintenance chemotherapy in patients with advanced disease is uncertain. MICHAELSON et al. (1983) treated some patients with MTC and 5-FU for up to one year and observed cumulative myelosuppression, azotemia possibly related to MTC, and microangiopathic hemolytic anemia. The results seemed no better than in patients who did not receive adjuvant chemotherapy. Other chemotherapy agents, which have occasionally produced responses in patients with extensive anal carcinomas, but which have not yet been studied systematically alone or in combination with radiation, have included bleomycin, CCNU, vincristine, adriamycin, and cis-platinum (CUMMINGS 1982).

4 Combination or Interaction?

The possible mechanisms of interplay between radiation and chemotherapy in this disease have occasioned considerable interest and speculation. In Figure 1 it can be seen that in all but one of the protocols where 5-FU, MTC, and radiation were combined, the clinical complete regression rate was 85% or more. In MICHAELSON'S (1983) study with low dose radiation therapy and chemotherapy however, the rate was only 50%. While there are many possible explanations for this difference (for example, different tumor stages at presentation, shorter interval between preoperative treatment and surgery etc.), it is also noteworthy that this group used sequential, rather than concurrent, chemotherapy and radiation therapy.

The addition of concurrent chemotherapy to radical radiation therapy in the Princess Margaret Hospital series was associated with an increase in local control rates, although the severity of the acute toxicity led to the adoption of split course techniques. Local control was achieved with radiation plus chemotherapy in 15 of 16 (94%) patients, whereas similar doses of radiation alone controlled primary carcinomas of similar clinical stage in only 15 of 25 (60%) patients (CUMMINGS et al. 1984). The effects of sequential chemotherapy and radical radiation have not been studied.

The important question of whether the chemotherapy and the radiation are acting additively or synergistically was examined by BYFIELD et al. (1982, 1983). They reviewed the literature on possible interactions between 5-FU and radiation, and reported their own studies in human adenocarcinoma cell lines in tissue culture (BYFIELD et al. 1982). They concluded that there was a time dependent enhancement of cell killing from combined 5-FU and x-rays, and that potentiation was found only with postradiation exposure of cells to 5-FU: prior exposure to 5-FU produced only

additive cell killing. The enhanced cell killing was maximized if the cells were exposed continuously to 5-FU following x-ray exposure for about 48 hours, well in excess of the cell cycle time. From related pharmacokinetic studies, they concluded that enhanced cell killing could not be achieved by bolus 5-FU administration, but that the cytocidal levels of 5-FU effective in the laboratory experiment were similar to those achieved by continuous intravenous infusions of 5-FU. Most of the clinical studies in patients with anal canal carcinoma have used doses of 1000 mg/m^2/24 hours for 4 days, equivalent to about 20 to 25 mg/kg/24 hours. BYFIELD et al. (1982) suggested that higher doses of 30 to 35 mg/kg/24 hours for 4 days should be considered for patients with locally advanced anal carcinomas, and that a cyclical schedule might be the most effective for patients with advanced disease. In clinical studies of cyclical radiation and 5-FU alone (Fig. 1), they noted excellent primary tumor regression rates, similar to those obtained by protocols using all three agents, and suggested that it might be advisable to omit MTC, a toxic alkylating agent with possible leukemogenic potential when combined with radiation. The minimum total radiation dose for cure using this cyclical schedule was considered to be 4000 cGy, and it was recommended that the rest period between cycles should be extended until all toxic effects (mainly mucosal and skin reactions) had subsided. The mechanism by which radiation and 5-FU interact is still uncertain, and the laboratory and clinical evidence does not establish the role of 5-FU as a "radiosensitizer". BYFIELD et al. (1982) speculated that exposing the cells to radiation might, in some way, enhance the cytocidal effects of 5-FU. In other words, radiation may be a chemosensitizer for 5-FU.

Laboratory studies of MTC and radiation have failed to demonstrate more than additive effects (ROCKWELL 1982). There have been no reports of laboratory experiments combining radiation and both 5-FU and MTC.

5 Conclusion

It is not possible to establish, from the clinical or laboratory evidence so far available, whether 5-FU, MTC and radiation act by addition or by supraadditive interaction in patients with anal cancer. Continued collaboration by clinical and laboratory investigators will be necessary to clarify these mechanisms. The success of empirically developed regimens, however, has made many more physicians aware of the possibility of preserving anal function in patients with anal carcinoma. For most patients it appears reasonable to commence treatment with either radiation therapy or with radiation plus chemotherapy, and to reserve radical excision with colostomy as a secondary treatment.

References

Boman BM, Moertel CG, O'Connell MJ, Scott M, Weiland LH, Beart RW, Gunderson LL, Spencer RJ (1984) Carcinoma of the anal canal. A clinical and pathological study of 188 cases. Cancer 54:114–125

Byfield JE, Barone RM, Sharp TR, Frankel SS (1983) Conservative management without alkylating agents of squamous cell anal cancer using cyclical 5-FU alone and x-ray therapy. Cancer Treat Rep 67:709–712

Byfield JE, Calabro-Jones P, Klisak I, Kulhanian F (1982) Pharmacologic requirements for obtaining sensitization of human tumor cells in vitro to combined 5-Fluorouracil or Ftorafur and x-rays. Int J Rad Oncol Biol Phys 8:1923–1933

Cantril ST, Green JP, Schall G, Schaupp WC (1983) Primary radiation therapy in the treatment of anal carcinoma. Int J Radiat Oncol Biol Phys 9:1271–1278

Cummings BJ (1982) The place of radiation therapy in the treatment of carcinoma of the anal canal. Cancer Treat Rev 9:125–147

Cummings BJ, Harwood AR, Keane TJ, Thomas GM, Rider WD (1980) Combined treatment of squamous cell carcinoma of the anal canal: radical radiation therapy with 5-Fluorouracil and Mitomycin C, a preliminary report. Dis Colon Rectum 23:389–391

Cummings BJ, Keane TJ, Thomas GM, Harwood AR, Rider WD (1984) Results and toxicity of the treatment of anal canal carcinoma by radiation therapy or radiation therapy and chemotherapy. Cancer 54:2062–2068

Flam SM, John M, Lovalvo LJ, Mills RJ, Ramalko LD, Prather C, Mowry PA, Morgan DR, Lau BP (1983) Definitive nonsurgical therapy of epithelial malignancies of the anal canal. Cancer 51:1378–1387

Frost DB, Richards PC, Montague ED, Giacco GG, Martin RG (1984) Epidermoid cancer of the anorectum. Cancer 53:1285–1293

Golden GT, Horsley JS III (1976) Surgical management of epidermoid carcinoma of the anus. Am J Surg 131:275–280

Michaelson RA, Magill GB, Quan SHQ, Leaming RH, Nikrui M, Stearns MW (1983) Preoperative chemotherapy and radiation therapy in the management of anal epidermoid carcinoma. Cancer 51:390–395

Nigro ND, Seydel HG, Considine B, Vaitkevicius VK, Leichman L, Kinzie JJ (1983) Combined preoperative radiation and chemotherapy for squamous cell carcinoma of the anal canal. Cancer 51:1826–1829

Nigro ND, Vaitkevicius VK, Considine B (1974) Combined therapy for cancer of the anal canal: a preliminary report. Dis Colon Rectum 17:354–356

Papillon J (1982) Rectal and Anal Cancers. New York, Springer-Verlag

Quan SHQ, Magill GB, Leaming RH, Hajdu SI (1978) Multidisciplinary preoperative approach to the management of epidermoid carcinoma of the anus and anorectum. Dis Colon Rectum 21:89–91

Rockwell S (1982) Cytotoxicities of Mitomycin C and x-rays to aerobic and hypoxic cells in vitro. Int J Radiat Oncol Biol Phys 8:1035–1039

Rousseau J, Mathieu G, Fenton J, Cuzin J (1973) Radiothérapie des cancers malpighiens de l'anus. J Radiol Electrol Med Nucl 54:622–626

Sischy B, Remington JH, Hinson EJ, Sobel SH, Woll JE (1982) Definitive treatment of anal canal carcinoma by means of radiation therapy and chemotherapy. Dis Colon Rectum 25:685–688

Stearns MW, Urmacher C, Sternberg SS, Woodruff J, Attiyeh F (1980) Cancer of the anal canal. Curr Probl Cancer 4:1–44

Wanebo JH, Futrell W, Constable W (1981) Multimodality approach to surgical management of locally advanced epidermoid carcinoma of the anorectum. Cancer 47:2817–2826

3 Extended Field Therapy

3.1 Total Body Irradiation for Bone Marrow Transplantation

GLENN P. GLASGOW

CONTENTS

LIST OF ABBREVIATIONS

TBI	Total Body Irradiation
ALL	Acute Lymphoblastic Leukemia
AML	Acute Myelogenous Leukemia
BMT	Bone Marrow Transplants
TMR	Tissue Maximum Ratio
PDD	Percentage Depth Dose
TAR	Tissue Air Ratio
CNS	Central nervous system
SSD	Source-to-Skin Distance
FHCRC	Fred Hutchinson Cancer Research Center

1 Introduction

Since the early days of radiotherapy, physicians have used total body irradiation (TBI) to treat advanced systemic and disseminated diseases, such as non-Hodgkin's lymphoma, chronic lymphocytic leukemia, lymphosarcoma, Ewing's sarcoma and other advanced generalized malignant diseases. Over the past decade, the main application of TBI has been in the conditioning regimen of patients receiving bone marrow transplantation, usually

GLENN P. GLASGOW, Professor
Mail Route 114B
Hines, IL 60141, USA

for leukemia. Several recent articles review both clinical applications and techniques of TBI (RIDER and VAN DYK 1983; GLASGOW 1982; SHANK 1983).

Achieving a uniform radiation dose to the total body is difficult. WEBSTER (1959) reviewed the physical considerations for the design of irradiators that would produce a homogeneous total body dose and concluded a minimum of four radioactive sources around the patient would be necessary. A few dedicated treatment rooms with four or more sources were built and used during the 1960's and 70's but such facilities were too expensive for most medical institutions. Two track mounted, mobile, parallel opposed ^{60}Co sources, with specially designed collimators, are used for TBI in the BMT program at the Fred Hutchinson Cancer Research Center (FHCRC) in Seattle, Washington (LAM et al. 1980) and by the Munich Cooperative Group for BMT (KOLB et al. 1979). From 1960 to 1974 a ^{60}Co moving field technique was used for TBI at the Princess Margaret Hospital in Toronto (CUMMINGHAM and WRIGHT 1962). This treatment method was succeeded by a ^{60}Co unit with only a 90 cm source-to-skin distance (SSD) but with a field 50 cm × 160 cm (VAN DYK et al. 1980b; LEUNG et al. 1981).

While specially designed irradiators offer obvious advantages, many total body irradiations must be performed with conventional teletherapy units. This chapter reviews the dosimetry of TBI performed with conventional teletherapy units to acquaint those unfamiliar with TBI with this method of radiotherapy.

2 Dosimetry

The dosimetry of TBI depends on some parameters that are a function of the treatment geometry and therapy unit and others that are a function of the patient's size and anatomical position during therapy.

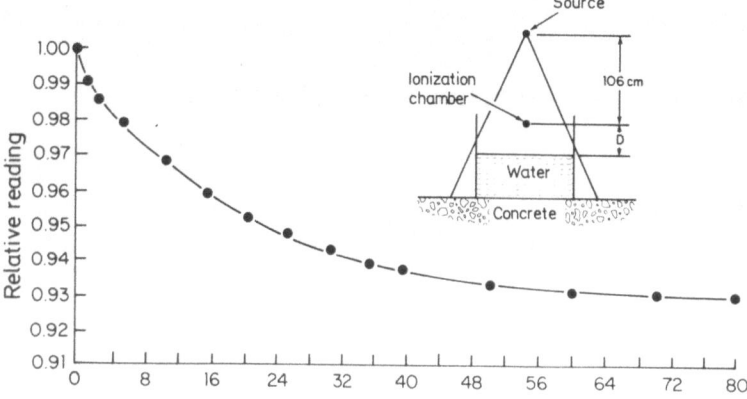

Fig. 1. The relative ionization chamber readings as a function of the distance (*D*) between the chamber and the backscattering medium. To achieve scatter free conditions for this large field cobalt irradiator D = 65 cm. (Redrawn from VAN DYK et al. 1980b)

2.1 Treatment Distance

Ideally, the distance from the source of radiation to the treatment plane should be several meters. The variation of the radiation intensity with the inverse square of the treatment distance requires a 3 m treatment distance to achieve a ± 5% uniformity in radiation intensity over a transverse length of 2 m; at 3 m the percentage depth doses essentially are those obtained from a source infinitely far away (WEBSTER 1959).

While there are reported techniques of TBI using treatment distances less than 3 m (SVENSSON et al. 1980; GLASGOW and MILL 1980; VAN DYK et al. 1980b), more uniform doses would be achieved if the treatment distances were at least 3 m, and this is possible in many facilities.

2.2 Field Size

The field size for TBI should be as large as possible. A therapy unit that projects a 40 cm × 40 cm field at 1 m will project at 3 m a field only 120 cm × 120 cm. Moreover, the useful treatment field may be substantially smaller than the projected light field, due to dose fall-off at the field edges. This has important implications for patient positioning within the radiation field (see below).

2.3 Dose Rate

The dose rate (rad per minute or monitor unit) of a teletherapy unit should be measured in the plane of treatment. MILLER et al. (1976) measured at 5% increase over the calculated inverse square dose rate (presumably for a large field) 16 cm from

a wall 3.52 m from a ^{60}Co source; VAN DYK et al. (1980b) noted similar dose increases on their large field cobalt irradiator; as in Fig. 1, the scattering medium had to be about 65 cm away from the dose measurement point in order to obtain scatter free conditions. The backscatter radiation from large fields incident on shielding barriers is more pronounced for ^{60}Co gamma rays than for the x-rays from higher energy linacs; AGET et al. (1977) measured only a 0.5% increase, from backscatter radiation, in the dose 20 cm from a concrete wall 4.5 m from a linac producing 25 MV x-rays.

2.4 Dose Ratio Parameters

The dose ratio parameters that are nominally independent of distance, i.e., TAR and TMR, are more useful for large field dosimetry than the PPD but their degree of independence with distance should be confirmed. For 10 MV, KAHN et al. (1980) measured TMR's for a 40 cm × 40 cm field at 100 cm that were within 1.5% of those measured for a 122 cm × 122 cm field containing a 40 cm × 40 cm phantom 4.1 m away. AGET et al. (1977) measured TMR's for 25 MV x-rays using a 30 cm × 90 cm phantom. At 4.5 m, for a depth of 15 cm, the TMR's were 2.4% higher than the TMR's measured at 15 cm depth at 1 m; greater differences were observed at greater depths. Hence, published tables of TAR and TMR for fields as large as 30 cm × 30 cm probably will agree, to within 3%, with values measured for the same field size at extended distances; the larger variations will occur at greater depths.

The dose ratio definitions assume the radiation is incident of a flat cubical phantom of sufficient dimensions to provide full scatter at the depth of

Fig. 2. Measured and calculated doses, D, in rad, as a function of lateral distance, d, in cm, from the mid-plane sagittal axis, in an anthropomorphic phantom, given a midplane pelvis dose of 900 rad at 200 cm SAD with ^{60}Co gamma-rays. Solid curves are eye-guides to the data. (From GLASGOW et al. 1980)

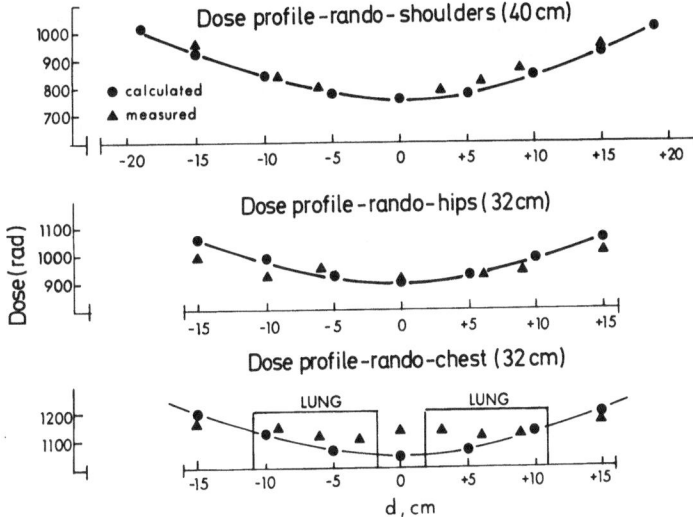

measurement. Patients do not present a uniform flat surface to the beam; moreover, the patients do not fill these large fields.

The dose distribution is a function of collimator field size or phantom size, whichever is smaller; for ^{60}Co scatter radiation to the central axis is negligible from material 50 cm to 60 cm away. LAM et al. (1979) observed, for ^{60}Co, that the relative doses measured at 5 cm depth intervals from the surface to 25 cm depth in a 25 cm × 25 cm tissue equivalent phantom increases asymptotically to their maximum value as the length of the phantom was increased to 65 cm.

HOCHHAUSER (1977), with BALK (1978) revised and measured cobalt TAR's for bilateral irradiation of elliptical phantom cross sections. TAR's measured at an SAD of 4 m in the elliptical pelvis of an anthropomorphic phantom with an equivalent square area of 31 cm × 32 cm perpendicular to the beam, were compared to TAR's for 30 cm × 30 cm field for a cuboidal treatment volume (GUPTA and CUNNINGHAM 1966). To about 14 cm depth the elliptical phantom TAR's are up to 6% lower than the TAR's measured in the cuboidal volumes; however, the TAR's converge at greater depths.

What equivalent square area does a patient present during TBI? Patient position during treatment must be considered to answer this question. For ^{60}Co TBI, GLASGOW et al. (1980) obtained good agreement between doses measured in an anthropomorphic phantom and those calculated using published TAR's for a 35 cm × 35 cm field (Fig. 2). Patients were crouched in a semi-fetal position and irradiated bilaterally in a 87 cm × 87 cm field at

220 cm SAD as shown in Fig. 3. KAHN et al. (1980) used the conventional 4 × A/P (area/perimeter) approximation for the side of an equivalent square for TBI with 10 MV x-rays and obtained ±2% accuracy in relating phantom dimensions to patient dimensions.

The key point is that the patient will produce less scatter than occurs in an infinite cubical phantom; this reduced scatter must be reflected in the dose calculations. For example, LAM et al. (1980)

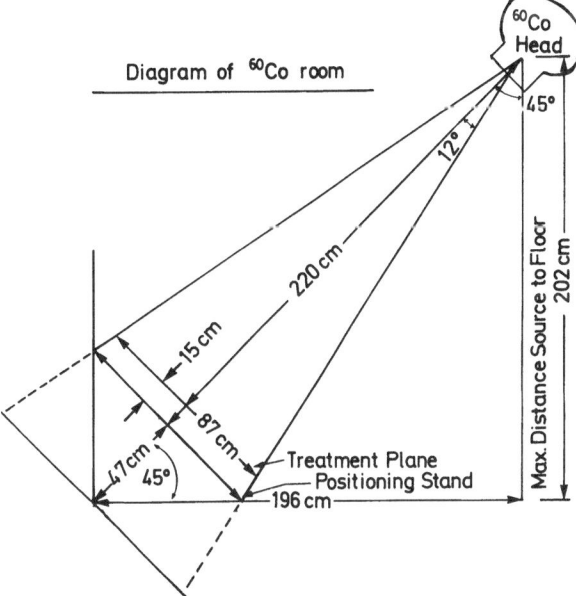

Fig. 3. Treatment geometry in a small (220 cm source axis distance 'SSD') therapy room. The 87 cm × 87 cm field is rotated so the 123 cm field diagonal coincides with the cephald-caudal dimension of the patient. (From GLASGOW and MILL 1980)

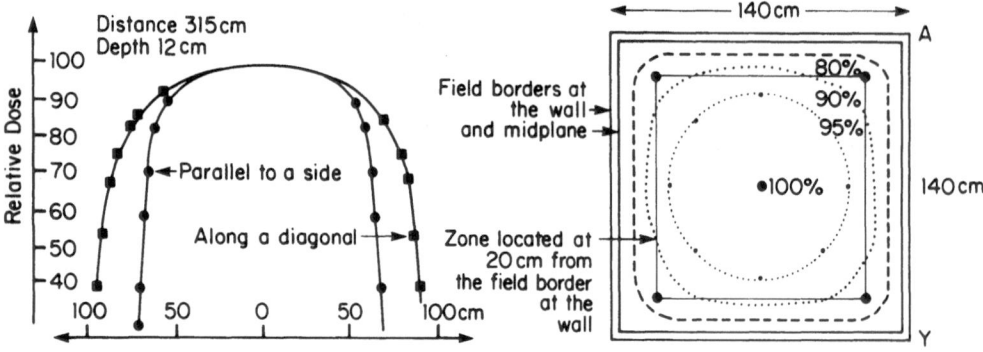

Fig. 4. a Dose homogeneity measured at 12 cm depth, along both the principal and diagonal axes, for about a 140 cm × 140 cm field 315 cm from a Theratron-80 cobalt 80 unit. **b** Dose homogeneity in the treatment plane at 12 cm depth. The useful treatment field is approximately defined by the 90% isodose curve. (Redrawn from JABLONSKI et al. 1979)

reviewing the dual cobalt sources dosimetry at the FHCRC, discovered an 8% dose discrepancy; the FHCRC dosimetry was based on square phantom TAR's and longitudinal patient area, whereas LAM et al. (1980) dosimetry was based on "long phantom measurements" that (apparently) included radiation scatter contributions not included in the FHCRC's dosimetry calculations.

2.5 Radiation Intensity Uniformity

Any radiation intensity non-uniformity is likely to be enhanced in the large fields used for TBI; hence, the "field flatnesses", must be measured in the treatment plane. For cobalt units, underdosing around the periphery of the field is common, as shown in Fig. 4 (JABLONSKI 1979). For linacs the oposite problem can exist, i.e., any "horns" produced by flattening filters can be enhanced and special filters may have to be designed to solve these problems (DUTREIX and BRIDIER 1979).

Non-uniformity can be used to advantage in achieving a uniform dose to the patient. For example, the thinner portions of the body can be placed in the periphery of a field where the dose is lower to achieve a more uniform total body dose. LAM et al. (1979) measured a 10% lower head dose relative to the central axis midline dose because of the reduced dose in the periphery of the cobalt field used for TBI. Conversely, a higher dose would be delivered to these thinner anatomical regions if there is a higher dose near the periphery

of the field. The desirability of dose uniformity will be discussed later.

2.6 Entry Doses

The effect of large field geometry on the entry doses and on the depth of maximum ionization should be measured. Table 1 shows the depth of maximum (d_m) measured for a 150 cm × 150 cm field at 400 cm for ^{60}Co unit, and for linacs with x-ray energies of 5.6 MV and 25 MV (DUTREIX and BRIDIER 1979). At all energies d_m was closer to the entry surface than during conventional therapy. JABLONSKI et al. (1979) measured d_{max} at 1.5 mm on their cobalt unit for 127 × 127 field at 3 m. At 10 MV, KAHN et al. (1980) observed a higher entry and build-up dose at 4.1 m than at 1.0 m, but the d_m of 2 cm was unchanged. As these effects are therapy unit and geometry dependent, it is important to measure the entry dose and the doses in the region of build-up to maximum ionization for the specific therapy unit, treatment aids, and geometry used in TBI. If the surface dose is too low, a lucite plate placed close to the patient will increase the skin dose. The skin doses and the doses in the region of build-up to maximum ionization are particularly important as the lym-

Table 1. Dose variation in build-up region field: 150 × 150 cm SSD (400 cm). (From DUTREIX and BRIDIER 1979)

	Cobalt 60 (mm)	5.6 MV (mm)	25 MV (mm)
Depth of maximum dose	2	6	20
Depth of 90% of the maximum dose	0.8	2.5	8

phatics near the skin surface and the marrow in the ribs, skull, and clavical can be underdosed. The use of bolus and "missing" tissue compensators will be discussed later.

2.7 Exit Dose

The skin and superficial tissue on the side of the patient from which the beam exits can receive a reduced dose if insufficient backscattering material is present (GOEDE et al. 1977). GAGNON and HORTON (1979) measured the exit dose, expressed as a percentage of the dose with full backscatter, as a function of distance from the exit surface. For ^{60}C, the dose reduction is greater the larger the field. For 25 MV x-rays this effect is independent of field size, and as little as 0.5 cm of backscatter material is sufficient to provide full backscatter to the exit surface.

3 Dose Prescriptions

The nominal dose prescription is related to the patient's position during therapy, and dose uniformity achieved. The points at which doses have been prescribed in TBI include the midline depth of the abdomen, the average midline depth of the head, neck, chest, and abdomen, and the half depth of the maximum width of the body.

KIM et al. (1980), in their review of TBI, concluded that the midline dose to the pelvis should be the reported dose; it is easy to calculate and is the dose most likely to be used to compare TBI dosimetry between facilities. This same report stresses that (for TBI) the radiotherapist must give a "point-by-point specification of the desired dose, including upper and lower limits for each organ or region".

The dose prescription should include and may be limited by the dose to critical organs. For example, GLASGOW and MILL (1980) initially treated five patients prescribing 10 Gy midline in the pelvis; they subsequently lowered the midline dose prescription to 9 Gy in order to limit the lung dose to less than 12 Gy.

3.1 Patient Positioning

Without tissue compensators, anterior-posterior irradiation will yield more uniform doses throughout the body than bilateral irradiation. SVENSSON et al. (1980) showed the superiority of anterior-posterior over bilateral positioning in phantom measurements using 4 MV x-rays at 2.79 m SSD. With compensated high energy beams, however, acceptable dose uniformity can be achieved with the convenience of bilateral irradiation of the reclining patient (see below).

Most reports of TBI have the patient lying either prone, supine, or in a crouched or semi-fetal position on a couch or stretcher. For bilateral irradiation patients can sit in a chair. GLASGOW and MILL (1980) used a treatment stand tilted at 45° relative to the floor to increase the SSD; the beam, angled toward the corner of the therapy room, is incident laterally on the patient as shown in Fig. 3.

LAWRENCE et al. (1980) improved dose uniformity by varying the patient's position during protracted TBI; for two thirds of the TBI the patients lay on their sides while for the remaining one third of the treatment they lay supine.

3.2 Dose Uniformity

The degree of acceptable dose non-uniformity using large field therapy is a clinical decision. Normally, one desires a uniform dose to the target volume; however, a degree of non-uniformity is inevitable during TBI and may be perfectly acceptable, e.g., the higher dose received by the legs during uncompensated bilateral parallel opposed treatments is of no serious consequence. However, the dose to the head and neck can be 10% to 20% higher than the mid-abdomen dose and compensation is required to avoid excessive mucosal reactions.

GALVIN et al. (1980) and KAHN et al. (1980) reviewed the dosimetry of external beam missing tissue compensators for 6 MV and 10 MV x-rays. Fig. 5 schematically depicts, for 10 MV x-rays, the relative thickness compensators made of thin lead strips attached to the therapy unit to achieve dose homogeneity using bilateral fields. AGET et al. (1977) used bolus adjacent to the patient to achieve a uniform dose with 25 MV x-rays, as shown in Fig. 6. In treating leukemia, the lack of skin sparing associated with the bolus technique is a theoretical advantage, since circulating leukemic stem cells could be present in the superficial vasculature. A dose uniformity of $\pm 10\%$ usually can be achieved by using one or other of these compensators systems. The effects of bone heterogeneities on megavoltage dose distributions are small and usually neglected in TBI.

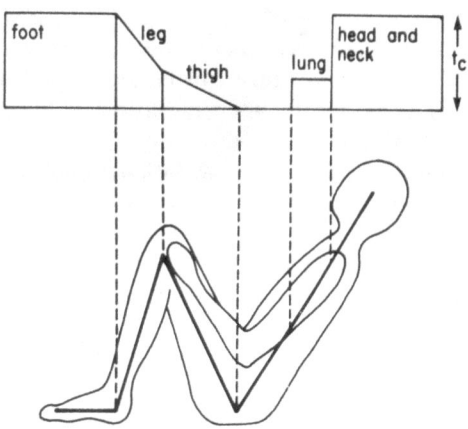

Fig. 5. A schematic diagram of anatomical areas requiring compensation during bilateral TBI in order to achieve a uniform dose. (Redrawn from Kahn et al. 1980)

3.3 Lung Dose

Knowledge of the dose to the lung during TBI, corrected for heterogeneities, is critical. The lung dose during TBI can be estimated from anthropomorphic phantom measurements or by numerous computational methods, such as the tissue-air-ratio method, the Batho-Young power law method, and others; their relative accuracy has been reviewed by Van Dyk et al. (1980a). The actuarial incidence of radiation pneumonitis as a function of absolute lung dose was reported by Van Dyk et al. (1981), based on their review of patients treated with half-body irradiations. For single fraction treatments, the onset of radiation pneumonitis occurs at about 750 cGy with an actuarial incidence of 5% at 820 cGy, 50% at 930 cGy, and 95% at 1060 cGy, with dose rates between 50 to 400 cGy min^{-1}.

Keane et al. (1981) reported "a definite relationship between the absorbed dose to the lung and the development of idiopathic interstitial pneumonia in patients receiving allogeneic bone marrow transplants"; their data, based on a review of TBI at five major centers performing low dose rate TBI are shown in Fig. 7. Both these data sets support a steep dose response relationship for radiation pneumonitis. However, the clinical syndrome of idiopathic interstitial pneumonitis was not significantly related to total radiation dose in the data of the International Bone Marrow Transplant Registry.

Lung dose can be lowered in several ways. During bilateral treatments, simply positioning the patient's arms by his side will decrease the dose to some of the lung. Shielding blocks are used by several of the BMT groups performing TBI (Aget et al. 1977; Galvin et al. 1980; Shank 1983). A lung dose of 800 rad may be optimal; this appears to be sufficient to suppress the immune system for successful engraftment following BMT, but has a minimum likelihood of causing radiation pneumonitis.

3.4 Dose Confirmation

Dose confirmation of TBI should consist of dose distributions measured in and on an anthropomorphic phantom as well as in vivo measurements in patients. The radiological physicist should de-

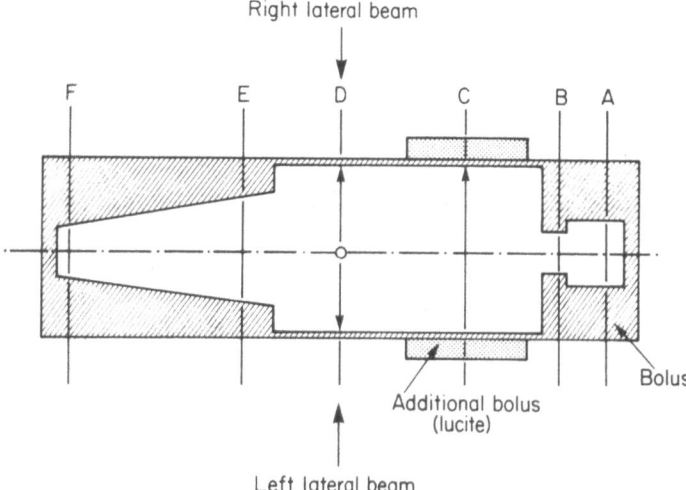

Fig. 6. A schematic diagram of the anatomical areas requiring bolus as compensation during anterior-posterior TBI to achieve a uniform dose. (Redrawn from Aget et al. 1977)

Fig. 7. A probit regression analysis of the estimated absolute lung dose versus the crude incidence of IIP for the centers using low dose rate TBI plus chemotherapy. The data points indicate the average absolute lung dose for each center and the error bars indicate the dose range. (Redrawn from KEANE et al. 1981)

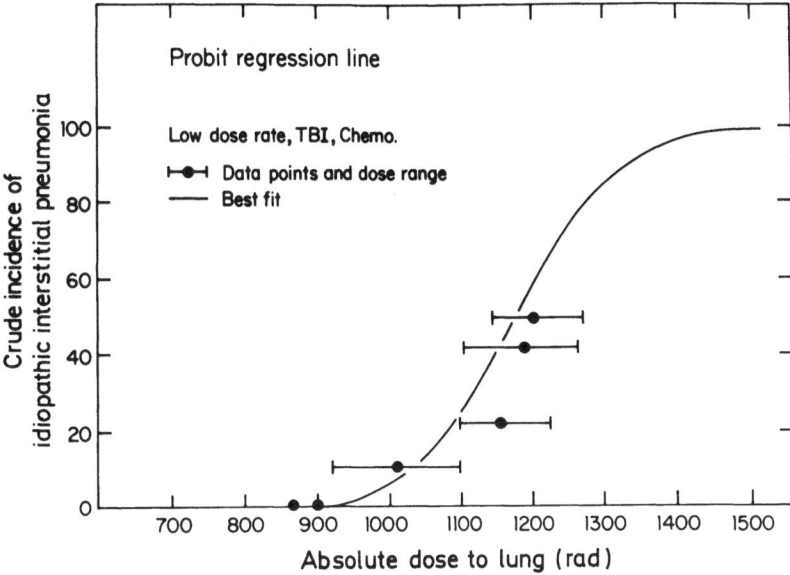

velop a method of calculating point doses during TBI and then confirm the dose calculational method using phantom and in vivo dosimetry. GLAS-GOW et al. (1980), using standard TAR's for a 35 cm × 35 cm field, and the inverse square law for radiation intensity, calculated lateral dose profiles for TBI with a cobalt unit; the calculated doses agreed well with the measured profiles, except within the lung and mediastinum (Fig. 2). Phantom measurements are required as in vivo measurements in patients are more limited in extent. However, the latter are used to confirm calculated doses for individual patients. In some cases of TBI requiring prolonged or fractionated treatment, the doses measured in vivo in the patient may be analyzed before completion of therapy to permit adjustment of the dose. Sites for in vivo measurements include the mouth, axilla, inner thighs, and rectum; parallel opposed entry and exit dose can be used to estimate the dose midway between the dosimeters.

den the supporting medical staff; patients frequently suffer nausea and vomiting during the latter period of therapy. Although linear accelerators have the capability of much higher dose rates than cobalt units, it may be predicted radiobiologically that single dose, high dose rate TBI would be therapeutically disadvantageous (PETERS et al. 1979; DUTREIX et al. 1979). The dose rate dependence of various lethal syndromes following TBI in mice has recently been reported (TRAVIS et al. 1985). These data comprise a much greater dose rate dependence, particularly below 5 cGy min^{-1}, of death due of the gastrointestinal syndrome, or late organ failure within one year of irradiation, compared with bone marrow ablation. The finding of the International Bone Marrow Tumor Registry (BORTIN et al. 1982) that the incidence of interstitial pneumonitis was significantly reduced when TBI was delivered at dose rates less than 4 cGy min^{-1}, is in concordance with these experimental data (See Chapter by BORTIN and HARTZ).

4 Radiobiological Considerations

The single fraction total body irradiation technique developed at the FHCRC in Seattle, Washington, used dose rates of about 5 to 8 cGy min^{-1} which are substantially lower than those used during conventional radiation therapy. However, there are obvious clinical difficulties with single fraction, protracted TBI. Treatment of several hours are uncomfortable for the patients and bur-

5 Conclusion

Total body irradiation involves many diverse dosimetric and radiobiological concepts. However, the lack of consensus on methods of dose specifications, dose uniformity, the use of missing tissue compensators, and other topics should not prevent the use of TBI when clinically warranted. Using conventional dosimetry concepts, measurements in anthropomorphic phantoms, and in vivo dosimetry, many questions about the dose throughout the patient can be answered. Conventional missing tissue compensators or bolus can be used to improve dose uniformity when required. The doses to critical organs should be estimated in all patients undergoing TBI to better define the relationship of dose, dose rate, and fraction to treatment outcome.

Acknowledgements. I wish to thank all of the authors and journal editors named in the table and figure captions for allowing me to include these data in this review. I particularly wish to express my appreciation to Mrs. CHERYL ZMAILA for her untiring efforts (and patience) exhibited during the preparation of this manuscript. Her valuable assistance made a difficult task easy.

References

Aget H, Van Dyk J, Leung PMK (1977) Utilization of a high energy photon beam for whole body irradiation. Radiol 123:747–751

Bortin MM et al. (1982) Factors associated with interstitial pneumonitis after bone marrow transplantation for acute leukemia. Lancet 1:437–439

Cummingham JR, Wright DJ (1962) A simple facility for whole body irradiation. Radiol 78:941–951

Dutreix A, Bridier A (1979) Total body irradiation techniques and dosimetry. Path Biol 27:373–378

Dutreix J, Wambersie A, Lonette M, Boisserie A (1979) Time factors in total body irradiation. Pathol Biol 27:365–369

Gagnon WF, Horton JL (1979) Physical factors affecting absorbed dose to the skin from cobalt-60 gamma rays and 25 MeV x-rays. Med Phys 6:285–290

Galvin JM, D'Angio GT, Walsh G (1980) Use of tissue compensators to improve the dose uniformity for total body irradiation. Int J Radiat Oncol Biol Phys 6:767–771

Glasgow GP (1982) The dosimetry of fixed, single source hemibody and total body irradiators. Med Phys 9:311–323

Glasgow GP, Mill WB (1980) Cobalt-60 total body irradiation at 220 cm source-axis-distance. Int J Radiat Oncol Biol Phys 6:773–777

Glasgow GP, Mill WB, Phillips GL, Herzig GP (1980) Comparative ^{60}Co total body irradiation (220 cm SAD) and 25 MV total body irradiation (370 cm SAD) dosimetry. Int J Radiat Oncol Biol Phys 6:1243–1250

Goede MR, Anderson DW, McCray KL (1977) Corrections to megavoltage depth dose values due to reduced backscatter thickness. Med Phys 4:123–126

Gupta SK, Cunningham JR (1966) Measurement of tissue-air-ratios and scatter functions for large field sizes for ^{60}Co gamma radiation. Br J Radiol 39:7–11

Hochhauser E (1977) Zum gewebe-luft-verhaltnis bei doppelseitiger ganzkorperbestralung. Strahlentherapie 153:820–824

Hochhauser E, Balk OA (1978) Tissue-air-ratios for whole body irradiation with cobalt-60 gamma rays. Br J Radiol 51:460–462

Jablonski O, Motta-Veyssiere CC, Guerin GR (1979) Irradiations corporelles totales-technique d'irradiation fractionnee par telecobalt. J Radiol 60:339–342

Keane TJ, Van Dyk J, Rider WD (1981) Idiopathic interstitial pneumonia following bone marrow transplantation: The relationship with total body irradiation. Int J Radiat Oncol Biol Phys 7:1365–1370

Khan FM, Williamson JF, Sewchand W, Kim TH (1980) Basic data for dose calculation and compensation. Int J Radiat Oncol Biol Phys 6:745–751

Kim TH, Khan FM, Galvin JM (1980) A report of the work party: Comparison of total body irradiation techniques for bone marrow transplantation. Int J Radiat Oncol Biol Phys 6:779–784

Kolb HL, Rieder I, Bobenberger U, Netzel B, Schaffer E, Kolb H, Thierfelder S (1979) Dose rate and dose fractionation studies in total body irradiation of dogs. Path Biol 27:370–372

Lam WC, Lindskoug BA, Order SE, Grant DG (1979) The dosimetry of cobalt 60 total body irradiation. Int J Radiat Oncol Biol Phys 5:905–911

Lam WC, Order SE, Thomas ED (1980) Uniformity and standardization of single and opposing cobalt 60 source of total body irradiation. Int J Radiat Oncol Biol Phys 6:245–250

Lawrence G, Rosenbloom Me, Hickling P (1980) A technique for total body irradiation in the treatment of patients with acute leukemia. Br J Radiol 53:894–897

Leung PMK, Rider WD, Webb HP, Aget H, Johns HE (1981) Cobalt-60 therapy unit for large field irradiation. Int J Radiat Oncol Biol Phys 7:705–712

Miller RJ, Langdon EA, Tesler AS (1976) Total body irradiation utilizing a single ^{60}Co source. Int J Radiat Oncol Biol Phys 1:549–552

Peters LJ, Withers HR, Cundiff JH, Dicke KA (1979) Radiobiological considerations in the use of total body irradiation for bone marrow transplantation. Radiol 131:243–247

Rider WD, Van Dyk J (1983) Total and partial body irradiation. In: Bleehen NM, Glatstein E, Haybittle JL (eds) Radiation Therapy Planning. Marcel Dekker, Inc., New York, Basel, p 559

Shank B (1983) Techniques of magna-field irradiation. Int J Radiat Oncol Biol Phys 9:1925–1931

Svensson GK, Larsen RD, Chen TS (1980) The use of a 4 MV linear accelerator for whole body irradiation. Int J Radiat Oncol Biol Phys 6:761–765

Travis EL, Peters LJ, McNeill J, Thames HD Jr, Karolis C (1985) Effect of dose-rate on total body irradiation: Lethality and pathologic findings. Radiotherapy & Oncology

Van Dyk J, Battista JJ, Rider WD (1980a) Half body radiotherapy: The use of computed tomography to determine the dose to lung. Int J Radiat Oncol Biol Phys 6:463–470

Van Dyk J, Leung DMK, Cunningham JR (1980b) Dosimetry considerations of very large cobalt-60 fields. Int J Radiat Oncol Biol Phys 6:753–759

Van Dyk J, Keane TJ, Kan S, Rider WD, Fryer CJA (1981) Radiation pneumonitis following large single dose irradiation: A reevaluation based on absolute dose to the lung. Int J Radiat Oncol Biol Phys 7:461–467

Webster EW (1959) Physical considerations in the design of facilities for the uniform whole-body irradiation of man. Radiol 75:19–31

3.2 Influence of Radiation Regimens on the Risk of Interstitial Pneumonitis in Leukemia Patients Treated with Allogeneic Bone Marrow Transplantation

Mortimer M. Bortin and Arthur J. Hartz

CONTENTS

The research reported here was supported by grant 40053 from the National Cancer Institute, DHHS, contract N01-AI-62530 from the National Institute of Allergy and Infectious Diseases, DHHS, contract BI6-084-US from the Commission of the European Communities and grants provided to the International Bone Marrow Transplant Registry by the Apple Family Foundation, A.J. Bitker Memorial Foundation, Jacob and Hilda Blaustein Foundation, Brotz Foundation, Henry W. Bull Foundation, Charles E. Culpeper Foundation, Fairchild Foundation, Lester Glen Family Foundation, William Randolph Hearst Foundation, Heller Foundation, William L. Law Foundation, Lederle Laboratories, Ambrose Monell Foundation, Samuel Roberts Noble Foundation, Elsa U. Pardee Foundation, Ann and Robert Pereles, Procter & Gamble Co., R.G.K. Foundation, Betty and Arthur J. Runft, Sandoz, Inc., Joan and Jack Stein, Swiss Cancer League and the Upjohn Company.

1 Background

Interstitial pneumonitis is the single most devastating complication of allogeneic bone marrow transplantation in leukemia patients. The magnitude of the problem can be judged from the results of a recent study of 932 leukemia patients reported to the International Bone Marrow Transplant Registry (Weiner et al. 1986). All patients were prepared for transplantation of bone marrow from HLA-identical siblings with chemotherapy and 920 also received total body irradiation. The incidence of interstitial pneumonitis was 29%, the case fatality rate was 84%, the mortality rate was 24% and the actuarial risk at two years was 35%!

Interstitial pneumonitis is a mysterious disease with no known cause, no effective preventive measures, and in most cases, no effective treatment. The clinical syndrome is characterized by dyspnea and non-productive cough. Roentgenograms of the chest exhibit unilateral or bilateral diffuse pulmonary interstitial infiltrates. Laboratory tests disclose hypoxemia and diminished diffusing capacity (Khouri et al. 1979; Myers et al. 1983; Sloane et al. 1983). The diagnosis usually is made on clinical grounds and is confirmed by lung biopsy or, all too often, at autopsy. The disease occasionally is fulminant with the interval from first symptom to death less than 24 hours, but usually it lasts from several days to several weeks or longer.

Direct or indirect evidence of a cytomegalovirus infection is present in from 30–60% of the cases in most large series (Winston et al. 1979; Meyers et al. 1983; Pino y Torres et al. 1982; Weiner et al. 1986). Other opportunistic pathogens such as *Pneumocystis carinii*, herpes simplex, herpes zoster, candida, aspergillus, etc. are found in perhaps 10–15% of the cases. In approximately half the cases, no pathogen is identified and the disease is classified as idiopathic. It is not known whether the opportunistic microorganisms found in the other half of the patients are etiologic agents or merely pulmonary superinfections in immunocompromised hosts whose lungs have been damaged by the underlying disease and its treatment.

Multiple interacting factors are thought to predispose to the development of interstitial pneumonitis including an immunosuppressed host, lung damage and the presence of opportunistic microorganisms (Bortin 1983). All three factors are

Mortimer M. Bortin, M.D., Professor
The Medical College of Wisconsin
Milwaukee, WI 53226, USA

Arthur J. Hartz, M.D., Ph.D.
Milton S. Hershey Medical Center
Hershey, PA 17033, USA

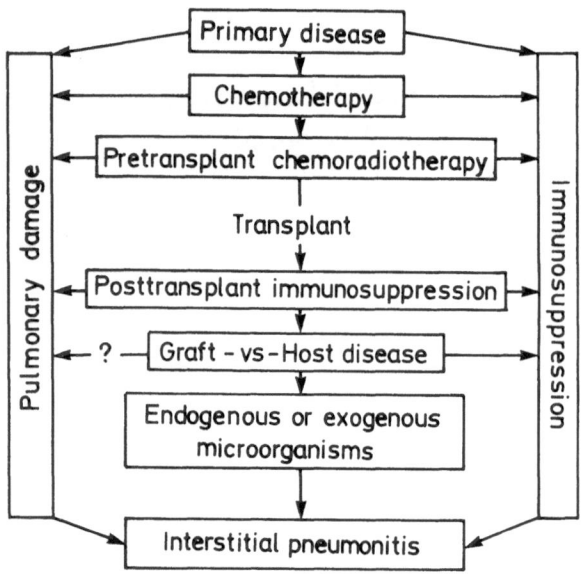

Fig. 1. Pathways for the pathogenesis of interstitial pneumonitis. (Modified from BORTIN 1983)

commonly present in marrow allografted leukemia patients accounting in large measure for the high incidence of this life-threatening complication.

The model in Fig. 1 shows some of the interactions that contribute to the pathogenesis of interstitial pneumonitis (BORTIN 1983). The model illustrates that any interpretation of the effect of radiation factors on interstitial pneumonitis also needs to take into account other factors that cause lung damage and/or immunosuppression, as well as the presence or absence of opportunistic pathogens.

In a recent analysis from the International Bone Marrow Transplant Registry (WEINER et al. 1986) more than 90% of 932 leukemia patients were given cyclophosphamide plus total body irradiation pretransplant for their immunosuppressive and leukemia cytoreductive effects and more than 70% of the patients were given methotrexate posttransplant to prevent or modify the severity of graft-vs-

host disease. The interaction between cyclophosphamide or methotrexate with irradiation is known to magnify the extent of lung damage produced by any one of the agents alone (PHILLIPS and FU 1978; CHAN et al. 1979). Thus, although the main thrust of this Chapter is on the role of radiation regimens on the incidence of interstitial pneumonitis, it must be born in mind that the etiology is multifactorial, and there are other independent and interacting factors that affect the risk of interstitial pneumonitis.

Shown in Table 1 are the six risk factors that were found to have significant associations with interstitial pneumonitis in multiple logistic analyses. Although the study was not a controlled clinical trial, there was sufficient variability in protocols between centers to allow extensive evaluation of the effect of radiation therapy. Results from this study and others are presented below.

2 Radiation Therapy Parameters

2.1 Dose-Rate and Dose

Dose-rate was the only significant factor ($P < 0.03$) related to the radiation regimen that was associated with the risk of interstitial pneumonitis (WEINER et al. 1986). The association was found only for patients given single-dose irradiation and methotrexate posttransplant to prevent graft-vs-host disease. There appeared to be a dose-response effect at dose-rates in the range from 2.0–6.0 cGy/min (Fig. 2). There was no further increment in the risk of interstitial pneumonitis with dose-rates between 6.0 and 108 cGy/min. This finding is consistent with the observations of TRAVIS et al. (1985) that the dose-rate for single dose total body irradiation must be less than 5 cGy/min to substantially reduce the risk of late radiation toxicity in mice subjected to total body irradiation. The data pre-

Table 1. Significant risk factors for interstitial pneumonitis in marrow allografted leukemia patients from multiple logistic analyses

Prognostic variable	Lower risk	Higher risk	Relative risk	P
Drug to prevent GVHD	Cyclosporine	Methotrexate	2.3	< 0.0002
Age of patient	≤ 21 yr	> 21 yr	2.1	< 0.0001
Karnofsky rating pre-Tx	100%	$< 100\%$	2.1	< 0.0001
Severity of GVHD	None to moderate	Severe	1.9	< 0.003
Interval Dx to Tx	≤ 6 mo	> 6 mo	1.6	< 0.002
Dose-rate of TBI	≤ 4.0 cGy/min	> 4.0 cGy/min	1.4	< 0.03 [a]

GVHD, graft-vs-host disease; Tx, transplantation; Dx, diagnosis; TBI, total body irradiation.
[a] For patients given methotrexate for prophylaxis of graft-vs-host disease

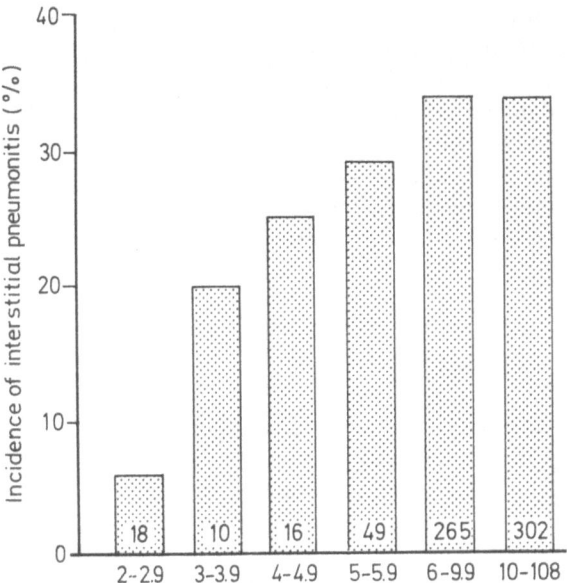

Fig. 2. Relationship between dose-rate of irradiation and the incidence of interstitial pneumonitis for the 660 patients who were treated with total body irradiation and methotrexate. The number within each bar indicates the number of patients in the group

sented in Fig. 2 must be interpreted with caution, since the observed effect of dose-rate on the risk of interstitial pneumonitis was evaluated independently of the total dose deliver (WEINER et al. 1986).

We (WEINER et al. 1986) found no association between lung dose of irradiation and interstitial pneumonitis (Fig. 3). At the extremes of total lung dose, the incidence of interstitial pneumonitis was 35% both in a group of 69 patients who received a mean lung dose of 5.6 Gy and in a group of 133 patients who received a mean lung dose of

12.8 Gy. SLOANE et al. (1983) likewise found no dose-response relationship between lung doses of 9.1–13.0 Gy and the incidence of interstitial pneumonitis.

It is possible that inaccuracies in measurement of lung dose and differences in methods of reporting between centers may have obscured a dose-response relationship. However, taken together, these data suggest that in this dose range the contribution of total body irradiation to the development of interstitial pneumonitis was overshadowed by other etiologic factors. This interpretation is supported by the discrepancy between total lung doses received with total body irradiation and the doses known to be tolerated when the thorax only is irradiated (e.g., BREUER et al. 1978). Further, interstitial pneumonitis is known to occur following allogeneic bone marrow transplantation, even in the absence of irradiation (WEINER 1987). As the dose of total body irradiation is increased, the contribution of radiation to the incidence of interstitial pneumonitis may become apparent. For example, in an attempt to reduce the probability of persistent leukemia in patients transplanted in relapse, the Seattle bone marrow transplant team (CLIFT et al. 1982) increased the dose of total body irradiation progressively from 14 Gy to 15.75 Gy to 17.5 Gy, all in seven daily fractions. At these three dose levels, the incidence of fatal pneumonitis was 0/19, 0/5 and 2/3, respectively.

2.2 Fractionation

PETERS et al. (1979) suggested on radiobiological grounds that fractionated total body irradiation would improve the tolerance of the lung for a given level of leukemia cell kill relative to a single dose at a high dose-rate. Subsequently, the Memo-

Fig. 3. Incidence of interstitial pneumonitis following mean lung doses of irradiation from 5.6–12.8 Gy. The number within each bar indicates the number of patients in the group

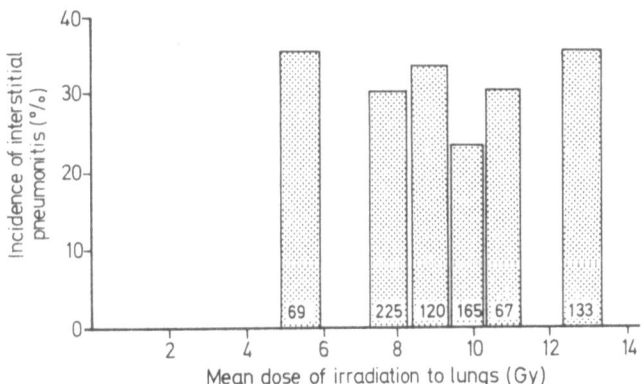

rial Sloan-Kettering bone marrow transplant team (SHANK et al. 1981) reported that fractionated total body irradiation was associated with a marked reduction in the incidence of interstitial pneumonitis. Their incidence was 70% (14/20) in patients given a lung dose of 10.0 Gy in a single fraction at a dose-rate of 5.0–7.0 cGy/min, and it decreased to 33% (16/48) with a fractionated regimen consisting of a total dose of 13.2 Gy in 11 equal fractions of 120 cGy administered over 4 days at a dose-rate of 10–19 cGy/min. Lung blocks were used to limit the total lung dose to approximately 9 Gy with electron beam boosts to the ribs and chest wall.

The Seattle team (MEYERS et al. 1982) in an uncontrolled study also found a decreased incidence of interstitial pneumonitis in allografted leukemia patients treated with fractionated total body irradiation (37%, 30/82) vs single dose (51%, 94/165); however, the difference was not statistically significant. In a controlled study comparing fractionated vs single-dose irradiation in 53 patients with acute nonlymphoblastic leukemia, the Seattle team found a 21% overall incidence of interstitial pneumonitis (THOMAS et al. 1982). They found no significant difference in the incidence of interstitial pneumonitis when single-dose (26%, 7/27) was compared with fractionated irradiation (15%, 4/26). In a larger but uncontrolled study, MEYERS et al. (1983) of Seattle reported that among allografted leukemia patients who received fractionated total body irradiation, the incidence of interstitial pneumonitis was 29% (91/315) in comparison with an incidence of 44% (132/299) among patients who received single-dose total body irradiation ($P < 0.001$). The difference was due primarily to a reduced incidence of idiopathic interstitial pneumonitis in the patients given fractionated total body irradiation. The incidence of cytomegalovirus-associated interstitial pneumonitis was similar in both groups.

Data from the International Bone Marrow Transplant Registry (WEINER et al. 1986) disclosed similar incidences of interstitial pneumonitis among patients given fractionated irradiation (30%, 100/334) compared with patients given single-dose total body irradiation (29%, 163/561). Because of the variety of radiation protocols followed, a subset comparison was made between two groups of patients who received either 10 Gy single dose or 12 Gy fractionated. These two lung doses were described by THOMAS et al. (1982) as radiobiologically equivalent. Animal studies (FIELD et al. 1976 and TRAVIS et al. 1983) indicate,

however, that the radiobiological effects on the lung are greater for 10 Gy in a single fraction vs 12 Gy in 4–8 fractions. We found the incidence of interstitial pneumonitis was 24% among the 121 patients who received a single lung dose of 10 Gy and 36% among the 70 patients who received a total lung dose of 12 Gy administered in 5 or 6 fractions. This difference was not statistically significant.

3 Summary

The complication of interstitial pneumonitis is one of the major causes for morbidity and mortality following allogeneic bone marrow transplantation in leukemia patients. Multiple independent and interacting factors predispose to the disease. Multiple logistic analyses of data from the International Bone Marrow Transplant Registry indicate that, within the range available for investigation, the only parameter of the radiation regimen that was a significant risk factor for interstitial pneumonitis was the dose-rate at which radiation was administered. And dose-rate was important only for patients given single-dose irradiation and methotrexate to prevent graft-vs-host disease. There was no significant influence of dose fractionation or the total dose delivered. The basis for the observed dose-rate effect is uncertain. The data suggest that low dose-rates of irradiation in patients treated with single-dose irradiation and methotrexate allows repair of lung damage that is sufficient to reduce the risk of interstitial pneumonitis. One may see a significant effect of the mode of delivery of total body irradiation – dose-rate in the case of single dose and size of dose per fraction – only at higher doses.

It should be emphasized that the analyses from the International Bone Marrow Transplant Registry were not based on prospective clinical trials. Although multivariate statistical techniques were used to adjust for other variables that may have influenced or biased the results, the results are subject to all the caveats of a retrospective analysis. Furthermore, the radiation lung doses may not be calibrated in the same way for all reporting institutions. Prospective and randomized controlled clinical trials using sophisticated radiation delivery systems and dosimetry are required to permit rigorous evaluation of the radiobiological concepts involved in optimizing the role of radiation in the context of bone marrow transplantation for leukemia.

Acknowledgements. Sincere thanks to the members of the Advisory Committee who participated in all of the International Bone Marrow Transplant Registry studies and on which we relied heavily for this report. (Members of the Advisory committee: ROBERT PETER GALE, M.D., Ph.D., Los Angeles, Chairman; FRITZ H. BACH, M.D., Minneapolis; A. JOHN BARRETT, M.D., MRC Path, London; DIRK W. VAN BEKKUM, M.D., Ph.D., Rotterdam; JAMES C. BIGGS, D. Phil. (Oxon) Sydney; KARL G. BLUME, M.D., Duarte; KAREL A. DICKE, M.D., Ph.D., Houston; ELIANE GLUCKMAN, M.D., Paris; JOHN M. GOLDMAN, M.D., London; ROBERT A. GOOD, M.D., Ph.D., St. Petersburg; ROGER H. HERZIG, M.D., Cleveland; RICHARD HONG, M.D., Madison; JOHN H. KERSEY, M.D., Minneapolis; HANS J. KOLB, M.D., Munich; ALBERTO M. MARMONT, M.D., Genoa; TOHRU MASAOKA, M.D., Osaka; HANS A. MESSNER, M.D., Toronto; RICHARD J. O'REILLY, M.D., New York City; RAY L. POWLES, M.D., London; ALFRED A. RIMM, Ph.D., Milwaukee; OLLE RINGDEN, M.D., Ph.D., Huddinge; JON J. VAN ROOD, M.D., Ph.D., Leiden; CIRIL ROZMAN, M.D., Barcelona; BRUNO SPECK, M.D., Basel; ROY S. WEINER, M.D., GAINESVILLE; FERRY E. ZWANN, M.D., Ph.D., Leiden) Thanks to Ms. D'ETTA W. KOSER, Ms. MARJORIE MITCHELL and Mr. TODD SIEFERT for help with data analysis and to Ms. KAREN WITKOWSKI for preparing the typescript. Finally, we thank Dr. LESTER J. PETERS who critically reviewed an earlier version of the manuscript and provided helpful suggestions.

References

Bortin MM (1983) Pathogenesis of interstitial pneumonitis following allogeneic bone marrow transplantation for acute leukemia. In: Gale RP (ed) Recent advances in bone marrow transplantation. Alan R. Liss, Inc., New York, pp 445–460

Bortin MM et al. (1982) Factors associated with interstitial pneumonitis after bone marrow transplantation for acute leukemia. Lancet 1:437–439

Breuer K et al. (1978) Irradiation of the lungs as adjuvant therapy in the treatment of osteosarcoma of the limbs. An E.O.R.T.C. randomized study. Eur J Cancer 14:461–471

Chan PYM et al. (1979) Pulmonary complications of combined chemotherapy and radiotherapy in lung cancer. In: Vaeth JM (ed) Combined effects of chemotherapy and radiotherapy on normal tissue tolerance. S. Karger, Basel, pp 136–144

Clift RA et al. (1982) Allogeneic marrow transplantation using fractionated total body irradiation in patients with acute lymphoblastic leukemia in relapse. Leukemia Res 6:401–407

Field SB et al. (1976) Effects of fractionated irradiation on mouse lung and a phenomenon of slow repair. Br J Radiol 49:700–707

Khouri NF et al. (1979) Pulmonary interstitial changes following bone marrow transplantation. Radiology 133:587–592

Meyers JD et al. (1982) Nonbacterial pneumonia after allogeneic marrow transplantation: a review of 10 years' experience. Rev Inf Dis 4:1119–1132

Meyers JD et al. (1983) Biology of interstitial pneumonia after marrow transplantation. In: Gale RP (ed) Recent advances in bone marrow transplantation. Alan R. Liss, Inc., New York, p 405

Peters LJ et al. (1979) Radiobiological considerations in the use of total-body irradiation for bone-marrow transplantation. Radiology 131:243–2477

Phillips TL, Fu KK (1978) The interaction of drug and radiation effects on normal tissues. Int J Radiat Oncol Biol Phys 4:59–64

Pino y Torres JL et al. (1982) Risk factors in interstitial pneumonitis following allogeneic bone marrow transplantation. Int J Radiat Oncol Biol Phys 8:1301–1307

Shank B et al. (1981) Hyperfractionated total body irradiation for bone marrow transplantation: Early results in leukemia patients. Int J Radiat Oncol Biol Phys 7:110–115

Sloane JP et al. (1983) Histopathology of the lung after bone marrow transplantation. J Clin Pathol 36:546–554

Thomas Ed et al. (1982) Marrow transplantation for acute nonlymphoblastic leukemia in first remission using fractionated or single-dose irradiation. Int J Radiat Oncol Biol Phys 8:817–821

Travis EL et al. (1983) Repair in mouse lung between multiple small doses of X-rays. Radiat Res 94:326–339

Travis EL et al. (1985) Effect of dose-rate on total body irradiation: lethality and pathologic findings. Radiotherapy & Oncology 4:341–351

Weiner RS et al. (1987) Interstitial pneumonitis following bone marrow transplantation. In: Gale RP, Champlin RE (eds) Recent advances in bone marrow transplantation. Alan R. Liss, Inc., New York, pp 507–523

Weiner RS et al. (1986) Interstitial pneumonitis following bone marrow transplantation: Assessment of risk factors. Ann Intern Med 104:168–175

Winston DJ et al. (1979) Infectious complications of human bone marrow transplantation. Medicine 58:1–31

3.3 Total Lymphoid Irradiation for Immunosuppression

Richard T. Hoppe and Samuel Strober

CONTENTS

ABBREVIATIONS

TLI	Total lymphoid irradiation
PHA	phytohemagglutinin
MLR	mixed lymphocyte reaction
DNCB	2,5-dinitrochlorobenzene
AIDS	acquired immune deficiency syndrome
ATG	anti-thymocyte globulin
SLE	systemic lupus erythematosus
CMV	cytomegalovirus

1 Experimental Background

1.1 Immunosuppressive Effects of Total Lymphoid Irradiation (TLI) in Patients Treated for Hodgkin's Disease

Total lymphoid irradiation (TLI) is a potent means of immunosuppression. The immunosuppressive effects of TLI in patients treated for Hodgkin's disease were detailed by Fuks et al. (1976) in an analysis of 227 treated and untreated patients with Hodgkin's disease. They observed a marked depression of the total peripheral blood

Richard T. Hoppe, M.D., Samuel Strober, M.D.
Stanford University
Stanford, CA 94305, USA

lymphocyte count during TLI which persisted for about two years, with gradual recovery to normal levels thereafter in most patients. Examination of lymphocyte populations in these patients revealed differential effects of TLI on specific lymphocyte subsets. For example, the majority of patients were noted to have a persistent decrease in the total number and percent of T-cells (T-lymphocytopenia) and in the same patients there was a compensatory increase in the total number and percent of B-cells (B-lymphocytosis). Therefore, in long term followup, most patients had normal total peripheral blood lymphocyte counts but had a reversal of the normal T/B cell ratio. Furthermore, when subsets of T-cells were examined in patients treated with TLI, a differential sensitivity of various T-cell subsets was observed (Posner et al. 1983). The T-lymphocytopenia was primarily due to a decrease in the number of helper T-cells with a persistence of normal or nearly normal numbers of suppressor T-cells. This resulted in a reversal of the normal helper:suppressor T-cell ratio to a value less than 1.0 compared to a value greater than 1.0 in normal controls or untreated patients with Hodgkin's disease.

Functional assays of lymphocytes revealed impaired ability to respond to mitogens such as phytohemagglutinin (PHA) and this persisted for at least ten years. The ability to respond to allogeneic cells in the mixed lymphocyte reaction (MLR) was markedly impaired at the completion of TLI but gradual recovery was observed more than two years after completion of therapy (Fuks et al. 1976). Impaired reactivity of lymphocytes in the *autologous* MLR was also noted in patients followed as long as 15 years (Engleman et al. 1980).

Total lymphoid irradiation also alters cutaneous delayed hypersensitivity reactions. Patients with untreated Hodgkin's disease often show defects in cell mediated immunity manifest by an impaired ability to respond to neo-antigens such as 2,5-dinitrochlorobenzene (DNCB) (Kaplan 1980). However, even those patients who have an intact ability to respond to a challenge with DNCB following sensitization, lose that ability following completion of TLI (Fuks et al. 1976). Although gradual recovery of DNCB reactivity is observed in the majority of these patients, nearly one-third will remain anergic.

Despite the degree and severity of the immunosuppression observed in vitro, only minimal potential immunological complications of any clinical significance have been reported in these patients (Kaplan 1980). The primary manifestation of this immune impairment is the development of infection with Herpes zoster which occurs in nearly one-third of patients. The likelihood of developing Herpes zoster is closely correlated with the duration of time since completion of TLI, with most infections occurring during the first two years of follow up. Even in these patients, the disease is usually limited to a single dermatome or two adjacent dermatomes and only rarely disseminates cutaneously or extracutaneously. Other opportunistic infections have not been reported in association with TLI. This is despite the fact that the effects of TLI on T-cell number and T-cell subsets are similar to those that have been reported in people with the acquired immune deficiency syndrome (AIDS) (Siegal 1984).

1.2 Animal Models for the Study of Total Lymphoid Irradiation

Following identification of the in vitro immunological abnormalities induced by TLI in man, a variety of animal models were developed to further define and exploit these immunosuppressive effects. Slavin et al. (1976) developed a technique for treating mice with TLI. Anesthetized mice were immobilized in a jig which provided shielding of the skull, lungs, long bones of the extremities, a portion of the pelvis, and the tail. The majority of the lymphoid tissue including that of the mediastinum, thymus, and mesentery was exposed to the radiation beam. Animals were treated with 250 Kv orthovoltage x-rays, 2 Gy per day, 5 days per week, to a total dose of 34 Gy. Adult BALB/c mice treated in this fashion developed changes in lymphocyte number, T- and B-cell percentages and functional immunologic impairment similar to that observed in patients treated with TLI for Hodgkin's disease.

Similar animal models were developed for other species and similar degrees of in vitro immune abnormality were demonstrated. Identical fractionation programs to those used in the mouse proved

feasible in other rodent species such as the rat. However, in larger mammals including dogs and non-human primates, hematologic tolerance did not permit the delivery of 34 Gy TLI in just 17 fractions. An alternative dose and fractionation program was identified which was associated with minimal morbidity and yet induced a similar degree of immune impairment to that seen with the 34 Gy program in smaller animals. This program consisted of the administration of 1 Gy fractions to TLI fields, 4 or 5 fractions per week, for a total cumulative dose of 18–20 Gy (Modry et al. 1983).

1.3 Transplantation Studies in Animals Treated With Total Lymphoid Irradiation

Following the development of animal models for TLI, attempts were made to utilize TLI as a means of immunosuppression to promote organ transplantation. When BALB/c (H-2d) mice were irradiated and then engrafted with skin from a histoincompatible C57BL/Ka (H-2b) mouse, graft survival increased five fold compared to unirradiated controls (Slavin et al. 1977). Subsequent studies in mice examined the ability of TLI to promote bone marrow engraftment as well as skin graft survival. Nearly all BALB/c mice treated with TLI followed by infusion of bone marrow cells from C57BL/Ka donors developed chimerism. These chimeric BALB/c mice showed no evidence of graft versus host disease (GVHD). When BALB/c mice pretreated with TLI received *both* bone marrow cells and skin grafts from C57BL/Ka donors, chimerism developed and permanent skin graft survival was demonstrated. These chimeric animals showed specific tolerance for C57BL/Ka skin grafts. Studies in rats demonstrated similar results (Slavin et al. 1978). In addition, these studies demonstrated permanent survival of heart allografts in TLI-treated rats infused with bone marrow cells from the heart donor despite major histocompatibility differences.

Experiments were performed to explain the lack of GVHD in TLI-mouse chimeras. These indicated that the induction of tolerance was mediated by nonspecific suppressor cells which developed after TLI but that the maintenance of tolerance was mediated by specific suppressor cells generated by the donor-host cell interactions (Strober et al. 1981).

In larger animals, although bone marrow chimerism could be induced following TLI treatment and bone marrow infusion (GOTTLIEB et al. 1980) permanent survival of organ grafts could not be demonstrated reliable with TLI either alone or in combination with bone marrow infusion. However, TLI in combination with other immunosuppressive modalities such as antithymocyte globulin (ATG), azathioprine, or cyclosporin-A appears to act synergistically and provide for long term graft survival in several large animal models (PENNOCK et al. 1981; MODRY et al. 1983).

1.4 The Use of Total Lymphoid Irradiation in Animal Models of Autoimmune Disease

A variety of animal models of autoimmune diseases have been examined with respect to the potential impact of TLI (HOPPE et al. 1984). These animal models include the immune-complex glomerulonephritis which develops in (NZB/NZW F_1 hybrid mice, the SLE-like syndrome of MRL/l mice, nephrotoxic serum nephritis in the inbred Lewis rat, adjuvant arthritis in the Lewis rat, collagen arthritis in rats, and chronic experimental allergic encephalomyelitis in juvenile strain-3 guinea pigs. Experimental data from two of these systems are reviewed in more detail.

NZB/NZW F_1 hybrid mice develop an autoimmune disease characterized by anti-nuclear antibodies and a fatal immune-complex glomerulonephritis which is similar to the nephritis observed in human systemic lupus erythematosus (SLE). KOTZIN and STROBER (1979) examined the impact of fractionated TLI (17 fractions of 2 Gy) on the development of nephritis in these animals. When animals with *low grade* proteinuria were irradiated, their survival six months after TLI was 90%. This compared to a six-month survival of only 25% in the control group. Deaths in all of the control animals were related to progressive renal disease. In another experiment, animals which had already developed *high grade* proteinuria were given TLI or sham irradiation. In the sham irradiated group there were no survivors six weeks later, compared to a survival of 75% in the TLI group. Among the irradiated animals which were still alive, nearly 80% had a reversal of the high grade proteinuria.

A useful animal model to test the potential efficacy of agents in the treatment of rheumatoid arthritis is adjuvant arthritis in rats. Adjuvant arthritis can be induced by a subcutaneous injection of mineral oil combined with Mycobacterium butyricum into one of the rat paws. SCHURMAN et al.

(1981) irradiated a group of rats with adjuvant arthritis utilizing either TLI (17 fractions of 2 Gy), paw irradiation (3 doses of 2 Gy) or both TLI and paw irradiation. Rats that were treated with TLI developed significantly less inflammation than the control group throughout the followup period. The inflammation and deformity measured in rats treated with paw irradiation alone was slightly reduced compared to the controls. The arthritis activity of animals treated with both TLI and low dose paw irradiation was the most dramatically altered.

2 Human Clinical Trials of Total Lymphoid Irradiation for Transplantation

The successful use of TLI in animal models of autoimmune disease and in animal-organ transplantation studies together with the relative lack of long term morbidity of TLI in patients treated for Hodgkin's disease led to the development of human clinical trials utilizing TLI as a means of immunosuppression. The major proving ground for TLI as a component of the immunosuppressive regimen for patients undergoing organ transplantation has been in the area of renal transplantation. Although fractionated TLI has been used in a small number of patients to promote bone marrow transplantation or heart transplantation, only renal transplantation has been investigated in a significant number of patients at several clinical centers.

The transplant group at the University of Minnesota was the first to report its results utilizing TLI as a component of the immunosuppressive regimen in patients undergoing renal transplantation (NAJARIAN et al. 1982). They selected patients who were at high risk for rejection based upon a history of prior rapid rejection of a renal graft. Patients underwent splenectomy at the time of initial renal transplant and therefore were asplenic at the time that TLI was administered. Patients were treated with TLI in 1–1.25 Gy fractions four or five days per week. After a total dose of 32 Gy was delivered, patients were placed on maintenance TLI programs with 1.25 Gy fractions delivered twice a week until an appropriate donor was identified. Total doses ranged from 10–40 Gy depending upon hematological tolerance and organ availability. Following TLI and renal transplantation patients were treated with maintenance azathioprine (1.0–1.5 mg/kg/day) and prednisone. Immunological studies following completion of TLI revealed a depletion of T-cells, predominantly in the helper-T-cell subset. In addition, there was functional impairment of residual T-cells documented by impaired response to mitogens. Among the 22 patients treated on this protocol, the two year graft function rate and two year patient survival rate were 72% and 75%, respectively, compared to 38% and 67% for the historical control group treated only with standard immunosuppression.

Investigators at the University of Leuven, Belgium, have utilized fractionated TLI prior to cadaveric renal transplantation in patients with type 1 diabetes and end-stage diabetic nephropathy. Prior to the initiation of TLI, bilateral nephrectomy and splenectomy were generally performed. Patients were treated with TLI, 1 Gy fractions, to a total dose of 20–30 Gy. Maintenance immunosuppression following TLI and renal transplantation consisted of prednisone, 15 mg per day. Prednisone was increased and azathioprine instituted whenever a rejection episode intervened (VANREN-TERGHEM et al. 1984). With a median follow up of approximately one year, functioning grafts were still in place in nine of ten patients. However, at least one rejection episode was observed in every patient who had been followed for more than two months. The median time to onset of the first rejection episode was more than three months, compared to only 18 days in a concurrent group of patients treated with conventional immunosuppression. Complications potentially related to irradiation in these patients included opportunistic infections with cytomegalovirus (CMV) and Herpes zoster, two instances of E-coli sepsis, mild bronchopneumonia, and a myocardial infarction. In vitro tests of immune function in the TLI group revealed more severe impairment of PHA-, Concanavalin-A, and pokeweed mitogen – induced blastogenesis, the mixed lymphocyte reaction, and cell-mediated lympholysis than in a control group which received standard immunosuppression. In addition, reversal of the normal T-helper:suppressor ratio was observed in the TLI group (WAER et al. 1984).

A collaborative program utilizing TLI prior to cadaveric renal transplantation was also developed at Stanford University and the Pacific Medical Center. The intent of this program was to combine TLI with ATG, reduce other means of chronic immunosuppressive therapy and thereby avoid some of the long term complications of immunosuppression (SAMPSON et al. 1985). An attempt was made to administer TLI in 1 Gy fractions, three

days per week, to a total dose of 20 Gy. Both the mantle and inverted-Y/spleen fields were to be treated each day. However, hematologic intolerance often necessitated interuption of therapy. This occurred more commonly than in the experience reported from the University of Minnesota and University of Leuven because most patients treated at those institutions had undergone splenectomy prior to initiation of TLI. When this occurred and treatment was later resumed, the mantle alone was treated with 1 Gy fractions, 4 or 5 days per week to a total cumulative dose of 20 Gy. This was followed immediately by treatment to the inverted-Y/spleen field, also with 1 Gy fractions, 4 days per week, to a total dose of 20 Gy. At the completion of TLI, patients received maintenance therapy of 1 Gy per week to the inverted-Y/spleen field until an acceptable organ donor was identified. Following TLI and renal transplantation patients were treated with six injections of ATG and then maintained on low dose prednisone (up to 0.14 mg/kg/day). Prednisone was increased and azathioprine instituted if a rejecion episode developed. Fourteen patients were treated in this fashion and twelve had good initial graft function. Four of these patients developed rejection episodes during the first year. Two were treated successfully, one patient lost his kidney graft, and one patient died from disseminated Herpes simplex during treatment for rejection with ATG. Two additional patients developed rejection episodes after the first year of follow up and these were both successfully treated. Overall, there were 10 intact and functioning renal grafts in the twelve evaluable transplanted patients. Complications observed during TLI in this group of patients included leukopenia, thrombocytopenia, flare of uremic pericarditis, mild nausea and fatigue. Following transplantation and institution of the other immunosuppressive agents, complications included opportunistic infections with Herpes zoster, Herpes simplex, and CMV.

3 Human Clinical Trials of Total Lymphoid Irradiation for Autoimmune Diseases

3.1 Rheumatoid Arthritis

The first autoimmune disease to be studied systematically with respect to the effects of TLI was rheumatoid arthritis. Concurrent trials were carried out at Stanford University and Harvard University (KOTZIN et al. 1981; TRENTHAM et al. 1981). Patients were selected for these trials who had severe rheumatoid arthritis with active synovitis and significant disability. They had to have been treated unsuccessfully with non-steroidal anti-inflammatory agents, gold, and penicillamine. All patients would have otherwise been candidates for cytotoxic therapy.

In the Stanford trial, TLI treatment consisted of 20 Gy in ten fractions of 2 Gy delivered in two weeks to the mantle field followed immediately by 20 Gy in three weeks (4 fractions of 1.5 Gy per week) to the inverted-Y/spleen field (KOTZIN et al. 1981). Patients were evaluated carefully on at least two occasions prior to initiation of therapy and serially thereafter with specific attention to joint tenderness, joint swelling, duration of morning stiffness, and a global comosite score which consisted of fourteen subjective and objective variables. In addition, patients underwent serial immunological monitoring. In the Stanford experience, improvement was generally reported within three months after completion of TLI with an average improvement of 61% in joint tenderness, 49% in joint swelling, 72% in morning stiffness, and 45% in the global composite score. Overall, nine of eleven patients had significant improvement (more than 35% improvement) in all four clinical parameters. Further follow up revealed that improvement persisted throughout the follow up period without any tendency for patients to develop a progression of disease to baseline levels (FIELD et al. 1983). Immunological evaluation of these patients after TLI revealed an impaired ability of their peripheral blood lymphocytes to respond to mitogens such as PHA and Con-A and also to allogeneic lymphocytes in the MLR. In addition, there was a significant inhibition of pokeweed mitogen induced immunoglobulin synthesis. Interestingly, after TLI there was no improvement in humoral responses associated with rheumatoid arthritis such as the presence of rheumatoid factor. Analysis of lymphocyte populations revealed a significant decrease in the total number of T-cells after TLI. Although there was a decrease in both the helper/inducer and suppressor/cytotoxic populations, a preferential effect on the helper/inducer population led to a reversal of the normal helper/inducer: suppressor/cytotoxic ratio with an excess of the suppressor/cytotoxic cells observed in patients after completion of TLI. Complications of treatment included mild systemic effects such as nausea and fatigue. local effects including dysphagia, xerostomia, and esophagitis. In addition, Herpes zoster occurred occasionally. One patient with Felty's syndrome developed an exacerbation of that syndrome during TLI and another patient with rheumatoid lung disease developed progression of pulmonary symptoms after completion of TLI. Occasional bacterial infections were noted either during or following treatment with TLI.

The Harvard treatment program utilized a higher dose and more protracted course of treatment (TRENTHAM et al. 1981). Patients received 30 Gy to the mantle field followed by a two week split, then 30 Gy to the paraaortic-spleen field, another two week split, and finally 30 Gy to the pelvic nodes. The improvement noted in these patients at six months was similar to that reported by the Stanford group. There appeared to be a tendency towards progression of disease in these patients by one year, although patients were still improved compared to their baseline level. In longer term follow up the Harvard group observed more significant infectious complications in their patients than was reported from Stanford.

In a subsequent study from Stanford, patients were randomized to treatment with 20 Gy TLI or a fractionated 2 Gy program (STROBER et al. 1985). In the 2 Gy program, patients received 0.2 Gy fractions to the mantle for a total dose of 2 Gy followed by 0.2 Gy fractions to the inverted-Y/spleen field to a total dose of 2 Gy. Patients treated with 20 Gy TLI showed significant improvements in joint tenderness, joint swelling, morning stiffness, and global composite score compared to pretreatment determinations. Patients treated with 2 Gy TLI showed progression of morning stiffness, essentially no change in joint tenderness or the global composite score, but significant improvement in joint swelling compared to pretreatment measurements. When the 20 Gy group was compared to the 2 Gy group, the higher dose program was significantly more beneficial with respect to joint tenderness, morning stiffness, and the global composite score. While the higher dose group had less joint swelling after TLI than did the low dose group, the differences were not statistically significant. Immunological monitoring showed that patients treated with the 2 Gy TLI program developed none of the immunological abnormalities previously identified after the higher dose TLI progrem.

3.2 Lupus Nephritis

A trial testing the efficacy of TLI for severe lupus nephritis has recently been reported from Stanford (STROBER et al. 1985). Patients were selected for this program who had nephritis which failed to respond to high dose prednisone or in whom prednisone could not be reduced below 0.5 mg/kg/day. TLI was administered according to the same protocol as was used in rheumatoid arthritis. Following completion of TLI, the serum albumin increased in all patients and the 24-hour urinary protein decreased in nine of ten patients. This was accompanied by a reduction in the serum anti-DNA antibodies or an increase in the serum complement in every patient. Significant improvements in the mean glomerular filtration rate and estimated renal plasma flow were also noted after the complation of TLI. In addition, eight of ten patients were receiving lower daily doses of prednisone at the time of last follow up compared to immediately before the initiation of TLI. The median follow up in this group of patients is 15 months.

4 Future Directions

The early promising results observed with TLI in organ transplantation and autoimmune disease trials, suggests a broad range of questions for future study. In the area of renal transplantation important considerations include the development of an optimal program of TLI with respect to total dose, fraction size, and timing of therapy. The optimal combination of TLI with other immunosuppressive therapies such as ATG, prednisone, azathioprine, cyclosporin-A, and monoclonal antibodies will also need to be defined. We will have to learn what minimal amount of chronic immunosuppressive therapy will be required to prevent late rejection of the engrafted organ. The introduction of TLI treatment programs for recipients of kidneys from living related donors will also be an important issue should cadaver studies continue to show promise.

The possible role of TLI prior to transplantation of other organs will also be explored. Data from animal models suggests an important potential role for fractionated TLI prior to bone marrow transplantation, although limited clinical experience has not confirmed these experimental data. The use of TLI prior to engraftment of other organs such as the heart, heart and lungs, or liver may also develop into clinical trials in the future.

Early clinical experience with TLI for the management of human autoimmune diseases suggests that the irradiation may alter the course of these diseases but not reverse all of their manifestations.

In rheumatoid arthritis, important issues include consideration of use of TLI earlier in the course of the disease, before many of the destructive joint changes have developed. In addition, the efficacy of TLI compared to cytotoxic therapies may have to be confirmed in a prospective randomized clinical trial. Important questions also remain regarding the duration of response following TLI and the development of alternative fractionation programs to provide for shorter treatment courses. In addition, there remains the basic question of why TLI works for these diseases. Studies are currently underway at Stanford looking at the kinetics of the changes of lymphocyte subpopulations both in the peripheral blood and in the synovium of patients being treated with TLI for rheumatoid arthritis. Based on these results, we may consider combining TLI with joint irradiation in studies analogous to those done in animals.

Other autoimmune diseases in addition to rheumatoid arthritis and lupus nephritis should be investigated to test the impact of TLI. A limited clinical experience testing TLI in advanced multiple sclerosis is being acquired at the New Jersey Medical College and a small number of patients have been treated for chronic progressive demyelinating neuropathy at the University of Colorado.

This is a fascinating, relatively new area of basic and clinical research in radiation therapy. Most of these studies are collaborative ventures between the radiation therapists, and immunologists, rheumatologists, transplant surgeons, and other specialists. Should these studies prove successful, it will herald the development of a totally new application of radiation in the management of human disease.

References

Engleman EG, Benike CJ, Hoppe RT, Kaplan HS, Berberich FR (1980) Autologous mixed lymphocyte reaction in patients with Hodgkin's disease: Evidence for a T-cell defect. J Clin Invest 66:149–158

Field EH, Strober S, Hoppe RT, Calin A, Engleman EG, Kotzin BL, Tanay AS, Calin HJ, Terrell CP, Kaplan HS (1983) Persistent improvement of intractable rheumatoid arthritis after total lymphoid irradiation. Arthritis and Rheumatism 26:937–946

Fuks Z, Strober S, Bobrove AM, Sasazuki T, McMichael A, Kaplan HS (1976) Long term effects of radiation on T and B lymphocytes in peripheral blood of patients with Hodgkin's disease. J Clin Invest 58:803–814

Gottlieb M, Strober S, Hoppe RT, Grumet FC, Kaplan HS (1980) Engraftment of allogeneic bone marrow without graft-versus-host disease in mongrel dogs using total lymphoid irradiation. Transplantation 29:487–491

Hoppe RT, Strober S, Kaplan HS (1984) Total lymphoid irradiation in the management of autoimmune diseases and organ transplantation. In: Phillips T and Pistenmaa DA (eds) Radiation Oncology Annual I, Raven Press, New York, p 205–232

Kaplan HS (1980) Hodgkin's disease, 2nd edn. Harvard University Press, Cambridge, Mass, p 366–441

Kotzin BL, Strober S (1979) Reversal of NZB/NZW disease with total lymphoid irradiation. J Exp Med 150:371–378

Kotzin BL, Strober S, Engleman EG et al. (1981) Treatment of intractable rheumatoid arthritis with total lymphoid irradiation. N Engl J Med 305:959–976

Modry DL, Strober S, Hoppe RT, Bieber CP, Pennock JL, Koretz S, Jamieson SW, Reitz BA, Stinson EB, Kaplan HS (1983) Total lymphoid irradiation: experimental models and clinical appliation in organ transplantation. Heart Transplantation 2:122–135

Najarian JS, Ferguson RM, Sutherland DER, Slavin S, Kim T, Kersey J, Simmons RL (1982) Fractionated total lymphoid irradiation as preparative immunosuppression in high risk renal transplantation. Clinical and immunlogical studies. Ann Surg 196:442–452

Pennock JL, Reitz BA, Bieber CP, Aziz S, Oyer PE, Strober S, Hoppe R, Kaplan HS, Stinson EB, Shumway NE (1981) Survival of primates following orthotopic cardiac transplantation treated with total lymphoid irradiation and chemical immune suppression. Transplantation 32:467–473

Posner MR, Reinherz E, Lane H, Mauch P, Hellman S, Schlossman SF (1983) Circulating lymphocyte populations in Hodgkin's disease after mantle and paraaortic irradiation. Blood 61:705–708

Sampson D, Levin BS, Hoppe RT, Bieber CP, Modry D, Girinski T, Kaplan HS, Strober S (1985) Clinical observations on the use of total lymphoid irradiation in human cadaver renal transplantation. Transplantation Proceedings 17:1299–1303

Schurman DJ, Hirshman HP, Strober S (1981) Total lymphoid and local joint irradiation in the treatment of adjuvant arthritis. Arthritis Rheum 24:38–44

Siegal FD (1984) Immune dysfunction in AIDS. Sem in Oncol 11:29–39

Slavin S, Reitz B, Bieber CP, Kaplan HS, Strober S (1978) Transplantation tolerance in adult rats using total lymphoid irradiation: permanent survival of skin, heart, and marrow allografts. J Exp Med 147:800–807

Slavin S, Strober S, Fuks Z, Kaplan HS (1976) Long-term survival of skin allografts in mice treated with fractionated total lymphoid irradiation. Science 193:1252–1254

Slavin S, Strober S, Fuks Z, Kaplan HS (1977) Induction of specific tissue transplantation tolerance using fractionated total lymphoid irradiation in adult mice: long-term survival of allogeneic bone marrow and skin grafts. J Exp Med 146:34–48

Strober S, Field E, Hoppe RT, Kotzin BL, Shemesh D, Engleman E, Ross JC, Myers BD (1985) Treatment of intractable lupus nephritis with total lymphoid irradiation. Ann Intern Med 102:450–458

Strober S, King DP, Gottlieb M, Hoppe RT, Kaplan HS (1981) Induction of transplantation tolerance after total lymphoid irradiation: cellular mechanisms. Federation Proc 40:1463–1465

Strober S, Tanay A, Field E, Hoppe RT, Calin A, Engleman EG, Kotzin B, Brown BW, Kaplan HS (1985) Efficacy of total lymphoid irradiation in intractable rheumatoid arthritis. A double-blind, randomized trial. Ann Intern Med 102:441–449

Trentham DE, Belli JA, Anderson RJ et al. (1981) Clinical and immunological effects of fractionated total lymphoid irradiation in refractory rheumatoid arthritis. N Engl J Med 305:976–982

Vanrenterghem Y, Waer M, Ang K, van der Schueren E, Gruwez J, Bouillon R, Michielsen P (1984) Cadaveric kidney transplantation in diabetics after total lymphoid irradiation (TLI). Transplantation Proc 16:636–639

Waer M, Vanrenterghem Y, Ang KK, van der Scheuren E, Michielsen P, Vandeputte M (1984) Comparison of the immunosuppressive effect of fractionated total lymphoid irradiation (TLI) vs conventional immunosuppression (CI) in renal cadaveric allotransplantation. J Immunol 132:1041–1048

3.4 Half Body Radiotherapy

Walter D. Rider

CONTENTS

1 Introduction and Evolution

"Necessity is the mother of invention and serendipity the handmaiden".

The Toronto philosophy in radiotherapy has, for several decades, been one of large volume irradiation in preference to the more classical teaching of "excisional therapy" using small volumes and high dose. In this respect our pattern of practice has been different and unique. However, it was based on critical retrospective reviews of "patterns of failure." In most sites where an improvement in survival was demonstrated, this was due to increased volume irradiated rather than increased dose; care was taken to exclude other variables,

Walter D. Rider, Professor
The Princess Margaret Hospital
Toronto, Ontario M4X 1K9, Canada

e.g., stage or grade, which might have been more responsible for any improvement than the therapy itself.

With this background it was not difficult to make the transition to using radiation as a systemic adjuvant, particularly because at that time chemotherapy was in its infancy. Thus a pilot study in Ewing's tumor suggested that 3 Gy total body irradiation as a single fraction was not only well tolerated but might have contributed to the improved survival (Jenkin et al. 1970). On the other hand the dose used was clearly too low to effect anything more than a 90% cell kill, if one is to believe radiobiology.

It was speculated that 8 Gy might give a cell kill of 99.9%, but how could that be delivered to the whole body without producing fatal haematologic complications? Further speculation suggested that (a) in slow growing tumors the "time to regrowth might be of sufficient length to afford significant palliation, and (b) that these tumors were unlikely to reseed from metastases in the weeks between the two half body irradiations" (Rider 1974).

Experimental data have demonstrated that survival from an otherwise lethal dose of total body irradiation is possible if some haemapoietic tissue is protected: it is assumed that the animal's irradiated bone marrow is reseeded from the protected volume.

Thus we had a hypothesis, all we needed was the courage and opportunity to try it. The opportunity was provided by a very special patient.

This lady was riddled with painful metastases from breast cancer and was nonresponsive to hormone manipulation. Her painful lesions were treated whenever there was cause, and various doses were used, ranging from 4 to 10 Gy as single treatments. Rarely did a week go by without us having to treat one or more of these exquisitely tender areas located, most often, in the subcutaneous tissues. After many such single treatments, she presented with intense pain in much of the lower half of her body, and demanded that she be treated in one sitting to save her the trouble of returning every week. Review of her previous irradiation suggested that the lowest dose that had relieved her pain was 6 Gy. We were given the consent of her only relative, her son, who is a physician, and proceeded to deliver, to the lower half of her body, 6 Gy ^{60}Co irradiation in a single exposure. The umbilicus was selected as the dividing mark between upper and lower half because it is so readily identifiable. The response was dramatic; her pain was relieved within 24 h. Her haematologic status was monitored very carefully for the next few months and showed practically no depression. Subsequently, her upper half was irradiated, also because of pain and with similar results.

Since our first publication in 1976, over 100 reports have now appeared in the literature on the subject of half body radiotherapy and describing its effectiveness as a palliative procedure.

2 Techniques

Generally speaking, our practice is to divide the body into two halves using the umbilicus as the landmark. However, this is, and can be modified to suit clinical circumstances. Thus "umbilicus to knees", mid-body, or the exclusion of the head are options not uncommonly used; much depends on the type of cancer being treated and the stage of the disease, but Murphy's Law in half body irradiation states that recurrences will appear in those areas shielded from the irradiation.

2.1 Equipment

Originally half body irradiation was carried out using a standard AECL Model 8 Cobalt 60 unit, and by extending the S.S.D. to encompass the desired volume (FITZPATRICK and RIDER 1976a, b). Because of the demand for this technique, a dedicated Cobalt 60 unit was built in our own workshop and named the "Hemitron". It can be used for all manner of large field therapy and is ideal for total body irradiation (LEUNG et al. 1981).

A review of the literature indicates that there are as many techniques as publications and all energies from Cobalt 60 to 20 MeV have been used.

Thus, it would appear that equipment, or energy, are not critical, but one thing is sure, the physics and dosimetry must be carefully considered if a uniform and homogeneous dose is to be delivered to the patient (RIDER and VAN DYK 1983).

2.2 Dose

As has been discussed in several publications (VAN DYK et al. 1981), the limiting dose for this technique is determined by pulmonary tolerance.

If single exposures at dose rates in excess of 25 cGy min^{-1} are used, the following doses of megavoltage irradiation should not be exceeded:

a) Lower Half: 10 Gy
b) Upper Half: 8 Gy. This dose must be calculated using sophisticated inhomogeneity corrections, preferably based on lung density measurements obtained by C.T. scanning.

Our experience in the use of fractionated half body irradiation is limited to a few patients, but it is an area worthy of further study. We have found that 14 Gy given as 1 Gy daily fractions (5 days per week) to the lower half has been safe, and well tolerated. Because of our worry about radiation pneumonitis, we have limited the dose to the upper half to 8 Gy (uncorrected for inhomogneity) using the same fractionation (1 Gy/day). It would be unwise to use N.S.D. or similar correction methods to extrapolate from our single fraction recommendations to "safe" doses for factionation.

Retreatment: We have retreated the lower half to 8 Gy on a number of occasions and found this to be safe. We have not retreated the upper half, but with appropriate lung shielding this should be possible.

Considerable clinical judgement must be exercised when considering H.B.I. after previous irradiation. All target tissues must be considered. On the other hand, previous areas of "spot irradiation" are rarely contraindications to H.B.I. provided that the area of lung included was small (e.g. 8 × 10 cm).

3 Toxicity

3.1 Acute

3.1.1 Radiation Sickness

This classical syndrome has been well described by us and others (RIDER and HASSELBACK 1968; DANJOUX et al. 1979). It occurs in about 80% of patients subjected to upper half body irradiation and about 10% following lower half body irradiation using the doses described above. Vomiting, usually without preceeding nausea, occurs within one hour of the start of radiation and is followed by lassitude and sleep; this picture recurs at intervals for 4–8 hours with each vomiting episode decreasing in severity until recovery, after which the patient is frequently very hungry. We have found antiemetics to be of no value, and indeed might be hazardous because of aspiration pneumonia in the sedated patient.

3.1.2 Gastrointestinal

A small number of patients will suffer a transient bout of diarrhea within hours of the irradiation and others will experience it within a few days.

3.1.3 Salivary Gland

Salivary function may be disturbed in 10–20% of patients. This may take the form of a dry mouth, as well as a painful parotiditis. Occasionally the eyes also become dry. These are self limiting complications of short duration.

3.1.4 Pyrexia

Pyrexia as a brief phenomenon has been observed.

3.1.5 Acute Pulmonary Distress

Acute pulmonary distress has been reported; two patients developed this syndrome within 100 minutes of irradiation and one died (DAWES 1979). We have not seen this picture in over 500 patients treated by upper half body irradiation and suspect that factors other than radiation pneumonitis accounted for the clinical picture.

3.2 Chronic

3.2.1 Haematologic

Our first concern, when we started this technique, was haematologic toxicity. It was soon learned that by monitoring the blood counts frequently, and, most importantly, by plotting them on a semilog graph it was possible to determine when it was safe to carry out the second half body irradiation. Semilog plotting of blood counts is far more

effective than "eye balling" a series of blood counts and highlights the hazardous circumstance. The observed blood counts, of course, may be modified by previous therapy, or from reduction of "bone marrow reserve" by the underlying disease. In the average case we found that an interval between the two half body irradiations of 5 weeks or more is required for haematologic safety.

It is still not clear whether bone marrow seeding from non-irradiated haematologic cells accounts for tolerance, or whether stem cells in the Haversian canals, which are considered to be resistant because of hypoxia (ALLALUNIS et al. 1984) are responsible for haematologic recovery. At the moment there seem to be no way in man of separating these hypotheses.

3.2.2 Pulmonary

Clearly the lungs are the most critical target organ for upper half body irradiation.

Originally few patients with an expected survival of greater than 90 days were treated, but as the spectre of haematologic intolerance faded we found that some patients lived longer than expected. Some of these survivors died of respiratory failure. An investigation of these patients was carried out (FRYER et al. 1978) which revealed a dose/response curve and a frighteningly high actuarial risk of radiation pneumonitis if the uncorrected dose to lung exceeded 7 Gy in a single fraction.

Subsequently a more detailed analysis was carried out (VAN DYK et al. 1981) in which C.T. derived lung density figures were used to determine the absolute dose absorbed in the lungs. This produced a realistic dose/response curve and demonstrated that for our technique 8 Gy absolute lung dose carried less than 5% risk of radiation pneumonitis.

VAN DYK noted a correlation between patient thickness (AP diameter) and a dose correction factor which could be applied to the uncorrected dose in order to give the absolute dose to lung. This nomogram is very useful when facilities for C.T. derived tissue densities are not available (VAN DYK et al. 1981).

When calculating the absolute lung dose account must be taken of all physical characteristics of the beam being used and the position and configuration of the patient. Thus the correction factor decreases with increasing energy, and lateral fields create greater variations in dose than AP:PA fields.

It is well to remember that the shape, size, and construction of the radiation room may make significant contributions to dosimetry.

Clinical picture of radiation pneumonitis. This syndrome is non-specific and can be mimicked by advancing cancer, pulmonary hypertension, and interstitial pneumonia. The most important factor in its recognition is the circumstances of previous irradiation to one or both lungs, and "clinical suspicion". Characteristically there is sudden onset of shortage of breath, a dry hacking cough and radiologic features of scattered areas of increased density throughout the irradiated lung tissue. The peak incidence is at about 90 days post-radiation but it can occur between 30 and 120 days; the interval to onset is not dose dependent within the range of 6 to 12 Gy (single fraction ^{60}Co). Withdrawal of steroid therapy may precipitate the syndrome. Unfortunately, lung biopsies are not pathognomonic, and the presence of opportunistic infections does not necessarily rule out the diagnosis. In fatal cases, death occurs within 10–14 days in 90% of cases irrespective of treatment. The rare non-fatal case resolves spontaneously; treatment makes no difference, although steroids are often prescribed; serial lung function studies are useful in monitoring the progress. C.T. scans in the prone and supine positions will sometimes demonstrate shift of the interstitial fluid presumably due to gravity.

Great care must be exercised in the diagnosis; the administration of chemotherapy on the assumption of "advancing cancer" can convert the nonfatal case into the fatal.

3.2.3 Renal and Hepatic

At the moment there is only one group of patients suitable for study of radiation effects on liver and kidney uncomplicated by the effects of the underlying malignancy. This is a group of 20 men who were subjected to midbody irradiation (MBI) as part of the primary management of prostatic cancer, when no evidence of metastases was proven.

MBI is defined as a large field extending from the level of the nipples to the midthighs. This volume was irradiated to 8 Gy as measured at the midplane in a single dose and no inhomogeneity corrections were used.

With a median observation time of 36 months, no abnormalities in hepatic or renal function have been observed by serial biochemical methods of assessment. These data suggest that a single dose of 8 Gy to liver and kidney is safe.

3.2.4 Neurologic

Only one neurologic complication, which could not be related to effects of cancer, has been observed, and this was under the unusual circumstances of a 65 year old male with Charcot-Marie-Tooth disease since adolescence. Within 1 week of irradiation to the uper half-body (8 Gy ^{60}Co) the patient went into a total motor neurologic decline, and suffered a transient radiation pneumonitis. The clinical picture was one of profound muscle weakness, with depression of all motor reflexes without any sensory changes being observed. Recovery was slow and gradual, until almost 4 months later when he returned to his preirradiation status. It is postulated that radiation suppresses oligodendrocyte division and consequently the production of myelin, which is integral to the conduction of nerve impulses (RIDER 1963) and that the radiation insult to the CNS was magnified because of a pre-existing defect in myelin production which accompanies Charcot-Marie-Tooth disease.

The pathogenesis of Charcot-Marie-Tooth disease and radiation myelopathy may have some common ground in that both may result from a process of demyelination.

3.2.5 Cataract

For patients who survive more than two years cataract is a distinct possibility, the price of which must be considered in the overall scheme of management. Recent data from the bone marrow transplant program at Seattle (DEEG et al. 1984) provides some evidence as to the dose/response but this is confused by the complexity of previous treatment (chemotherapy, and steroids) as well as the effects of graft versus host disease. These authors claim a benefit from fractionated irradiation over a single dose.

In our bone marrow transplant program, T.B.I. as a single fraction of 5 Gy (^{60}Co at 60 cGy/min) has been employed for the past 5 years (RIDER and MESSNER 1983); four asymptomatic early cataracts have been detected in about 100 patients at risk.

3.2.6 Leukemia

We have treated 6 patients with upper and lower half body irradiation to 4 Gy in the management of late stage rheumatoid arthritis. These patients had run the gamut of „rheumatic therapy" including steroids, aspirin, gold alkylating agents, immunosuppression. etc. Four of these patients were serologically confirmed rheumatoid arthritis, and two were not. Two patients have developed fatal acute myeloid leukemia within two years of irradiation, and both were typical rheumatoid arthritics. The association of increased risk of leukemia in patients treated by irradiation for ankylosing spondylitis, many years ago, is currently under re-evaluation; it is suspected now that ankylosing spondylitis and other "rheumatoid" diseases, as treated by current methods, have a higher incidence of leukemia than the normal population, even without the confounding issue of irradiation. It is well know that alkylating agents alone carry a leukemic risk.

At the moment, half body irradiation (total lymphoid irradiation) is not recommended until further investigation has elucidated the mechanisms involved.

3.2.7 Fertility

This important aspect in the quality of survival cannot be assessed on our data, and may never become an issue unless the half body technique is extended into pediatric oncology. There are some indications that this may well happen in the future.

Our somewhat anecdotal experience suggests that the ovaries in adolescent patients are relatively radioresistant; thus we have four children born to two patients following total body irradiation (3 Gy) used in the management of Ewing's tumor. Both patients have survived 18 years, and the children are normal. One girl who was irradiated to the whole abdomen with 20 Gy in 20 fractions at the menarche (for recurrent and metastatic dysgerminoma), proceeded to a delayed onset of menses, but some five years later was delivered of a normal child. The combination of multi-drug chemotherapy and half body irradiation will almost certainly result in permanent sterility if the patient survives.

4 Combination of Chemotherapy and Half Body Irradiation

This is a thorny problem in the practice of oncology in North America and will remain so as long as medical oncologists fail to be party to multidisciplinary management when the diagnosis of cancer is first made.

In our experience haematologic recovery is complete after half body irradiation, such that it is possible, with rare exceptions, to administer chemotherapy without dose modifications.

When chemotherapy is given first, and to maximum tolerance, the situation is quite different. In such cases, it is usually best to avoid half body radiotherapy as a "last resort"; the risks of complications far outweigh the chances of benefit to the patient.

The above comments do not negate the use of half body irradiation when it is integrated with chemotherapy in the overall management of malignant disease from the beginning.

5 Half Body Radiotherapy and Radiosensitizers

On first principles, half body radiation, as a single fraction, combined with a hypoxic cell radiosensitizer, given as an intravenous bolus, should be a good method of testing the virtue of radiosensitizers. However, it is a difficult study to carry out because assessment of response, be it subjective or objective, is fraught with so many variables. Nonetheless, the concept should not be ignored.

6 Future Prospects

The somewhat serendipitous introduction of half body irradiation in 1971 defied most of the tenets of "good radiotherapy". However, the relief of pain from metastases in bone proved to be significant and the morbidity (after recognition of radiation pneumonitis) was low. Because of the frequency of breast and prostate cancers our major experience has been with these two.

In the 100 publications in the literature to date, half body radiotherapy has been attempted in one form or another in practically all types of malignancy. Many papers record its use in lung cancer in an adjuvant setting with conflicting results. Some good results have been claimed in multiple myeloma (ROWLAND et al. 1983).

It is clear that the full potential has not been evaluated; there is room for innovative studies using fractionation as well as single doses.

A few anecdotes might point the way to future studies:

a) A female of 60 years of age was treated for stage 3A non-Hodgkin's lymphoma by two half body doses of 5 Gy each, because she lived far from haematology services which would have been required had chemotherapy been used. More than 8 years later she is free of disease and is a model of cost effectiveness.

b) A male of 48 years was investigated for haematuria revealing a tumor of the bladder neck invading the prostate producing a fixed mass of 8–10 cm diameter. Histologic sections revealed an anaplastic carcinoma with no features to indicate its site of origin, either bladder or prostate. Bone scan was negative but bipedal lymphography was convincingly positive in all nodes demonstrated. In our experience this syndrome carried a 90% mortality within 2 years whether it is considered to be a carcinoma of prostate or bladder and hormone manipulation is ineffective.

He was treated by half body radiotherapy, 8 Gy to the lower and 6 Gy (uncorrected) to the upper. The patient failed to return for follow-up assessment regarding a "boost" to the primary site until 4 months after treatment. Examination under anesthesia and cystoscopy at that time revealed no evidence of disease. A year later a repeat lymphogram was perfectly normal and 6 years later he remains free of disease. The boost dose was never given.

c) A male aged 63 presented with squamous cell carcinoma of left main bronchus with positive nodes on mediastinoscopy and a 10 cm metastatic mass in the right scapula with bone destruction. Liver scan was considered positive for metastases. He was treated by upper half body irradiation, excluding the head, in 1 Gy fractions daily to 20 Gy with a concomitant 5 FU infusion during the first 4 days of irradiation (1.0 gm/m^2 continuous daily × 4). About day 70 he developed interstitial pneumonia which resolved spontaneously over the next 30 days. By 90 days his chest was radiologically clear, the scapular mass had vanished, and his liver scan was reported as "probably normal". Approximately 6 months post treatment he presented with a mass in the left tendo-Achillis which on biopsy was squamous cell carcinoma. This metastases was treated by 1 Gy fractions × 20 daily without chemotherapy and showed no response. The patient died of cerebral metastases 12 months post treatment without signs of recurrence in upper half body irradiation volume.

7 Animal Studies

Dogs suffer from a variety of non-Hodgkin's lymphoma, many of which are of high grade of malignancy and advanced stage, e.g., V A and B. Recently in cooperation with the Veterinary College at the Guelph University, Ontario, we have treated a small series of dogs with half body irradiation; 7 Gy to each half with a month's interval between the two HBIs. Remissions have occurred in most dogs, but recurrences have also developed. The patterns of radiation sickness, haematologic change and x-ray studies of the lungs are quite different from man. We hope, in the future, to assess the value of half body radiotherapy in the less malignant lymphomas which are, histologically, more comparable to those in humans, e.g. Stage IV. This is an attempt to evaluate the prospects of using this technique in man. If it proves to be successful, it would have tremendous cost effectiveness.

8 Conclusions

Half body radiotherapy is a technique with tremendous potential that has not been fully realized in the decade since it was introduced. Clearly much work has still to be done in order to define dose, fractionation and possible combination with chemotherapy and possibly radiosensitizers.

Acknowledgements. Although it is a single author report, it is evident from the references that many people at Princess Margaret Hospital have contributed their time and talents in radiation oncology and clinical physics. I acknowledge a deep gratitude to all my colleagues, past and present, who have contributed to this experience. I would be remiss not to single out Dr. PETER FITZPATRICK for his sterling contribution, and likewise to my secretary, Mrs. SARAH ROBINSON, for her efforts.

References

Allalunis MJ, Turner AR, Chapman JD (1982) Misonidazole enchances cyclophosphamide toxicity to bone marrow. Int J Radiat Oncol Biol Phys 8:655–658

Danjoux CE, Rider WD, Fitzpatrick PJ (1979) The acute radiation syndrome. A memorial to William Michael Court-Brown. Clin Radiol 30:581–584

Dawes PJ (1979) Acute pulmonary distress following high dose irradiation of the upper half body. Br J Radiol 52 (623):876–879

Deeg JH, Flournoy N, Sullivan KM, Sheehan K, Buckner CD, Sanders JE, Storb R, Witherspoon RP, Thomas ED (1984) Cataracts after total body irradiation and bone marrow transplantation: a sparing effect of dose fractionation. Int J Radiat Oncol Biol Phys 10:957–964

Fitzpatrick PJ, Rider WD (1976a) Half body radiotherapy of advanced cancer. J Can Assoc Radiol 27:75–79

Fitzpatrick PJ, Rider WD (1976b) Half body radiotherapy. Int J Radiol Oncol Biol Phys 1:197–207

Fryer CJH, Fitzpatrick PJ, Rider WD, Poon P (1978) Radiation pneumonitis: experience following a large single dose of radiation. Int J Radiat Oncol Biol Phys 4:931–936

Jenkin RDT, Rider WD, Sonley MH (1970) Ewing's sarcoma. A trial of adjuvant total body irradiation. Radiology 96:151–155

Leung PMK, Rider WD, Webb HP, Johns HE (1981) Cobalt 60 therapy unit for large field radiation. Int J Radiat Oncol Biol Phys 7:705–712

Rider WD (1963) Radiation damage to the brain. A new syndrome. J Can Assoc Radiol 14:67–69

Rider WD (1974) Innovations in radiation therapy. JAMA 227:183–184

Rider WD, Hasselback R (1968) The symptomatic and haematological disturbances following total body radiation of 300 rad gamma ray irradiation. In: Guidelines to radiological health. U.S. Publ Health Serv Publ No 999-RH-33 p. 139–144

Rider WD, Messner HA (1983) Magna-field irradiation: work in progress in bone marrow transplantation at the Princess Margaret Hospital, Toronto. Int J Radiat Oncol Biol Phys 9:1967

Rider WD, Van Dyk (1983) Total and partial body irradiation. In: Bleehen N, Glatstein E, Haybittle JL (eds) Radiation Therapy Planning. Marcel Dekker, New York and Basel, p. 559–694

Rowland CG, Garrett MJ, Crowley C (1983) Half body radiation in plasma cell myeloma. Clin Radiol 507–510

Van Dyk J, Keane TJ, Kan S, Rider WD (1981) Dose-response curve for radiation pneumonitis based on absolute dose to lung. Int J Radiat Oncol Biol Phys 7:461–467

Weiden PL, Wright SE (1972) Vincristine neurotoxicity. New Engl J Med 286:1369–1370

3.5 Targeted Radionuclides

STEVEN A. LEIBEL

CONTENTS

1 Introduction

Radiolabeled antibodies with specificity against tumor-associated antigens offer an exciting opportunity in oncology. Targeted radionuclides may have application in the diagnosis, staging, and treatment of malignancy as well as in the follow-up of previously treated patients. This review will focus on the use of radiolabeled antibodies to deliver radiation therapy. The historical observations leading to the current interest in targeted radionuclides will be summarized. Tumor antigens which serve as the target for radiolabeled antibodies and pertinent aspects of antibody preparation will be reviewed. The rationale for radioimmunotherapy is based on the ability of radioimmunoglobulin to selectively target to tumor both in patients and in experimental animals. From this research clinical trials have emerged, and the results of these preliminary studies will be presented.

This investigation was supported by PHS Grant Number CA21439 awarded by the National Cancer Institute, DHHS.

STEVEN A. LEIBEL, M.D., Associate Professor
University of California, School of Medicine
San Francisco, CA 94143, USA

1.1 Historical Background

The concept of using radiolabeled antibodies to detect cancer was originated by Pressman (PRESSMAN and KEIGHLEY, 1948). PRESSMAN and KORNGOLD (1953) and BALE et al. (1955) showed that labeled antibodies against Wagner osteosarcoma and Walker carcinoma could be successfully targeted to these allogeneic tumors in rats. SPAR et al. (1967) conducted diagnostic and therapeutic studies using ^{131}I-labeled antibodies to human fibrinogen. This pursuit was based on the rationale that fibrin and fibrinogen were deposited in areas of tumor ischemia and necrosis. Interest in this approach was limited because of inconsistent results and lack of tumor specificity (DELAND and GOLDENBERG 1983). The isolation of tumor-associated antigens by GOLD and FREEDMAN (1965) led to renewed enthusiasm in exploring targeted radionuclides. Targeting of radiolabeled polyclonal antibodies to tumor-associated antigens for imaging was first described by Quinones et al. (1971) who used ^{125}I labeled rabbit anti-human chorionic gonadotropin (hCG) immunoglobulin G (IgG) to scan a human testicular choriocarcinoma growing in the cheek pouch of a Syrian hamster. GOLDENBERG et al. (1978) reported the successful diagnostic imaging of tumors in patients using radiolabeled affinity-purified polyclonal antibodies to carcinoembryonic antigen (CEA). Clinical trials in which radiolabeled polyclonal antibodies were used for the treatment of patients were pioneered by ORDER et al. (1980a, b).

A major advance in this field has been the ability to produce monoclonal antibodies using the hybridization technique of KOHLER and MILSTEIN (1975). Several groups have achieved successful tumor imaging using radiolabeled monoclonal antibodies to a variety of specificities (MACH et al. 1981; FARRANDS et al. 1982; EPENETOS et al. 1982; and LARSON et al. 1983a). Clinical trials employing radiolabeled monoclonal antibodies for therapy have been initiated (LARSON et al. 1983b; EPENETOS et al. 1984).

1.2 Tumor-Associated and Tumor-Specific Antigens

Tumor antigens serve as the target for radiolabeled antibody in radioimmunotherapy. They have been referred to as "tumor-associated" and "tumor-specific". Many of the tumor-associated antigens that have been described are present in normal tissues, but are inappropriately expressed in malignancy. Within this category are the oncofetal antigens (Alexander 1972) including CEA, alphafetoprotein (AFP) and ferritin. Gamma globulin in plasma cell dyscrasias, hormone-like substances in small cell lung carcinoma and renal cell carcinoma, and the pregnancy-associated tumor antigen, hCG, are also included within this grouping. They exemplify increased synthesis or inappropriate expression of normal cell products. "Tumor-specific" antigens are those which are restricted to a single malignancy. Although tumor-specific antigens have been demonstrated in animal malignancies, they have been difficult to identify in malignancies in humans (Goldenberg 1976) except in B-cell lymphomas (Pauwels and Cleton 1984).

Antigens best suited as targets for radiolabeled antibody are those that are expressed on the cell surface or that are shed into the stroma and interstitial space surrounding the tumor cell (DeLand and Goldenberg 1983). Tumor antigens need not be tumor-specific for preferential targeting (Order and Leibel 1984). In fact, tumor-associated antigens may be more advantageous targets than tumor-specific antigens; tumor-specific antigens may be limited in concentration and subject to modulation, whereas tumor-associated antigens found in the stroma surrounding tumor cells quantitatively provide more target for radioimmunoglobulin (Order 1982).

1.3 Antibodies for Radioimmunotherapy

Immunoglobulin G is the type of immunoglobulin employed in current research in radioimmunotherapy. This antibody can be subdivided using proteolytic enzymes; with papain digestion, for example, IgG can be divided into three molecules: two Fab fragments which are involved in antigen binding, and the Fc fragment which is involved with monocyte binding and complement activation. Although immune fragments have some features which are of value in radioimmunoimaging (Pauwels and Cleton 1984) they are not as useful as the whole immunoglobulin molecule in radioim-

munotherapy (Order 1982). Their value in radioimmunotherapy is limited because the fragment is cleared from the body with a much shorter half-life.

The antibody preparation may be polyclonal or monoclonal. Polyclonal-derived antibody is 15–25% specific for the antigen used for immunization and will recognize a number of different antigenic sites on the antigenic moiety. The antibody can be further purified using affinity chromatography, resulting in an antibody with greater than 70% immunospecific reactivity (Goldenberg et al. 1978). Homogeneous monoclonal antibodies that recognize a single antigenic specificity can be raised in large quantity using hybridoma methodology (Kohler and Milstein 1975). Radiolabeled polyclonal antibodies have been used in the clinical trials to be described. The use and limitations of monoclonal antibodies in radioimmunotherapy will be discussed later in this review.

2 Radioimmunotherapy

2.1 Rationale for Radioimmunotherapy

2.1.1 Tumor Imaging

Successful scanning with radiolabeled polyclonal antibodies and with affinity-purified polyclonal and monoclonal antibodies against a number of specificities including anti-CEA, anti-AFP, anti-hCG, and antiferritin has been achieved both in experimental models and in the clinic (Goldenberg and DeLand 1982). The presence of circulating antigen does not preclude tumor localization (Rhodes et al. 1983). Radioimmunoimaging with polyclonal and intact antibodies or fragments of monoclonal antibodies has been found to successfully localize a number of malignancies (Table 1). The demonstration that radiolabeled antibodies with specificity against tumor-associated antigens could successfully localize in tumor led to the development of phase I–II studies using polyclonal antibody labeled with therapeutic doses of [131]I.

2.1.2 Antiferritin IgG

The antibody used most frequently in radioimmunotherapy has been antiferritin IgG. Ferritin is found in normal tissues including the heart, spleen, liver, and bone marrow (Munro and Linder 1978). The thymus-derived lymphocytes in

Table 1. Malignancies successfully imaged with radiolabeled antibody

Primary Tumor	Reference
Colorectal carcinoma	DeLand and Goldenberg 1983; Mach et al. 1983
Melanoma	Larson et al. 1983a, b
Ovarian carcinoma	Leibel et al. 1981; DeLand and Goldenberg 1983; Epenetos et al. 1985
Testicular carcinoma	Goldenberg et al. 1983
Choriocarcinoma	Bagshawe et al. 1980; Goldenberg et al. 1980b
Intrahepatic biliary carcinoma	Ettinger et al. 1978
Hepatoma	Order et al. 1980a
Hodgkin's disease	Order et al. 1980b
Neuroblastoma	Order et al. 1981
Non-oat cell lung carcinoma	DeLand and Goldenberg 1983; Moylan et al. 1985
Breast carcinoma	Wright et al. 1979; Epenetos et al. 1982; DeLand and Goldenberg 1983
Medullary carcinoma of the thyroid	Berche et al. 1982
Prostate carcinoma	Goldenberg and DeLand 1982
Renal cell carcinoma	Belitsky et al. 1978
Pancreas carcinoma	DeLand and Goldenberg 1983
Gastric carcinoma	Berche et al. 1982; DeLand and Goldenberg 1983
Cervical carcinoma	DeLand and Goldenberg 1983

Hodgkin's disease synthesize and secrete ferritin (Sarcione et al. 1977), and ferritin may be crystallized and purified from Hodgkin's tumor tissue (Eshhar et al. 1974). Lymphoscintigraphy (Order et al. 1975) and radionuclide scans following intravenous administration of ^{131}I antiferritin IgG (Order et al. 1981) in patients with Hodgkin's disease demonstrated that radiolabeled antibody selectively targeted tumor but not normal tissues including those with high concentrations of ferritin such as the spleen. Ferritin, an oncofetal tumor-associated antigen, has been identified in a number of other malignancies including hepatoma, neu-

roblastoma, acute myelogenous leukemia, monocytic leukemia, multiple myeloma, and carcinomas of the lung, breast, and pancreas (Leibel 1983).

The selection of the radionuclide ^{131}I was based on its known efficacy in the treatment of both hyperthyroidism and thyroid carcinoma. Polyclonal antibody is easily labeled with ^{131}I without affecting the antigen-binding properties of the antibody.

2.1.3 Experimental Hepatoma Model

Using the H4-II-E rat hepatoma model which synthesizes and secretes ferritin, Rostock et al. (1983) compared non-specific ^{131}I-labeled IgG with ^{131}I-labeled rabbit antiferritin antibody. A threefold increase in tumor deposition with antiferritin compared with nonspecific IgG demonstrated that specificity of antiferritin was necessary to achieve tumor deposition. Radiolabeled antiferritin uptake could be blocked by pretreatment with non-labeled antiferritin antibody. Radiolabeled antiferritin IgG did not bind to normal tissues to a greater degree than did nonspecific radioimmunoglobulin.

The term "biologic window" has been used to describe the features that allow preferential tumor targeting including: 1) a tumor vasculature lacking smooth muscle and competent walls; 2) a quantitatively higher concentration of tumor-associated antigen at the tumor site; and 3) slower blood flow through the tumor (Rostock et al. 1984a). As predicted by the biologic window theory, tumor size, vascularity, and ferritin content correlate with tumor localization. Rostock et al. (1984a, b) demonstrated in the hepatoma model that smaller tumors synthesize and secrete ferritin at a higher rate, and have a greater vascular cross section than larger tumors. As tumors increase in size both a reduction in vasculature and ferritin secretion occurs. Coincident with the decrease in ferritin production and vasculature, a reduction in tumor targeting takes place.

Isotopic immunoglobulin may have other antitumor activity in addition to local irradiation from isotope deposition. As demonstrated in an ovarian cancer model, the Fc portion of the IgG molecule may bind host macrophages leading to macrophage cytotoxicity (Order et al. 1974). Because it is foreign to the host, bound heterologous antibody can also elicit an antigenic response resulting in macrophage processing with T and B lymphocytes, leading to anti-antibody production (Order 1984).

2.2 Clinical Trials Employing Radiolabeled Polyclonal Antibody

Polyclonal radiolabeled antibodies were introduced into clinical trials by Order and his colleagues in 1979. Studies for the treatment of primary hepatic malignancy, Hodgkin's disease, and non-oat cell lung carcinoma have been carried out at Johns Hopkins Hospital, University of California San Francisco, Thomas Jefferson University Hospital, and Albert Einstein Medical Center, Philadelphia, under the aegis of the Radiation Therapy Oncology Group (RTOG).

2.2.1 Primary Hepatic Malignancy

Hepatoma. The identification of ferritin as a tumor-associated antigen both on the tumor cell surface and in the stroma of hepatoma (BECK and BOLLACK 1974) and the poor response of hepatoma to conventional therapy (FRIEDMAN 1983) led to the development of clinical trials employing ^{131}I antiferritin antibody. A series of phase I–II studies were introduced for patients with nonresectable hepatoma (with or without metastatic disease) who were previously untreated or who failed to respond to chemotherapy. At the time of initiation of these studies, no knowledge existed as to the methodology of delivery, dosimetry, toxicity, or efficacy of isotopic immunoglobulin, and their purpose was to determine guidelines for its clinical application. The study design was modified as insight into the use of isotopic immunoglobulin unfolded.

The initial phase I–II trial was a single-dose escalation study to gain knowledge of the dosimetry and toxicity of radiolabeled antibody administration. Patients received external radiation therapy to the whole liver to a dose of 2100 rad in 7 fractions, integrated with intravenous doxorubicin (15 mgm), and 5-FU (500 mgm). This was followed in one month by two monthly cycles of doxorubicin (60 mgm/m²) and 5-FU (500 mgm/m²), and followed one month later by ^{131}I labeled rabbit antiferritin IgG in single escalating doses of 50 mCi, 100 mCi, and 150 mCi. The observation that patients were progressing during the two cycles of chemotherapy led to the omission of the second round of chemotherapy, and the induction regimen of external irradiation and chemotherapy was followed in one month by radiolabeled antibody.

The dose escalation study showed that 30 mCi was sufficient to saturate the tumor, and doses up to 150 mCi resulted in increased free circulating radiolabeled antibody and total body irradiation but not a higher dose to the tumor. The tumor-effective half-life for ^{131}I rabbit antiferritin IgG was 4 to 5 days (LEICHNER et al. 1983). Based on tumor dose kinetic studies, the administered dose of ^{131}I

was reduced to the tumor saturation dose of 30 mCi; and to extend the tumor-effective half-life over a longer period of time, a second dose of 20 mCi was given 4 to 5 days later. Toxicity was limited to thrombocytopenia and less frequently leukopenia occurring 4–6 weeks after treatment, with recovery by 8 weeks. The degree of hematologic toxicity was proportional to the administered mCi dose of ^{131}I (ETTINGER et al. 1982).

Cyclic radioimmunotherapy was next introduced using antibody derived from different animal species to permit retreatment without inappropriate immune reaction. The final protocol integrated the most effective species of ^{131}I antiferritin IgG (rabbit, pig, monkey, and bovine) with doxorubicin (15 mg) and 5-FU (500 mg) given on the day before antibody treatment. The rationale for using this approach was to potentiate the dose rate effect of ^{131}I (SHERMAN et al. 1982) and to implement the observation that chemotherapy enhanced the response to antiserum therapy in experimental tumor models (LEIBEL et al. 1981). Escalating doses of doxorubicin and 5-FU were evaluated and the final schedule was chosen on the basis of the observed hematologic toxicity with higher drug doses. Chemotherapy and radioimmunotherapy were administered cyclically every two months, the time required for hematologic recovery between cycles (Fig. 1).

Dosimetry. Radiation dose calculations to the tumor and normal tissues were estimated employing the method of absorbed fractions of the Medical Internal Radiation Dose Committee of the Society of Nuclear Medicine (LEICHNER et al. 1983). A tumor dose of 1,000 to 1,200 rad at a dose rate of 5 rad/hour was deposited following a dose of 30 mCi of ^{131}I labeled antiferritin IgG on day 0 and 20 mCi on day 5 (Table 2). ^{131}I anti-ferritin IgG deposited 8.4 µCi/g to the tumor and a comparison of mean activities deposited per gram in tumor with normal tissue revealed a tumor to liver ratio of 4.8 to 1 (Table 3) (LEICHNER et al. 1984). A linear relationship was demonstrated between tumor volume and the maximum activity of ^{131}I-labeled polyclonal antiferritin deposited in the tumor for hepatomas with a volume of less than 2000 cc. For larger tumors (2290 to 3020 cc) the tumor to liver ratio was 1.6. These findings are consistent with those in the experimental hepatoma model (ROSTOCK 1984a).

In the phase I–II studies, ^{131}I-labeled rabbit anti-AFP was compared with ^{131}I antiferritin IgG. ^{131}I anti-AFP deposited 2.7 µCi/gram to the tumor, with a tumor to liver ratio of 1.0; and the combination of antiferritin and anti-AFP deposited a tumor activity in the tumor of 7.3 µCi/gram, with a tumor to liver ratio of 2.9. Treatment with anti-AFP antibody did not lead to tumor regression, and its use was discontinued. The use of affinity-purified antibody and antibody fragments resulted in a reduced tumor-effective half-life and

Induction therapy										
Days	1	2	3	4	5	6	7	8	9	10
Liver irradiation (Gy) +	3	3	–	3	3	–	–	3	3	3
Adriamycin, 15 mg	+	–	–	+	–	–	–	+	–	+
5FU, 500 mg	+	–	–	+	–	–	–	+	–	+

1 month
Self Care (Karnofsky 60% or greater)
Stratify
AFP ⊕ vs AFP ⊖

Randomize

Adriamycin, 60 mg/m² and 5FU, 500 mg/m²   ¹³¹I Antiferritin IgG

Repeat q 3 weeks   30 mCi (day 0), 20 mCi (day 5)
+
Adriamycin, 15 mg and 5FU, 500 mg, (day-1)

Repeat q 2 months

Two cycles minimal treatment, each arm of study from time of randomization:
25% volumetric progression of tumor = protocol failure
30% volumetric regression = partial response

Fig. 1. Treatment schema of phase III randomized prospective trial (RTOG 83-19) comparing adriamycin and 5-FU to ¹³¹I labeled antiferritin IgG plus adriamycin and 5-FU in the treatment of hepatoma. All patients receive induction therapy consisting of external irradiation with alternate day doxorubicin and 5-FU. Patients are stratified by AFP titer

Table 2. Radiation dose estimates for ¹³¹I-labeled antiferritin, anti-AFP, antiferritin + anti-AFP, and anti-CEA. Dose calculations for antiferritin and anti-AFP are for administered activities of 30 mCi on day 0 and 20 mCi on day 5; for anti-CEA 20 mCi on day 0 and 10 mCi on day 5. (From LEICHNER et al. 1984)

Antibody	Effective half-life (days)		Radiation dose (rads)		
	Tumor and liver	Total body	Tumor	Liver	Total body
Antiferritin[a]	4.6	3.5	1100	230	45
Anti-AFP	4.4	3.6	350	350	50
Antiferritin + Anti-AFP	4.2	3.3	960	330	50
Anti-CEA	4.0	3.6	620	140	30

[a] Antiferritin dose estimates are for tumor volume less than 2290 cm³

was not superior to polyclonal antibody (LEICHNER et al. 1984).

Method of Administration. Antiferritin antibody was prepared from splenic tumor infiltrates of patients with Hodgkin's disease and labeled with iodine-131 using the lactoperoxidase method with a specific activity of 8–10 mCi/mgm. Sterility and pyrogen testing were carried out before antibody treatment was administered.

Table 3. Mean activities per gram (µCi/g) in tumor and liver tissues and tumor to liver ratios. (From LEICHNER et al. 1984)

Antibody	No. of patients	Tumor volumes (cm³)	Mean (range)		
			Mean activity		Tumor-to-liver ratios
			Tumor	Liver	
Antiferritin	18	220–1700	8.4	1.8	4.8
	4	2290–3020	2.6	1.6	1.6
Anti-AFP	5	145–2705	2.7	2.7	1.0
Antiferritin + Anti-AFP	3	780–1326	7.3	2.6	2.9
Anti-CEA	5	467–1275	4.7	1.1	4.4

Table 4. Results of treatment of 105 patients with hepatoma

Response

Following external irradiation and chemotherapy (38 patients evaluable) – 22.8%

Following ^{131}I antiferritin (66 patients evaluable) – 48%

Tumor volume <2290 cm^3 (58 patients) 4 complete, 24 partial responses;
≥ 2290 cm^3 (8 patients) 2 partial responses

Median survival

NonAFP producing (59 patients) – 7 months

No previous treatment; no metastases (20 patients) –10$^1/_2$ months

AFP producing (46 patients) – 5 months

Toxicity (210 patient administrations [with and without chemotherapy])

	Grade 3	Grade 4
Thrombocytopenia	17%	7%
Leukopenia	10%	2%

Patients were given 10 drops of Lugol's solution orally 2 to 3 times daily during the week before antibody administration in order to block thyroid uptake of free ^{131}I. This regimen was continued throughout treatment and two weeks after therapy. Testing of skin and eyes was performed 24 hours before radiolabeled antibody administration to ensure that the patient was not allergic to the materials. Because of the potential radiation hazards to others, the patient was confined to a specially prepared room. Hospitalization was required for 8 to 10 days to allow the radioactivity to diminish to levels which permitted the patient to be discharged. Because of the need for self-care, entry into these studies was limited to patients who exhibited a Karnofsky Performance Status of at least 60. Each dose was administered as a bolus through a running intravenous catheter which was maintained during the first 24 hours as a precaution against potential allergic reactions.

Treatment Results. ORDER and his colleagues (1985) have reported the outcome of 105 patients with hepatoma treated with ^{131}I antigens in the phase I–II trials. The results of treatment are summarized in Table 4. Forty-eight percent of 66 evaluable patients had an objective response defined as a 30% or greater reduction in tumor volume using computerized tomographic (CT) volumetric analysis. Responses occurred twice as frequently in patients with non-AFP-producing tumors as in those with AFP-bearing tumors. This result may

be due to the ineffectiveness of very low dose rate irradiation in rapidly proliferating AFP-producing tumors (MARCHESE et al. 1984). A median survival of 7 months was achieved in 59 patients whose tumor did not produce AFP. Deletion of patients with metastases, failure of previous treatment, or both, revealed a 10$^1/_2$ month median survival (20 patients). The median survival of 46 patients with AFP-producing tumors was 5 months for previously treated or untreated patients. Other investigators have also observed a relationship between AFP production, tumor aggressiveness, and prognosis (MATSUMOTO et al. 1982). Thrombocytopenia was the major toxicity and was enhanced when doses of doxorubicin greater than 15 mg, and 5-FU greater than 500 mg, were delivered together with radiolabeled antibody. Toxicity became more severe as the number of cycles increased and bone marrow reserve diminished. There was no renal toxicity or anaphylaxis associated with ^{131}I antiferritin administration.

Randomized Study. The expected median survival for patients with hepatoma is 3–4 months. The findings of the phase I–II studies with isotopic IgG, while encouraging, cannot be directly compared with those of other series because of potential differences in patient selection and distribution of prognostic groups (FRIEDMAN 1983). A randomized prospective study has been initiated under the sponsorship of the RTOG comparing full-dose chemotherapy given every 3 weeks, with ^{131}I antiferritin IgG preceded by chemotherapy given every 2 months (Fig. 1). All patients receive initial external irradiation and chemotherapy. It is too early in the study to present findings at this time.

Intrahepatic Biliary Carcinoma. The general principles outlined for hepatoma have been applied to intrahepatic biliary carcinoma except that the antibody was derived against CEA. Dose kinetic studies revealed that a schedule of 20 mCi on day 1, and 10 mCi on day 5 resulted in tumor-specific activity deposition (4.7 µCi/g) similar to that of larger doses, but with reduced total body irradiation and a tumor to liver ratio of 4.4 (LEICHNER et al. 1984) (Tables 2 and 3). Seven of 14 patients with intrahepatic biliary carcinoma achieved objective responses.

2.2.2 Hodgkin's Disease

Ferritin is a tumor-associated protein that has been found in Hodgkin's disease (SARCIONE et al. 1977). A phase II study of ^{131}I antiferritin in pa-

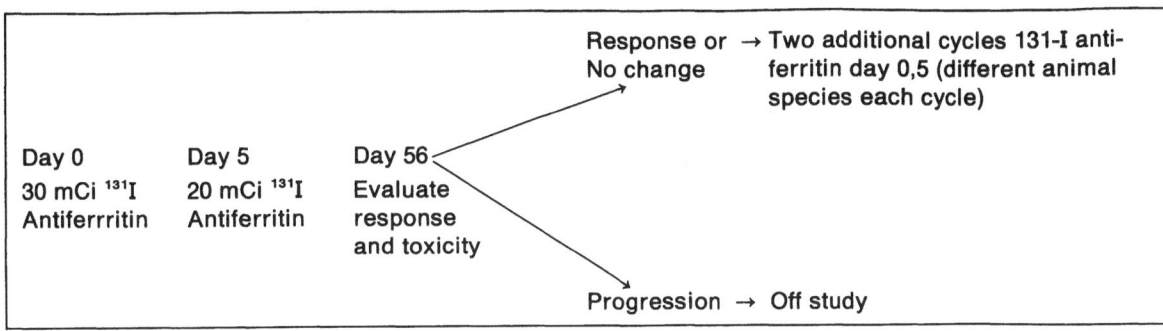

tients with advanced Hodgkin's disease who relapsed after treatment with at least two combination chemotherapy regimens (MOPP and ABVD) was carried out by the RTOG and reported by LENHARD and his colleagues (1985) (Fig. 2). Patients were treated with 30 mCi of ^{131}I antiferritin IgG on day 0 and with 20 mCi given 5 days later. Additional cycles were planned at 8-week intervals using antibody derived from different animal species. Sixteen of 37 patients (43%) had an objective, measurable response following 1–2 cycles of treatment (Table 5). Symptomatic response, often with complete resolution of symptoms, occurred in 17 of the 22 (77%) patients who had "B" symptoms at the time of initial treatment. The median survival of all patients measured from the time of entry into the study was 53 weeks. In this clinical setting of heavily treated relapsed patients the responses observed were comparable or superior to those reported in other phase II trials with single agents. Thrombocytopenia was the major toxicity seen, with 18 of 36 patients having platelet depression to below 100,000/cu mm. Four patients had thrombocytopenia below 20,000/cu mm. Recovery of platelet counts was slow and in many instances led to delays in the initiation of the second cycle. There were no fatal or life-threatening hemorrhages.

2.2.3 Non-Small Cell Lung Carcinoma

Isotopic immunoglobulin as an adjuvant to external radiation therapy is being investigated for patients with non-small cell bronchogenic carcinoma. The rationale for its use is to eradicate occult metastases and to deliver additional regional therapy. Carcinoembryonic antigen and ferritin have been identified as tumor-associated antigens in these tumors (GROPP et al. 1978).

Preliminary results of this study were reported by MOYLAN and his colleagues (1985). Fifty-one patients with unresectable primary tumors and no

Fig. 2. Treatment schema of phase I–II study (RTOG 83-09) of ^{131}I antiferritin antibody for the treatment of advanced Hodgkin's disease

Table 5. Hodgkin's disease therapeutic results

	Objective		Subjective (B symptoms)	
Number evaluable	37		22	
Complete response	1	43%	17	77%
Partial response	15			
No response/progression	21		5	

evidence of metastatic disease have been entered into this study and 32 patients have received at least 1 cycle of radiolabeled anti-CEA or antiferritin. Patients were initially treated with split-course radiation therapy receiving 3000 rad in 10 fractions over 2 weeks to fields encompassing the primary lesion and mediastinal lymph nodes. After a 2-week break, an additional boost of 2100–2400 rad in 7–8 fractions was delivered. Different fractionation schemes were employed in a few patients. Three weeks after external irradiation, the patients received 20 mCi of radioimmunoglobulin on day 0, and 10 mCi on day 5. This low-dose schedule was designed to allow out-patient therapy. If patients manifested no evidence of toxicity or distant metastases, isotopic immunoglobulin administration was repeated every 2 months using different animal species. Most patients received antiferritin antibody, 4 received anti-CEA, and 1 received both preparations.

Complete responses were seen in 4 patients, and 11 patients achieved partial responses (defined by a 50% or more decrease in tumor size). The overall response rate was 47%. At the time of reporting, the one-year survival was approximately 40%, with 17 patients remaining alive. Toxicity included moderate myelosuppression which was cumulative

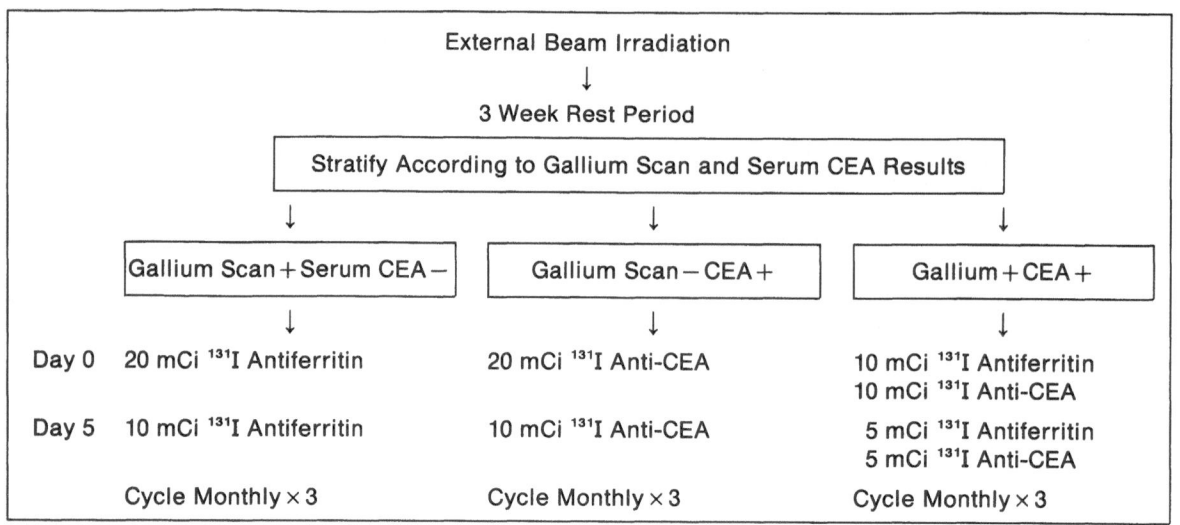

Fig. 3. Treatment schema of phase II study (RTOG 81-03) for the treatment of unresectable non-small cell bronchogenic carcinoma. Patients with positive gallium scans and normal CEA titers are treated with ^{131}I antiferritin. Patients whose gallium scans are negative with elevated serum CEA titers receive ^{131}I anti-CEA. Patients who display both gallium positivity and elevated CEA titers receive an admixture of both ^{131}I antiferritin and ^{131}I anti-CEA

following 3 cycles of treatment. An unexpected increased incidence of radiation pneumonitis was encountered. Non-fatal radiation pneumonitis occurred in 11 of the 51 accessioned patients. Three of the patients with pneumonitis received external radiation alone. Because of contralateral hilar involvement, it was necessary to encompass the larger volumes of normal lung tissue in the boost portals of these patients. Eight patients developed pneumonitis following radioimmunoglobulin administration. In 5 patients this complication was observed after the first cycle of antibody. The enhanced risk of radiation pneumonitis may have been due to nonspecific lung deposition of radiolabeled antibody related to pulmonary inflammation and infection (ROSTOCK et al. 1983).

Since January 1984 the frequency of antibody injection has been changed from every 2 months to monthly. Efforts are being made to characterize the antigenic profile of non-small cell bronchogenic carcinoma in regard to avidity for antiferritin and anti-CEA based on serum and tumor CEA levels and gallium positivity (CLAUSEN et al. 1974) of the primary lung tumor. Treatment in a new phase II study (Fig. 3) is predicated on the results of these analyses.

2.3 Monoclonal Antibodies

Monoclonal antibodies are advantageous in having high specificity for a unique target, in potentially increasing tumor antibody deposition, and in reducing nonspecific total body irradiation. Monoclonal antibody may, in addition, have a longer tumor-effective half-life because of its higher titer of specific antibody. However, several factors restricting the use of monoclonal antibody have become apparent. Tumor-associated antigens are heterogenously expressed on tumor cell surfaces (BURCHIEL 1983), are subject to modulation (OLD et al. 1968), and may be expressed in different quantities during various stages of the cell cycle (BURCHIEL 1983). Because of the unique specificity of monoclonal antibodies, a "family" of antibodies to a number of antigenic specificities might be required to achieve tumor saturation and adequate radiation doses. A second limiting factor is the species of derivation. At this time the mouse is the only species available for large scale hybridoma monoclonal antibody production, and the number of administrations of monoclonal antibody may be restricted because of immunologic toxicity. CARRASQUILLO et al. (1984) found that 78% of patients with melanoma who received a single dose of whole monoclonal antibody for scanning developed anti-mouse antibodies. While Fab fragments are considered to be less immunogenic than whole antibody, 47% of patients in Carrasquillo's series receiving one or more injections were found to have anti-mouse antibody titers. Serum antibody titers to mouse immunoglobulin may be measured as early as 6 to 10 days after monoclonal antibody administration (SEARS et al. 1982). The presence of anti-mouse antibody may lead to allergic reactions, rapid clearing of antibody, and marked reduction in tumor uptake. Human-derived monoclonal antibody would allow multiple administrations without the restriction of immunogenicity, although an allotype allergy could occur.

Another major limitation is that mouse monoclonal antibody does not bind the ^{131}I label as avidly as polyclonal-derived antibody. The dehalogenation of mouse monoclonal antibody leads to ^{131}I accumulation in the stomach and other organs rather than persistence at the tumor target (ORDER 1982). The identification of new radiolabels and methods of attaching these labels to monoclonal antibodies is necessary before monoclonal antibody therapy can proceed.

The experience using monoclonal antibody therapy has been very limited compared with that using polyclonal antibody. CARRASQUILLO et al. (1981) reported 10 patients with advanced melanoma treated with ^{131}I labeled Fab monoclonal antibody fragments against the melanoma oncofetal tumor-associated antigen p97. Patients received individual doses of 4 to 342 mCi and cumulative doses of 132 to 861 mCi. Three patients receiving cumulative doses of 374 to 861 mCi of ^{131}I anti-p97 Fab antibody were evaluable. One of two patients with hepatic metastases had transient stabilization of disease following therapy; the third patient with metastatic inguinal and pelvic lymphadenopathy achieved an objective response but tumor regrowth occurred three months later. The development of anti-mouse antibody frequently prevented subsequent treatment and resulted in a decreased effective half-life secondary to neutralization of antibody. Severe bone marrow toxicity was seen in patients receiving higher doses of ^{131}I.

EPENETOS et al. (1984) at the Hammersmith Hospital have reported three patients successfully treated with intracavitary therapy using anti-HMFG2 monoclonal antibody labeled with 20 mCi of ^{131}I. One patient had a malignant pleural effusion secondary to poorly differentiated adenocarcinoma; one had ovarian carcinoma with peritonealized disease and ascites; and a third patient had a malignant pericardial effusion and tumor mass from a bronchogenic carcinoma. Cytologic examination of the patients with the peritoneal and pleural effusions revealed clearing of malignant cells; and CT scan in the third patient showed a decrease in size of the tumor mass with resolution of the pericardial effusion after therapy.

3 Current Concepts and Future Directions

The use of radiolabeled antibody in both the diagnosis and treatment of malignant disease holds considerable promise. From early studies several important concepts have emerged. Tumor-specific antigens are not required to achieve preferential targeting. Dosimetric quantitation of radiolabeled antibody can be determined and tumor dose kinetic studies can be used to derive proper dose scheduling. While preliminary therapeutic results are encouraging, the field of radioimmunotherapy is in its infancy and there are many issues which remain to be addressed in order to optimize radiolabeled antibody therapy. The most appropriate antigen targets, the class and type of antibody or antibody combination, and the most suitable radionuclide for therapy need to be defined. Questions such as which tumors are most suitable for treatment and what dose and dose schedule are optimal need to be studied. The integration of radioimmunotherapy with other therapies requires further investigation. Prospective trials will be required to determine optimal therapeutic programs which will ultimately lead to the integration of radioimmunotherapy into clinical practice.

Many of these issues are currently being pursued. While the beta emission of ^{131}I is suitable for radioimmunotherapy, the physical half-life of ^{131}I (8 days) is prolonged relative to the biologic lifetime of the antigen-antibody tumor cell complex (4 days) (DeNARDO et al. 1985). Once the antigen-antibody complex leaves the tumor, or complexes are formed in the blood from circulating antigen, they are scavenged by the reticuloendothelial organs which receive the remaining radiation dose. An ideal radionuclide for radioimmunotherapy would be one that has a physical half-life of 1 to 3 days. The radionuclide should not interfere with the immunoreactivity of the antibody and should allow for outpatient administration. Phase I studies of yttrium-90-labeled antiferritin have recently begun. Yttrium-90 is a pure beta emitting isotope with a half-life of 64.4 hours. The biochemical ability to increase specific labeling activity (mCi/mg IgG) will allow for the selective delivery of significantly higher tumor dose rates and total doses to the tumor without concurrent total body irradiation. If not limited by toxicity, this will represent a major advancement in radioimmunotherapy. Other labels being explored include copper-67 (DeNARDO et al. 1983) and an alpha particle emitter, astatine-211 (SCHEINBERG et al. 1982).

Initial experience with ^{131}I monoclonal antibodies indicated that rapid dehalogenation occurred *in vivo*. This restriction should be overcome with new radiolabels that have been developed. However, limited species of origin (murine) for monoclonal antibody and rapid immunosensitization are problems that remain to be solved. The development of human monoclonal antibodies for clinical therapy without major sensitization problems would represent an additional major therapeutic advancement (Olsson and Kaplan 1980).

Single photon emission computerized tomography (SPECT) has proven to be a major advancement in the imaging of neoplasms with radiolabeled antibodies (Berche et al. 1982). SPECT allows three-dimensional reconstruction of the distribution of the radiopharmaceutical in a manner similar to that provided by CT scanning. The ability to quantitate the pharmacokinetics of radiolabeled antibodies *in vivo* using computerized integrated SPECT scanning is being applied to the development of models for radioimmunotherapy dosimetry and treatment planning. Quantitative radionuclide studies will allow the clinician to predetermine which radiolabeled antibody or combination of antibodies would be best suited for the treatment of a specific tumor. The residence times of the radionuclide at the tumor and in critical organs can be estimated by linking serial quantitative images through kinetic models. This allows determination of the cumulative amount of radioactivity integrated over time and the volume of tissue in which it is distributed. Total radiation dose and dose rate to the tumor and other organs in the body can then be calculated (DeNardo et al. 1985).

Acknowledgements. The author gratefully acknowledges Mrs. Cindy Nakada, Ms. Daisy Ho, and Mrs. Eleanor Haas for their excellent secretarial and editorial assistance.

References

Alexander P (1972) Foetal antigens in cancer. Nature 235:137–181

Bagshawe KD, Searle F, Lewis J, Brown P, Keep P (1980) Preliminary therapeutic and localization studies with human chorionic gonadotropin. Cancer Res 40:3016–3017

Bale WF, Spar IL, Goodland RL, Wolfe DE (1955) In vivo and in vitro studies of labeled antibodies against rat kidney and walker carcinoma. Proc Soc Exp Biol Med 89:564–568

Beck G, Bollack C (1974) Synthesis of ferritin in cultured hepatoma cells. Fedn Exp Biol Soc 47:314–317

Belitsky P, Ghose T, Aqino J (1978) Radionuclide imaging of metastase from renal cell carcinoma by ^{131}I-labeled antitumor antibody. Radiology 126:515–517

Berche C, Mach J-P, Lumbroso JD, Langlais C, Aubry F, Buchegger F, Carrel S, Rougier P, Parmentier C, Tubiana M (1982) Tomoscintigraphy for detecting gastrointestinal and medullary thyroid cancers: First clinical results using radiolabeled monoclonal antibodies against carcinoembryonic antigen. Br Med J 285:1447–1451

Burchiel SW (1983) Expression and detection of human tumor-associated antigens: Implications for radioimmunoimaging and radioimmunotherapy. In: Radioimmunoimaging and Radioimmunotherapy, Burchiel SW and Rhodes BA (eds), Elsevier Science Publishing Co., pp 13–23

Carrasquillo JA, Krohn KA, Beaumier P, McGuffin RW, Brown JP, Hellstrom KE, Hellstrom I, Larson SM (1984) Diagnosis of and therapy for solid tumors with radiolabeled antibodies and immune fragments. Cancer Treat Rep 68:317–328

Clausen J, Edeling C-J, Fogh J (1974) ^{67}Ga binding to human serum proteins and tumor components. Cancer Res 34:1931–1937

DeLand FH, Goldenberg DM (1983) In vivo cancer diagnosis by radioimmunodetection. In: Radioimmunoimaging and Radioimmunotherapy, Burchiel SW, Rhodes BA (eds), Elsevier Science Publishing Co., pp 329–343

DeNardo GL, DeNardo SJ (1983) Perspectives on the future of radioimmunodiagnosis and radioimmunotherapy and cancer. In: Radioimmunoimaging and Radioimmunotherapy, Burchiel SW, Rhodes BA (eds), Elsevier Science Publishing Co., pp 41–62

DeNardo SJ, DeNardo GL, Peng J-S, Colcher D (1983) Monoclonal antibody radiopharmaceuticals for cancer radioimmunotherapy, Burchiel SW, Rhodes BA (eds), Elsevier Science Publishing Co., pp 409–417

DeNardo GL, Raventos A, Hines HH, Scheibe PO, Macey DJ, Hays MT, DeNardo SJ (1985) Requirements for a treatment planning system for radioimmunotherapy. Int J Radiat Oncol Biol Phys 11:335–348

Epenetos AA, Britton KE, Mather S, Shepherd J, Granowska M, Taylor-Papadimitriou J, Nimmon CC, Durbin H, Hawkins LR, Malpas JS, Bodmer WF (1982) Targeting of iodine-123-labelled tumour-associated monoclonal antibodies to ovarian, breast, and gastrointestinal tumours. Lancet 2:999–1006

Epenetos AA, Courtenay-Luck N, Halnan KE, Hooker G, Hughes JMB, Krausz T, Lambert J, Lavender JP, MacGregor WG, McKenzie CJ, Munro A, Myers MJ, Orr JS, Pearse EE, Snook D, Webb B, Burchell J, Durbin H, Kemshead J, Taylor-Papadimitriou J (1984) Antibody-guided irradiation of malignant lesions: Three cases illustrating a new method of treatment. A report from the Hammersmith Oncology Group and the Imperial Cancer Research Fund. Lancet 1:1441–1443

Epenetos AA, Shepherd J, Britton KE, Mather S, Taylor-Papadimitriou J, Granowska M, Durbin H, Nimmon CC, Hawkins LR, Malpas JS, Bodmer WF (1985) [123]I radioiodinated antibody imaging of occult ovarian cancer. Cancer 55:984–987

Eshhar Z, Order SE, Katz DH (1974) Ferritin, a Hodgkin's disease associated antigen. Proc Nat Acad Sci USA 71:3956–3960

Ettinger DS, Dragon LH, Klein J, Sgagias M, Order SE (1979) Isotopic immunoglobulin in an integrated multimodal treatment program for a primary liver cancer: A case report. Cancer Treat Rep 63:131–134

Ettinger DS, Order SE, Wharam MD, Parker MK, Klein JL, Leichner PK (1982) Phase I–II study of isotopic immunoglobulin therapy for primary liver cancer. Cancer Treat Rep 66:289–297

Farrands PA, Perkins AC, Pimm MV, Hardy JD, Embleton MJ, Baldwin RW, Hardcastle JD (1982) Radioimmunodetection of human colorectal cancers by an anti-tumour monoclonal antibody. Lancet 2:397–400

Friedman MA (1983) Primary hepatocellular cancer-present results and future prospects. Int J Radiat Oncol Biol Phys 9:1841–1850

Gold P, Freedman SE (1965) Specific carcinoembryonic antigens of the human digestive system. J Exp Med 122:467–481

Goldenberg DM (1976) Oncofetal and other tumor-associated antigens of the human digestive system. Curr Topics Pathol 63:289–342

Goldenberg DM, DeLand FH (1982) Review. History and status of tumor imaging with radiolabeled antibodies. J Biol Resp Mod 1:121–136

Goldenberg DM, DeLand F, Kim E, Bennett S, Primus FJ, van Nagell JB Jr, Estes N, DeSimone P, Rayburn P (1978) Use of radiolabeled antibodies to carcinoembryonic antigen for the detection and localization of diverse cancers by external photoscanning. N Engl J Med June 22:1384–1388

Goldenberg DM, Kim EE, DeLand F, Spremulli E, Nelson MO, Gockerman JP, Primus FJ, Corgan RL, Alpert E (1980a) Clinical studies on the radioimmunodetection of tumors containing alpha-fetoprotein. Cancer 45:2500–2505

Goldenberg DM, Kim EE, DeLand FH, van Nagell JR Jr, Javadpour N (1980b) Radioimmunodetection of cancer using radioactive antibodies to human chorionic gonadotropin. Science 208:1284–1286

Gropp C, Havemann K, Lehmann F-G (1978) Carcinoembryonic antigen and ferritin in patients with lung cancer before and during therapy. Cancer 42:2802–2808

Kohler G, Milstein C (1975) Continuous cultures of fused cells secreting antibody of predefined specificity. Nature 256:495–497

Larson SM, Brown JP, Wright PW, Carrasquillo JA, Hellstrom I, Hellstrom KE (1983a) Imaging of melanoma with ^{131}I-labeled monoclonal antibodies. J Nucl Med 24:123–129

Larson SM, Carrasquillo JA, Krohn KA, Brown JP, McGuffin RW, Ferens JM, Graham MM, Hill LD, Beaumier PL, Hellstrom KE, Hellstrom I (1983b) Localization of ^{131}I-labeled p97-specific fab fragments in human melanoma as a basis for radiotherapy. J Clin Invest 72:2101–2114

Leibel SA (1983) Radioimmunotherapy (chapter 27). Modern Radiation Oncology, Gilbert HA (eds), JB Lippincott Co., pp 581–606

Leibel SA, Klein JL, Sgagias M, Leichner P, Order SE (1981) The integration of tumor associated antigens in cancer management. Sem Oncol 8:92–102

Leichner PK, Klein JL, Fishman EK, Siegelman SS, Ettinger DS, Order SE (1984) Comparative tumor dose from ^{131}I-labeled polyclonal antiferritin, anti-AFP, and anti-CEA in primary liver cancer. Cancer Drug Delivery 1:321–328

Leichner PK, Klein JL, Siegelman SS, Ettinger DS, Order SE (1983) Dosimetry of ^{131}I-labeled antiferritin in hepatom: Specific activities in the tumor and liver. Cancer Treat Rep 67:647–658

Lenhard RE Jr, Order SE, Spunberg JJ, Asbell SO, Leibel SA (1985) Isotopic immunoglobulin: A new systemic therapy for advanced hodgkins disease. J Clin Oncol 3:1296–1300

Mach J-P, Buchegger F, Forni M, Ritschard J, Berche C, Lumbroso JD, Schreyer M, Girardet C, Accolla RS, Carrel S (1981) Use of radiolabelled monoclonal anti-CEA antibodies for the detection of human carcinomas by external photoscanning and tomoscintigraphy. Immunol Today 2:239–249

Mach J-P, Buchegger F, Forni M, Ritschard J, Carrel S, Haskell CM (1983) Radiolabeled polyclonal and monoclonal antiCEA antibodies for the in vivo detection of human colorectal carcinoma. In: Radioimmunoimaging and radioimmunotherapy, Burchiel SW, Rhodes BA (eds), Elsevier Science Publishing Co., pp 345–356

Marchese MJ, Hall EJ, Hilaris BS (1984) Encapsulated iodine-125 in radiation oncology. I. Study of the relative biological effectiveness (RBE) using low dose rate irradiation of mammalian cell cultures. Am J Clin Oncol 7:607–611

Matsumoto Y, Suziki T, Asad I, Ozawa K, Tobe T, Honjol I (1982) Clinical classification of hepatoma in Japan according to serial changes in serum alpha-feto protein levels. Cancer 49:354–360

Moylan DJ, Order SE, Zinreich E, Leibel SA, Spunberg J, Asbell SO, Klein JL, Leichner P, Ettinger D, Powers G (1985) Phase I trial of radiolabeled antibody as an adjuvant to radiation therapy for unresectable non-small cell bronchogenic carcinoma: A radiation therapy oncology group study. Cancer Treat Rep

Munro HN, Linder MC (1978) Ferritin: Structure, biosynthesis and role in iron metabolism. Physiol Rev 58:317–396

Old LJ, Stockert E, Boyse EA, Kin JH (1968) Antigenic modulation and loss of TL antigen from cells exposed to TL antibody: Study of the phenomenon in vitro. J Exp Med 127:523–539

Olsson L, Kaplan HS (1980) Human hybridomas producing monoclonal antibodies of predefined antigenic specificity. Proc Natl Acad Sci USA 77:5429–5431

Order SE (1982) Monoclonal antibodies: Potential role in radiation therapy and oncology. Int J Radiat Oncol Biol Phys 8:1193–1201

Order SE (1984) Radioimmunoglobulin therapy of cancer. Comp Ther 10:9–18

Order SE, Bloomer WD, Jones AG, Kaplan WD, Davis MA, Adelstein J, Hellman S (1975) Radionuclide immunoglobulin lymphangiography: A case report. Cancer 35:1487–1492

Order SE, Kirkman R, Knapp R (1974) Serologic immunotherapy: Results and probable mechanism of action. Cancer 34:175–183

Order SE, Klein JL, Ettinger D, Alderson P, Siegelman S, Leichner P (1980a) Phase I–II study of radiolabeled antibody integrated in the treatment of primary hepatic malignancies. Int J Radiat Oncol Biol Phys 6:703–710

Order SE, Klein JL, Ettinger D, Alderson P, Siegelman S, Leichner P (1980b) Use of isotopic immunoglobulin in therapy. Cancer Res 40:3001–3007

Order SE, Klein JL, Leichner PK (1981) Antiferritin IgG antibody for isotopic cancer therapy. Oncology 38:154–160

Order SE, Leibel S (1984) Radiolabelled antibodies in the treatment of primary liver cancer. Applied Radiology 15:67–73

Order SE, Stillwagon GB, Klein JL, Leichner PK, Siegelman SS, Fishman EK, Ettinger DS, Haulk T, Kopher
K, Finney K, Surdyke M, Self S, Leibel S (1985) [131]I
antiferritin, a new treatment modality in hepatoma. Clin
Oncol 3:1573–1582

Pauwels EKJ, Cleton FJ (1984) Radiolabelled monoclonal
antibodies: A new diagnostic tool in nuclear medicine.
Radiother Oncol 1:333–338

Pressman D, Keighley G (1948) The zone of activity of
antibodies as determined by the use of radioactive tracers:
The zone of activity of nephritoxic anti-kidney serum.
J Immunol 59:141–146

Pressman D, Korngold L (1953) The in vivo localization
of anti-wagner-osteogenic-sarcoma antibodies. Cancer
6:619–623

Quinones J, Mizejewski G, Beierwaltes H (1971) Choriocarcinoma scanning using radiolabeled antibody to chorionic
gonadotropin. J Nucl Med 12:69–75

Rhodes BA, Burke DJ, Breslow K, Reed K, Austin R, Burchiel SW (1983) Effects of circulating antigen on antibody
localization in vivo. In: Radioimmunoimaging and Radioimmunotherapy, Burchiel SW, Rhodes BA (eds), Elsevier Science Publishing Co., pp 25–39

Rostock RA, Klein JL, Leichner PK, Kopher KA, Order
SE (1983) Selective tumor localization in experimental
hepatoma by radiolabeled antiferritin antibody. Int J Radiat Oncol Biol Phys 9:1345–1350

Rostock RA, Klein JL, Kopher KA, Order SE (1984a) Variables affecting the tumor localization of ^{131}I-antiferritin
in experimental hepatoma. Am J Clin Oncol 6:9–18

Rostock RA, Klein JL, Leichner PK, Order SE (1984b)
Distribution of and physiologic factors that affect [131]I
antiferritin tumor localization in experimental hepatoma.
Int J Radiat Oncol Biol Phys 10:1135–1141

Sarcione EJ, Smalley JR, Lema MJ, Stutzman L (1977)
Increased ferritin synthesis and release by hodgkin's disease peripheral blood lymphocytes. Int J Cancer
20:339–346

Scheinberg DA, Strand M, Gansow OA (1982) Tumor imaging with radioactive metal chelates conjugated to
monoclonal antibodies. Science 215:1511–1513

Sears HF, Atkinson B, Mattis J, Ernst C, Herlyn D, Step-
lewski Z, Hayry P, Koprowski H (1982) Phase-I clinical
trial of monoclonal antibody in treatment of gastrointestinal tumours. Lancet 1:762–765

Sherman DM, Carabell SC, Belli JA, Hellman S (1982) The
effect of dose rate and adriamycin on the tolerance of
thoracic radiation in mice. Int J Radiat Oncol Biol Phys
8:45–51

Spar IL, Bale WF, Marrack D, Dewey WC, McCardle RJ,
Harper PV (1967) ^{131}I-labeled antibodies to human fibrinogen. Cancer 20:865–870

4 Restricted Field Therapy

4.1 Intraoperative Radiotherapy

Timothy J. Kinsella, William F. Sindelar, Joel E. Tepper, Zelig Tochner, and Tyvin A. Rich

CONTENTS

1 Introduction

Intraoperative radiotherapy (IORT) is an area of renewed clinical interest in the treatment of locally advanced tumors of the abdomen, pelvis and retroperitoneum. The strategy of IORT is quite simple. It involves the use of a large dose of radiation delivered, at the time of surgical exploration, to a tumor or tumor bed and potential areas of locoregional spread. The use of IORT may improve the therapeutic ratio of tumor control to normal tissue toxicity for two major reasons. First, the extent of tumor can be more precisely defined at surgery and directly irradiated. Second, all or part of sensitive normal tissues or organs may be ex-

cluded from the treatment volume by operative mobilization, customized lead shielding, and/or the selection of appropriate electron beam energies. In theory, these are definite advantages compared to conventional external beam irradiation where the tumor (or target) volume can be difficult to define, even with contrast CT scanning, and where the total radiation dose is often limited by the tolerance of adjacent normal tissues incidentally incorporated within the external beam treatment volume.

The concept of IORT is similar in some aspects to the use of interstitial or intracavitary radiation where a large dose can be delivered to a specified tumor volume with relative sparing of adjacent tissue. IORT may have an advantage over brachytherapy techniques by providing a more homogenous dose distribution especially to large volumes (>5 cm), although the dose rate used for IORT (usually 200–1000 cGy/min) may be less biologically advantageous. The idea for IORT is not new. Finisterer described a technique of "eventration" treatment in 1915 which combined laparotomy and intraoperative orthovoltage irradiation to a locally advanced gastric carcinoma (FINSTERER 1915). Two decades later, Eloesser from Stanford University reported short-term local control with acceptable normal tissue toxicity in 4 of 6 patients with locally advanced GI cancers using low energy x-rays at exploration (ELOESSER 1937). Although there were a few small clinical series using IORT in the 1940's and 1950's, technical limitations of x-ray equipment and energy retarded further development of IORT.

The recent era of IORT began in the 1960's and its development is credited to Abe and co-workers at Kyoto University in Japan (ABE et al. 1980). In general, their approach to IORT has involved gross surgical resection followed by delivery of 2,000–4,000 cGy to the tumor bed using high energy electrons generated by a betatron. When resection is not possible, higher doses of radiation are delivered to the intact tumor at exploration and often combined with external beam irradiation. At

Timothy J. Kinsella, M.D.
William F. Sindelar, M.D. Ph.D.
Zelig Tochner, M.D.
Building 10, National Institutes of Health
Bethesda, MD 20892, USA

Joel E. Tepper, M.D., Associate Professor
Massachusetts General Hospital
Boston, MA 02114, USA

Tyvin A. Rich, M.D., Assistant Professor
6723 Bertner Avenue
Houston, TX 77030, USA

present, over 1,500 patients have been treated with IORT in Japan (ABE, TAKAHASHI 1981; ABE 1984). Approximately 30 Japanese institutions are now involved in IORT.

More recently, several U.S. centers have initiated clinical trials using IORT with some promising preliminary results (GOLDSON 1978; TEPPER, SINDELAR 1981; SINDELAR et al. 1983; GUNDERSON et al. 1983; KINSELLA et al. 1983; RICH et al. 1984; KINSELLA, SINDELAR 1985; TEPPER et al. 1986).

Approximately 600 patients have been treated at 5 U.S. centers using various combinations of IORT, external beam irradiation and surgery. Investigators at Howard University and the National Cancer Institute (NCI) use IORT in a manner similar to the Japanese, giving high doses ($\geq 2,000$ cGy) of electrons to the tumor bed and areas of loco-regional spread following gross surgical resection. The general approach to IORT at the Massachusetts General Hospital (MGH), Mayo Clinic, and Joint Center for Radiation Therapy (JCRT) is to combine conventional fractionated external beam irradiation (4,500–5,000 cGy) with an IORT boost (1,500–2,000 cGy) using high energy electrons (MGH and Mayo) or 300 KV x-rays (JCRT). A number of other U.S. institutions have started to use IORT and the Radiation Therapy Oncology Group is developing clinical trials.

2 General Concepts of Tumor and Normal Tissue Response to IORT

The radiation tolerance of most normal tissues to conventional fractionated external beam radiation is quite well defined. Information on normal tissue tolerance to large single doses of radiation as used in IORT is quite limited. Clearly, a first principle of IORT is to exclude as many normal tissues as possible from the radiation beam. However, the practical clinical use of IORT necessitates the inclusion of some adjacent normal tissues and it is necessary to establish tolerance limits applicable to IORT for tissues such as major blood vessels and nerves that are not normally dose-limiting with conventional radiotherapy. The available preliminary information from these studies is reviewed in later sections of this chapter.

Reliable information on an IORT dose-tumor response relationship is also lacking in contrast to data for conventionally fractionated external beam therapy, where a dose of 4,500–5,000 cGy over 5 weeks is considered adequate to provide high levels of control of microscopic residual disease following gross surgical resection of most solid tumors. For gross residual or unresectable disease, higher doses of fractionated radiation (6,000–7,500 cGy over 7–10 weeks) may control small tumors (< 5 cm), but are often ineffective in permanently controlling larger tumors. A second goal of the clinical IORT studies will be to establish "equivalent" IORT dose guidelines for use alone or combined with external beam therapy. While it has been estimated that an IORT dose equivalent factor may be 2–3X less than an external beam dose with conventional fractionation, this factor is based on an extrapolation from experimental tumor data. Carefully controlled clinical trials are needed to study the validity of this estimated IORT dose equivalent factor.

3 Experimental Normal Tissue Studies with IORT

The initial experimental work on normal tissue tolerance to IORT was performed by Abe and Arakawa who subjected dogs to laparotomy and intraoperative single-dose irradiation (ABE, ARAKAWA 1967). They determined that the major retroperitoneal blood vessels could be irradiated with no significant acute toxicity, but that hallow viscera such as the GI tract had to be excluded from the radiation field. While this study established the early clinical guidelines for use of IORT in Japan, a comprehensive study of both acute and late radiation effects on normal tissues in the abdomen and retroperitoneum was not undertaken until approximately 7 years ago, when investigators at the National Cancer Institute and elsewhere began a series of experimental studies on normal tissue tolerance to large single doses of IORT. Several recent reports have addressed the findings of some of these normal tissue studies in detail (SINDELAR et al. 1982a; SINDELAR et al. 1982b; TEPPER et al. 1983; SINDELAR et al. 1983; GILETTE and HOOPES 1983; GILETTE et al. 1983; KINSELLA et al. 1985b; KINSELLA et al. 1985c; BARNES et al. 1987).

A major concern in the use of IORT to treat tumors which involve the retroperitoneum has been potential acute and late radiation damage to *major blood vessels*. Since these blood vessels are relatively fixed structures and often are contiguous with the tumor, establishing their tolerance is central to the clinical application of IORT. Fortunately, it appears that major blood vessels will maintain their structural integrity with long-term follow-up (up to 5 years) even following doses as high as 5,000 cGy. Histological studies have shown few histopathological changes in these vessels treated to 3,000 cGy or below. Above 3,000 cGy, subintimal and medial fibrosis is evident within 1 year following IORT in both the aorta and vena cava and loss of elastic elements in the walls of large arteries can be observed. Hyalinization of the walls of large veins has not resulted in significant narrowing or occlusion. Additionally, premature atherosclerosis has not been observed.

As expected, the bowel does not tolerate the large doses used in IORT. Within months following a dose of 2,000 cGy, an irradiated segment of small intestine developed mucosal ulceration and atrophy, fibrosis of the muscularis and loss of coordinated peristalsis. With higher doses delivered to a segment of functional small intestine, the gross and microscopic changes were more marked and resulted in obstruction or perforation. However, in a surgically bypassed defunctionalized loop of small intestine, structural integrity was maintained following IORT doses up to 4,500 cGy. Irradiation of the *large intestine* showed similar histopathological changes with obstruction developing after 2,000–3,000 cGy and perforation after 4,500 cGy. Clearly, it appears that the bowel is a dose-limiting structure for IORT and in the clinical setting, functional bowel must be excluded from the IORT field.

The tolerance of *liver and bile duct* to IORT is important to study since IORT may have clinical application for some locally advanced upper abdominal tumors. Todoroki treated the liver hilum of rabbits and reported hepatic parenchymal atrophy and necrosis as well as marked biliary fibrosis using a single dose of > 3,000 cGy (TODOROKI 1978). At the NCI, irradiation of the extrahepatic bile duct in dogs resulted in fibrosis with eventual stenosis at all doses over 2,000 cGy (SINDELAR et al. 1982a). Secondary changes of biliary cirrhosis were evident within a few months of developing significant bile duct stenosis.

The tolerance of the *genitourinary tract* to IORT has also been studied using the experimental dog model (SINDELAR et al. 1982b and 1984; GILETTE, HOOPES 1983a). The kidney showed changes of parenchymal atrophy and necrosis with doses of > 2,000 cGy. A ureter tolerated a dose of 2,000 cGy, but fibrosis and progressive obstruction developed following > 3,000 cGy. The bladder wall maintained structural integrity up to 5,000 cGy, although contraction resulted in ureterovesical junction narrowing or obstruction in some dogs receiving > 3,000 cGy (KINSELLA et al.

1985c). From these studies, it appears necessary to exclude the ureter from an IORT field especially if the dose exceeds 2,000 cGy. While part of a kidney may be included within an IORT field, a nephrectomy is recommended if it is necessary to include an entire kidney. Finally, irradiation of part of the bladder wall seems reasonable, especially if it does not include the ureterovesical junction.

Peripheral nerves are uncommonly injured with conventional fractionated external irradiation (KINSELLA et al. 1980). However, a preliminary analysis of a clinical IORT study of retroperitoneal sarcomas revealed that some patients developed severe pain with evidence of motor and/or sensory changes in the distribution of an irradiated nerve within 6–8 months of IORT. Non-invasive studies on these patients could not differentiate between nerve entrapment (perineural fibrosis) or direct nerve injury. An experimental dog study involving irradiation of the femoral and sciatic nerve documented dose-related leg paresis with a threshold for clinical nerve injury as low as 2,500 cGy (KINSELLA et al. 1985b). Histological study of the irradiated nerves in these dogs reveals primary nerve injury manifest as loss of nerve fibers without evidence of vascular occlusion or thrombosis.

In addition to assessing the tolerance of intact normal tissues, it is of equal importance to determine the tolerance of *surgically manipulated normal tissues* to IORT. When IORT is used following surgical resection, it is often necessary to irradiate surgically manipulated tissues (e.g. vascular anastomoses, bypassed intestine) which lie within or immediately adjacent to the tumor bed. Some experimental studies evaluating the tolerance of surgically manipulated tissues have been reported.

The tolerance of *arterial anastomoses* was studied by transsecting the abdominal aorta and performing an end-to-end anastomoses followed by immediate IORT (TEPPER et al. 1983). The anastomoses healed adequately following doses up to 4,500 cGy, although progressive histological changes of subintimal and medial fibrosis were evident at doses > 3,000 cGy. The fibrosis resulted in stricture at the anastomosis site in some dogs, occasionally progressing to total occlusion. However, clinical arterial insufficiency has not been observed in these dogs followed for up to 5 years because of the development of collateral vessels.

In a similar fashion, the tolerance of *gastrointestinal suture lines* and *biliary-enteric anastomoses* were studied (TEPPER et al. 1983; SINDELAR et al. 1983). The suture line of a defunctionalized Roux-

En-Y intestinal loop remained intact, although with longer follow-up, the irradiated bowel showed progressive fibrosis and narrowing. Applying this approach to the anastomosis between transsected bile duct and a defunctionalized loop of small bowel resulted in failure to heal the anastomosis with the lowest dose, of 2,000 cGy.

The results of these experimental studies on intact and surgically manipulated normal tissues should serve as a general framework for the clinical application of IORT. Longer follow-up on some of these studies and additional work on normal tissue tolerance are needed. The tolerance of mediastinal structures to IORT is currently undergoing study at the NCI. Preliminary analysis suggests that intact mediastinal structures will tolerate IORT to doses of 2,000 cGy without significant clinical sequellae (BARNES et al. 1987).

4 Clinical Approach to IORT

4.1 General Principles of IORT

A "team approach" is an essential ingredient for the design and implementation of clinical IORT (KINSELLA and SINDELAR 1985a). Not only do the radiation oncologist and surgeon need to communicate and participate freely in this clinical effort, but a major support staff consisting of physicists, kanesthesiologists, nurses and radiation technologists is necessary. Cooperation of diagnostic radiology and pathology are also needed to make important clinicopathological correlations of tumor control and normal tissue injury following IORT.

4.2 Technical Aspects of IORT

The technical complexity of IORT demands considerable modification of the standard physical and dosimetric approaches used in external beam therapy. High energy electrons have been used most commonly in the clinical IORT studies both in Japan and the U.S. A depth-dose distribution for high energy electrons (12–20 MeV) compared to a 10 MeV photon beam is illustrated in Fig. 1. By proper selection of IORT electron energy, a large tumor volume (> 5 cm) can be treated homogeneously (± 10%) with relative sparing of subjacent normal tissues at greater depth. The depth-dose distribution for a filtered 300 KV orthovoltage beam similar to that used at the Joint Center

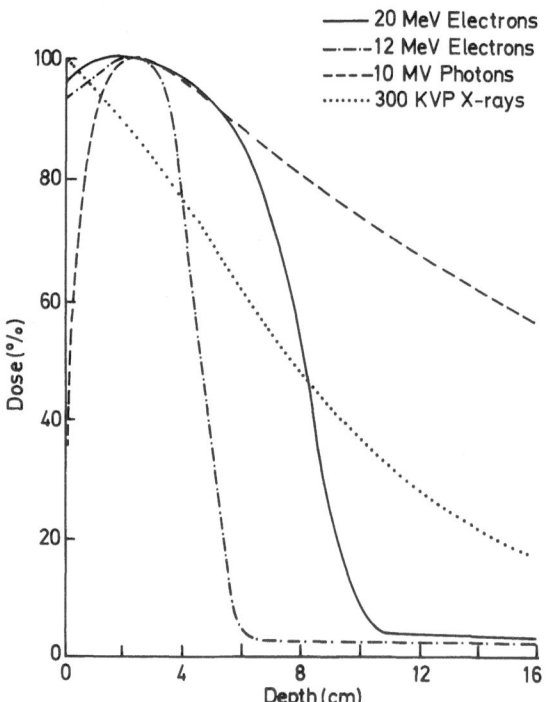

Fig. 1. A depth-dose distribution for 12 and 20 MeV electrons compared to orthovoltage (300 KV) x-rays and 10 mV photons

for Radiation Therapy is also plotted in Fig. 1. The advantages to orthovoltage IORT are that the x-ray unit is less expensive and more mobile, requires less room shielding than a linear accelerator used to generate high energy electrons, and the beam characteristics are suitable for irradiation of a resected tumor bed (RICH et al. 1984). However, the dose distribution is quite inhomogenous, particularly at depths of > 5 cm, which limits its usefulness for treating large unresectable tumors. Another potential drawback to orthovoltage IORT is the increased bone absorption which may increase late radiation damage to irradiated bone; but to date, this has not been encountered.

The initiation of an IORT program requires a significant amount of device fabrication. This entails development of an applicator system; adapting the applicator system to the treatment machine; designing the shapes and sizes of the applicator cones; and developing an IORT field verification system. The design of the applicator cones and adaptor system clearly affect the IORT field dosimetry and this must be documented prior to clinical use.

The applicator system used at the NCI is shown in Fig. 2. The IORT adaptor is basically a box which slides into the head of the linear accelerator,

Fig. 2. The IORT applicator system used at the National Cancer Institute. The IORT adaptor is attached to the head of the linear accelerator which includes a TV verification system. The docking adaptor and lucite cones attach to the bottom of the IORT adaptor

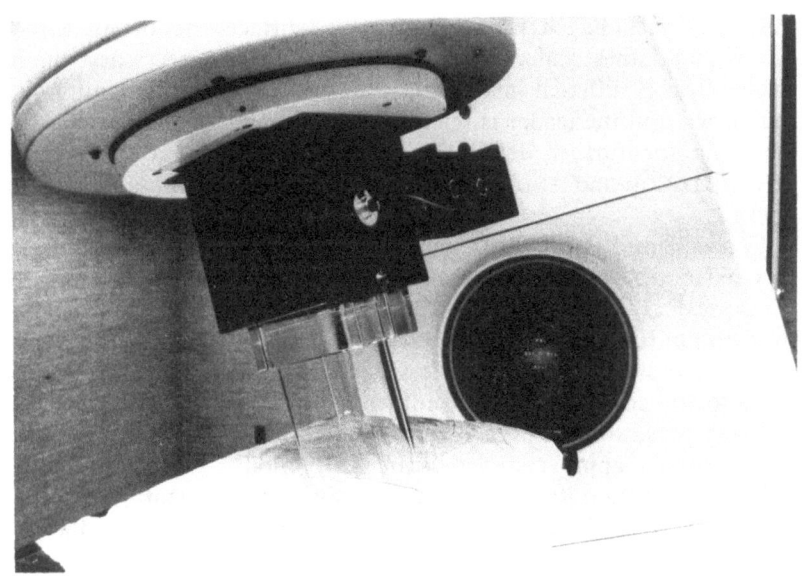

replacing the block tray holder. A TV camera and lights for the TV system mount on the side of the box. A mirror slides in and out of the adaptor box, allowing the TV camera to focus on the area to be treated. Further details on this applicator system are included in recent publications (FRAASS et al. 1983; FRAASS et al. 1985). Electron beam IORT is performed using specially constructed lucite applicator cones which extend from the adaptor attached to the linear accelerator to abut on the tumor or tumor bed within the patient. The IORT cones serve 3 major functions: collimation of the electron beam, delineation of the treatment volume, and displacement of normal tissues. The peripheral dose (immediately outside of the lucite cones) has been reported to be between 10–30% of the given dose (BIGGS et al. 1981; McCULLOUGH and ANDERSON 1982). The additional use of a stainless steel shield (1.6 mm thick) can reduce the peripheral dose by a factor of 5X (FRAASS et al. 1985). Both the applicator cones and shields are gas sterilized and handled as sterile surgical equipment during the IORT procedure.

A detailed set of isodose curves is available for each applicator cone for the available electron energies to facilitate selection of appropriate applicators during surgery. The shape of the cones is dependent on the area to be treated. In general, round or "squircle" shaped (one square end and one circular end) are preferred over rectangular and square applicators, particularly for use in the upper abdomen or pelvis. The treatment end of the cone may be beveled (15–30° angle) to facilitate treatment along sloping surfaces such as the pelvic

side wall. A limited number of lucite cones are necessary to treat most abdominal, pelvic and retroperitoneal tumor sites. The cone size usually ranges from 6–15 cm in diameter with lengths of 30–40 cm to treat deep-seated tumors.

With large tumor volumes, two or more IORT fields may be required, necessitating field matching. Proper and consistent matching of the electron fields is a major concern. Although methods have been proposed to improve field matching at the surface of a patient, the use of these methods for IORT would be quite complicated. As a compromise, a set of general rules have been established at the NCI where multiple IORT fields are used in each patient (FRAASS et al. 1985). For matching IORT fields, the square end of the squircle cone is used or a straight border is created using customized lead wafers. The match line of the first IORT field is marked with surgical clips and an appropriate gap based on electron energy field size and field shape is used to maximize dose homogeneity between fields. For example, in matching two rectangular fields, if 12 MeV electrons are used, the inner edges of the matching fields are abutted while for 20 MeV electrons, a 2 mm gap between the inner edges is used. A TV or mirror verification system is very helpful for field matching since it allows visualization of the clips of the first field (inner edge) in relationship to the new field edge.

Several other technical factors are of importance to ensure quality assurance for IORT. In general, IORT doses are quoted to the 90% isodose line with a typical dose range of 1,500–3,000 cGy. Complete dosimetry for each applicator cone is necessary including data on depth dose, surface dose, field flatness and x-ray contamination. Dosimetry from 3 different institutions using IORT is published and the reader is referred to these publications for further detail (BIGGS et al. 1981; McCULLOUGH and ANDERSON 1982; FRAASS et al. 1985).

A specialized IORT table such as that recently devised at the NCI is of great value for IORT (FRAASS et al. 1985). Standard operating room tables do not have the fine vertical, lateral, and longitudinal motions which are necessary to dock the cone to the adaptor. While radiotherapy couches provide these motions, they cannot tilt, making many surgical approaches very difficult. By modifying the base of a standard operating room table, the fine vertical, lateral and longitudinal motions are possible as well as pitch and roll motions.

4.3 Surgical Aspects of IORT

The surgeon must provide adequate exposure for IORT in addition to performing whatever surgery is necessary for the patient's clinical condition, be the procedure a resection, palliative by-pass or simple exposure of a tumor or tumor bed. The surgical approaches used at the NCI for IORT involving various abdominal, pelvic, and retroperitoneal structures are outlined and illustrated in detail elsewhere (SINDELAR et al. 1987). Since self-contained methods for maintaining surgical exposure are necessary for IORT, the type of incision and extent of normal tissue mobilization are typically more generous than might be needed for the same operation without IORT. For example, exposure of the pancreas for IORT may require complete mobilization of the stomach, reflection or division of the gastrocolic omentum, mobilization of the duodenum and retraction of the liver edge.

Retroperitoneal and central abdominal tumors can be approached with a midline incision to deliver IORT. In the upper abdomen, including approaches to gastric, pancreatic and biliary carcinomas, a bilateral subcostal or high transverse incision can allow for easier delivery of IORT. For carcinomas involving the esophagogastric junction and proximal stomach, a left thoraco-abdominal incision may be required to provide adequate exposure for IORT. Exposure of pelvic tumors is usually quite difficult and generous incisions are required.

In the operating room, the dimensions of the tumor volume are determined and the appropriate cones are selected to cover the volume and adapt to the patient's anatomy. If patient transport is necessary, the incision may be closed with a running continuous suture or may be simply packed open. Safe and expeditious transport of the anesthetized patient between the operating room and radiation rooms requires planning and coordination between the surgeon, anesthesiologist and nursing staff. Although continuous mechanical ventilation is possible during transport, the patient is usually ventilated by hand to ensure adequate continuous respiratory support. Remote continuous electrocardiographic monitoring, as well as blood pressure monitoring, are performed. An emergence drug box, a portable defibrillator and a portable suction device also accompany the patient.

The radiation treatment room needs to be fully equipped as a temporary operating room with adequate staff and surgical instruments to deal effectively with potential surgical emergencies such as acute hemorrhage from an unsecured blood vessel or disruption of a gastrointestinal anastomosis. Adequate exposure of the tumor or tumor bed for cone placement may necessitate further surgical intervention in the radiation treatment room. Additionally, it can be difficult to position a cone without further retraction of incision edges, costal margins, major viscera and other structures. At the NCI, the Thompson retractor system which attaches to the IORT table has been found to be well suited for IORT. The group at the Joint Center for Radiation Therapy has found the Bookwalter retractor suitable. Adequate and continuous remote monitoring of the patient during IORT delivery is a major concern of the anesthesiology staff. Closed circuit television is helpful to monitor the patient as well as to view the anesthesia machine and gas flow gauges to check for proper functioning.

A dedicated IORT suite can dispense with the need to transport patients and reduce some of the technical complexity of IORT. However, the considerable expenditure of resources for a dedicated suite at more than a few select institutions does not appear reasonable until further information on the clinical utility of IORT is available.

5 Results of Clinical Studies Using IORT

The clinical studies of IORT both in Japan and the U.S. have concentrated on locally advanced malignancies of the abdomen, pelvis and retroperitoneum. While over 1,500 patients have been treated in Japan and approximately 600 in the U.S., conclusive data on the benefit of IORT are still lacking. Preliminary results indicate that it is technically feasible to use IORT alone or combined with a major surgical procedure and the acute morbidity is quite acceptable (ABE, TAKAHASHI 1981; SINDELAR et al. 1983; TEPPER et al. 1984; KINSELLA and SINDELAR 1985a; SINDELAR et al. 1987). However, Phase III trials at the NCI and elsewhere are still too early to determine whether IORT alone or combined with external beam radiation is clearly superior to conventional therapy in terms of local control and normal tissue toxicity.

For certain tumor sites such as a locally advanced rectal carcinoma which extends through the rectal wall, the addition of external beam radiation following gross resection appears to improve local control with acceptable normal tissue toxicity (WITHERS et al. 1981). However, in other tumor sites, such as gastric and pancreatic carcinomas, there is little information to support the use of conventional post-operative external radiation. Although most clinical studies of IORT are considered as Phase I or Phase II investigations, control patients will be necessary in the near future to clarify any benefit to IORT (KINSELLA and SINDELAR 1985a). Since the issues of local failure following surgery and the technical considerations of IORT vary by tumor site, the available results of IORT are best discussed according to tumor site.

5.1 Gastric Carcinoma

Abe and Takahashi have the largest single-institution clinical experience at Kyoto University and have a prospective control group (ABE, TAKAHASHI 1981). Patients received surgery alone (110 patients) or surgery with IORT (84 patients) depending on the day of the week that surgery was performed. The IORT dose varied from 2,800–4,000 cGy and was delivered as a single IORT field covering the tumor bed and regional nodes. A survival advantage to combined modality therapy was evident by actuarial analysis at 5 years in Stage II (extension to the muscular gastric wall) and Stage IV (extension through serosa and positive loco-regional nodes) patients. A slight survival improvement was found in Stage III (positive nodes) patients and no survival difference was seen in Stage I (confined to the mucosa and submucosa) patients, which represent a good prognosis group. Within the Stage IV patients, combined modality

treatment resulted in 5/27 survivors at 5 years compared to 0/18 survivors with surgery alone at 2 years. No significant complications were reported. Unfortunately, no analyses of local control or patterns of failure were performed.

Although the Japanese study suggests an advantage to combined surgery and IORT in certain patient groups with gastric cancer, the possibility exists that similar results could have been obtained with post-operative external beam irradiation. A randomized prospective trial is ongoing at the NCI in patients with resectable gastric carcinoma who have extension through the serosa, positive loco-regional nodes, or gross residual disease. Patients are randomized to IORT (2,000 cGy and intravenous misonidazole at 3.5 gm/m^2) or post-operative external beam irradiation (5,000–5,400 cGy over 5–6 weeks). Of 64 patients evaluated, only 29 have been found operable, with most patients having multiple positive lymph nodes and extension through the serosa (Stage IV in the Japanese staging system). With variable follow-up to 4 years in this small group of patients, there appears to be no clear difference in local control nor survival between the two treatment arms. Two patients who had an extended gastrectomy with partial pancreatectomy have developed fistulas within the IORT field (SINDELAR et al. 1983; KINSELLA and SINDELAR, Unpublished Results).

5.2 Pancreatic Carcinoma

While up to one-half of patients with pancreatic carcinoma have loco-regional disease at presentation, the treatment results of most single and combined modality therapy shows little curative potential (HERTER et al. 1982; WHITTINGTON et al. 1981; GASTROINTESTINAL TUMOR STUDY GROUP 1979). Only 15% of patients can undergo curative resection and local failure has been reported in up to 50% of resected patients (TEPPER et al. 1976). With locally advanced, unresectable disease, the use of high dose external beam radiation with or without 5-fluorouracil results in clinical local control in less than 50% of patients and only a rare long-term survivor. Thus, for patients with localized pancreatic cancer, the use of IORT combined with resection or high dose external beam radiation has the potential to improve local control and possibly to improve survival.

The use of IORT alone for unresectable pancreatic cancer has shown little benefit. In an early pilot study of 19 patients with pancreatic cancer at Howard University, the median survival was < 6 months, although their patients frequently had liver metastases at presentation (10/19 patients) and would be predicted to have very limited survival (GOLDSON et al. 1981). Similar survival results are reported from a larger Japanese study (108 patients), although patients did report pain relief after IORT to > 2,000 cGy (ABE, TAKAHASHI 1981). Unfortunately, there was no analysis of the extent nor duration of the pain relief. One-quarter of patients did experience hematochezia believed secondary to IORT-induced duodenal mucositis.

At the Massachusetts General Hospital, the combination of external beam radiation (5,000 cGy) and IORT (1,500–2,000 cGy) in patients with unresectable pancreatic carcinoma produced a median survival of 16.5 months which compares favorably with the 6–9 month median survival in similar patients using other treatment regimens (WOOD et al. 1982; SHIPLEY et al. 1984). While these results in a small group of patients are impressive, it is important to point out that some of these patients were selected to receive IORT if they did not develop peritoneal seeding or distant metastases within the 6–10 week interval between the two explorations, possibly selecting for patients with a more favorable natural history. Even with the combination of external beam and IORT, clinical local failure occurred in 45% (7/16 patients). Significant IORT complications were found with gastric outlet obstruction in one patient and upper GI bleeding in two other patients. Both the Mayo Clinic and the NCI are involved in prospective trials combining IORT and external beam irradiation with concomitant 5-fluorouracil in patients with unresectable pancreatic cancer in an attempt to confirm the MGH results.

A second NCI trial in pancreatic carcinoma is designed to assess the role of IORT (2,000 cGy plus intravenous misonidazole) in resectable pancreatic carcinoma who have positive loco-regional lymph nodes, positive microscopic margins or gross residual disease. A control group receives conventional post-operative radiation therapy (5,000 cGy). Because of the low resectability rate, patient accrual has been slow (24 patients) and preliminary analysis shows no difference in overall and disease-free survival.

5.3 Rectal Carcinoma

The use of external beam radiation in patients with resectable but high-stage rectal carcinomas (Stage B_2 and C) appears to reduce local failure from up to 40% to less than 15% of patients (WITHERS et al. 1981). With gross residual disease, local control with the use of post-operative external beam irradiation is only 50% (GUNDERSON et al. 1983). In an attempt to improve local control in patients with gross residual or unresectable rectal carcinoma, investigators at the MGH are using a combined modality approach consisting of preor post-operative external beam irradiation (5,000 cGy), surgery and an IORT "boost" of 1,000–1,500 cGy depending on the surgical findings (GUNDERSON et al. 1983; TEPPER et al. 1986). Fifty-one patients have completed the entire treatment, including 29 patients with primary unresectable rectal cancer and 22 patients with recurrent rectal cancer. With a minimum of 24 months of follow-up, there appears to be an improvement in local control and survival compared to historical controls treated with surgery and external beam radiation only. Only 2 of 29 patients (7%) with unresectable cancer failed locally compared to 10 of 22 patients (45%) with locally recurrent disease. Sixteen of the primary unresectable patients and six of the locally recurrent patients remain disease-free. A detailed analysis of complications showed that approximately one-quarter of patients had significant soft tissue complications being somewhat higher in patients treated for recurrent tumors (40% complication rate) compared to patients with primary tumors (15%) (TEPPER et al. 1985). Although the overall complication rate was comparable to a historical control population treated with surgery and external beam irradiation, pelvic pain in the absence of apparent recurrent tumor was reported in three patients treated for recurrent tumors who received IORT.

5.4 Genitourinary Cancer

A combination of IORT and post-operative external beam irradiation has been used in 57 patients with early stage bladder carcinoma (not penetrating into the bladder wall) by a group of Japanese investigators (MATSUMOTO et al. 1981). Following clinical staging, appropriate patients underwent laparotomy with open cystotomy and delivery of 2,500–3,000 cGy using 4–6 MeV electrons. There was no attempt at fulguration nor resection. Most patients received post-operative radiation to 3,000–4,000 cGy to the entire bladder. These investigators report 80% local control at 5 years which compares favorably to the results of Van der Werf Messing using a radium needle implant with or without additional external irradiation (VAN DER WERF MESSING 1978). Only one serious complication involving bilateral hydronephrosis was reported and this patient required urinary diversion. Additionally, 14 patients with localized prostate cancer have been treated using a perineal approach with IORT. With variable follow-up, 13 of 14 patients have local control with no major complication to the bladder, urethra or rectum (TAKAHASHI et al. 1985).

5.5 Cervix Cancer

Since the para-aortic lymph nodes may be pathologically involved in up to 70% of patients with advanced cervix cancer, the use of IORT seems to be an interesting approach in these patients. Goldson and co-workers at Howard University and Georgetown University have treated over 40 patients with IORT using a single rectangular field encompassing the para-aortic chain from the renal vessels to the aortic bifurcation (GOLDSON et al. 1978; DELGADO et al. 1984). Care is taken to avoid any overlap with the external beam pelvic field. For patients with pathologically negative nodes on frozen section, a dose of 1,000 cGy is used while 2,500 cGy plus external beam irradiation is delivered to grossly involved nodes. Some patients received an IORT boost to the pelvic side wall. Of the initial 22 patients treated, 16 patients are alive with a median follow-up of 1 year. Complications from this approach include two patients with arterial bleeding requiring re-exploration, one patient with a unilateral ureteral obstruction, and one patient with pelvic pain believed secondary to retroperitoneal fibrosis (DELGADO et al. 1984). The Japanese have reported on a group of 21 cervix cancer patients, but give no detailed information on local control or complications (ABE et al. 1981).

5.6 Sarcomas

Retroperitoneal soft tissue sarcomas have a marked tendency to recur locally following resection (up to 70%), reflecting the nature of these tumors to widely infiltrate adjacent vital structures such as nerves and major blood vessels (CODY et al. 1981). The use of post-operative external beam irradiation may provide local control, but can result in significant morbidity. In a recent review of 31 patients treated at the NCI for retroper-

itoneal sarcoma with surgery and 5,000–5,500 cGy post-operatively, local control was found in 75% of patients, but severe bowel injury occurred in 25% (GLENN et al. 1985).

At present, investigators at the NCI are involved in a prospective randomized trial of wide excision, 2,000 cGy IORT to the tumor bed followed by 4,000 cGy external beam therapy. The control arm receives wide excision and external beam therapy to 5,000–5,500 cGy. A preliminary analysis of 35 randomized patients in this trial shows a difference in local control (78% versus 45%), but no difference in overall (36 months median) or disease-free (20 months median) survival (KINSELLA et al. 1983; KINSELLA et al. 1986). However, there appears to be less bowel injury in the IORT patients (1 case of severe enteritis compared to 5 cases in the control arm) at this time. Three IORT patients have developed a severe pain syndrome believed to be related to peripheral nerve entrapment with fibrosis or actual radiation-induced demyelination. This latter injury is potentially worrisome and is being studied experimentally in the dog.

Soft tissue sarcomas at other sites have also been treated with IORT. Abe and co-workers have treated 28 patients with a combination of excision and IORT to 3,000–4,500 cGy (ABE, TAKAHASHI 1981). They report good local control (11/15 patients) and survival (21/28 patients), although no information is provided on extent of resection, tumor grade, stage, duration of follow-up nor complications of treatment. Investigators at the MGH have treated 12 sarcoma patients with pre-operative external beam radiation (5,000 cGy), wide excision and IORT to 1,000–2,000 cGy (GUNDERSON et al. 1982; SUIT et al. 1985). With limited follow-up, 9 of 12 patients show local control with no significant complications. Finally, a limited experience at NCI in bone sarcomas of the pelvic girdle (5 patients) suggests an improvement in local control with combined surgery (hemipelvectomy) and IORT (4 of 5 with local control) compared to a historical series where 5 of 6 patients failed locally following surgery alone (HOEKSTRA et al. 1987).

5.7 Other Sites

IORT has been used occasionally for tumors at other anatomical sites, including the lung, mediastinum and brain. The clinical data are limited and no assessment of treatment results and complications are possible at this time. Experimental work using the dog model and a clinical Phase I study are under investigation at the NCI to study normal tissue tolerance of mediastinal and pulmonary structures, as well as local control of locally advanced non-small cell lung cancer.

References

Abe M, Arakawa M (1967) Fundamental studies on surgical irradiation. Histological and hematological changes following irradiatin during laparotomy of dogs. Japanese Soc Cancer Ther 2:271–278

Abe M, Takahashi M, Yabumoto E et al. (1980) Clinical experiences with intraoperative radiotherapy in locally advanced cancers. Cancer 45:40–48

Abe M, Takahashi M (1981) Intraoperative radiotherapy: The Japanese experience. Int J Radiat Oncol Biol Phys 7:863–868

Abe M (1984) Intraoperative radiation therapy for gastrointestinal malignancy. In: DeCosse JJ, Sherlock P (eds). Clinical management of gastrointestinal cancer. Cancer Treatment and Research, Vol 18, Martinus Nijhoff Press, Boston, pp 327–351

Barnes M, Pass H, DeLuca A et al. (1987) Response of the mediastinal and thoracic viscera of the dog to intraoperative radiation therapy. Int J Radiat Oncol Biol Phys 13:371–378

Cody HS, Turnbull AO, Fortner JG, Hajdu SI (1981) The continuing challenge of retroperitoneal sarcomas. Cancer 47:2147–2157

Delgado G, Goldson AL, Ashayer E et al. (1984) Intraoperative radiation in the treatment of advanced cervical cancer. J Obst Gyn 63:246–252

Eloesser (1937) The treatment of some abdominal cancers by irradiation through the abdomen combined with cautery excision. Ann Surg 106:645–652

Finsterer H (1915) Zur Therapie inoperabler Magen- und Darmkarzinome mit Freilegung und nachfolgender Röntgenbestrahlung. Strahlentherapie 6:205–213

Fraass BA, Harrington FS, Kinsella TJ, Sindelar WF (1983) Television system for verification and documentation of treatment fields during intraoperative radiation therapy. Int J Radiat Oncol Biol Phys 9:1409–1411

Fraass BA, Miller R, Kinsella TJ et al. (1985) Intraoperative radiation therapy at the National Cancer Institute: Technical innovations and dosimetry. Int J Radiat Oncol Biol Phys 11:1299–1311

Gastrointestinal Tumor study Group (1979) Comparative therapeutic trial of radiation with or without chemotherapy in pancreatic carcinoma. Int J Radiat Oncol Biol Phys 5:1643–1647

Gilette EL, Hoopes PJ (Abstract: 1983a) The progression of renal damage in intraoperatively irradiated canine kidneys. Proceedings of 7th International Congress of Radiation Research

Gilette EL, Hoopes PJ, Withrow SJ (Abstract: 1983b) Aortic changes following intraoperative electron or fractionated X-irradiation. Proceedings of the 7th International Congress of Radiation Research

Glenn J, Sindelar WF, Kinsella TJ et al. (1985) Results of multimodality therapy of resectable soft-tissue sarcomas of the retroperitoneum. Surgery 97:316–325

Goldson A (1978) Preliminary clinical experience with intraoperative radiotherapy. J Natl Med Assoc 70:493–496

Goldson AL, Delgado G, Hill LT (1978) Intraoperative radiation of the para-aortic nodes in cancer of the uterine cervix. Obstet Gynecol 52:713–717

Goldson AL, Ashaueri E, Espinoza MC et al. (1981) Single-dose intraoperative electrons for advanced stage pancreatic cancer: Phase I pilot study. Int J Radiat Oncol Biol Phys 7:869–874

Gunderson LL, Shipley WU, Suit HD et al. (1982) Intraoperative irradiation: A pilot study combining external beam photons with "boost" dose intraoperative electrons. Cancer 49:2259–2266

Gunderson LL, Gohen AM, Dosoretz DE et al. (1983) Residual unresectable or recurring colorectal cancer: External beam irradiation and intraoperative electron beam boost ± resection. Int J Radiat Oncol Biol Phys 9:1597–1606

Herter FP, Cooperman AM, Ahlborn TN, Antinori C (1982) Surgical experience with pancreatic and periampullary cancer. Ann Surg 195:274–281

Hoekstra HJ, Sindelar WF, Kinsella TJ (1987) Surgery with intraoperative radiotherapy for sarcomas of the pelvic girdle. Cancer

Kinsella TJ, Weichselbaum RR, Sheline G (1980) Radiation injury of cranial and peripheral nerves. In: Gilbert H, Kagan R (eds) Radiation Damage to the Nervous System: Delayed Therapeutic Hazards, Raven Press, New York, pp 145–151

Kinsella TJ, Sindelar WF, Rosenberg SA, Glatstein E (Abstract: 1983) Wide excision combined with intraoperative radiation therapy and external beam therapy in retroperitoneal soft tissue tumors. Int J Radiat Oncol Biol Phys 9 (Supple):92

Kinsella TJ, Sindelar WF (1985a) Intraoperative radiation therapy In Devita VT, Hellman S, Rosenberg SA (eds). Principles and Practice of Oncology, 2nd Edition, Lippincott, Philadelphia, pp 2293–2304

Kinsella TJ, Sindelar WF, DeLuca AM et al. (1985b) Tolerance of peripheral nerve to intraoperative radiotherapy (IORT): Clinical and experimental studies. Int J Radiat Oncol Biol Phys 11:1941–1946

Kinsella TJ, Sindelar WF, DeLuca AM et al. (Abstract, 1985c). Tolerance of the bladder to intraoperative radiotherapy: An experimental study. Int J Radiat Oncol Biol Phys 11:187

Kinsella TJ, Sindelar WF, Glatstein E, Rosenberg SA (Abstract, 1986). Preliminary results of a prospective randomized trial of intraoperative (IORT) and low dose external beam radiotherapy vs high dose external beam radiotherapy as adjuvant therapy in resectable soft tissue sarcomas of the retroperitoneum. Int J Radiat Oncol Biol Phys 12:100

Matsumoto L, Kakizoe T, Mikuriyama S et al. (1981) Clinical evaluation of intraoperative radiotherapy for carcinoma of the urinary bladder. Cancer 47:509–513

McCullough EC, Anderson JA (1982) The dosimetric properties of an applicator system for intraoperative electron-beam therapy utilizing a Clinac 18 accelerator. Med Phys 9:261–268

Rich TA, Cady B, McDermott WV, Kase KR, Chaffey JT, Hellman S (1984) Orthovoltage intraoperative radiotherapy: A new look at an old idea. Int J Radiat Oncol Biol Phys 10:1957–1965

Shipley WU, Wood WC, Tepper JE et al. (1984) Intraoperative electron beam irradiation for patients with unresectable pancreatic carcinoma. Ann Surg 200:289–296

Sindelar WF, Tepper J, Travis EL (1982a) Tolerance of bile duct to intraoperative irradiation. Surgery 92:533–540

Sindelar WF, Tepper J, Travis EL, Terrill R (1982b) Tolerance of retroperitoneal structures to intraoperative radiation. Ann Surg 196:601–608

Sindelar WF, Kinsella TJ, Tepper J et al. (1983) Experimental and clinical studies with intraoperative radiotherapy. Surg Gynecol Obstet 157:205–219

Sindelar WF, Hoekstra H, Kinsella TJ (1987) Surgical approaches and techniques in intraoperative radiotherapy for intra-abdominal, retroperitoneal, and pelvic neoplasms. Surgery

Suit HD, Mankin HJ, Wood WC, Proppe KH (1985) Preoperative, intraoperative and postoperative radiation in the treatment of primary soft tissue sarcoma. Cancer 55:2659–2667

Takahashi M, Okada K, Shibanoto Y et al. (1985) Intraoperative radiotherapy in the definitive treatment of localized carcinoma of the prostate. Int J Radiat Oncol Biol Phys 11:147–151

Tepper J, Nardi GL, Suit HD (1976) Carcinoma of the pancreas: Review of the MGH experience from 1963–1973. Analysis of surgical failure and implications for radiation therapy. Cancer 37:1519–1524

Tepper J, Sindelar W (1981) Summary of the workshop on intraoperative radiation therapy. Cancer Treat Rep 65:911–918

Tepper JE, Sindelar W, Travis EL et al. (1983) Tolerance of canine anastomoses to intraoperative radiation therapy. Int J Radiat Oncol Biol Phys 9:987–991

Tepper JE, Gunderson LL, Orlow E et al. (1984) Complications of intraoperative radiation therapy. Int J Radiat Oncol Biol Phys 10:1831–1839

Tepper JE, Cohen A, Wood WC et al. (1986) Intraoperative electron beam radiotherapy in the treatment of unresectable rectal cancer. Arch Surg 121:421–423

Todoroki T (1978) The late effects of single massive irradiation with electrons of the liver hilum in rabbits. Japanese J Gastroenterol Surg 11:169–177

Todoroki T, Iwasaki Y, Okamura T et al. (1980) Intraoperative radiotherapy for advanced carcinoma of the biliary system. Cancer 46:2179–2184

Van der werf Messing B (1978) Cancer of the urinary bladder treated by interstitial radium implant. Int J Radiat Oncol Biol Phys 4:373–378

Whittington R, Dobelbower RR, Mohiuddin M et al. (1981) Radiotherapy of unresectable pancreatic carcinoma: A six-year experience with 104 patients. Int J Radiat Oncol Biol Phys 7:1639–1644

Withers RH, Cuasay L, Mason KA et al. (1981) Elective radiation therapy in the curative treatment of cancer of the rectum and rectosigmoid colon. In: Stroehlein JR, Romsdahl MM (eds), Gastrointestinal Cancer, Raven Press, New York, pp 351–362

Wood W, Shipley WU, Gunderson LL et al. (1982) Intraoperative irradiation for unresectable pancreatic carcinoma. Cancer 49:1272–1275

4.2 Precision Pencil-Beam Radiation Therapy for Pituitary Adenomas

Kevin W. Mead

CONTENTS

1 Introduction

The treatment of pituitary adenomas by any surgical approach or by the use of the implantation of radioactive sources carries three disadvantages. Firstly, there is a small mortality rate for each procedure. Secondly, there is some morbidity because of the important structures adjacent to the gland and thirdly the methods are such that it is often difficult to achieve selective destruction of the adenoma with preservation of normal pituitary function.

On the other hand, precision high dose external radiotherapy can adequately control a functioning adenoma and leave the normal pituitary tissue almost intact. Although some degree of hypopituitarism has been reported to follow external radiotherapy for carcinoma of nasopharynx, pituitary adenoma and other tumors in this region, the degree of hypopituitarism is usually quite small and replacement therapy satisfactory. It should also be noted that in these reports the hypothalamus has usually been included in the irradiated volume. Techniques using small volumes completely avoiding the hypothalamus and its blood supply, may reasonably be expected to produce fewer side-effects on hypothalamic-pituitary function.

The dose required to ablate a normal pituitary is very high; that required to control adenomas is much less and probably lies between 50 and 100 Gy in 25 fractions over 5 weeks. Because it is possible to deliver a more even dose to the contents of the sella with external beams, external beam radiotherapy represents a more controlled technique and is therefore preferred.

This chapter describes techniques developed and used during the past 17 years, discusses their anatomical basis, and analyzes the results of treatment.

2 Anatomical Considerations

The occulomotor nerve pierces the roof of the cavernous sinus just antero-lateral to the posterior clinoid. At this point, it is a little more than 1 cm from the midline. Where it passes the anterior clinoid it is 1.5 cm from the midline.

The 4th, 5th and 6th cranial nerves are usually 1.5 cm from the midline but may be closer, though they are always separated from the pituitary gland by the carotid artery and cavernous sinus (McLachlan 1968). The figure of 1.5 cm from the midline is a safe assumption on which to base a therapy technique.

The optic nerve and chiasm are separated from the diaphragma by the chiasmatic cistern. They are usually 8 to 10 cm from the center of the sella. A CT scan, preferably with Metrizamide contrast, before treatment is essential to avoid treating an empty sella in which the chiasm may be situated.

The chiasm receives its blood supply from five arteries (anterior cerebral, anterior communicating, posterior communicating, internal carotid, and superior hypophysial), whereas the proximal part of the optic nerve is supplied by two arteries only, the superior hypophysial and the ophthalmic. All the blood supply to the optic nerve therefore comes from below it while two of the sources of supply to the chiasm are from above (anterior cerebral and anterior communicating). Thus, the total blood supply to the optic nerve is more limited in direction of origin than is that

Kevin W. Mead, Professor
Prince of Wales Hospital
Randwick, N.S.W. 2031, Australia

to the chiasm and it is, therefore, more likely to be included completely in any treatment volume. In addition, as the nerve and ophthalmic artery are enclosed in a bony canal, edema and swelling of the nerve could cause pressure on the ophthalmic artery or even obstruct the central retinal artery which comes from the ophthalmic artery in or close to the bony optic canal. On the other hand, the chiasm is free to expand in the fluid of the interpeduncular cistern.

These anatomical features require that we focus our attention particularly on avoiding the optic nerve where it enters the optic canal as well as on the chiasm, hypothalamus, and motor nerves in the cavernous sinus. Reports of unilateral radiation optic nerve damage support an explanation based on these antomical features (Bloom and Kramer 1984). Though the optic foramina should be excluded from the full dose of radiation, the front of the fossa just below and between them must be treated in many cases as some adenomas extend forward and undercut the tuberculum sellae.

As patients with pituitary secreting adenomas are more susceptible to radiation injury than are normal patients (Aristizabal et al. 1979) it is con-

sidered unsafe to deliver more than 60 Gy to any structures adjacent to the pituitary and to limit the dose to the chiasm and optic nerves at their entry into the optic foramina to 50 Gy at a dose rate of 200 cGy per day. The treatment volume is approximately spherical or ovoidal to correspond to any eccentricity of the pituitary adenoma. The arrangement of fields, if possible, should be such that the entrance path is not above a horizontal plane through the sella thus avoiding the important structures above the gland.

3 Techniques

Three different high dose techniques will be described and their suitability for various tumors discussed.

The first consists of using seven small fields to deliver 100 Gy with a 1.2 cm field to the pituitary fossa for Cushing's pituitary disease (Fig. 1).

The second delivers 50 Gy to a pituitary adenoma which has caused enlargement of the sella with a boost to the lower half to a total of 75 Gy for patients with acromegaly and for prolactinomas, again using seven fields (Fig. 2).

The third consists of a similar field arrangement boosting the center of the tumor to 75 Gy for inoperable chromophobe adenomas (Fig. 3).

Fig. 1. Seven field arrangement for pituitary Cushing's disease

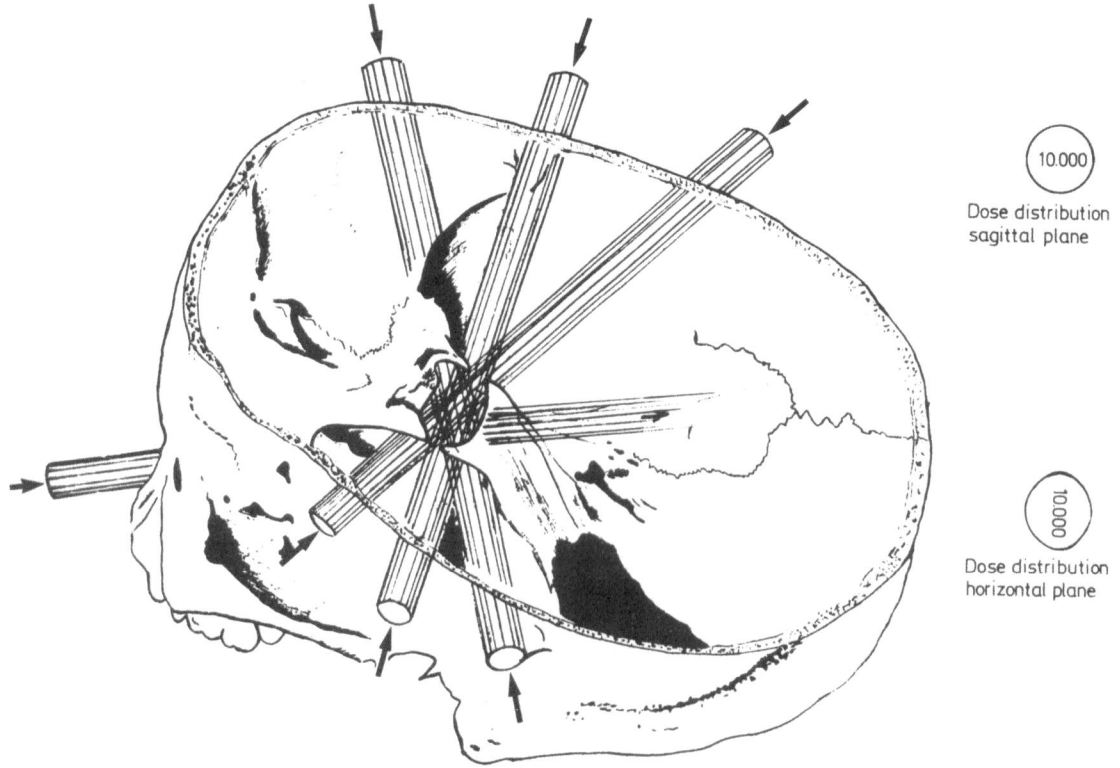

10.000

Dose distribution
sagittal plane

10.000

Dose distribution
horizontal plane

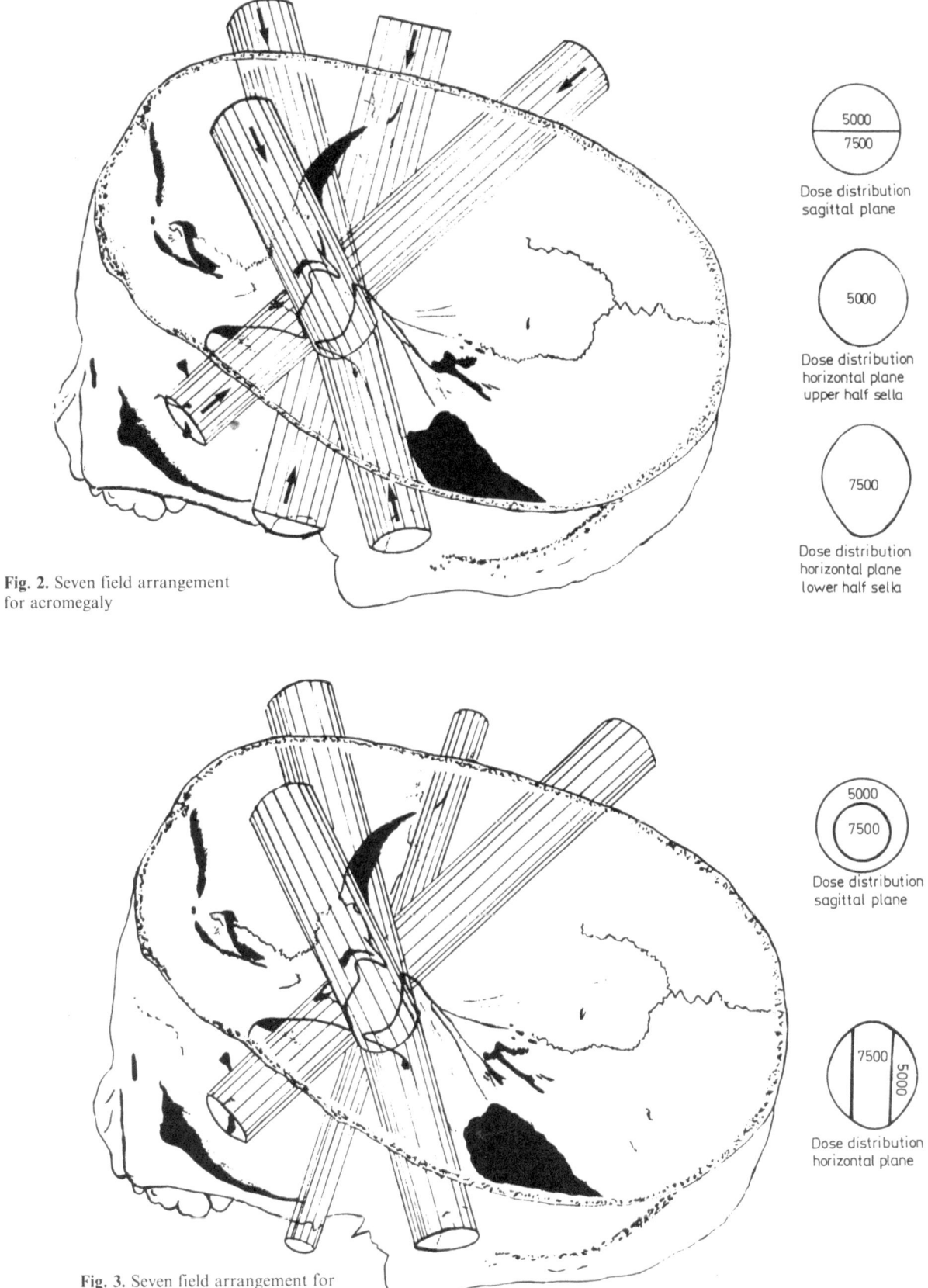

Fig. 2. Seven field arrangement for acromegaly

5000
————
7500

Dose distribution sagittal plane

5000

Dose distribution horizontal plane upper half sella

7500

Dose distribution horizontal plane lower half sella

5000

7500

Dose distribution sagittal plane

7500 | 5000

Dose distribution horizontal plane

Fig. 3. Seven field arrangement for inoperable chromophobe adenoma

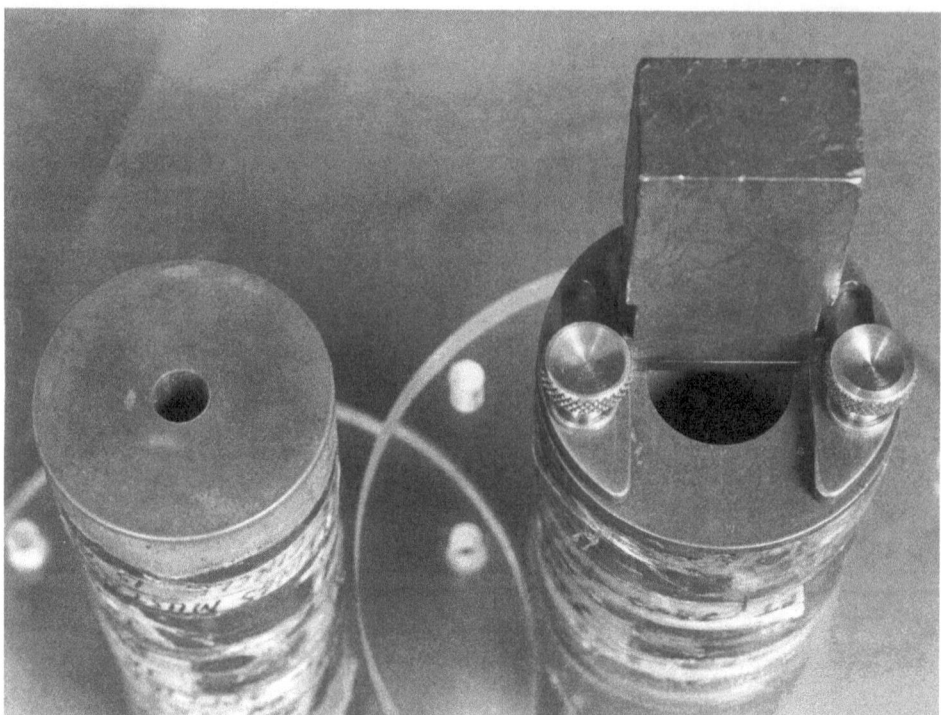

Fig. 4. Circular field collimators

Conventional linear accelerators producing beams of 4 or 10 MeV were used, and circular treatment collimators were attached to the shadow tray (Fig. 4). All techniques require precise patient immobilization achieved with custom casts and a bite block or other external methods.

These techniques were employed in treating various groups of patients as outlined below. The total series comprises 134 patients treated between 1968 and 1982.

3.1 Cushing's Disease

The field arrangement (Fig. 1) consists of two lateral fields, four lateral oblique and one transsphenoidal, each 1.2 cm in diameter. All fields are below the diaphragma and as they are circular there is no corner to project either upwards towards the chiasm or forwards to the optic foramen. The transsphenoidal field transverses no structures of importance before reaching the gland and exits below the hypothalamus through the interpeduncular fossa and mid brain. It passes below the optic nerves and chiasm. The maximum tumor dose is 100 Gy and the rapid fall off ensures that the dose at the chiasm is less than 50 Gy. This has been confirmed by thermo-luminescent dosimetry in a phantom man in which the capsules were placed at sites of interest, the cavernous sinus, chiasm, prefixed chiasm, pituitary, hypothalamus and optic foramen. The accuracy of the fields is verified in the following way. Small lead markers are sutured to the skin in each temporal region so that the line joining them passes precisely through the center of the sella (Fig. 5). These markers can then be seen in the port films in the center of the lateral fields (Fig. 6). The transsphenoidal field is verified by ensuring that its center is equidistant from each skin marker and on the line joining them (Fig. 7).

In the oblique port films the sella can be seen within the small circular field but accuracy is verified geometrically in the following manner. The port film of the oblique field shows the position of the field relative to the positions of the lead markers. In order for the central axis of the field to bisect the line joining the skin markers (i.e., the center of the sella), two conditions must be met: (1) The ratio of the distances B'P' and P'A' on the film should be as shown in Fig. 8. (2) The line joining the images of the markers should bisect the image of the field. This verification is accurate to 1 mm. An example is seen in Fig. 9. The couch can be moved in the vertical or linear direction as required to rectify any error shown in any of these port films before treatment is given.

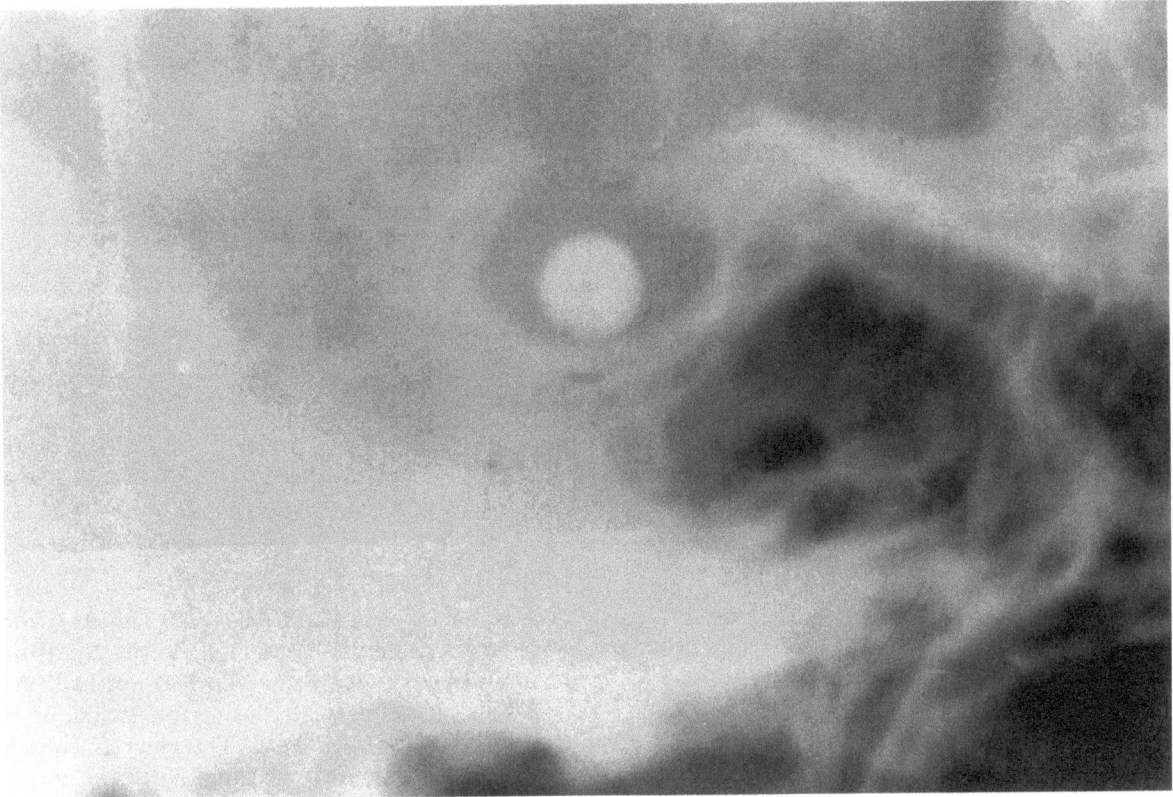

Fig. 5. Planning radiograph showing markers overlying center of sella

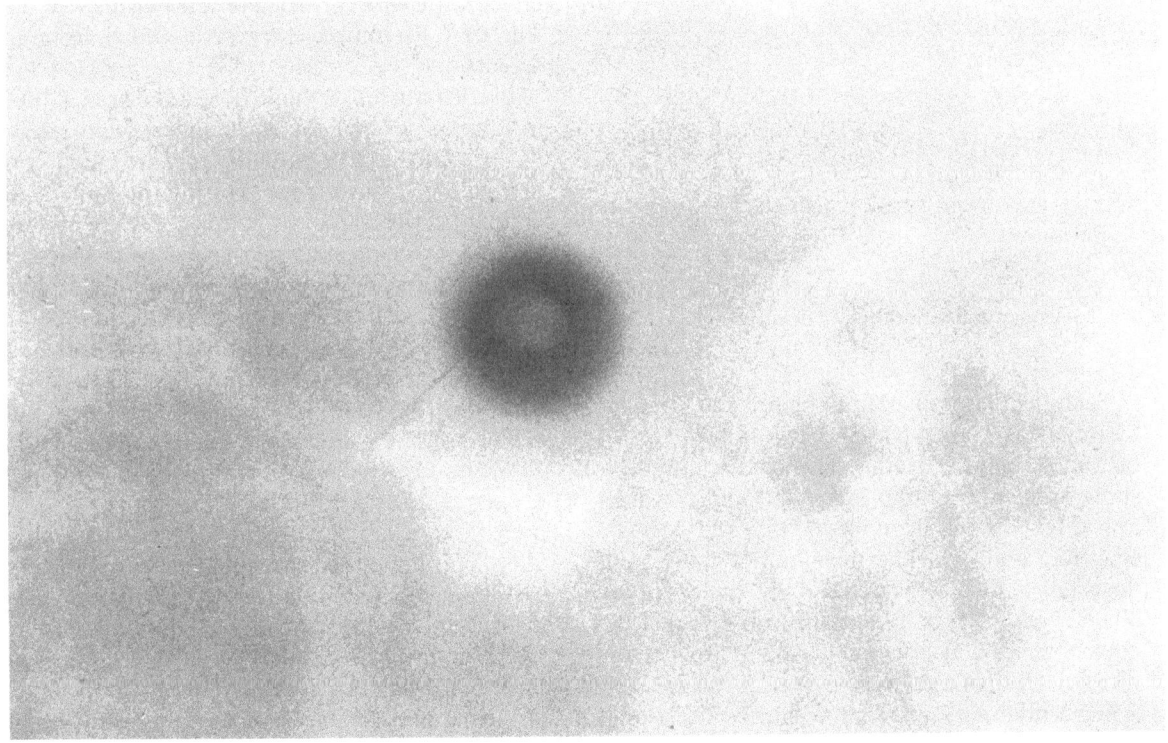

Fig. 6. Port film of lateral field

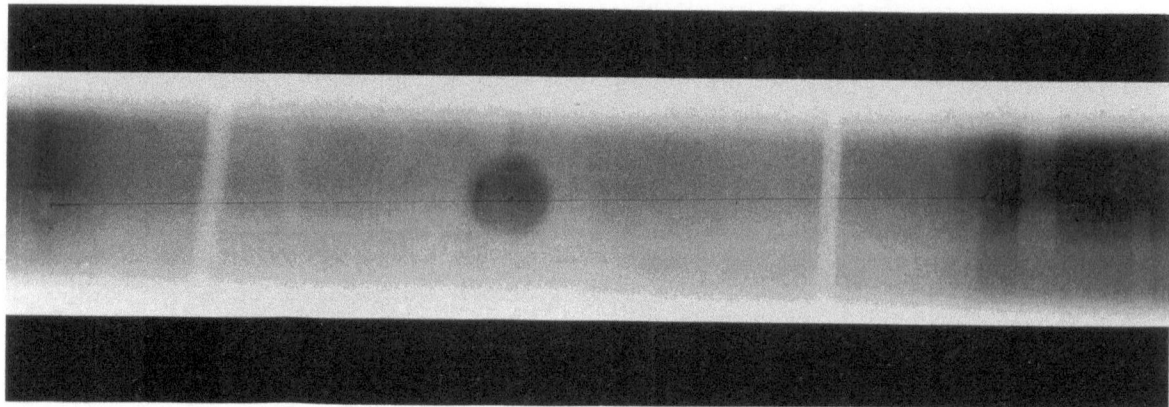

Fig. 7. Port film of transsphenoidal field

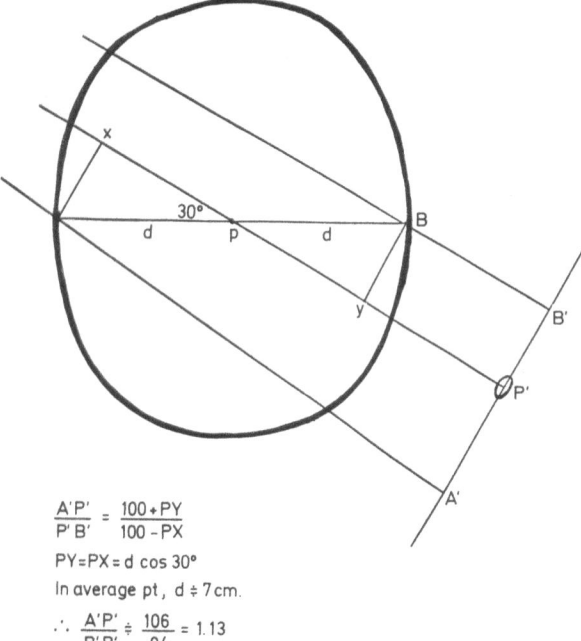

$$\frac{A'P'}{P'B'} = \frac{100 + PY}{100 - PX}$$

$$PY = PX = d \cos 30°$$

In average pt, $d \doteq 7\,cm.$

$$\therefore \frac{A'P'}{P'B'} \doteq \frac{106}{94} = 1.13$$

Fig. 8. Geometrical verification of oblique field

Each field is verified, both before and after each treatment is given, so that small adjustments can be made before treatment and that any error shown in the after film is known, and can be allowed for later in the course. One field is treated each day and, with the maximum 100 Gy tumor dose given in 5 weeks, the daily tumor dose is 400 cGy and the daily entrance dose is 600 cGy. However, each field is small and is treated only three of four times over 5 weeks. These fields achieve minimal treatment volumes. The isodose diagram in the horizontal and sagittal planes are shown in Fig. 10.

3.1.1 Results

Twenty-eight patients (8 males; 20 females) with pituitary Cushing's disease ranging in age from 8 to 60 (median 48) years who had not had previous surgery were treated using this technique to tumor doses of 60–100 Gy. The clinical features of pituitary-dependent Cushing's disease are so characteristic that clinical cure is fairly obvious. The biochemical criteria of cure were a return to normal of the 24 hour urinary 17 oxogenic steroids, the plasma cortisol, and the plasma A.C.T.H. The time to complete response varied from 1 to 4 years.

In 19 patients, a high dose was used (100 Gy in 5 weeks, except for two children who received 75 Gy). Of these 19 patients, 16 were cured, 1 improved and 2 have failed. During the same period and with the same technique, 9 patients were treated to 60 Gy and of these 5 were cured. Of the 4 failures, 3 were given an additional 40 Gy and 2 of these have been cured. Thus, in this small group of 9, 7 have been cured by radiotherapy. Of the total group of 28 patients, 23 have been cured (82%), 1 improved, and 4 failed to repond (Table 1). The follow-up period varied from 2 to 14 years. Of the 26 patients followed for 5 years or longer, the cure rate at 5 years was 85%. One patient, considered cured at 5 years, has relapsed later. This patient was treated to 60 Gy only. This sustained cure rate contrasts with surgical results in which the long term success rate falls progressively or is not available (ZERVAS 1984). Figure 11 shows the clinically evident improvement in one of the cured patients.

Six patients with Nelson's syndrome have been treated with the same technique to 60–100 Gy,

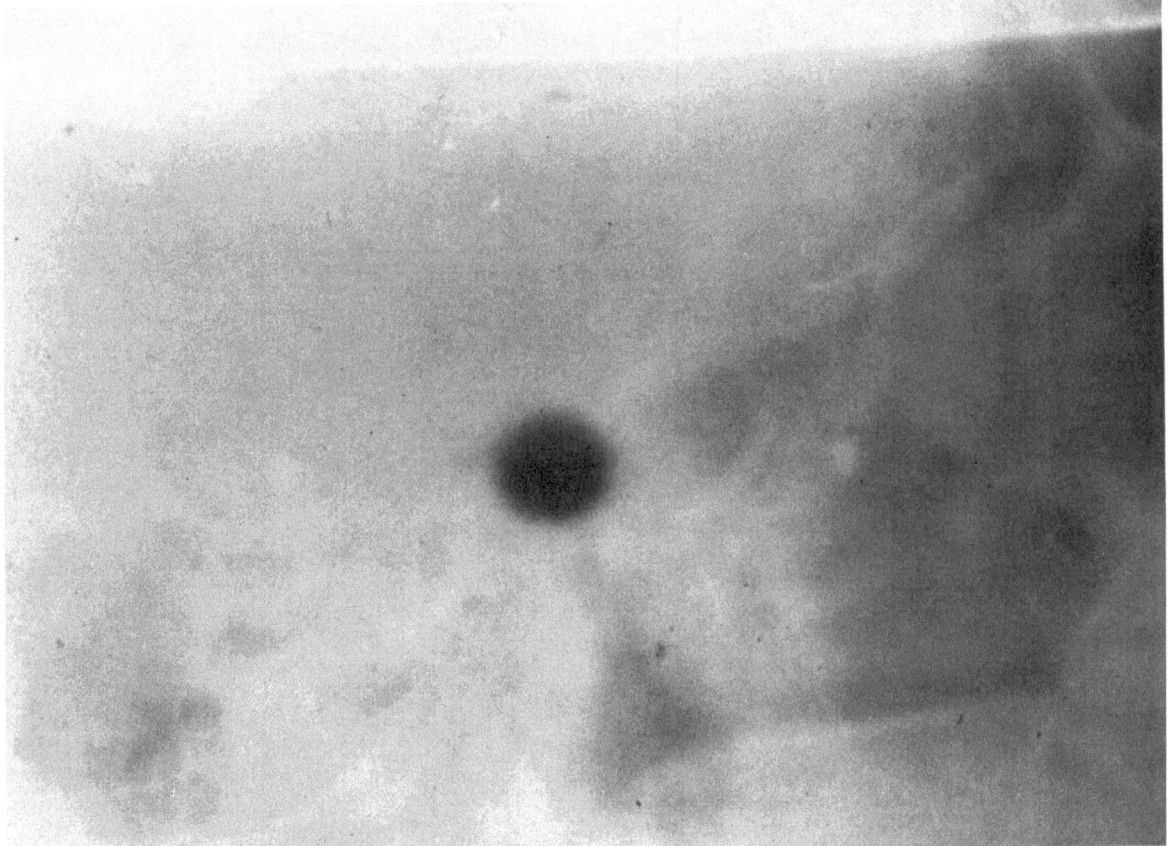

Fig. 9. Port film of oblique field

though the fields have usually been slightly larger as the adenoma in these instances is known sometimes to be invasive. The outcome in this small group is satisfactory (4 are cured, 1 failed, and 1 was lost to follow-up), but the number is too small to draw general conclusions.

The optimal dose level for Cushing's disease is still uncertain, but the excellent results obtained with the high dose technique suggest an advantage in its use. RAHN et al. (1980) has reached a similar conclusion and achieved excellent results using the gamma radiosurgical unit. The absence of complications is attributed to the small volume and great care in delivering the treatment. With a dose of 100 Gy at the center of the sella, the chiasm and optic nerves receive approximately 30 Gy, the cavernous sinus 50 Gy, and the hyothalamus less than 2 Gy, all in 25 fractions. In pituitary dependent Cushing's disease the tumor and the sella are small, and the high dose small volume technique is logical. Radiotherapy is particularly attractive as the basophil tumor is less well defined and less easily found at surgery than is the eosinophil ad-

enoma (WILSON and DEMPSEY 1978). The sustained results of the treatment used in this series with no visual complications and only 3 cases of hypopituitarism strongly favor the technique used as the treatment of choice. Although the response to radiotherapy is slow, medical treatment is usually successful during this period.

3.2 Acromegaly

LAWRENCE et al. (1971) reviewed the results of radiation treatment for acromegaly and reported that with conventional doses complete control can be achieved in 70% of patients within 2 years. A higher figure than this has been achieved with the proton beam (KLIMAN et al. 1984). As the facility to irradiate with charged particles is available in very few centers, an alternative technique with megavoltage x-ray equipment was used in this series of patients who had not previously undergone any type of surgical treatment.

A total of 30 patients (13 males; 17 females), ranging in age from 27–70 years (median 41 years),

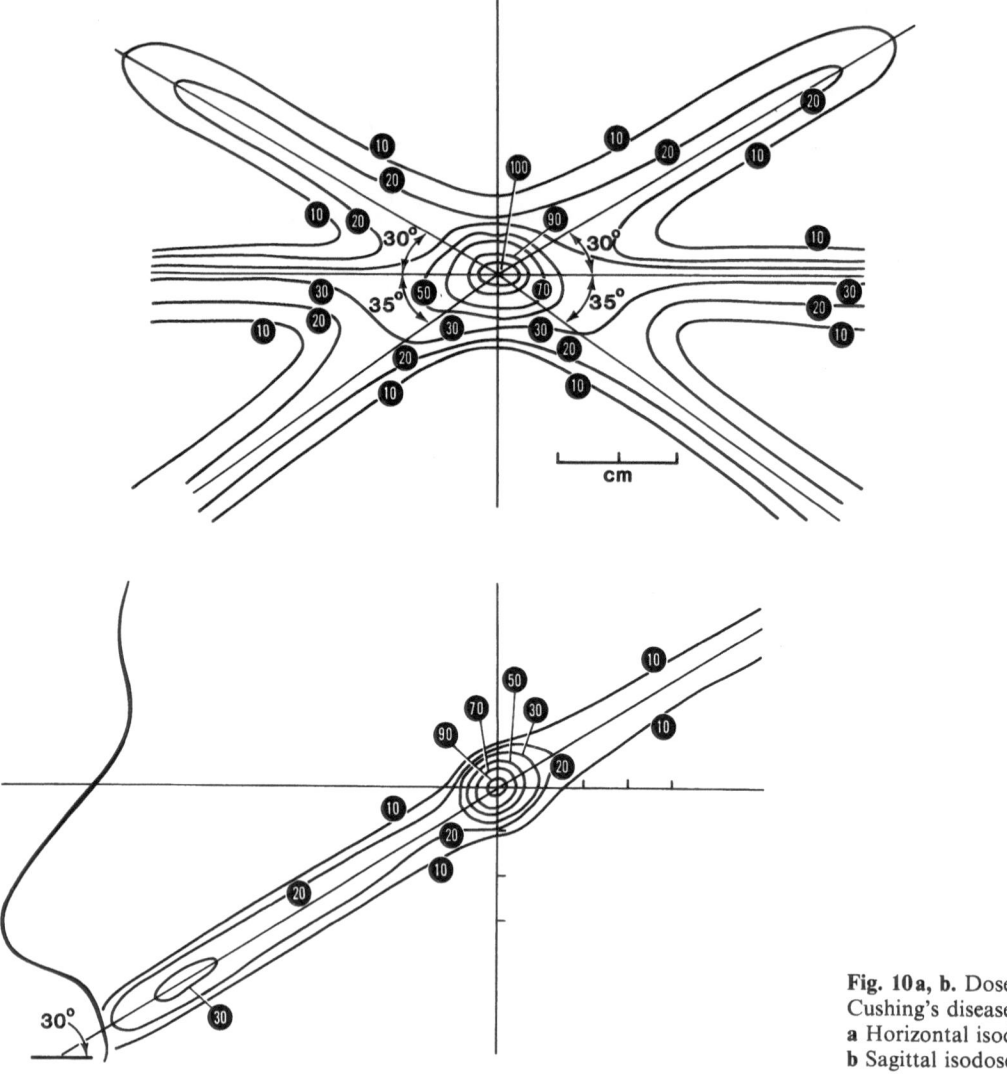

Fig. 10a, b. Dose distribution of
Cushing's disease technique.
a Horizontal isodose diagram.
b Sagittal isodose diagram

Table 1. Cushing's – Status at 2 to 14 years since treatment

10,000 to a 1 cm sphere	Number	Cured	Complications	Hypopituitarism
(10)	19	16	0	2
6,000 + 4,000 to a 1 cm sphere				
(t + 4)	9	7	0	1
Total	28	23 (82%)	0	3

have been treated. Eleven patients with small pituitary fossae were treated by the method described already using 7 fields to a small volume and a dose of 100 Gy. Of these, 8 have been cured. The 3 failures are attributed to the use of a treatment volume too small for the size of the tumor. A second series of 9 patients were treated with a larger field, usually 2.5 or 3 cm in diameter, to ensure coverage of the whole adenoma and to this volume

Fig. 11. Photograph of Cushing's patient before and 12 ▷ months after radiotherapy

Fig. 12. Port film of a lateral semicircular boost field for acromegaly

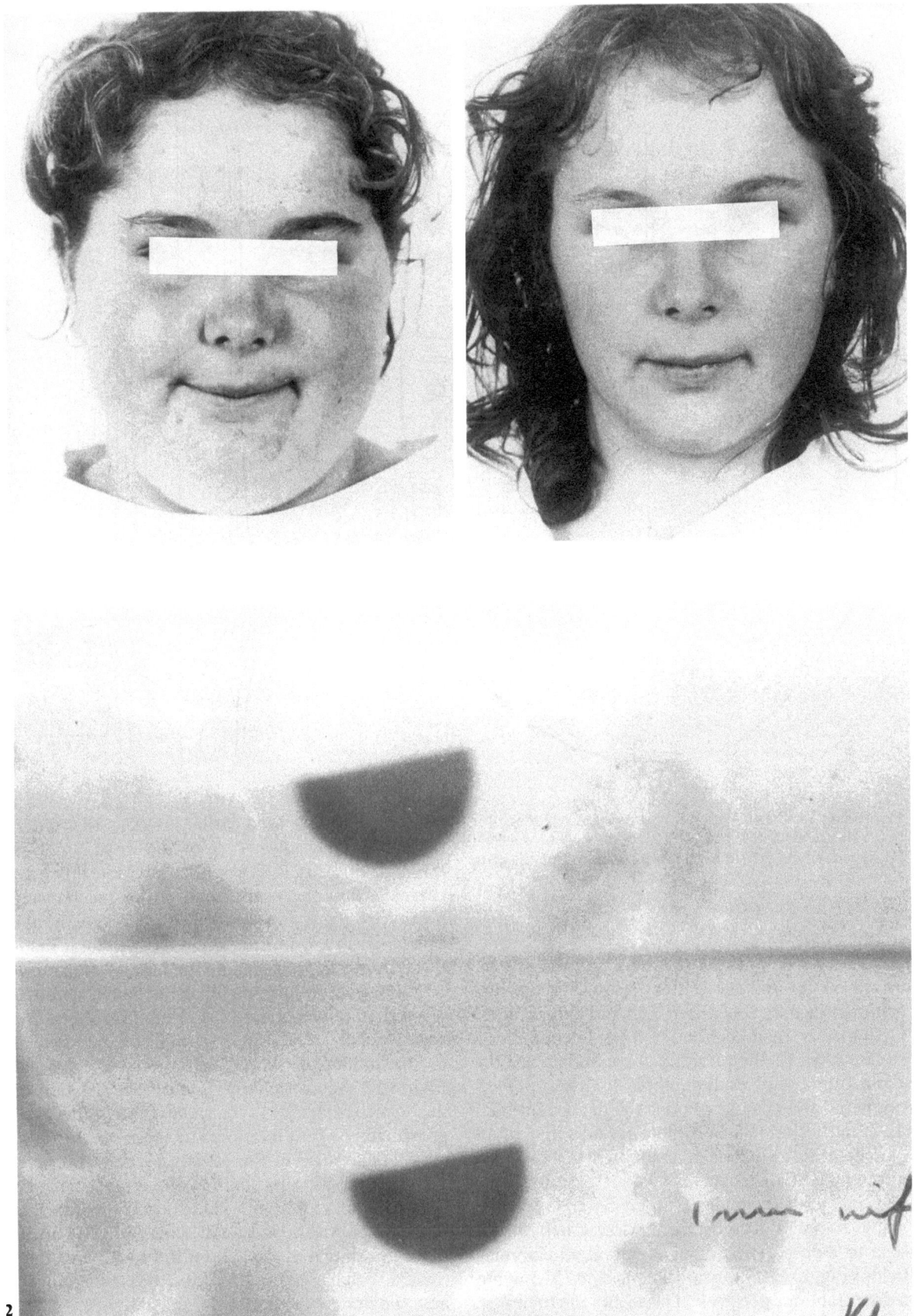

2

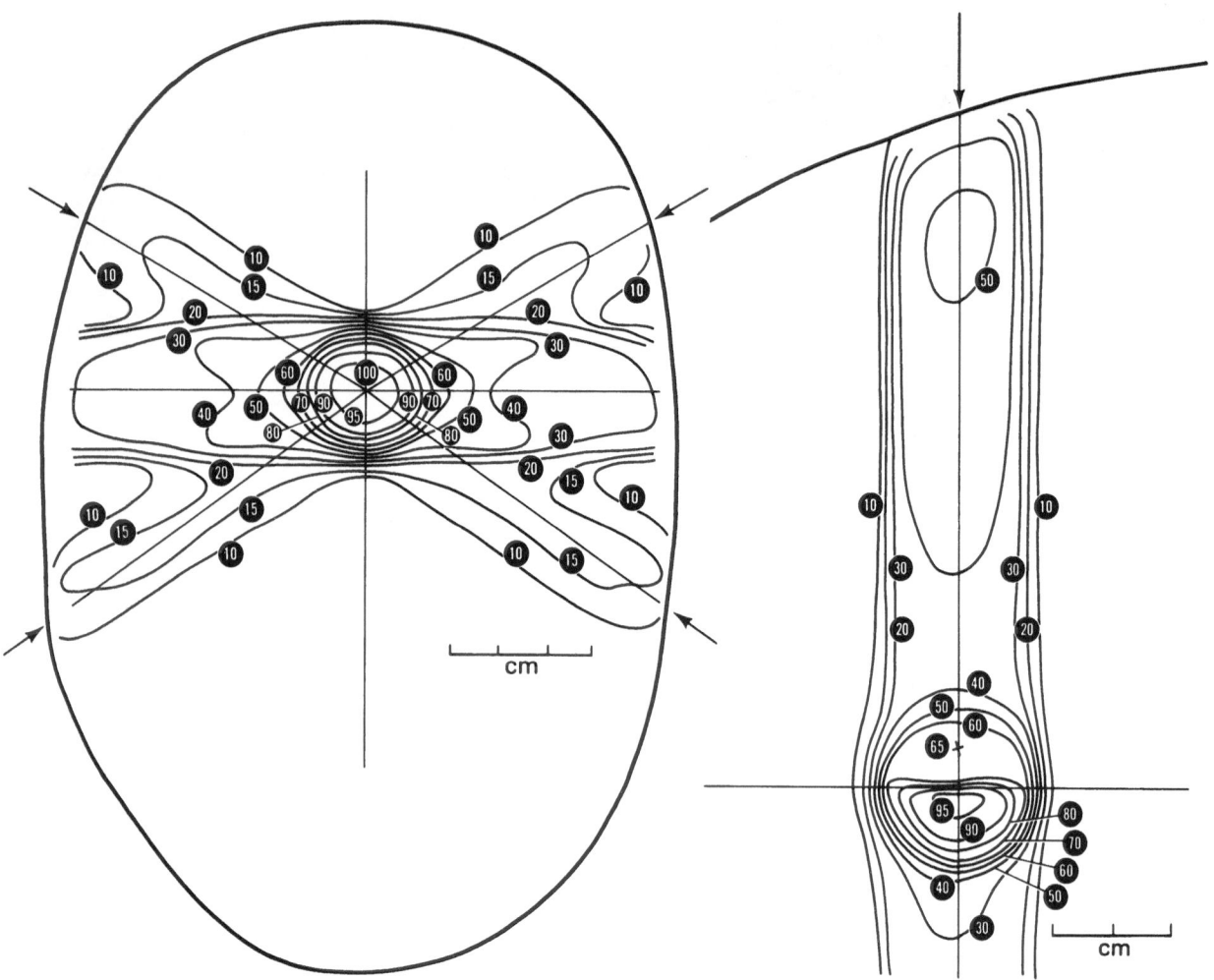

Fig. 13a, b. Dose distribution for acromegaly technique for field arrangement in Fig. 2. **a** Horizontal isodose diagram (+ superior field 2.5 cm circle), **b** sagittal isodose diagram (superior field)

was added a central boost. The larger volume received 50 Gy and the center 75 Gy. Success was achieved in only 6 of these, and the failures were attributed to the likelihood that the adenoma was situated low in the pituitary fossa. Whatever the explanation, the result in these two groups was not better than can be obtained with conventional dose and technique. In a more recent series of 10 patients, the technique was adapted to boost the lower half of the fossa using four oblique fields and one vertical circular field giving 50 Gy to the whole tumor and boosting the lower half of the sella to a dose of 75 Gy using lateral semicircular fields (Fig. 2). The overall time is 5 weeks, giving 5 dose fractions per week. This technique therefore

differs from those used earlier in which the center, rather than the lower half of the fossa, received the high dose. It is essential to exclude the optic nerves within the optic canals from the boosted portion of the tumor volume (the 75 Gy volume). The upper margin of the lateral semicircular fields must, therefore, not include the base of the anterior clinoids. The movement of the couch required when the pre-treatment port check film shows the beam is not in perfect position can be effected to the millimeter with conventional equipment. Figure 12 shows such an alteration of position of the semicircular field which has been shifted approximately 1 mm inferiorly to come off the optic nerves. The dose in the cavernous sinus must be kept below 55 Gy by limiting the diameter of the vertical field to 2.5 cm. The isodose diagrams in the horizontal and saggital planes for this technique are shown in Fig. 13. Of the 10 patients thus treated, 8 have been cured and this technique is now the one preferred for acromegaly.

Table 2. Acromegaly – Status at 2 to 15 years since treatment

Thousand rads	Number	Cured	Compli-cations	Hypo-pituitarism
⑩	11	8	0	1
5 / (7.5) / 5	9	6	0	1
5 / 7.5	10	8	0	1
Total	30	22 (73%)	0	3

The overall results of the acromegaly series are summarized in Table 2; 22 of 30 patients have been cured, with a range of time to complete response from 1 to 10 years. This technique has also been used for prolactinomas though the numbers are too few to allow any firm conclusions. The use of bromocryptine could modify any surgical or radiotherapeutic approach to prolactinomas in the future.

3.3 Chromophobe Adenoma

Of the 60 patients with chromophobe adenoma treated during this period, most were irradiated postoperatively after subtotal excision giving 50 Gy in 20 fractions over 4 weeks with a 3 field technique. In patients with larger inoperable tumors, a central boost to 75 Gy in 5 weeks was given as illustrated in Fig. 3. Of the 3 patients, 1 died with persistent tumor after 12 months, and the other 2 are alive and well more than 5 years after treatment. The overall recurrence rate at 5 years for the chromophobe group is 10% (MEAD 1981).

4 Complications

No serious complications have been encountered in this entire series in spite of the high doses delivered. This is attributed to the use of small fields, specially made applicators and meticulous attention to beam direction including the use of port verification films before and after every treatment.

Indeed, the techniques described cannot be recommended unless such care is taken to achieve dose precision.

In the patients with secreting tumors treated to high doses (greater than 75 Gy) and followed up for 2–14 years, the incidence of hypopituitarism is approximately 10%. Although this incidence may increase with time, hypopituitarism usually follows radiotherapy within 5 years of treatment. It is likely that the low incidence of this side effect is associated with the small volumes irradiated, avoiding the hypothalamus directly and also most of its blood supply. Reporting a 20 year experience with proton beam therapy for acromegaly, KLIMAN et al. (1984) has found an incidence of only 9% supporting an explanation based on the avoidance of irradiation to the hypothalamus. The achievement of pregnancy in 3 patients in this series following high dose radiotherapy confined to the pituitary gland also supports this view.

There have been no visual complications in any of the patients treated with the high dose techniques. None had been treated previously by surgery or radiotherapy. This is an important factor in the avoidance of radiation complications.

Those patients who have undergone surgery and radiotherapy for chromophobe adenoma usually needed hormone replacement and frequently were found to have persisting visual field defects. In no instance did either of these clinical findings worsen following radiotherapy unless the tumor recurred.

5 Summary

Techniques are described which enable the delivery of a high dose of radiation to pituitary adenomas with safety, using conventional linear accelerators. Long-term results are given. The anatomical basis for the field selection is also discussed.

Acknowledgement. I gratefully acknowledge that the geometrical method of accuracy vertification was contributed by Dr. D. WALKER, Physicist, Queensland Radium Institute.

References

Aristizabel SA, Boone ML, Laguna JF (1979) Endocrine factors influencing radiation injury to central nervous system. Int J Radiat Oncol Biol Phys 5.349–353, 1979
Bloom B, Kramer S (1984) Conventional radiation therapy in the management of acromegaly. In: Mc L.Black P, Zervas NT, Ridgway EC, Martin JB (eds) Secretory tumors of the pituitary gland. Progress in endocrine re-

search and therapy, Vol. 1, Raven Press, New York, p 189

Kliman B, Kjellberg RN, Swisher B, Butler W (1984) Proton beam therapy of acromegaly: a 20 year experience. In: Mc L.Black P, Zervas NT, Ridgway EC, Martin JB (eds) Secretory tumors of the pituitary gland. Progress in endocrine research and therapy, Vol. 1, Raven Press, New York

Lawrence AM, Pinsky SM, Goldfine ID (1971) Conventional radiation therapy in acromegaly: A review and reassessment. Arch Intern Med 128:369

McLachlan MSF (1968) applied anatomy of the pituitary gland and fossa: A radiological and histopathological study based on 50 necropsies. Brit J Radiol 41:782

Meed KW (1981) High dose radiotherapy for pituitary tumours. Australian Radiol 25:229

Rahn T, Thoren M, Hall K, Backlund EO (1980) Sterotactic radiosurgery in Cushing's syndrome: Acute radiation effects. Surg Neurol 14:85

Wilson CB, Dempsey LC (1978) Transsphenoidal microsurgical removal of 250 pituitary adenomas. J Neurosurg 48:13

Zervas NT (1984) Surgical results for pituitary adenomas: Results of an international survey. In: Mc L.Black P, Zervas NT, Ridgway EC, Martin JB (eds) Secretory tumors of the pituitary gland: Progress in endocrine research and therapy, Vol. 1, Raven Press, New York, pp 379–381

4.3 Stereotaxic Interstitial Brachytherapy for Malignant Brain Tumors

Philip H. Gutin and Steven A. Leibel

CONTENTS

1 Introduction

Results of recent studies of patients with glioblastoma multiforme show that when these lesions recur after irradiation, they do so most commonly within 2 cm of the original site (Hochberg and Pruitt 1980). Moreover, metastases from malignant gliomas within the central nervous system are uncommon (Erlich and Davis 1978) and systemic metastases are rare (Alvord 1976). Yet, despite the localized nature of many malignant brain tumors, the principal experimental thrust in their treatment has been systemic chemotherapy, a modality for which the traditional target has been metastatic disease (Gutin and Levin 1983).

Results published by the Brain Tumor Study Group (BTSG) show that patients harboring primary malignant brain tumors who received more than 50 Gy of radiation to the whole brain sur-

Philip H. Gutin, M.D., Associate Professor
Steven A. Leibel, M.D., Associate Professor
School of Medicine
University of California
San Francisco, CA 94143, USA

vived 20.5 weeks longer than patients treated by surgery only (Walker et al. 1978). Walker et al. (1979) analyzed the BTSG data more critically and showed stepwise increments in survival in patients cohorts receiving 50, 55, or 60 Gy. Even after irradiation to 60 Gy, however, local tumor recurrence was the rule, and this dose cannot be much escalated because doses of radiation greater than 60 Gy put patients at a significant risk for developing brain necrosis (Sheline et al. 1980).

Because of the localized nature of primary brain tumors, intensive local treatment techniques such as hyperthermia, intratumoral chemotherapy, or interstitial brachytherapy would seem to be the appropriate modalities for the treatment of these lesions. Given that radiation therapy has been the most effective modality, brachytherapy becomes a logical local treatment for brain tumors either as a "boost" immediately after maximal external beam treatment for primary treatment or for reirradiation of recurrent gliomas.

2 History

In 1914, Frazier (Frazier 1920) implanted radium sources into brain tumors harbored by 32 patients, and over the next 40 years numerous reports of brachytherapy for brain tumors with mixed results were published (Bernstein and Gutin 1981). Greater accuracy and sophistication were achieved in brain tumor brachytherapy with the availability of Leksell stereotaxic systems that allowed the implantation of isotopes into brain tumors without open craniotomy using stereotaxic ventriculography and angiography for guidance. Talairach et al. (1955) in Paris and Mundinger et al. (1978, 1984) in Freiburg pioneered the techniques of stereotaxic interstitial brachytherapy and have gained enormous experience with a variety of brain tumors, predominantly the lower grade gliomas. These tumors were commonly treated with permanently-implanted, low activity iridium-192 (^{192}Ir) sources.

3 Present

The computerized tomographic (CT) scanner has made interstitial radiation of brain tumors an attractive treatment modality because it is possible preoperatively to estimate tumor size, consistency, and location. The availability of a number of integrated CT-stereotaxic systems allows the calculation of a trajectory to any tumor target(s) seen on the CT scan and makes possible the extraordinarily accurate placement of the radioactive source at the target(s) through an often distant, small burr hole in the skull (Mackay et al. 1982; Heilbrun et al. 1983). Other developments that have led to the recent interest in brain tumor brachytherapy are the availability of new, safer, and possibly more effective isotopes such as iodine-125 (^{125}I) and the maturation of neuro-oncology into a clinical science with emphasis on long-term follow-up review and rigid criteria of response to therapy (Levin et al. 1977).

4 Removable High Activity Iodine-125 Implants for Recurrent Gliomas

4.1 Rationale

The European groups have used brain tumor brachytherapy primarily to treat low grade gliomas, tumors for which we prescribe external beam treatment (Leibel et al. 1975). At our institution we have focused on the more malignant brain tumors. Over the past 4 years we have used CT-stereotaxic techniques to implant gold-198 (^{198}Au), ^{192}Ir, and ^{125}I sources into 141 patients with primary and metastatic malignant brain tumors. Most patients have been implanted with removable, high activity ^{125}I sources for the irradiation of recurrent malignant gliomas or as an adjuvant interstitial "boost" dose to residual malignant gliomas after surgical reduction and conventional external beam radiation therapy. In this chapter the clinical results obtained for brachytherapy for recurrent malignant gliomas will be described. The interstitial "boost" adjuvant treatment protocol will be described, but results are too preliminary to be discussed at this writing.

4.2 Patient Selection

Patients with recurrent malignant gliomas as large as 6 cm in the largest dimension were treated with brachytherapy if lesions were localized with distinct margins on CT scans. Diffusely infiltrative tumors, tumors with subependymal spread, or multifocal tumors were not treated with this technique. Because of the limited biological reserve of previously irradiated posterior fossa structures, only supratentorial tumors were implanted.

Between January 1, 1980 and September 1, 1984, 53 patients with malignant gliomas that had recurred after surgery and conventional radiation therapy were implanted with removable high activity ^{125}I sources. Most patients had been treated with various chemotherapeutic agents. Patients ranged in age from 5 to 61 years. Twenty-two patients harbored glioblastomas, 29 anaplastic astrocytomas, and two anaplastic ependymomas.

4.3 Isotope

Although ^{198}Au and ^{192}Ir have been used extensively for interstitial irradiation of brain tumors (Bernstein and Gutin 1981; Mundinger and Weigel 1984; Szikla 1979), we prefer ^{125}I because the characteristic X rays have a far lower energy (27–35 keV) than the gamma-rays from other isotopes used for brachytherapy. The lower energy makes it easier to protect personnel (Liu and Edwards 1979) and, because of tissue attenuation, limits to some extent the radiation exposure of normal brain surrounding the lesion (Krishnaswamy 1978). There is some evidence that the relative biological effectiveness of ^{125}I is greater than unity (Kim and Hilaris 1975; Freeman et al. 1982), although we have reported the results of experiments in which this effect was not found (daSilva et al. 1984).

^{125}I is available commercially as a standard low activity (0.5 mCi) source. A large number of these sources would have to be implanted into fast growing, malignant brain tumors to deliver dose rates that would stop the growth of these tumors. Thus, high activity ^{125}I sources (30 to 50 mCi) were supplied by special order from the manufacturer (Medical Products Division, 3 M Co., St. Paul, Minnesota).

A well ionization chamber with a sensitivity of 2.3×10^{11} A°/mg radon equivalent for the higher photon energies was used to calibrate sources. Because an absolute calibration factor is not yet available for ^{125}I and the inherent difficulty of dosimetry around ^{125}I sources (Krishnaswamy 1978), chamber readings were related to the activity stated by the manufacturer.

4.4 Implantation Technique

A CT scan with contrast enhancement was obtained before the procedure and measurements of the tumor were made. A target was chosen at the center of roughly spherical tumors, while sources were positioned along the axis of elongated (prolately ellipsoidal) tumors. Most often two, three, or four catheters, each containing several sources, were implanted. The location and the size of the tumor determined whether the radiation dose was delivered to the periphery of the area of contrast enhancement seen on CT scans or to a volume beyond it. Catheters were loaded with a sufficient number of ^{125}I sources to deliver approximately 10 Gy/day (30–50 cGy/hr) to the area considered to be the tumor margin.

Implantations were performed under local anesthesia in adults (Fig. 1) and under general anesthesia in children. The Leksell stereotaxic system modified for use with the CT scanner was used to position the sources (MacKay et al. 1982) (Leksell stereotaxic apparatus manufactured by Downs Surgical Inc., 2500 Park Central Boulevard, Decatur, Georgia) in the initial phases of the study, but recently we have used the Brown-Roberts-Wells stereotaxic system (Brown-Roberts-Wells sterotaxic apparatus manufactured by Trentwells, Inc., Southgate, California) (HEILBRUN et al. 1983). Sources were held in afterloaded coaxial silicone catheters that have been described (GUTIN and DORMANDY 1982). The advantages of this system are that implanted high-activity sources can be removed after the desired dose has been delivered and that catheters hold the sources at the correct target positions in the often necrotic tumor centers.

The availability of integrated stereotaxic and CT scanner systems (MacKay et al. 1982; MUNDINGER et al. 1978; OSTERTAG et al. 1980) has made the implantation of isotopes into tumors at open craniotomy suboptimal. It is frequently difficult to expose a glioma at craniotomy well enough to be able to appreciate its geometry, and this inability makes the implantation of a suitable isotope array nearly impossible. However, CT-stereotaxy allows precise implantation of sources into targets selected from CT scans, which show the exact shape and dimensions of a tumor. Because a craniotomy wound may take more than an hour to close, surgeons and nurses would be exposed unnecessarily to high levels of radiation. Stereotaxic implantation of isotopes can be performed through small skin incisions and burr or twist drill holes in the skull, which can be closed with facility.

Patients were isolated in private rooms while the sources were in place and were cared for by nurses trained in radiation safety. A radiation physicist monitored the rooms carefully and determined the safe exposure times for nurses and visitors. A helmet lined with lead foil sufficient to shield ^{125}I X rays almost totally was worn by the patient when visitors or medical personnel entered the room.

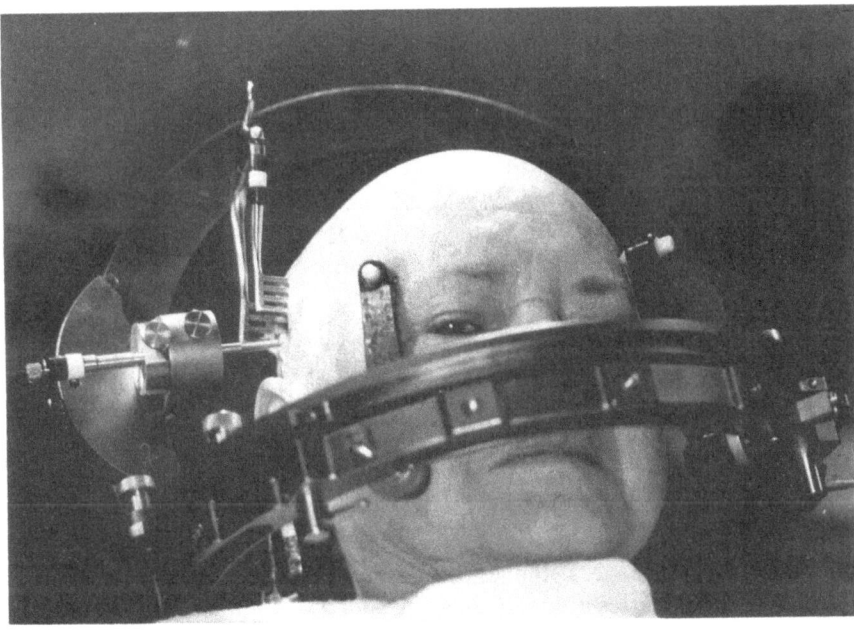

Fig. 1. Photograph showing one of several catheters being implanted into a right parietal anaplastic astrocytoma using the CT stereotaxic guidance system. The surgery is performed under local anesthesia

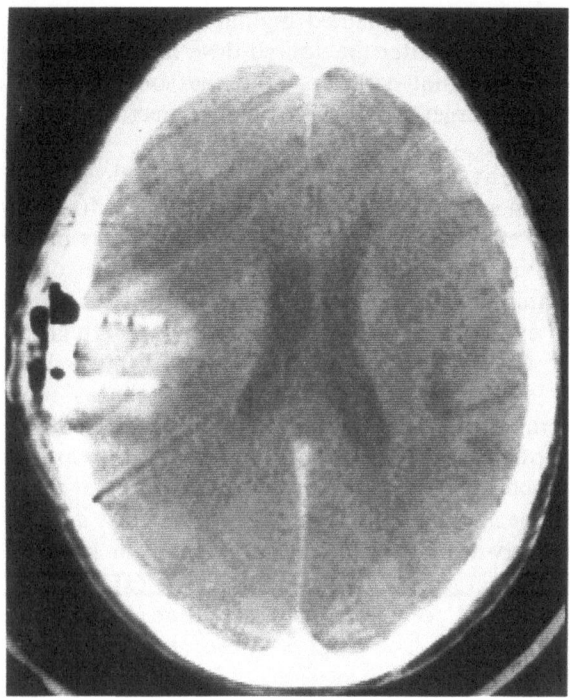

Fig. 2. Computed tomographic scan localizing the position of ¹²⁵I sources in two of four catheters implanted into the tumor harbored by the patient shown in Fig. 1. The other catheters can be seen on another slice

4.5 Dosimetry

After sources were implanted, a CT scan was performed to confirm that sources had been placed accurately (Fig. 2), and orthogonal radiographs were taken to determine source relationships. A computer program converted position data and source strengths into dose rate contours in any plane. The implantation time for the desired dose was calculated, and sources were removed in a simple procedure under local anesthesia at the appropriate time. Dose rate contours were converted by the computer to total dose plots, which were scaled to match the magnification and to allow superimposition on radiographs and postimplantation CT scans.

A computer program, kindly provided by Dr. Volker Sturm and Dr. Wolfgang Schlegel of the University of Heidelberg, is now available for planning ¹²⁵I brachytherapy based on CT scan images (Schlegel et al. 1982). Targets in the tumor are chosen and isodose contours are quickly plotted on axial images and in any reformatted plane to assess coverage of the lesion. Because of anisotropy, ¹²⁵I sources are treated as line sources

with the angle of implantation taken into account in the dosimetry plots (Fig. 3). Obviously, dosimetry determined with the computer program will be more accurate that dosimetry based on orthogonal skull X rays, upon which tumor cannot be visualized.

4.6 Patient Evaluation

Postoperatively, corticosteroid doses were adjusted as needed to improve neurological function and to reduce the symptoms of increased intracranial pressure. Because improvement caused by steroids can mimic response to interstitial irradiation, doses were increased only when required to treat clear clinical deterioration. In addition, attempts were made to reduce the steroid dose every 6 to 8 weeks if the patient was clinically stable or improving. Anticonvulsant agents were used when medically indicated.

Patients were evaluated by neurological examinations and CT scanning at intervals of 8 weeks, when possible, and graded on a scale of −2 to +2 (deterioration to improvement) (Levin et al. 1977). Patients were considered evaluable if they were alive and available for their first evaluation 8 weeks after implantation. Response was defined as a definite improvement in at least one criterion in the same evaluation period if the corticosteroid dose was unchanged or decreased. Progression of disease was defined as definite deterioration in at least one criterion if the corticosteroid dose was unchanged or increased. Stable disease was defined as no change in either criterion if the corticosteroid dose was unchanged or decreased. Time to progression was measured from the day of implantation until progression was documented.

4.7 Results

4.7.1 Response to Treatment

One to four catheters, each containing one to three high-activity ¹²⁵I sources, were implanted and delivered 30–120 Gy (most recently 80 Gy) minimum tumor dose. Dose rates were between 20–100 cGy/hr; most commonly they were 40 cGy/hr. Results of 45 implantation procedures in 43 patients are currently evaluable. Of the 10 non-evaluable patients, three died of non-neurological causes, one developed a brain abscess that required reoperation, and one was lost to follow-up. The other

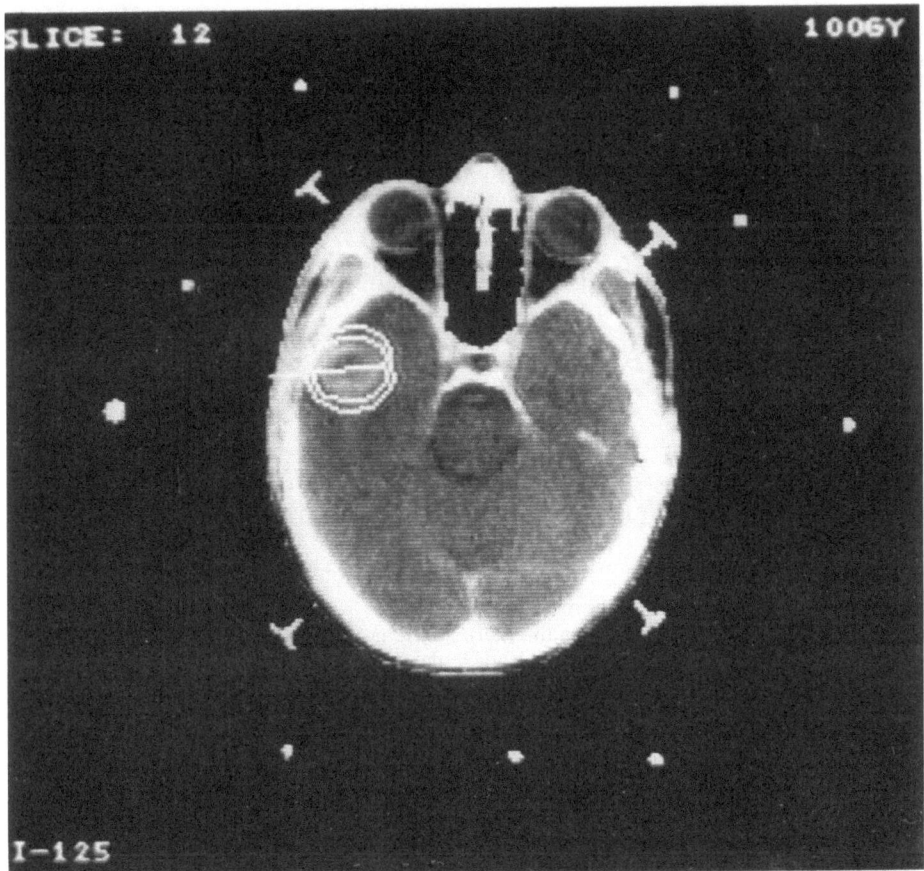

Fig. 3. CT scan image used for the treatment planning for a left temporal glioblastoma. One of several catheter trajectories and the composite isodose configurations can be seen in the upper left center of the image. The patient's head is held in the stereotaxic array, and target coordinates can be calculated based on the array of localizing rods, seen as dots on the scan, around the head

five non-evaluable patients have not returned for their first evaluation.

Twenty-two of the implantations into recurrent malignant gliomas produced responses that have persisted for as long as 17 months. Seven implantations produced stabilization of disease for 3–15 months, and in 16 patients implantation did not halt progression of disease. As defined by our criteria, progression is not necessarily a harbinger of poor survival because, as defined by clinical and radiologic criteria, deterioration is frequently the direct result of focal radiation necrosis in the tumor and peritumoral brain (GUTIN et al. 1984) (see below). Such changes have been described after permanent implantation of ^{192}Ir sources into brain tumors and are certainly to be expected with high focal doses of radiation in brain previously irradiated to tolerance (OSTERTAG et al. 1979). Focal necrosis cannot be distinguished from tumor regrowth using the results of CT scan and neurologic examination as criteria for the evaluation of responses to treatment. We are studying the use of positron emission tomography (PATRONAS

et al. 1982) and magnetic resonance imaging for this purpose.

4.7.2 Reoperation

Fourteen patients treated with interstitial brachytherapy for recurrent malignant gliomas have undergone craniotomy 5–18 months after implantation. To reduce cerebral edema and mass effect and to differentiate focal radiation necrosis from tumor regrowth, an exploration was performed to resect contrast-enhancing lesions seen on CT scans (Fig. 4). Six of these patients had shown progression of disease at evaluation first their at 2 months

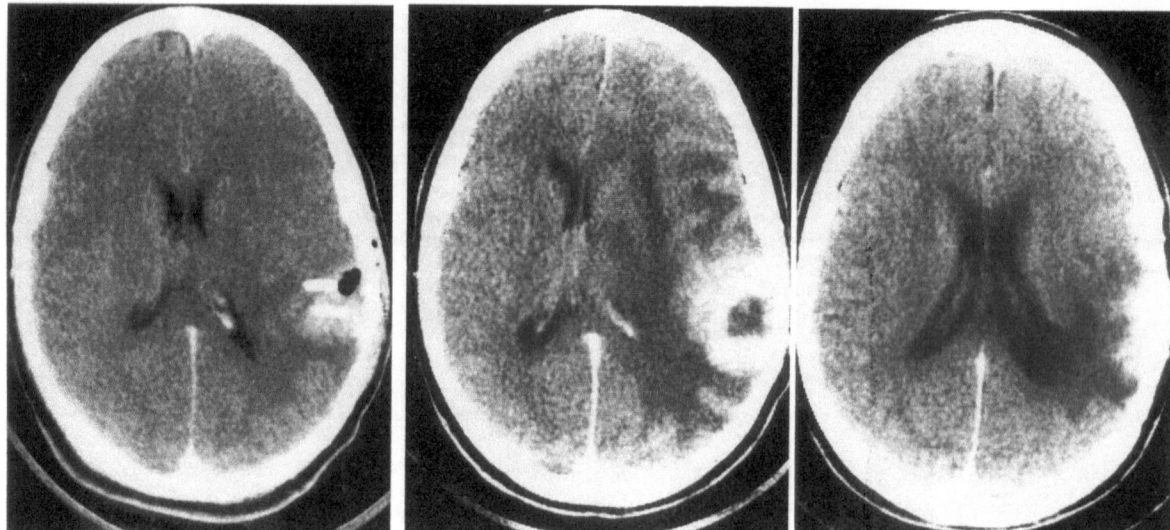

Fig. 4. CT scans showing a recurrent right parietal anaplastic astrocytoma at the time of implantation (*left*), and four months (*center*) and 16 months (*right*) after brachytherapy with a minimum tumor dose of 80 Gy. Because of the marked persistent worsening seen after implantation (center), exploratory craniotomy was performed four months after the implantation procedure. A large amount of tissue was resected, which was found to be mostly necrotic material at histopathologic examination. Some tumor tissue was also identified at histopathologic examination. The patient is stable and off steroid therapy 19 months after the implantation procedure was performed

alive and without obvious progession at 13–18 months after implantation; tumor recurred in the eighth patient. The long-term survival in this group suggests that tumor cells present in mixed specimens may have a low growth potential, and their presence is not predictive of rapid regrowth. We have begun studies of these cells cultured *in vitro* (ROSENBLUM et al. 1978). In many instances, tumor cells will not form colonies, a fact that may predict a good result.

after implantation, six were responders for 2–13 months, and two had stabilized for 5 and 11 months before signs of deterioration were apparent. The histopathology of the operative specimens showed pure necrotic tissue in three patients, predominantly tumor in three, and a mixture of tumor and necrotic tissue in eight. Of the patients treated for recurrent malignant glioma, those in this reoperated group had the longest survival: 11 of 14 patients remain alive 10–48 months (mean 30 months) after brachytherapy.

The histopathology of resected tissue was somewhat predictive of outcome. Two of three of the patients from whom tissue that was primarily tumor was obtained at reoperation died at 17 and 20 months after brachytherapy, and the other is alive with gross recurrence at 12 months. The three patients with purely necrotic tissue at reoperation are alive without disease progression at 10–37 months after brachytherapy. Curiously, the eight patients from whom tissue was a mix of tumor cells and necrotic tissue have done well with seven

4.7.3 Survival

Because standard neuro-oncological endpoints – CT scan and neurological examination – cannot distinguish tumor regrowth from focal radiation necrosis, survival is the most rigorous criterion of response to therapy. The median survival after implantation in the entire group of patients treated for recurrent malignant gliomas is now more than one and one-half years with over half the patient group still surviving. This result is far better than that produced by our best chemotherapy regimens used to treat recurrent tumors (GUTIN and LEVIN 1983). However, such a comparison is biased in favor of brachytherapy because those patients treated with brachytherapy were selected on the basis of favorable tumor geometry. Nevertheless, many patients were classified as being "endstage" because they had received aggressive chemotherapy for recurrence before being implanted. In addition, because we did not recognize the possible complication of radiation necrosis initially, resection of the necrotic mass was not performed until relatively late in the series. A case control study is underway to eliminate bias in comparison of the forms of treatment and these results will be reported elsewhere.

Because brachytherapy can induce focal brain necrosis, the neurological deficit may be induced or exacerbated; the nature and extent of the deficit appears to depend on the location of the tumor and the volume treated. Reoperation can sometimes arrest deterioration allowing steroids to be withdrawn (GUTIN et al. 1984), although some patients may remain steroid dependent for prolonged periods. A minority of patients are unable to care for themselves, but many return to work, school, or homemaking activities.

In summary, our experience with brachytherapy for brain tumors that recur after radiation therapy indicates that it is not unreasonable to predict a long-term survival for a patient harboring a well-circumscribed tumor that is implanted correctly. However, focal radiation necrosis should be anticipated and managed surgically.

5 Adjuvant Interstitial "Boosts" for Malignant Gliomas

It is enormously difficult to cure any recurrent tumor. Control of the disease at initial treatment is obviously preferred. For this reason we have begun a protocol study under the auspices of the Northern California Oncology Group. The protocol is based on the implantation of patients with removable ^{125}I "boosts" immediately after localized external-beam irradiation. WALKER et al. (1979) found stepwise increments in survival in patient groups receiving 50, 55, or 60 Gy of external beam irradiation after surgery. While higher doses of external beam irradiation might lead to further increments of survival, the risk of developing large volume radiation necrosis would become unacceptable. Our implanted "boost" is designed to increase the radiation dose to the tumor while sparing surrounding normal brain tissue. The risk of focal radiation necrosis to the patients receiving "boosts" is unknown, but, based on our experience with patients in the series discussed here, this complication should be surgically manageable. It is not possible to predict for the individual patient the extent of neurological deficit that might be caused by such aggressive therapy.

Currently, 45 patients have been placed on this protocol. It is too early to evaluate the results. However, the addition of brachytherapy to the regimen will have to yield significantly superior results over those obtained in patients receiving identical therapy without the boost to justify the risk of increased deficit and the expense of the brachytherapy procedure.

6 Hyperthermia and Brain Tumor Brachytherapy

Because focal brain injury remains one of the most serious problems in brain tumor brachytherapy, it seems prudent to seek ways to lower the interstitially delivered radiation dose required for local tumor control. Local hyperthermia, delivered along with brachytherapy, may be helpful in this regard (MANNING et al. 1982). Interstitially implanted microwave antennae or localized current field needle electrodes are the best devices currently available for the delivery of heat to deep tumor targets. Such hardware can be placed accurately into brain tumors during the procedure in which sources are implanted. Because fewer microwave antennae than localized current field electrodes must be implanted to heat a given volume, the microwave system is the more attractive. Strohbehn and his coworkers (STROHBEHN et al. 1979; COUGHLIN et al. 1983) have developed an interstitial microwave hyperthermia system for human use operated at 915 MHz. Although a few patients with brain tumors have been treated with brachytherapy and hyperthermia at various institutions, many technical problems remain to be overcome, and most research is still at the preclinical level (LYONS et al. 1984).

References

Alvord EC Jr (1976) Why do gliomas not metastasize? Arch Neurol 33:73–75

Bernstein M, Gutin PH (1981) Interstitial irradiation of brain tumors: a review. Neurosurgery 9:741–750

Coughlin JCT et al. (1983) Interstitial hyperthermia in combination with brachytherapy. Radiology 148:285–288

DaSilva V et al. (1984) Relative biological effectiveness of ^{125}I sources in a murine brachytherapy model. Int J Radiat Oncol Biol Phys 10:2109–2111

Erlich SS, Davis RL (1978) Spinal subarachnoid metastasis from primary intracranial glioblastoma multiforme. Cancer 42:2854–2864

Frazier CH (1920) The effects of radium emanations upon brain tumors. Surg Gynecol Obstet 31:236–239

Freeman ML et al. (1982) Studies with encapsulated ^{125}I sources. II. Determination of the relatively biological effectiveness using cultured mammalian cells. Int J Radiat Oncol Biol Phys 8:1355–1361

Gutin PH, Dormandy RH Jr (1982) A coaxial catheter system for afterloading radioactive sources for the interstitial irradiation of brain tumors. Technical note. J Neurosurg 56:734–735

Gutin PH, Levin VA (1983) Surgery, radiation and chemotherapy in the treatment of malignant brain tumors. In: Thompson RA, Green JR (eds) Controversies in neurology. Raven Press, New York, pp 67–86

Gutin PH et al. (1984) Brachytherapy of recurrent malignant brain tumors with removable high-activity iodine-125 sources. J Neurosurg 60:61–68

Heilbrun MP et al. (1983) Preliminary experience with the Brown-Roberts-Wells (BRW) computerized tomographic stereotaxic guidance system. J Neurosurg 59:217–222

Hochberg F, Pruitt A (1980) Assumptions in the radiotherapy of glioblastoma. Neurology 30:907–911

Kim JH, Hilaris BJ (1975) Iodine-125 source in interstitial tumor therapy. AJR 123:163–169

Krishnaswamy V (1978) Dose distribution around a ^{125}I seed source in tissue. Radiology 126:489–491

Leibel SA et al. (1975) The role of radiation therapy in the treatment of astrocytomas. Cancer 35:1551–1557

Levin VA et al. (1977) Criteria for evaluating patients undergoing chemotherapy for malignant brain tumors. J Neurosurg 47:329–335

Liu J, Edwards FM (1979) Radiation exposure to medical personnel during iodine-125 seed implantation of the prostate. Radiology 132:748–749

Lyons BE et al. (1984) Localized hyperthermia in the treatment of malignant brain tumors using an interstitial microwave antenna array. IEEE-BME 31:53–62

MacKay AR et al. (1982) Computed tomography-directed stereotaxy for biopsy and interstitial irradiation of brain tumors: Technical note. Neurosurgery 11:38–42

Manning MR et al. (1982) Clinical results of a phase I trial employing hyperthermia alone or in combination with external beam or interstitial radiotherapy. Cancer 49:205–216

Mundinger F et al. (1978) Treatment of small cerebral gliomas with CT-aided stereotaxic curietherapy. Neuroradiology 16:564–567

Mundinger F, Weigel K (1984) Long-term results of stereotactic interstitial curietherapy. Acta Neurochir Supp 33:367–371

Ostertag CB et al. (1979) CT-changes after long-term interstitial iridium-192-irradiation of cerebral gliomas. In: Szikla G (ed) Stereotactic cerebral irradiation. Elsevier, Amsterdam, pp 149–155

Ostertag CB et al. (1980) Stereotactic biopsy of brain tumors. Surg Neurol 14:275–283

Patronas NJ et al. (1982) Work in progress: ^{18}F-Fluorodeoxyglucose and positron emission tomography in the evaluation of radiation necrosis of the brain. Radiology 144:885–889

Rosenblum ML et al. (1978) Development of a clonogenic cell assay for human brain tumors. Cancer 41:2305–2314

Schlegel W et al. (1982) CT images as the basis of operation planning in stereotactical neurosurgery. Proceedings of the 1st International Symposium on Medical Imaging and Image Interpretation, pp 172–177

Sheline GE (1980) Therapeutic irradiation and brain injury. Int J Radiat Oncol Biol Phys 6:1215–1228

Strohbehn JW et al. (1979) An invasive microwave antenna for locally induced hyperthermia for cancer therapy. J Microwave Power 14:339–350

Szikla G (ed) (1979) Stereotactic cerebral irradiation. Elsevier, Amsterdam

Talairach J et al. (1955) A new method of treatment of inoperable brain tumours by stereotaxic implantation of radioactive gold – a preliminary report. Br J Radiol 28:62–74

Walker MD et al. (1978) Evaluation of BCNU and/or radiotherapy in the treatment of anaplastic gliomas. A cooperative clinical trial. J Neurosurg 49:333–343

Walker MD et al. (1979) An analysis of dose-effect relationship in the radiotherapy of malignant gliomas. Int J Radiat Oncol Biol Phys 5:1733–1740

4.4 Photodynamic Therapy

THOMAS J. DOUGHERTY

CONTENTS

1 Historical Introduction

The use of light absorbing chemicals to cause photoreactions in biological systems dates back to at least 1900 when Raab reported a lethal effect on paramecium exposed to light and an acridine dye. Since that time numerous examples of the "photodynamic effect" have been reported for a wide range of photosensitizers both in vitro and in vivo (for a review see SPIKES and STRAIGHT 1967). In most cases oxygen is required in addition to a photosensitizer and light. The mechanism generally accepted for inactivation of biological systems is an energy transfer process from the excited triplet state of the sensitizer to oxygen, producing singlet oxygen which causes irreversible oxidation of some essential cellular component.

While a number of photosensitizers can be considered for localization and possible therapy of tumors, the porphyrins have received most attention since the observation of Policard in 1924 that certain malignant tumors in animals and man demonstrated a reddish fluorescence attributed to accumulation of endogenous porphyrins resulting from secondary infection by hemolytic bacteria.

In 1966 Lipson, Gray and Baldes reported the first use of hematoporphyrin derivative, Hpd, to treat cancer. While the primary purpose of their study was tumor detection, Lipson realized the potential for selective destruction of tumors containing Hpd by making use of its photodynamic properties. A patient with a large ulcerating recurrent breast tumor was treated by multiple Hpd injections and local exposure of the tumor to filtered light from a Xenon arc lamp (spectrum not specified) (LIPSON et al. 1966). While the lesion remained after several weeks of repeated treatment, objective evidence of response was found. No further therapy using this method was reported by this group or any others until the 1970's.

For a photosensitizer to be widely clinically useful it should be non-toxic in clinically useful doses, be selectively taken up and/or retained in malignant tissue, be activated by penetrating light (>600 nm), and be relatively photochemically efficient. The active fraction of hematoporphyrin derivative, which appears to be dihematoporphyrin ether (DHE), meets these criteria reasonably well (DOUGHERTY et al. 1984).

In 1975 Dougherty and colleagues reported complete eradication of transplanted mouse mammary tumors without excessive damage to the surrounding skin using systemic Hpd, activated by red light (600–700 nm) from a Xenon arc lamp. Neither the light nor Hpd alone as applied resulted in any gross effects on tumor or skin. After toxicology and preclinical studies were completed, a clinical trial was begun by this group in 1976.

Also in 1976 Kelly and Snell reported specific Hpd uptake in malignant and pre-malignant lesions of the bladder and reported treatment of a single case of bladder cancer using Hpd and light from a mercury lamp directed into the bladder via a glass light guide. Tumor destruction was found only in the illuminated areas of tumor. No

THOMAS J. DOUGHERTY, Ph.D.
Roswell Park Memorial Institute
Buffalo, NY 14263, USA

further work has been reported by this group. Since 1976 and especially since 1980 numerous studies of Hpd photoradiation applied to a wide variety of tumors have been initiated and reported (see below).

2 Hematoporphyrin Derivative (Hpd) and Its Active Component

Dougherty et al. have tested numerous porphyrins as in vivo photosensitizers of the SMT-F tumor transplanted in DBA/2 mice, e.g. hematoporphyrin, protoporphyrin, uroporphyrin, etc. Among these, only tetraphenylporphine sulfonate (TPPS), hematoporphyrin derivative (Hpd), and its active component DHE have been found to be active in this system although other compounds are active in vitro (see below). Hematoporphyrin itself has been reported to be active in vivo by some investigators (TOMIO et al. 1983) and inactive by others (DOUGHERTY 1983a). It is now known that various preparations of hematoporphyrin may contain material similar to the active material in Hpd and when this is removed, in vivo activity disappears (DOUGHERTY 1983b).

While TPPS was found to be at least as active as Hpd, its low rate of serum clearance (BELLNIER 1982) and reported neurotoxocity (KENNEDY 1983) have precluded it from being tested clinically.

When Hp is acetylated it yields monoacetate (20–30%), di-acetate (50–60%), and unchanged Hp (5–20%). In addition the mono-and di-dehydration products of Hp are formed. None of the components of this acetate mixture are active in photosensitizing tumors (BERENBAUM et al. 1982). However, when dissolved for injection in dilute sodium hydroxide solution or slightly acidic saline, the acetate groups are rapidly hydrolyzed producing a mixture of porphyrins very active as a tumor localizer and photosensitizer and termed here hematoporphyrin derivative (Hpd). In 1981 Dougherty separated Hpd by gel exclusion chromatography and identified a new fraction representing approximately 45% of the mixture. This material was found to be responsible for the tumor photosensitizing ability of Hpd (DOUGHERTY et al. 1983). In addition, it appeared to provide a higher therapeutic ratio in animals (tumor vs skin) than the Hpd mixture. A common name suggested for this compound is dihematoporphyrin ether (DHE).

This material has a strong tendency to self-associate in aqueous solutions even in the presence of albumin at a concentration similar to that found in serum (~ 30 mg/ml). Grossweiner has estimated that 15–20% of this material remains unbound to serum protein in patients (1984). In fact, spectroscopy of sera taken from patients 0.5 to 3 hr after receiving DHE indicated considerable self-association of the porphyrin whereas at longer times it appeared to be mainly dissociated (probably bound to serum protein). It is this strong tendency for self-association that may be responsible for long periods of retention of Hpd and DHE in tumors. Phagocytosis of DHE by macrophages, Kupfer cells, mast cells, and cells of the reticuloendothelial system has been demonstrated (BUGELSKI et al. 1981). There is preliminary evidence that tumor endothelial cells may also take up DHE and may be an important site of tumor activation by PDT (DOUGHERTY and WITYK 1984).

DHE in aqueous solutions demonstrates no fluorescence. However, in tetrahydrofuran, a solvent that caused disaggregation, the typical red porphyrin fluorescence was seen. Further, bright fluorescence was seen in tumors in animals or humans, similar to that found for Hpd. The actual fluorescent yield of DHE has not yet been determined; for Hpd it is 2–3% (DOIRON et al. 1979).

Also, when aggregated, DHE does not generate singlet oxygen, being less than one-quarter as efficient as Hp at similar concentrations in water (DOUGHERTY et al. 1983). Therefore, it is reasonable to assume that DHE aggregates, while they may be important in tumor uptake and retention, are not responsible as such for the fluorescence or photosensitizing effect of DHE, which apparently must first disaggregate (and/or metabolize) within the tissue to be effective.

The uptake of DHE and Hpd in the DBA/2 Ha mouse tissue indicates that compared to Hpd, only half the injected amount of DHE is necessary to achieve similar tissue levels, e.g. 3–5 µg/g tumor (SMT-F) 3 to 24 hr following 10 mg/kg Hpd or 5.0 mg/kg DHE intraperitoneally (DOUGHERTY et al. 1984).

The distribution of Hpd in various organs and tissues of the mouse delineated by visual fluorescence is not consistent with the distribution determined using radioactivity tagged porphyrins. For example, while little fluorescence is apparent in liver, kidney, and spleen after systemic Hpd injection, these organs take up more [3]H- or ^{14}C-Hpd than any other tissues (GOMER and DOUGHERTY 1979). While in principle it could be argued that porphyrin metabolites are responsible for this discrepancy, animals receiving Hpd and illumination of the peritoneal cavity (red light) die of liver damage (see below). Thus it is more likely that fluorescence in these organs cannot be observed due to the high absorptivity by the blood for both the activating light (usually blue) and the fluorescent light (630, 690 nm). Thus, even though these organs do not fluoresce, great care should be exercised to prevent their exposure to the therapeutic light when tumors are treated in areas near or involving them.

Because of the tendency of Hpd and DHE to be retained in skin, patients receiving these materials are cautioned to remain out of bright sunlight for a minimum of 30 days.

It appears that Hpd uptake in at least some spontaneous tumors in animals and man is considerably higher than that measured in the rodent tumors. For example, a spontaneous, primary adamantinoma tumor removed from a pet dog 72 hr post 5.0 mg/kg Hpd demonstrated considerably brighter fluorescence than that seen in a transplanted SMT-F tumor in the DBA/2 mice 24 hr after receiving the same dose of Hpd and the porphyrin level of approximately 50 µg/g tumor was more than ten times that of the SMT-F tumor (DOUGHERTY 1983a). WHAREN et al. (1983) used superficial tissue fluorescence of frozen biopsy samples to determine porphyrin levels in normal brain tissue and three glioblastomas in humans and in a transplanted rat glioblastoma. Porphyrin levels measured in two astro-oligodendrogliomas (Grade III), one removed 24 hr and the other 48 hr post injection of 5.0 mg/kg Hpd, were 2.5 µg/g and 0.1 µg/g respectively, indicating a possibly rapid clearance of Hpd from these types of tumors. This is quite unlike the results in transplanted mammary tumors reported by GOMER and DOUGHERTY (1979), which showed little clearance over many days.

3 Toxicology

Direct drug toxicity was determined in Albino Swiss mice (Ha/ICR) by injecting the porphyrin intraperitoneally and maintaining the animals in the dark (DOUGHERTY and DOUGLASS 1983). The LD_{50} dose at 24 hr post injection for Hpd in both male and female mice was 275 mg/kg. At 14 days the LD_{50} values were 230 mg/kg and 180 mg/kg for male and female mice respectively. Multiple doses (50 mg/kg every day for 5 days) or 25 mg/kg every other day for 10 days yielded no deaths. On a weight basis, DHE is approximately twice as toxic as Hpd with LD_{50} values near 130 mg/kg.

Death in all cases was attributed to liver and kidney necrosis. Necrosis of splenic and thymic lymphocytes was also observed. Bone marrow was unaffected.

Both porphyrins were considerably more toxic when animals were exposed to light. Following shaving of the entire back, the mice were exposed for 5 hr to full spectrum xenon light (6 mW/cm^2) with IR filtered out, immediately following systemic injection of various doses of Hpd or DHE. Skin irritation and erythema on ears and feet was apparent at the higher drug doses immediately after exposure. Moribund animals appeared to be hypoxic. The LD_{50} found both at 1 and 14 days post treatment was 7.5 mg/kg. The values for DHE were approximately 4 mg/kg. Death of animals in this group could not be attributed to any specific organ damage and was considered to be due to a shock syndrome. Similar studies were done with rats (receiving 20 mg/kg Hpd) but no deaths occurred in these animals, indicating a possible relationship to size or relative surface area exposed.

Since some applications of PDT include intra-abdominal exposure, toxicity of Hpd + light was carried out for a variety of rabbit organs exposed surgically. In some cases the Brown-Pearce tumor was implanted into the organ one or two weeks prior to treatment. The animals received 5.0 mg/kg Hpd 48 to 72 hr prior to surgical exposure and treatment. Five days later the animals were sacrificed and all exposed organs and tumor examined histologically. It was found that, in general, stomach, small intestine, liver, pancreas, kidney and bladder demonstrated slight to no effects at light doses of 70–100 Joules/cm^2 (630 ± 5 nm) whereas higher light doses produced more extensive damage. Also at 72 hr or longer post injection light exposure was less damaging than at earlier times. The tumor underwent necrosis at all doses (30 Joules/cm^2 or higher) and time intervals studied.

4 Efficacy Studies in Experimental Animals

HAYATA and colleagues (1983) have carried out a pre-clinical study of PDT in treating intrabronchial squamous cell carcinoma induced in dogs. They also determined that they could detect the majority of these tumors by observing the Hpd fluorescence induced by violet light from a Krypton laser. In these cases the exciting light was delivered via a single quartz fiber in the biopsy channel of the bronchoscope fitted with appropriate filters and an image intensifier to observe the fluorescing (red) light. Normal bronchial mucosa and tumors in dogs not receiving Hpd were not seen to be fluorescent. This method has also proven feasible in detecting occult lung tumors in humans (BALCHUM et al. 1982; CORTESE et al. 1979; HAYATA et al. 1982b; KING et al. 1982) as well as in delineating tumors and dysplasia in the bladder (BENSON et al. 1982).

For treatment of these tumors, the red light from an argon-dye laser system (approximately 630 nm) was directed through the fiber in the biopsy channel of the bronchoscope. The tumors received 60 to 240 Joules/cm^2 48 hr following 2.5 to 3.0 mg/kg Hpd. Complete response was documented histologically in the three animals treated this way. Only minor normal tissue effects were seen. Tumors in control animals (60 or 120 Joules/cm^2 light without Hpd) and tissues in normal animals receiving Hpd but no light were found to undergo no histological changes.

GOMER and co-workers (1983a) examined acute eye toxicity in rabbits following PDT. A dye laser system (635 ± 5 nm) similar to that used by Hayata was the source of light which was directed onto a 1 cm^2 area of the retina through the cornea of pigmented rabbits. Rabbits received Hpd (1 to 10 mg/kg) 48 hr prior to a 15 min exposure (40 to 400 mW/cm^2). Using a variety of methods (fundus photography, fluorescein angiography and histological examination) it was found that light alone at power levels below 200 mW/cm^2 (180 Joules/cm^2) produced no damage whereas higher doses (400 Joules/cm^2) led to damage ranging from edema to retinal detachment even outside the treatment field. Following Hpd at 2.5 mg/kg (the usual dose used in humans) treatment damage was minimal at light doses up to 45 Joules/cm^2 (40 mW/cm^2) whereas following 10 mg/kg extensive damage was seen, even at the lowest light dose (45 Joules/cm^2). It was concluded that since the safe range for normal tissue damage occurred within the usual dose range used to treat tumors in humans that this method might be applicable to treatment of a variety of ocular tumors (see below).

To determine the safety of PDT in treatment of bladder tumors, normal bladders in dogs were exposed to a variety of light doses (630 nm) three days after a systemic injection of DHE (2.5 mg/kg) by NSEYO and POTTER (1983). Using a 1 cm^2 spot size from the light fiber within the bladder (fiber placed via a rigid cystoscope), doses as high as 360 Joules/cm^2 were used. At this dose, a lesion was produced which extended to the muscle layer (examined 5 days post treatment) but was not sufficient to have caused a fistula. At doses from 100 to 360 Joules/cm^2 only superficial lesions were produced. In some cases the bladder was first irritated chemically, or an ulceration was induced by biopsy prior to Hpd administration. No enhancement of damage was seen in these areas. In some cases, whole bladder illumination (30 Joules/cm^2) was used without producing evidence of irreversible damage.

JOCHAM and colleagues (1981) have used PDT to treat the Brown-Pearce carcinoma transplanted into the bladder of rabbits. They have demonstrated both selective uptake of Hpd in the bladder tumors as well as the ability to destroy the tumor without damage to normal urothelium. In some cases the tumor was put into the neck of the bladder and treated with a light fiber which produced spherical illumination. In combination with a dispersing medium they demonstrated the ability to eradicate these tumors even in the neck of the bladder without damage to normal tissue. Light doses were 100–200 Joules/cm^2 (approximately 630 nm): the Hpd dose was not stated but presumably was 5.0 mg/kg given two days prior to treatment as in their detection studies.

5 In Vivo Action Spectrum

Since tunable dye lasers are most commonly used for PDT, it is important to determine the wavelength most effective in producing tumoricidal effects with Hpd or DHE. The reason for using red light for activation rather than shorter wavelengths which actually are absorbed more strongly by these porphyrins is that the red is considerably more penetrating through tissue (see below). In solution the maximum wavelength for absorption of Hpd is near 620 nm whether or not serum albumin is added. However, when absorbed onto or into cells, the maximum red absorption is near 630 nm. The action spectrum for control of the transplanted SMT-F tumor in DBA/2 mice was determined by DOUGHERTY and colleagues (1983). Using standard conditions (75 mW/cm^2, 30 min, 1 day post 7.5 mg/kg Hpd or 5.0 mg/kg DHE) and varying only the wavelength, it was determined that maximum response occurred at 630 nm. In an earlier study this group had also determined that maximum normal skin response of Hpd in albino mice occurred at the same wavelength.

Shortly after PDT (immediate to one day, depending on conditions) tumors in experimental animals became hemorrhagic (e.g. subcutaneous SMT-F tumor in the mouse) or in some cases totally blanched (e.g. Green melanoma in rabbit eye). When effectively treated, the tumor mass becomes non-palpable or non-observable usually within a matter of a few days. Complete eradication is possible depending on treatment conditions. It has been demonstrated that oxygen levels in experimental tumors drop rapidly during PDT treatment (BICHER et al. 1981; HETZEL et al. 1984). When examined histologically, the earliest changes occur in and around the tumor vasculature with red cell congestion and some enucleation of cells adjacent to the vessels. At later times obvious red cell extravasation is seen along with apparent total destruction to tumor cells (BUGELSKI et al. 1981).

It has been shown autoradiographically that tritium-labeled Hpd with the SMT-F tumor or the Sarcoma 180 mouse tumor is located in the vascular stroma at a level five times that in or around the tumor cells (BUGELSKI et al. 1981). A similar pattern can be observed by fluorescence microscopy of frozen sections of these tumors. However, a common characteristic of these experimental animal tumors is their poor vascularity. It is unclear if similar drug distribution and vascular damage occur in tumors in humans.

6 In Vitro Studies

Several groups have studied the uptake of Hpd in normal cells in culture for comparison with cells of malignant tissue origin (ANDREONI et al. 1983; BERNS et al. 1982; CHANG and DOUGHERTY 1978; CHRISTENSEN et al. 1983; COPPOLA et al. 1980; HENDERSON et al. 1983; MOAN et al. 1981). In general, these have failed to show selective uptake by transformed cells.

Many of the data indicate the central role of cellular membrane as the site of damage resulting from porphyrins and light. This damage may be a result of cross-linking of membrane protein reported by DUBBELMAN et al. (1980) and GIROTTI (1976). However, HILF et al. (1984) have demonstrated inactivation of mitochondrial membrane enzymes as an early event in cells exposed to light in vitro following Hpd uptake in vivo.

Recently several investigators have demonstrated a "tightly bound" porphyrin fraction in cells exposed to Hpd or DHE. Its fraction of total porphyrin increases with time of incubation to a maximum of 50–60% at 24 hr. HENDERSON et al. (1983) and BELLNIER and LIN (1983) have demonstrated increased photosensitivity of cells containing "tightly bound" porphyrin compared to those with "loosely bound" (i.e. removed by washing in media) porphyrin. It is expected that these in vitro conditions may be better correlated with the in vivo situation. KESSEL and CHOU (1983) and CHRISTENSEN et al. (1983) have demonstrated enhanced uptake in vitro of DHE compared to the other components of Hpd. The DHE appears to correspond to the "tightly bound" fraction of Hpd since it is the only Hpd component not removed from cells by washing following even long-term exposure (CHRISTENSEN et al. 1983).

While very little of the Hpd in cells is taken up by the nucleus, effects of photoradiated porphyrins on DNA can be measured. Single strand breaks have been demonstrated by MOAN and BOYE (1981) in NHIK 3025 cells exposed to hematoporphyrin and light, but the frequency is low compared to ionizing radiation and does not correlate with cell survival. Also, sister chromatid exchange has been demonstrated by MOAN et al. (1980) and by GOMER et al. (1983). On the other hand, Hpd + light has been found not to produce mutants in CHO cells using light doses sufficient to produce survival similar to that produced by X-irradiation which produced a high degree of mutation in these cells (GOMER et al. 1983b). It has also been reported that Hpd + light is negative in the Ames test for mutagenicity in bacteria (KENNEDY 1983).

7 Mechanism of Action

Questions regarding Hpd and DHE uptake and distribution in animal tissue, cellular target sites, tissue target sites, and mechanism of tissue distribution following PDT have been addressed for several years by several groups. However, until recently few definitive data were available. As pointed out above, effects of PDT on mitochondria, cellular membranes and DNA have been found although the initial target(s) are still uncertain.

In a study by BUGELSKI et al. (1981) the distribution of ^{3}H-Hpd matched the distribution of labeled albumin. At longer periods (over 6 hr) the porphyrin was cleared from most normal tissue with certain exceptions. No change was seen in the tumor from 3 hr to over a several day period although dilution occurred presumably due to cell proliferation. Within the tumor the porphyrin was found to be primarily associated with vascular stroma (macrophages, mast cells, possibly fibroblasts). The relative density of porphyrin in stroma to that in tumor cells was approximately 5:1. In the liver, hepatocytes appeared to retain little if any porphyrin, but Kupfer cells retained high levels. The porphyrin appears to be associated with reticuloendothelial cells in general in all tissues. Fluorescence microscopy of experimental mouse tumors indicates that fluorescence occurs intracellularly in cells associated with the vascular stroma. While some of these are likely macrophages, it is unclear if other cells, e.g. the endothelium of the tumor vasculature, also retain the material. It is also unclear if such cells in the tumor behave fundamentally differently from cells in normal tissues.

Little is known about Hpd distribution within tissues and spontaneous tumors in man other than most are seen to be fluorescent following Hpd injection. In general, with equal doses per weight of injected drug, tumors in humans and spontaneous tumors in dogs are much more fluorescent than are the transplanted tumors in rodents studied to date.

As indicated above, the porphyrin in the experimental mouse tumors appears to be associated primarily with the vascular stroma. In fact, the earliest histological effects of Hpd + light occur in this area. BUGELSKI et al. (1981) examined tumors by electron microscopy at various times following treatment. The earliest change which could be observed was blebbing of tumor cells adjacent to the microvasculature. The endothelium appeared to be intact at this point. At longer periods tumor cells more remote from the vessels demonstrated blebbing and endothelial cells were seen to be retracted and damaged and red cells had extravasated. Finally, massive extravasation and tumor cell destruction was observed.

Such data raised the question of the role of direct tumor cell destruction, such as that studied in vitro (see above), and destruction of the vasculature in the overall process of tissue destruction following PDT.

HENDERSON et al. (1984) have studied this question by examining tumor cell survival following PDT in vivo, using the EMT-6 mouse tumor system, an in vivo to in vitro colony formation survival assay. Tumors were treated using DHE and 630 nm light with doses which produced destruction of tumor bulk in all animals and 52% long-term cures. No significant tumor cell inactivation was found following PDT in vivo when tumors were explanted immediately after completion of treatment. However, when tumors were allowed to remain in situ for varying lengths of time (1–10 hr) following treatment, tumor cell death was found to occur rapidly and progressively. This delayed cell death was similar to that caused by shut down of the tumor blood circulation by simply killing the mouse. Thus, at least in this system, death of tumor cells seemed to be the result of vascular damage by PDT rather than of direct photodynamic damage. While it is possible that sublethal damage to tumor cells combined with vascular destruction is necessary for cure of the tumor, this has not yet been demonstrated. Recently, Henderson was found that the subcutaneously implanted L1210 mouse leukemia is destroyed by PDT through what seems to be primary tumor cell destruction. The situation in patients is likely to be a combination of both vascular and tumor cell effect.

Singlet oxygen is likely to be involved in in vitro destruction of cells containing porphyrins (WEISHAUPT et al. 1976) (see above). While no comparable experiments have been carried out in vivo, it is likely that singlet oxygen may be involved at least as an initially formed cytotoxic species. It has been demonstrated that if tumors in the legs of mice are shut off from oxygen by leg-clamping that the usual destructive effect of Hpd + light is prevented (WEISHAUPT and DOUGHERTY 1983).

Recent results indicate a synergistic interaction between PDT and heat in experimental animal systems (WALDOW and DOUGHERTY 1984). A reasonable means of heat delivery may be to use the Nd-YAG laser concurrent or subsequent to delivery of 630 nm light.

8 Dosimetry of Light in Tissue

An important parameter determining the extent of tumor necrosis is the penetrability of the necessary visible light through tissue. SVAASAND et al. (1983; SVAASAND and ELLINGSEN 1983) have considered this question theoretically and made measurements of penetration of various wavelengths in various tissues in experimental animals and tissues. For a diffusion dominant, one dimensional case (surface illumination)

$$\Phi = \Phi_{0e}^{-\alpha X}$$

where Φ = space irradiance

Φ_0 = irradiance at surface

α = total attenuation coefficient

$(\beta/\zeta)^{1/2}$

β = absorption coefficient

ζ = diffusion coefficient

X = distance   (1)

Measured values for δ (mm) = I/α, which is the attenuation distance or the depth at which the incident intensity falls off to I/ε or approximately 37% range from 1 to 4 mm. When fibers are inserted into the tumor for interstitial PDT, the equation for space irradiance in the diffusion dominant case is

$$\Phi = \Phi_0 \frac{(a)}{(r)} \, e^{-\alpha(r-a)} \qquad (2)$$

where r = radial distance in tissue

a = radius of fiber

Histological examination of tumors removed after treatment by PDT indicates necrosis extending to a depth of 5 to 10 mm from the surface (point of light application). Coagulation necrosis of tumor obstructing bronchi following PDT has been demonstrated by inserting special fibers which allow for lateral light distribution (see below). Such fibers have been demonstrated to cause necrosis within a radius of 9–10 mm from the point of insertion (DOUGHERTY 1983).

While many of early clinical studies were carried out with a filtered xenon arc lamp with a fairly broad spectral output of 600–700 nm, such systems are rarely used today, although they may have some application for superficial skin lesions. Most clinical studies use lasers in order to take advantage of the high coupling efficiency to optical fibers which allow light to be delivered conventiently to many areas.

A variety of delivery fibers are available: those with an optically flat end with lenses to produce a spot of homogeneous intensity generally used to treat cutaneous or subcutaneous tumors; fibers with various lenses on the ends to further expand the spot, and those with diffusers of various lengths which produce a cylindrical pattern along the diffuser length and are generally used within a lumen or for interstitial PDT. Fibers without lenses or diffusers should not be used since they produce inhomogeneous spots or hot spots when used interstitially.

9 PDT for Treatment of Cancer in Humans

Since the early clinical reports from Roswell Park Memorial Institute describing the efficacy of PDT for treatment of cutaneous and subcutaneous lesions (DOUGHERTY et al. 1978; DOUGHERTY et al. 1979), many additional reports have been published from the U.S. and abroad. The following is a compilation of the current state of these studies.

9.1 Cutaneous and Subcutaneous Tumors

Results are summarized in Table 1. Note that the percent responses are approximated since not all

Table 1. Clinical results from various centers – skin cancers

Type	Approx. no of patients/ sites	Response (%)			Longest followup without recurrence (to date) (years)
		CR	PR	NR	
Metastatic breast cancer	120/>1000	60–70	20–30	10	4
Basal cell carcinoma	15/50	70–80	20–30	0	4
Squamous cell carcinoma	5/10	20	70–80	10	1
Malignant melanoma	50/>1000	50	30	20	1
Mycosis fungoides	5	20	60	20	1
Kaposi's sarcoma	5/>100	80	20	0	3
Bowen's disease	2/10	100	–	–	1.5

CR, Complete Response (disappearance of tumor or biopsy proven); PR, At least 50% reduction in tumor volume; NR, Less than 50% reduction in tumor volume

References: DOUGHERTY (RPMI), J. Natl. Cancer Inst. 62:231, 1979. FORBES, et al. (Univ. Adelaide), Med. J. Aust. 2.489, 1980. KENNEDY (Ontario Cancer Found.), Porphyrin Photosensitization, Plenum Press (New York), 1983. Porphyrin Localization and Treatment of Tumors, eds. D.R. DOIRON and C.J. GOMER, ALAN R. LISS (New York), 1984. TOKUDA (Tokyo Med. Coll.), Lasers and Hematoporphyrin Derivative in Cancer, Igaku-Shoin (Tokyo/New York), 1983. WILE, et al. (U.C. Irvine), Lasers in Surg. Med. 2:163, 1982.

investigators used the same criteria of response and not all reported their data as indicated here.

A number of points must be made regarding these data. Most patients had received multiple therapies prior to PDT including ionizing radiation in the majority of cases. The tumors ranged in size from a few mm to more than 10 cm and in pigmentation from slight color to black (highly pigmented melanoma). In most cases the light source was a laser emitting at approximately 630 nm, but some patients were treated with other light sources making direct comparisons difficult. In general, however, the dose rate was 15 to 100 mW/cm² to total delivered light doses of 20 to 120 Joules/cm². Many patients, especially those with large tumors treated aggressively, experienced moderate to severe pain. This invariably occurred when overlying or adjacent skin necrosed forming deep eschars, and did not occur at the lower dose range. The superficial tumors (1–3 mm) responded completely at the lower dose range generally preserving the normal skin. Other side effects besides the generalized photosensitivity were increased sensitivity to PDT in previously irradiated (ionizing) fields in patients who received Adriamycin up to a few months prior to PDT. Also, patients with inflammatory breast cancer frequently were unusually sensitive to treatment.

Patients with small, superficial tumors can be benefitted by PDT even if the lesions are widespread and in areas previously treated with ionizing radiation. Optimum conditions for treatment are 3.0 mg/kg Hpd, 1.5 to 2.0 mg/kg DHE, 20–35 Joules/cm² (630 nm) for Hpd and 30–72 Joules(cm² for DHE delivered 2 to 5 days post injection. Higher light doses destroy normal skin as well as tumor. Patients with large tumors (> 1 cm) are generally benefitted only if the tumors are relatively few and localized. These tumors are best treated aggressively by a combination of superficial treatment (> 70 Joules/cm²) confined to the tumor as much as possible and interstitial PDT. Some must be treated repeatedly following sloughing or debriding of dead tissue. As a general rule, a depth of tumor 0.5 to 1.0 cm from the light source will be destroyed by a given treatment whether applied superficially or interstitially. Therefore, multiple interstitial treatments with multiple fibers (500 mW/cm length of diffuser) are necessary to destroy tumors of large volume. While the occasional patient may benefit from this aggressive approach, debulking of tumor is not the best application of PDT.

9.2 Lung Cancer

Overall results are summarized in Table 2. The first patient to receive PDT for lung cancer was treated by Hayata and Kato at the Tokyo Medical College in early 1980 (Hayata et al. 1982a). Nearly four years post treatment this patient was cancer free upon autopsy following a heart attack.

The most often used procedure was to inject 2.5–3.0 mg/kg Hpd three days prior to endoscopic PDT. In some cases the patients were anesthetized and in some cases mildly sedated. Light from the laser (near 630 nm) was delivered through 200 µM or 400 µM quartz fibers placed into the channel and directed at the lesion externally for smaller tumors or inserted into the mass for large or obstructing tumors. It has been found recently that the fibers with diffusing tips described above, which allow lateral light distribution, are most convenient for treating intraluminal tumors. While it is difficult to determine light dosimetry accurately because of the wide variation in size and shape, doses of approximately 50–100 Joules/cm² have been effective for treatment of most lesions.

Hayata and colleagues (1984a) have recently reported results in 73 cases of lung cancer. They recommend PDT for early stage cases involving superficial or intramural invasion. When tumor has invaded beyond normal muscular or cartilage layers light delivery may be inadequate, especially if diffusing fibers are not used.

Balchum et al. (1984) achieved a major advance in the treatment of partially or totally obstructing lung tumors by illuminating the tumors via a quartz fiber with a special light distribution end three days after 3.0 mg/kg Hpd. In most cases the fiber, with a lateral diffusing end of 1–2 cm, was inserted directly into the tumor. The power at 630 nm was 400 mW/cm of diffusing length. Treatment time was approximately 8.5 min, thus producing 200 Joules per cm of diffuser. For smaller lesions, the same fiber was held within the remaining lumen adjacent to the tumor. Patients were re-bronchoscoped three days post PDT and tumor debris and firm exudate emoved. If residual tumor was found (11/35 cases) PDT was repeated. Clean-up bronchoscopy was carried out three days later. If indicated by dyspnea, clean-up bronchoscopy was done as early as eight or 24 hr post PDT and whenever necessary thereafter. Thirty-three of the 35 patients with endobronchial tumors had complete opening of the lumen to its full extent with no visible remaining tumor although biopsies frequently were positive at the clean-up procedure.

Table 2. PDT clinical results from various centers – lung cancer

Institution	No. of patients	Patient category	Method	Response			Complete opening	Adverse experiences
				CR	PR	NR		
RPMI	17	Very advanced	S	–	13	2	–	Exudate, fever, abscess – 14
	34	Advanced	S	7	10	17	–	Exudate – 6 hemoptysis – 5(?)
	5	Advanced	I	–	–	–	5	–
USC	70	Advanced	I	–	–	–	70	–
Tokyo Med. Coll.	107	Advanced	S	30	77	0	–	Exudate
	46	100% obstructed	S/I	–	–	–	28	–
	13	Early	S	10	3	0	–	–
Mayo Clinic	19	Early	S	7	8	a		Sunburn – 3 Cough – 4 Obstruction (temporary) 4
Other	50	–	–	–	–	–	–	–
Total	311			54	111	19	103	

[a] 4 lost to followup
S, Superficial treatment; I, Interstitial treatment

Maximum followup: RPMI – 1 yr; USC – 1 yr; Tokyo med. Coll. – 4 yr, Mayo Clinic – 2 yr.

References: VINCENT and DOUGHERTY, Chest 85:29–33, 1984. BALCHUM, et al., Lasers in Surgery and Medicine 4:13–30, 1984. HAYATA, et al., Chest 86:169–177, 1984; Lasers and Hematoporphyrin Derivative in Cancer, ed. Y. HAYATA and T.J. DOUGHERTY, Igaku-Shoin (Tokyo/New York), 1983. CORTESE and KINESE, Chest 86:8–13, 1984.

One other patient was opened partially. One patient with a benign, fibrous mass was unresponsive.

In an earlier study by BALCHUM (1983) and others it had been noted that some patients were put at considerable risk following PDT due to heavy secretions which could further obstruct or result in obstructive pneumonia. This problem is obviated by selecting patients who are non-terminal and who have reasonable respiration upon mild exertion and by routine bronchoscopy three days after PDT to remove debris and secretions. In only a few patients was an earlier re-bronchoscopy necessary due to respiratory distress. In this way PDT can be carried out safely and effectively for palliation.

Hayata and colleagues have applied PDT to make in anoperable patients operable in cases where surgery had been precluded because of extension of the disease. They have also been able to reduce the extent of surgery in some cases by using PDT preoperatively (1982; KATO et al. 1983). Recent studies reported by CORTESE and KINSEY (1984) and HAYATA et al. (1984) demonstrate that early stage lung cancers may be effec-

tively treated by PDT and may be a useful technique to delay surgery in patients at high risk for new tumors.

HAYATA et al. (1984b) and CORTESE and KINSEY (1984) have recently reported results of PDT for treatment of carcinoma-in-situ or early stage endobronchial tumors. Seventeen of 32 patients demonstrated a complete response to treatment. Followup ranged from one to four years.

9.3 Cancer of the Esophagus

The rationale for use of PDT in esophageal cancer is similar to that for treatment of lung cancer, i.e., early stage disease can be treated locally with little risk and advanced cases may receive palliation. It should be emphasized that PDT provides the clinician with another modality which should be appropriately worked into the overall management of the patient along with other modalities. The guiding principle is that PDT is more localized and selective than some of the other treatments but cannot be expected to entirely eliminate large, bulky tumor, especially outside the lumen or in lymph nodes.

Table 3. PDT clinical results from various centers – bladder cancer

Institution	No. of patients/ sites	Patient category	Method	Response (to 2 yr)			Adverse experiences
				CR	PR	NR	
RPMI	4	Very advanced	WB	1	3	–	Bladder shrinkage – 2
Mayo clinic	14	CIS/TCC	WB/F	11	–	3	None
WILT (Santa barbara)	6	CIS/TCC	WB/F	4	2	–	Temporary bladder shrinkage – 1 Sunburn – 2
Kanazawa university	9 (46)	CIS/TCC	F	(28)	(8)	(10)	None
	18	CIS/TCC	WB/F	18	–	–	Temporary bladder shrinkage, 3–4 mo followup
Tokyo medical college	11	CIS/TCC	F	8	3	–	None
Total	62 (93)			(70)	(16)	(13)	

WB, whole bladder treatment; F, focal treatment

References: NSEYO, et al., J. Urol. XXVI(3):274–280, 1985. BENSON, et al., J. Urol. 130:1090–1095, 1983. HISAZUMI, et al., J. Urol. 130:685–687, 1983. HISAZUMI, et al., J. Urol. 131:884–887, 1984. OHI, et al., Lasers and Hematoporphyrin Derivative in Cancer, Igaku-Shoin (Tokyo/New York), 1983.

To date approximately 30 patients with esophageal cancer have received PDT (AIDA and HIRASHIMA 1983; MCCAUGHAN et al. 1984; NAVA 1983; TIAN 1983). Most patients had advanced disease and previously had received therapy (surgery, radiation therapy). Palliation was achieved in most instances, and survival occasionally has exceeded one year. Although the tumor sloughs and dysphagia may be relieved within a few days, there may be severe mediastinal pain for the first few days. As with bronchogenic cancer the endoscopic fiber transmitting the 630 nm light should have a diffusing end.

9.4 Bladder Cancer

PDT may become the treatment of choice for multi-centric superficial cancer of the bladder since it may provide a greater degree of selectivity than other treatments. BENSON et al. (1982) has demonstrated a high degree of selectivity of Hpd for dysplasia and carcinoma in situ in the bladder. To date approximately 62 bladder cancer patients have been treated by PDT ranging from CIS to invasive carcinoma (Table 3). Both sessile and pedunculated tumors have been treated. Hpd dose was 2.5 mg/kg, the wavelength was 630 nm from dye laser systems delivered endoscopically. In these cases the light dose has ranged from 150 to 360 Joules/cm^2 for treatment of individual lesions. The non-responding tumors were those receiving only 50 Joules/cm^2 regardless of size.

BENSON (1984) has equivalent results from treating patients at 3 hr or 48 hr post injection. All other studies report treatment at 48 to 72 hr post injection.

To date only a few patients have been treated by whole bladder illumination following Hpd or DHE. All patients had previously received resection, radiation and chemotherapy. Following light doses to the whole bladder of 35 to 100 Joules/cm^2, shrinkage was observed. Dose ranges of 10–25 Joules/cm^2 and careful control of bladder volume and pressure during treatment has reduced this problem. HISAZUMI (1984) found that bladder shrinkage was related to the bladder volume prior to treatment and recommends that the bladder volume be at least 150 cc if PDT is to be used. Prior treatments and/or prolonged extensive distention alone may produce fibrosis and shrinkage (REUTER et al. 1982).

9.5 Gynecological Tumors

The application of PDT in this type of tumor has not been extensive but is impressive. In 1982 WARD et al. (1982) reported treatment of five cases of recurrent vaginal cancer by PDT. Also SOMA et al. (1982) reported a single case of PDT for primary vaginal carcinoma and more recently has treated 13 cases. Patients received 2.5 to 5.0 mg/kg Hpd generally two to three days prior to PDT which was performed by surface illumination in most cases at a dose rate of 25 to 100 mW/cm^2 and a total dose of approximately 200–300 Joules/cm^2. Many of the lesions reported by Ward were large (>3 cm in depth) and were treated by multiple interstitial placements of the fiber at doses of approximately 600 Joules per insertion where thermal effects are likely to be substantial. However, SOMA and NUTAHARA (1983) have successfully eradicated large lesions using only surface illumination of up to 500 Joules/cm^2 at a low dose rate of 25 mW/cm^2 where thermal effects would be of little consequence (see below). In several cases, initial treatment gave only partial response. These cases were retreated within one to three weeks resulting in complete responses. RETTENMAIER et al. (1984) recently reported six cases with recurrent cervical, vaginal, and endometrial tumors using total delivered light doses of only 30–40 Joules/cm^2. Two of these patients demonstrated a complete response to treatment. Aside from the usual treatment photosensitivity, no side effects were noted. Excellent re-epithelialization was seen after tumor necrosis and sloughing which occurred generally over three to four weeks.

9.6 Cancers of the Head and Neck

Wile and co-workers studied various head and neck tumors (WILE et al. 1982; WILE et al. 1984). Nineteen sites in 16 patients were treated for recurrent squamous cell carcinoma: five demonstrated complete response (up to one year currently) and 10 showed partial responses. In most cases patients were given 3.0 mg/kg Hpd, 72 hr prior to light doses in the range of 25–90 Joules/cm^2. Also, TAKETA and IMAKIIRE (1983) have reported six cases of squamous cell carcinoma including laryngeal carcinoma, cancer of the nasopharynx, tongue and vocal cords. In most cases a reduction in tumor mass was found but generally the biopsies remained positive in the deeper portion of the tumors involving areas beneath the mucosa.

9.7 Other Tumors

PDT is currently being investigated for treatment of a variety of other types of tumors, but results are still very preliminary. For example, LAWS et al. (1981) and McCULLOCH et al. (1984) have applied PDT in the treatment of brain tumors.

One of the most promising new areas for application of PDT is in treatment of intraocular tumors such as malignant melanoma of the choroid and retinoblastoma. Early results of MURPHREE et al. (1984) have shown that malignant melanoma of the choroid responds to PDT (3.0 mg/kg Hpd) when the light is applied both through the cornea and through the sclera. Similar results have been obtained by BRUCE (1984). Long-term followup in these patients is not yet available although there

Table 4. Summary of response of various tumors to PDT (to 1984)

Tumor type	No. of patients or (sites)	Response			Longest followup to date (years)
		CR	PR	NR	
Skin (met. breast, basal cell, squamous, melanoma)	(219)	(147)	(29)	(43)	4
Endobronchial-late stage	262	106[a]	136	20	1.5
Endobronchial-early stage	32	17	10	–	4.5
Bladder – superficial	(70)	(38)	(16)	(13)	2
Head/neck-recurrent	49	9	26	14	2
Gyn – recurrent	11	4	5	2	2
Esophagus – advanced	17	0	11[b]	6	1

[a] Complete opening to wall of lumen following physical removal after PDT
[b] Partial relief of obstruction

is one case of recurrence at approximately one year after PDT of a choroidal melanoma treated by L'ESPERANCE and DOUGHERTY (1983). The proper light dose and means of delivery are still under investigation. In general patients treated by Bruce have been treated by high power densities (up to 600 mW/cm^2) whereas GOMER et al. (1983) have limited the dose rate to 200 mW/cm^2 where they have demonstrated that little damage occurs to ocular structures in rabbits. The high degree of pigmentation of some of the melanomas raises the possibility of a significant contribution by thermal effects to the overall results. Table 4 summarizes the overall results of PDT reported from different centers in the past five years.

Phase III, randomized, controlled clinical trials of PDT for treatment of endobronchial tumors and superficial bladder tumors now are in progress.

10 Summary

Photodynamic therapy is a new, experimental method of treating malignant tumors by utilizing the relatively selective retention of the photosensitizer (hematoporphyrin derivative or dihematoporphyrin ether) and its ability to elicit an efficient photodynamic reaction upon activation with penetrating light. Application of this therapy to tumors in the bronchus, bladder, skin and several other sites has demonstrated both safety and efficacy even in advanced cases. Eradication of early stage tumors in the bronchus and bladder has been demonstrated. Selective retention of the photosensitizers in tumors is apparently related to the relatively large size of the aggregates of these materials resulting in phagocytosis by reticuloendothelial cells as well as slow clearance from tumor interstitial fluid with uptake in lipophylic components of cells. Upon light activation, generally delivered from lasers via fiber optics, the sensitizers generate singlet oxygen, the apparent cytotoxic agent, causing both vascular damage and injury to tumor cells.

References

Aida M, Hirashima T (1983) Cancer of the esophagus. In: Hayata Y, Dougherty TJ (eds) Lasers and Hematoporphyrin Derivative in Cancer. Igaku-Shoin, Tokyo New York, p 57–64

Andreoni A, Cubeddu R, DeSilvestri S et al. (1983) Effects of laser irradiation on hematoporphyrin-treated normal and transformed thyroid cells in culture. Can Res 43:2076–2080

Balchum O (1983) Unpublished results

Balchum O, Doiron DR, Huth G (1984) Photoradiation therapy of endobronchial lung cancer using the photodynamic action of hematoporphyrin derivative. Lasers Surg Med 4:13–30

Balchum OJ, Doiron DR, Profio AE et al. (1982) Fluorescence bronchoscopy for localizing early bronchial cancer and carcinoma in situ. In: Recent Results in Cancer Research. Springer-Verlag, Berlin Heidelberg, p 98–120

Bellnier DA (1982) In vitro photoradiation – Hematoporphyrin derivative accumulation and interaction with ionizing radiation. PhD thesis, State University of New York at Buffalo

Bellnier D, Lin C (1983) Photodynamic destruction of cultured human bladder tumor cells by hematoporphyrin derivative: Effects of porphyrin molecular aggregation. Photobiochem Photobiophys 6:357–366

Benson RC Jr, Farrow GM, Kinsey JH et al. (1982) Detection and localization of in situ carcinoma of the bladder with hematoporphyrin derivative. Mayo Clin Proc 57:548–555

Benson RC Jr (1984) The use of hematoporphyrin derivative (Hpd) in the localization and treatment of transitional cell carcinoma (TCC) of the bladder. In: Doiron DR, Gomer CJ (eds) Porphyrin Localization and Treatment of Tumors. AR Liss Inc, New York, p 795–804

Berenbaum MC, Bonnett R, Scourides PA (1982) In vivo biological activity of components of hematoporphyrin derivative. Br J Cancer 45:571–581

Berns MW, Dahlman A, Johnson FM et al. (1982) In vitro cellular effects of hematoporphyrin derivative. Can Res 42:2325–2329

Bicher HI, Hetzel FW, Vaupel P et al. (1981) Microcirculation modifications by localized microwave hyperthermia

and hematoporphyrin phototherapy. Biblthca Anat 20:628–632

Bruce RA (1984) Photoradiation of choroidal malignant melanomas. In: Doiron DR, Gomer CJ (eds) Porphyrin Localization and Treatment of Tuors. AR Liss Inc, New York, p 777–784

Bugelski PJ, Porter CW, Dougherty TJ (1981) Autoradiographic distribution of hematoporphyrin derivative in normal and tumor tissue of the mouse. Can Res 41:4606–4612

Chang C, Dougherty TJ (1978) Photoradiation therapy: Kinetics and thermodynamics of porphyrin uptake and loss in normal and malignant cells in culture. Radiat Res 74:498 (one page only-abstract)

Christensen T, Sandquist T, Feren K et al. (1983) Retention and photodynamic effects of hematoporphyrin derivative in cells after prolonged cultivation in the presence of porphyrin. Br J Cancer 48:35–43

Coppola A, Viggiani E, Salzarulo L et al. (1980) Ultrastructural changes in lymphoma cells treated with hematoporphyrin and light. Amer J Path 99:175–192

Cortese DA, Kinsey JH, Woolner LB et al. (1979) Clinical application of a new endoscopic technique for detection of in situ bronchial carcinoma. Mayo Clin Proc 54:635–641

Cortese DA, Kinsey JH (1984) Hematoporphyrin derivative phototherapy in the treatment of bronchogenic carcinoma. Chest 86:8–13

Doiron DR, Profio E, Vincent RG et al. (1979) Fluorescence bronchoscopy for detection of lung cancer. Chest 76:27–32

Dougherty TJ (1983a) Unpublished results

Dougherty TJ (1983b) Hematoporphyrin as a photosensitizer of tumors. Photochem Photobiol 38:377–379

Dougherty TJ (1984) Photodynamic therapy (PDT) of malignant tumors. In: Davis S (ed) Critical Reviews in Oncology/Hematology 2(2):83–116

Dougherty TJ, Boyle DG, Weishaupt KR et al. (1983) Photoradiation therapy – Clinical and drug advances. In: Kessel D, Dougherty TJ (eds) Porphyrin Photosensitization, Plenum Press, New York London, p 3–14

Dougherty TJ, Douglass HO Jr (1983) Unpublished results

Dougherty TJ, Grindey GB, Fiel R et al. (1975) Photoradiation therapy. II. Cure of animal tumors with hematoporphyrin and light. J Nat Cancer Inst 55:115–121

Dougherty TJ, Kaufman JE, Goldfarb A et al. (1978) Photoradiation therapy for the treatment of malignant tumors. Can Res 38:2628–2635

Dougherty TJ, Lawrence G, Kaufman JH et al. (1979) Photoradiation in the treatment of recurrent breast carcinoma. J Natl Cancer Inst 62:231–237

Dougherty TJ, Potter WR, Weishaupt KR (1984) The Structure of the active the active component of hematoporphyrin derivative. In: Andreoni A, Cubeddu R (eds) Tumor Phototherapy. Plenum Press, New York London, p 23–35

Dougherty TJ, Wityk KE (1984) Unpublished results

Dougherty TJ, Wityk KE, Malone PB (1983) Unpublished results

Dubbelman TMAR, DeGoeij AFPM, VanSteveninck J (1980) Protoporphyrin-induced photodynamic effects on transport processes across the membrane of human erythrocytes. Biochem Biophys Acta 595:133–139

Girotti AW (1976) Photodynamic action of protoporphyrin. IX. On human erythrocytes: Cross-linking of membrane proteins. Biochem Biophys Res Comm 72:1367–1374

Gomer CJ, Doiron DR, Jester JV et al. (1983a) Hematoporphyrin derivative photoradiation therapy for the treatment of intraocular tumors. Examination of acute normal ocular tissue toxicity. Can Res 43:721–727

Gomer CJ, Dougherty TJ (1979) Determination of ^{3}H- and ^{14}C-hematoporphyrin derivative distribution in malignant and normal tissues. Can Res 39:146–151

Gomer CJ, Rucker N, Banerjee A et al. (1983b) Comparison of mutagenicity and induction of sister chromatid exchange in Chinese hamster cells exposed to hematoporphyrin derivative photoradiation, ionizing radiation or ultraviolet radiation. Can Res 43:2622–2627

Grossweiner L (1984) Personal communication

Hayata Y, Kato H, Konaka C et al. (1982a) Fiberoptic bronchoscopic laser photoradiation for tumor localization in lung cancer. Chest 82:10–14

Hayata Y, Kato H, Konaka C et al. (1983) Fiberoptic bronchoscopic photoradiation in experimentally induced canine lung cancer. Cancer 51:50–56

Hayata Y, Kato H, Amemiya R et al. (1984a) Indications of photoradiation therapy in early stage lung cancer on the basis of post-PRT histological findings. In: Doiron DR, Gomer CJ (eds) Porphyrin Localization and Treatment of Tumors. AR Liss Inc, New York, p 747–758

Hayata Y, Kato H, Konaka C et al. (1984b) Photoradiation therapy with hematoporphyrin derivative in early and stage I lung cancer. Chest 86:169–177

Hayata Y, Kato H, Ono J et al. (1982b) Fluorescence fiberoptic bronchoscopy in the diagnosis of early stage lung cancer. In: Recent Results in Cancer Research, Springer-Verlag, Berlin-Heidelberg, p 121–130

Henderson BW, Bellnier DA, Ziring B et al. (1983) Aspects of the cellular uptake and retention of hematoporphyrin derivative and their correlation with the biological response to PRT in vitro. In: Kessel D, Dougherty TJ (eds) Porphyrin Photosensitization, Plenum Press, New York, p 129–138

Henderson BW, Dougherty TJ, Malone PB (1984) Studies on the mechanism of tumor destruction by photoradiation therapy (PRT). In: Doiron DR, Gomer CJ (eds) Porphyrin Localization and Treatment of Tumors. AR Liss Inc, New York, p 601–612

Hetzel FW, Farmer H (1984) Dose effect relationships in a mouse mammary tumor. In: Doiron DR, Gomer CJ (eds) Porphyrin Localization and Treatment of Tumors. AR Liss Inc, New York, p 583–590

Hilf R, Smail DB, Murant RS et al. (1984) Hematoporphyrin derivative-induced photosensitivity of mitochondrial succinate dehydrogenase and selected cytosolic enzymes of R3230AC mammary adenocarcinomas of rats. Can Res 44:1483–1488

Hisazumi H (1984) Personal communication

Jocham D, Staehler G, Chaussy Ch et al. (1981) Laserbehandlung von blasentumoren nach photosensibilisierung mit hematoporphyrin-derivat. Urologe A 20:340–343

Kato H, Konaka C, Ono J et al. (1983) Effectiveness of Hpd and radiation therapy in lung cancer. In: Kessel D, Dougherty TJ (eds) Porphyrin Photosensitization. Plenum Press, New York, p 23–39

Kelly JF, Snell ME (1976) Hematoporphyrin derivative: A possible aid in the diagnosis and therapy of carcinoma of the bladder. J Urol 155:150–151

Kennedy J (1983) Unpublished results

Kessel D, Chou T (1983) Tumor-localizing components of porphyrin preparation hematoporphyrin derivative. Can Res 43:1994–1999

King EG, Doiron D, Man G et al. (1982) Hematoporphyrin derivative as a tumor marker in the detection and localization of pulmonary malignancy. In: Recent Results in Cancer Research. Springer-Verlag, Berlin-Heidelberg, p 90–96

Laws ER, Cortese DA, Kinsey JH et al. (1981) Photoradiation therapy in the treatment of malignant brain tumors. A phase I (feasibility) study. Neurosurg 9:672–678

L'Esperance F, Dougherty TJ (1983) Unpublished results

Lipson RL, Gray MJ, Baldes EJ (1966) Hematoporphyrin derivative for detection and management of cancer. Proc IX Internat Cancer Congr, p 393 (one page-abstract)

McCaughan JS, Hicks W, Laufman L et al. (1984) Palliation of esophageal malignancy with photoradiation therapy. Cancer 54(12):2905–2910

McCulloch GAJ, Forbes IJ, Lee See K et al. (1984) Phototherapy in malignant brain tumors. In: Doiron DR, Gomer CJ (eds) Porphyrin localization and treatment of Tumors. AR Liss Inc, New York, p 707–717

Moan J, Boye E (1981) Photodynamic effect on DNA and cell survival of human cells sensitized by hematoporphyrin. Photobiochem Photobiophys 2:301–307

Moan J, Steen HB, Feren K et al. (1981) Uptake of hematoporphyrin derivative and sensitized photoinactivation of C3H cells with different oncogenic potential. Cancer Lett 14:291–296

Moan J, Waksvik H, Christensen T (1980) DNA single-strand breaks and sister chromatid exchanges induced by treatment with hematoporphyrin and light or by x-rays in human NHIK 3025 cells. Can Res 40:2915–2918

Murphree AL, Doiron DR, Gomer CJ et al. (1984) Hematoporphyrin derivative photoradiation treatment of ophthalmic tumors. Presented at the Clayton Foundation Symposium on Porphyrin Localization and Treatment of Tumors, Santa Barbara, CA, April

Nava H (1983) Unpublished results

Nseyo U, Potter WR (1983) Unpublished results

Policad A (1924) Etudes sur les aspects offerts par des tumeur experimentales examinee a la lumiere de woods. CR Hebdomadaires Soc Biol 91:1422–24

Raab C (1900) Über die wirkung fluoreszirenden stoffe auf infusoria. Z Biol 39:524–526

Rettenmaier M, Berman M, DiSaia P et al. (1984) Gynecologic uses of photoradiation therapy. In: Doiron Dr, Gomer CJ (eds) Porphyrin Localization and Treatment of Tumors. AR Liss Inc, New York, p 767–715

Reuter HJ, Kohen RJ, Reuter MA (1982) Transurethral Resection. In: Atlas of Urologic Endoscopic Surgery. WB Saunders Co, Philadelphia, PA, p 1–167

Soma H, Akiya K, Nutahara S et al. (1982) Treatment of vaginal carcinoma with laser photoirradiation following administration of haematoporphyrin derivative. Report of a case. Ann. Chirurgiae Gynaecologiae 71:133–136

Soma H, Nutahara S (1983) Cancer of the female genitalia. In: Hayata Y, Dougherty TJ (eds) Lasers and Hematoporphyrin Derivative in Cancer. Igaku-Shoin, Tokyo New York, p 97–109

Spikes JD, Straight R (1967) Sensitized photochemical processes in biological systems. Ann Rev Phys Chem 18:409–436

Svaasand LO, Doiron DR, Dougherty TJ (1983) Temperature rise during photoradiation therapy of malignant tumors. Med Phys 10:10–17

Svaasand LO, Ellingsen R (1983) Calibration of applications of non-ionizing electromagnetic radiation. Part 2. Experimental results. Report #RB/PE029, Division of

Physical Electronics, University of Trondheim, Norway, Norwegian Institute of Technology

Taketa C, Imakiire M (1983) Cancer of the ear, nose and throat. In: Hayata Y, Dougherty TJ (eds) Lasers and Hematoporphyrin Derivative in Cancer, Igaku-Shoin, Tokyo New York, p 70–78

Tian M (1983) Unpublished results

Tomio L, Zorat PL, Corti L et al. (1983) Effect of hematoporphyrin and red light on AH-130 solid tumors in rats. Acta Radiol [Oncol] 22(1):49–53

Waldow SM, Dougherty TJ (1984) Interaction of hyperthermia and photoradiation therapy. Radiat Res 97:380–385

Ward BG, Forbes IJ, Cowled PA et al. (1982) The treatment of vaginal recurrences of gynecologic malignancy with phototherapy following hematoporphyrin derivative pretreatment. Am J Obstet Gynecol 142:356–357

Weishaupt KR, Dougherty TJ (1983) Unpublished results

Weishaupt KR, Gomer CJ, Dougherty TJ (1976) Identification of singlet oxygen as the cytotoxic agent in photoinactivation of a murine tumor. Can Res 36:2326–2329

Wharen RE Jr, Anderson RE, Laws ER Jr (1983) Quantitation of hematoporphyrin derivative (Hpd) in human gliomas, experimental central nervous system tumors, and normal tissues. Neurosurg 12:446–450

Wile AG, Dahlman A, Burns RG (1982) Laser photoradiation therapy of cancer following hematoporphyrin sensitization. Lasers Surg Med 2:163–168

Wile AG, Novotny J, Mason GR et al. (1984) Photoradiation therapy for head and neck cancer. In: Doiron DR, Gomer CJ (eds) Porphyrin Localization and Treatment of Tumors, AR Liss Inc, New York, p 681–691

5 New Imaging Technologies and Radiotherapy

5.1 CT in Radiation Therapy Treatment Planning

GEORGE T.Y. CHEN

CONTENTS

1 Introduction

Precise knowledge and control of the amount of radiation delivered to specifically defined regions in the patient are essential for state-of-the-art radiotherapy (STEWART et al. 1978). Computerized tomography (CT) is an important component in precision dose delivery. The introduction of CT in the mid 1970's and the concurrent availability of supermini-computers has resulted in a synergistic effect which is revolutionizing radiation therapy treatment planning. The combination of these two technologies offers the potential of greater precision in radiation therapy through improved three dimensional assessment of disease, localization of normal critical structures, inhomogeneity corrected dose calculations and precise field alignment. These improvements can result in more confident irradiation of the tumor with maximal spar-

ing of adjacent normal structures. This chapter provides an overview of the capabilities of three dimensional treatment planning systems today and reports on current research and development in this area likely to be of clinical benefit in the near future. A number of recent references provide the interested reader with additional information (WRIGHT and BOYER 1983; GOITEIN 1982a; LING 1982; CUNNINGHAM et al. 1984).

2 Hardware Requirements

We begin with considerations in CT scan data acquisition and computer hardware common to advanced treatment planning systems.

2.1 CT Scan Acquisition

Treatment planning in three dimensions requires the availability of sequential images generated from diagnostic quality CT scanners. Diagnostic and therapeutic scans share a number of common needs. These include a) the ability to scan with thin slices b) a method to locate the axial scan position on a radiograph like image (Scanogram or Scoutview) c) a need for accurate CT numbers for quantitative use, and d) fast scan and reconstruction times. Additionally, therapy scans should be performed in the treatment position, on a flat bed similar to the therapy couch, with the external body contour being visible, and with external markers (when needed) to locate surface landmarks or structures of interest (e.g. palpable nodes).

With most CT hardware capable of fast scans (5 sec or less), it is possible for the patient to hold his breath during the scan process. This condition provides the best diagnostic quality images where motion artifacts are minimized. At what point in the process should the patient suspend respiration? MAH and HENKELMAN (1984) observed that during respiration, anatomical points within the lung

The submitted manuscript has been authored by a contractor of the U.S. Government under contract No. W-7405-ENG-48. Accordingly, the U.S. Government retains a nonexclusive, royalty-free license to publish or reproduce the published form of this contribution, or allow others to do so, for U.S. Government purposes.

GEORGE T.Y. CHEN, Ph.D.
University of Chicago
Chicago, IL 60637, USA

move 1 cm or more, and lung density variations are as large as 8%. In their study, CT scans were taken at various points within the respiration cycle, and corresponding dose distributions were calculated. They concluded that a scan taken with breathing suspended at mid-respiration results in a dose distribution which differs by a few percent from the time averaged dose. Very slow scan times (in excess of 20 seconds) proposed by others for treatment planning result in blurred images which are of little diagnostic or tumor localization use. Therefore, if only one series of scans is to be taken, the recommended technique is suspended respiration at the mid-point of normal shallow breathing.

Since accurate localization of the tumor and normal structures is essential in precision radiation therapy, the CT scans must be taken with optimal diagnostic technique. This generally implies intravenous and oral contrast when indicated. These agents assist in accurate delination of the tumor and identification of adjacent critical structures, but may interfere with dose calculations, as will be discussed later.

The most direct approach has been for the radiotherapy department to have a close working relationship with the diagnostic radiology department, and have sufficient access to the scanner to provide studies suitable for accurate treatment planning. Such collaborative arrangements have been in effect for a number of years at the Royal Marsden Hospital (BERRY et al. 1983), where radiation technologists set up the patient in the CT scanner to insure proper patient positioning. An alternative to utilization of the radiology department CT facilities is a dedicated scanner within the radiation therapy department. Commercial firms recently have offered third generation CT scanners adapted for treatment planning and simulation. Still others have approached this problem through the in-house construction of a CT scanner designed for simulation and radiation therapy planning, (SMITH 1980). Regardless of approach, the objective is to obtain volumetric anatomic information.

2.2 Treatment Planning Computers

The development of sophisticated treatment planning computer programs has been aided by the availability of moderately priced powerful minicomputers, typically 32-bit machines. The primary advantage of such machines has been their ability to perform calculations on the large matrices associated with CT data. Complex and large computer programs may be written without the programming overhead of overlaying sections of the computer code to fit within the environment of a restricted computer memory. The wide availability of such machines has increased the need to share software development.

The second key hardware component of state of the art treatment planning systems has been the introduction of raster graphics to treatment planning. These devices permit the visualization of the CT data, and other graphically oriented information such as reformatted sagittal or coronal images of sequential axial scans, isodose contours superimposed on CT scans, radiographic images generated from volumetric CT data, and three dimensional graphics for anatomical and dose display. Examples of these images will be given later.

The desirability of calculating dose in three dimensions, and calculating several plan variations in order to choose the optimal plan has resulted in interest in the integration of array processors in treatment planning and display hardware (CURRAN and STERNICK 1984). These devices permit increase in calculational speed by factors of 10 or greater.

Several institutions with an investment in a central computing facility and graphics capabilities have treatment facilities spread over a distance of up to several miles. To facilitate the transmission of treatment planning images over such distances, these institutions have relied on microwave links from the computing facility and the remote treatment site (GOITEIN 1982b).

Few institutions have more than one or two full time computer scientists dedicated to refining treatment planning programs. Yet with the additional capabilities provided by improved hardware, the need for software development has dramatically increased. To accelerate program development, groups have been formed to share software for radiation therapy treatment planning (KIJEWSKI 1984).

3 Treatment Planning Process

In essence, the CT scanner and computer are used as a simulator. The target volume is defined on CT data and angulation of beams is chosen. Following this, dose distributions are calculated throughout the entire three dimensional volume, and doses to target and critical organs are analyzed. The capabilities common to advanced treat-

Table 1. Features of advanced treatment planning systems

– Based on volumetric CT or MRI data
– Capability to outline three dimensional structures
– Produces beam's eye view of structures
– Three dimensional display capabilities
– Dose calculation with inhomogeneity corrections
– Quantitative Dosimetric Analysis
– Design of beam modifying devices

ment planning systems are listed in Table 1. Several groups throughout the country are actively developing software directed towards achieving these capabilities. We now examine some of these capabilities in more detail.

3.1 Target Definition

Studies have shown that CT is an important adjunct in tumor volume definition (GOITEIN et al. 1979; HOBDAY et al. 1979). LICHTER et al. (1983) summarized the findings of 11 studies on the impact of CT on treatment planning. Overall, ap-

proximately 40% of plans were altered, 30% because of suspected inadequate target volume definition, 5% to reduce the volume treated, and the remainder because of a change of intent or modality of treatment (LICHTER et al. 1983). The three dimensional localization of tumor and adjacent radiation sensitive organs is clearly needed in precise radiotherapy.

The target definition process begins with taking contiguous CT scans through the region of interest. The data are then transferred via magnetic tape or other data link directly into the treatment planning computer. The study is viewed on a raster graphics display unit and target contours are interactively entered by the radiotherapist via a digitizing device. Representative contours of the target and normal adjacent structures on one such slice are shown in Fig. 1. The contours of radiation sen-

Fig. 1. Axial CT scan with target contour encompassing pancreatic tumor. The liver and kidneys are also contoured, for later use in dosimetric analysis

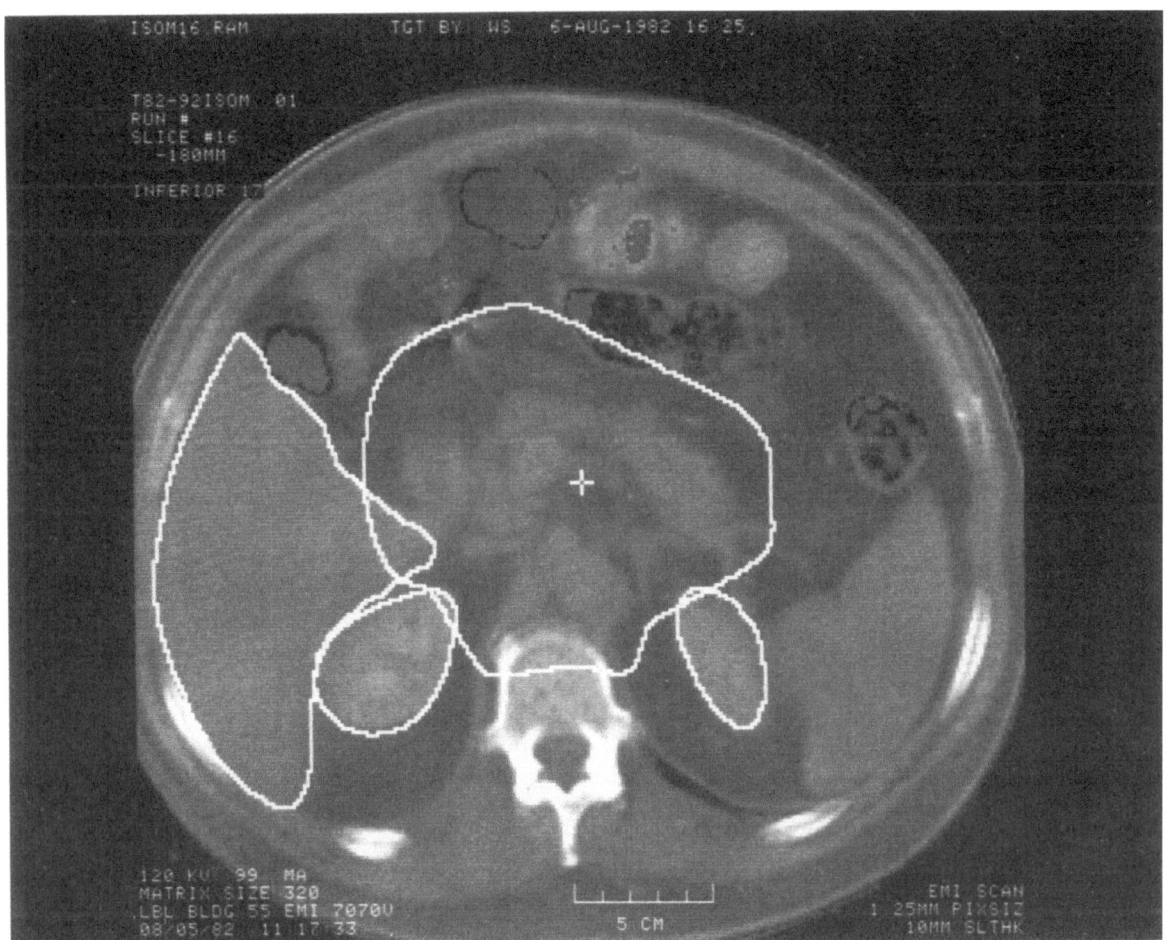

sitive organs are also digitized and later used in dosimetric analyses. Several advanced systems present the radiotherapist with simultaneous axial, coronal, and sagittal images, on which he may enter contours in any plane. This capability allows one to delineate a structure through interpolation in a plane other than axial, where such a structure may be more easily identified (GOITEIN et al. 1983). In addition to closed contours, landmarks may be entered for later use in portal alignment.

The target contours drawn by the radiotherapist reflect the volume he wishes to treat to a specific dose level. Conedown volumes must also be entered if a complete dosimetric analysis is required. In entering the target contour, margins are included for microscopic disease, uncertainties due to daily variations in patient setup, involuntary organ movement, and weight loss. In a recent study (CHEN et al. 1984a) tumor and kidney movement in the irradiation of abdominal tumors was estimated. Sequential CT scans of 10 patients, performed over several weeks, were used in documenting organ movement relative to bony landmarks. Movements in the craniocaudal axis were generally within 2 cm but extreme excursions of 3 cm were observed in isolated patients. In the AP and lateral axis, movement was generally 1 cm or less. These and similar data at other sites are needed in determining the appropriate margins for specific regions of the body.

Target entry is a physician-labor-intensive step in treatment planning. To reduce the effort of this step requires the ability to edit, erase or modify contours easily, and to create contours through interpolation (GOITEIN et al. 1983). Automatic contouring is possible for certain organs if a high contrast boundary exists between the organ and surrounding tissue. Autocontouring techniques are usually adequate for outlining the external body contour, lungs, and some bones. However, in general, these algorithms are unsuitable for internal organs such as kidneys or liver.

3.2 Beam Angle Selection

Following the definition of target volume and normal adjacent structures, beam entry angle and a collimator must be selected for each port. Graphic techniques to display the relative positions of tumor and adjacent anatomy are essential tools in determination of an appropriate beam entry angle. Beam selection criteria for determining an entry angle include: a) minimizing or excluding critical structures from the radiation path, b) minimizing

the pathlength to the target c) determining paths where inhomogeneities have the least perturbing effect and d) considering multiple fields which produce a uniform tumor dose. A beam's-eye view of the target and critical structures is helpful in this task.

For example, the target and kidneys outlined in a patient with pancreatic carcinoma are shown in axial, sagittal and coronal view in Fig. 2. Contours on the coronal and sagittal reconstruction define the target and kidney from the beam's eye view. Circular symbols show the position of landmarks defining the lateral edges of the vertebral column. This image provides the treatment planning team with collimator shape and portal alignment aids for an anterior and lateral irradiation of the target volume. The sagittal and coronal images are averaged over approximately one half of the body to produce an image similar to a diagnostic x-ray radiograph. The vertical resolution of this image is limited since the slice thickness used in this CT study is 1 cm. Images of the head and neck generated from CT scans taken with 0.2 cm slice thickness produce good quality simulated "x-ray" image.

Anatomical relationships may also be displayed through surface representations. Fig. 3 shows an abdominal target volume and the kidneys in two formats, a shaded surface representation and a wire frame image. This beam's eye view is useful in integrating the separate contours. A "transparency mode" in the shaded surface mode allows the viewer to look through structures to see what is behind an object. The objects may be interactively rotated, as shown in Fig. 3b.

Most field arrangements used in current radiation therapy practice are "coplanar". The central rays of the beams all lie in the same plane. There has been recent interest in visualization of structures and calculation of dose from fields shich may be non-coplanar (GOITEIN 1982c). Non-coplanar fields may provide a beam's eye view of the target where critical structures are lateral to the irradiated field. It has been shown that such beams can be confidently set up with a CT derived radiograph, on which the position of the radiation field is overlayed. Such non-coplanar fields appear to be most useful in the head and neck region.

3.3 Inhomogeneity Density Data

CT can provide information on the size, shape, and electron density of inhomogeneities which perturb radiation beams. Two approaches to incor-

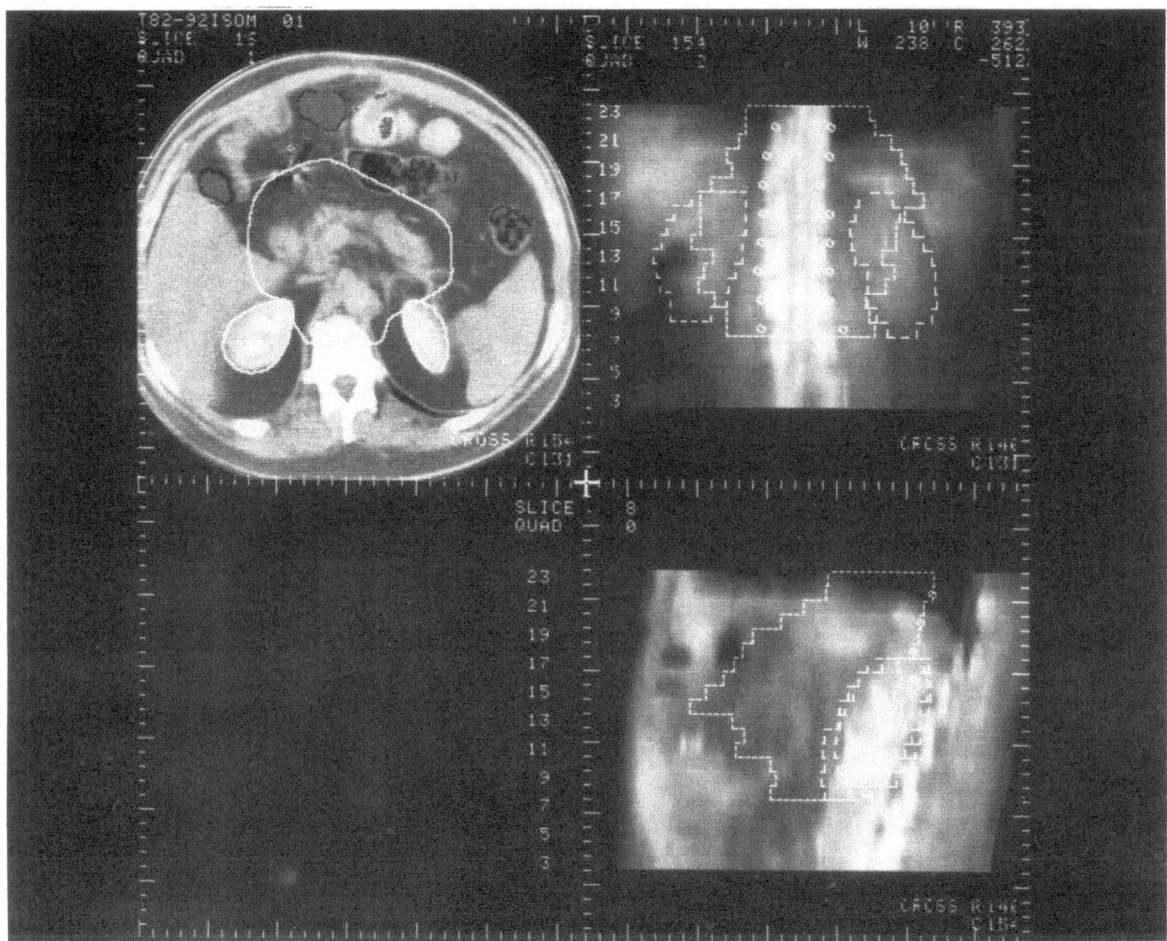

porating density information in treatment planning have been in use: a) the heterodense structures are contoured, and an average tissue density is assigned to points within the contour and b) the CT data are used on a pixel by pixel basis where the density is determined from the CT number of each pixel through a calibration curve. To approach the desired dose accuracy, pixel by pixel dose calculations coupled with new algorithms are likely to be required.

Photons are near – exponentially attenuated, and an error in the determination of the effective depth to the point of calculation generally produces a modest dose perturbation. For 4 MeV photons, a 1 cm error in effective depth results in a 5% dose error. For higher energy photons, this error is slightly smaller (about 4% for 20 MeV photons). If multiple fields are used, the effect of an inhomogeneity in the path of the beam is reduced. Pixel by pixel inhomogeneity corrections to treatment plans provide modest refinements in

Fig. 2. Multiplanar reconstructions of sequential axial images. The upper left quadrant displays the axial CT image. The right half of the figure show AP and lateral simulated "x-rays" generated from axial scans. Superimposed on theses images are the beam's eye view of the target and kidney contours

megavoltage dose calculations. On the other hand, the influence of inhomogeneities on electron and other charged particle beams is substantial, and sophisticated density corrections with these beams are necessary.

CT numbers are a measure of the linear attenuation coefficient of each pixel at diagnostic photon energies, and therefore are not solely a measure of the electron density. To integrate CT quantitatively into treatment planning, experimental calibration curves based on measured electron density of tissue equivalent phantom materials have been used. Such curves are sufficiently accurate for photon and electron treatment planning purposes

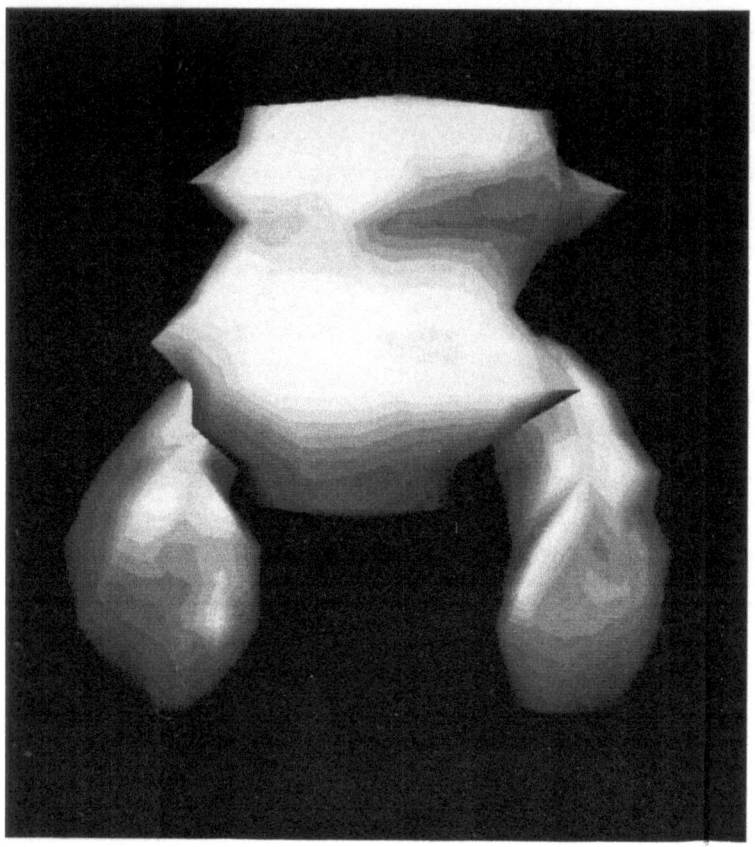

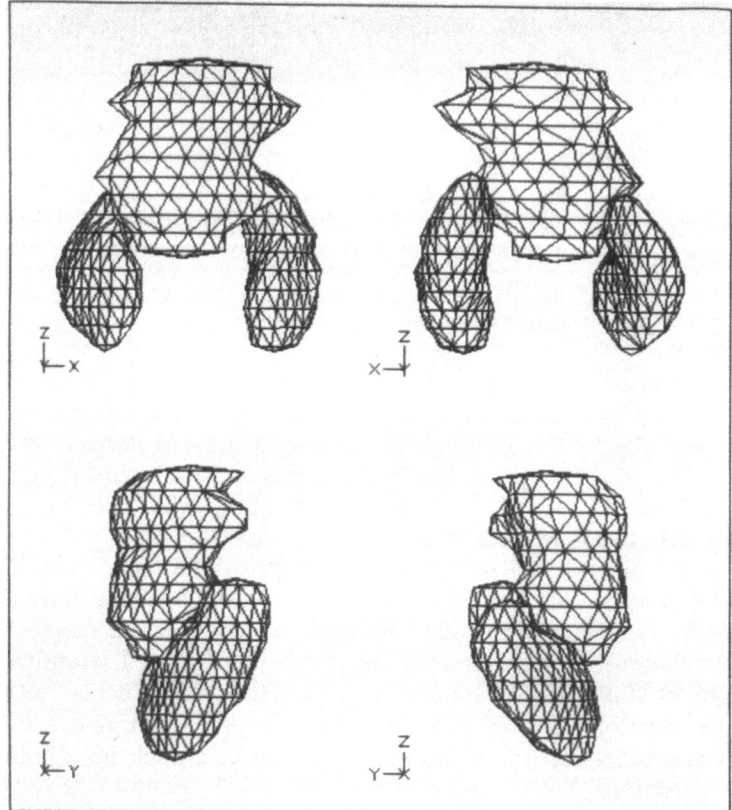

Fig. 3. a Surface display of a pancreatic target volume and kidneys. **b** Wire frame representations of the same target and kidneys viewed from AP, PA, left and right lateral viewpoints

(CHEN et al. 1979; BATTISTA 1980). When using calibration curves relating CT number and effective water equivalent thickness, the data should be experimentally measured for each scanner, as they are dependent upon scanner characteristics and scan parameters.

3.4 CT Data Preparation

The improved accuracy of dose calculations through the use of pixel by pixel heterogeneity corrections is dependent upon accurate CT numbers. In using CT quantitatively, CT number drift, beam hardening effects, partial volume sampling, presence of artifacts, and the transient nature of some inhomogeneities (such as gas in the GI tract) must be minimized.

To achieve accuracy and a more realistic treatment plan representative of fractionated radiotherapy, CT data often needs to be edited before dose calculations are performed. The need for this data preparation is strongly dependent upon treatment site. In particular, the presence of gas and contrast agents in the GI tract are the primary reason for such editing. The presence of these materials will interfere with an accurate treatment plan. Specifically, contrast in the scan will attenuate the photon beam in a manner similar to bone, and gas in the GI tract will result in a dose overshoot. Since contrast is not present during therapy and gas patterns change quasi-randomly, a dose calculation including these materials is not recommended.

One method to eliminate these materials is to identify the regions of contrast or gas, contour these regions, and replace the pixel values within the contoured region to water equivalent CT numbers. This editing process may be performed by a dosimetrist and limited to those CT slices which include the target, if coplanar treatment plans are generated. A more general approach is required for non-coplanar beams.

The elevation of CT numbers from intravenous contrast is highly dependent on the scan time and bolus injection point. The density elevation is organ specific, with greatest accumulation appearing in the kidneys. The apparent density increase of organs which have preferential uptake of contrast material may be as great as 10%. No unambiguous method for CT number correction of these contrast enhanced tissues is universally appropriate. If the perturbations appear to be extremely large, the editing of its CT numbers to more typical numbers is appropriate.

3.5 Dose Calculation Algorithms

The ICRU Commission on Radiation Units and Measurements has suggested that dose delivery in radiotherapy should be accurate to 5%. After unfolding uncertainties in delivering dose to a point in water, CUNNINGHAM (1983) cites that this implies an accuracy of about 3.8% for procedures for correcting dose for tissue inhomogeneities. New algorithms for dose computation have been introduced in an attempt to improve the accuracy of dose calculations, with the aim of integrating CT data into the process. Several reviews of this topic have recently appeared (PURDY 1983; CUNNINGHAM 1983). The expected improvement in accuracy has been quoted to be as large as 10% when compared with non-inhomogeneity corrected calculations. In treatment planning, the lung is the most important inhomogeneity, and phantom studies have indicated that 30% errors may be introduced if no corrections are made. If simple dose corrections for lung are made, the absolute difference between dose calculations and measurement is reduced to 5% or better. In other simpler and more homogeneous sites, such as abdomen or brain, dose calculation algorithms agree with dosimetry to within approximately 3–4%.

SONTAG (1979) reported a dose algorithm which includes not only the primary beam dose from a direct path from source to calculation point, but also the size, shape and position of structures not along the primary ray. His equivalent tissue-air ratio method lends itself particularly well to input using CT data, and its use rarely gives rise to errors greater than 5%. WONG et al. (1984) have proposed a "delta volume model" for three dimensional photon dose calculations which involves ray tracing of the first scattered photons. These more complex algorithms result in greater computation times, perhaps by factors of 10–50 (CURRAN and STERNICK 1984), requiring array processors or other specialized computation hardware if computation times are to be clinically acceptable.

3.6 Dose Display

The need for three dimensional appreciation of dose distributions was recognized as early as 1939 by Mayneord. Routine displays of the three dimensional dosimetric data have not been possible until recently. A number of methods are under development to display three dimensional dose information to the therapist. Display of isodose contours in the axial plane, superimposed on a grey level CT image may be complemented with displays in the sagittal and coronal planes. To compare rival plans, side by side display of different distributions on the raster graphics display unit is useful. Three dimensional representations of dose surfaces simultaneously superimposed on anatomical surfaces show promise, as do the color schemes developed at the Massachusetts General Hospital which combine dose with anatomy. All these techniques have been used experimentally, but it is still too early to determine which method will be most effective in presenting three dimensional dose information. It is likely that in the next few years, additional new and innovative approaches will be developed for dose display.

3.7 Dose Volume Histograms

The graphic display of isodose contours or surfaces superimposed on anatomy is qualitative, and a quantitative parameter related to irradiation of an organ is desirable. The quantitative evaluation of treatment plans is of interest in elucidating a number of points: a) feasibility of delivering the prescribed dose to target while irradiating adjacent critical tissues to a dose below tolerance, b) assessment of relative plan merit in comparison with other proposed plan variations and c) in research to estimate partial organ radiation tolerance. Quantitative treatment plan scoring has been an elusive and difficult task for both radiation therapist and physicist. This is due in part to the lack of quantitative techniques for such analysis and the lack of data on normal tissue tolerance if only a portion of the organ is irradiated. Three dimensional dosimetry provides additional insight into this problem. The dose to a specific organ or structure may be histogrammed if the three dimensional dose matrix has been calculated and the contours outlining the structure have been defined. Dose volume histograms have been used in treatment plan evaluation in conventional radiotherapy (Chin et al. 1981), in the assessment of partial organ tolerance (Austin Seymour 1984), and in treatment planning assessment (Chen et al. 1984b).

A representative dose volume histogram is shown in Fig. 4. In its differential form the abscissa displays the dose, either in Gy or percent target volume. The ordinate represents the percentage of organ irradiated. In integral form, the dose volume histogram displays that fraction of the organ irra-

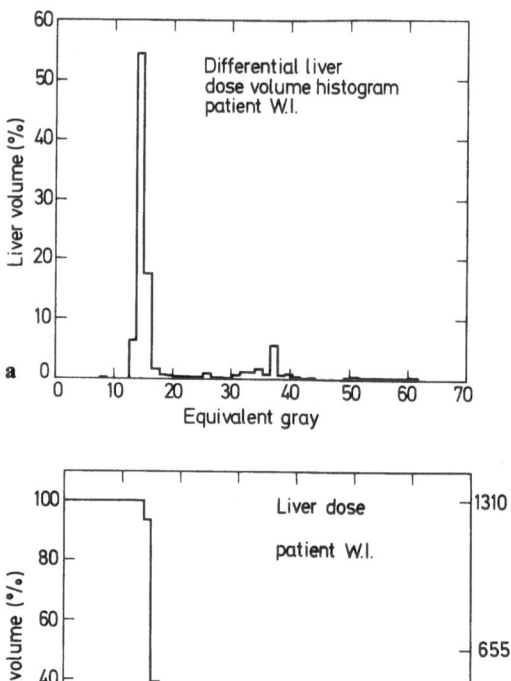

Fig. 4. a Differential dose volume histogram of liver for patient irradiated for carcinoma of the pancreas. In addition, the whole liver was irradiated to 15 GyE prophylactically. **b** Integral dose volume histogram. Approximately 20% of the liver was irradiated to a dose of 20 GyE or greater

diated (on the ordinate) in excess of the specified dose on the abscissa.

Dose volume histograms for a specific organ calculated with various field configurations or radiation types may be overlayed onto one plot. From such a representation, one may judge the relative merit of a plan by examining which dose volume curve irradiates the least amount of a critical structure to the lowest dose (Chen et al. 1984b).

Dose volume histogram analysis in conjunction with clinical findings may also be used to estimate partial organ radiation tolerance. Austin, Seymour (1984) examined the liver dose in 10 patients irradiated with heavy charged particles for pancreatic carcinoma. In addition to partial irradiation of the liver in the treatment of the pancreatic mass, the whole liver was irradiated with the intent of controlling metastases. One of the patients given 21 Gray Equivalent (GyE) to the liver in 3 GyE fractions subsequently developed radiation liver damage. A comparison of this patient's dose volume histogram for the liver with other patients who did not develop clinical liver damage suggests that no more than $1/3$ of the liver should receive a dose in excess of 30 GyE.

A three dimensional analysis of the dose matrix through dose volume histograms may prove to be useful in the determination of partial organ radiation tolerance. However, one limitation of these plots as currently developed, is that the dose per fraction, considered to be important in complications analysis, is not a parameter considered in the histogram. Dose volume histograms also imply a dose response which is uniform throughout the organ; the presence of a more critical or radiation sensitive part of a structure is not taken into account. It is therefore necessary to consider both three dimensional isodose distributions dose per fraction corrections and quantitative data such as dose volume histograms in plan analysis.

3.8 Compensator Design

By specifying a desired dose level within the target on a two dimensional surface perpendicular to the beam axis, one may design a three dimensional compensator. Compensators have been routinely used in photon radiation therapy to offset variations of dose due to external contour changes, and in the heavy charged particle therapy, where both external contours and tissue inhomogeneities are taken into account. Recently, the Princess Margaret Hospital/Ontario Cancer Institute has begun fabricating compensators with a computer controlled milling machine to provide inhomogeneity corrected dose distributions for cobalt-60 irradiations in hemi-body therapy and in mantle treatments for lymphoma (TAKIZAWA et al. 1984). An improvement in dose homogeneity to the lung can be achieved with a compensating filter, where the standard deviation from a homogeneous dose is reduced from 14% to 3%.

4 Conclusions

It is clear that initially, the process of three dimensional radiation therapy will be costly. A major source of costs lie in the labor intensive efforts of the radiotherapist in defining a three dimensional target volume and in the physicist's developing alignment aids, multiple dose distributions,

and inhomogeneity corrected compensators. Although "user-friendly" software will streamline some aspects of the complex process of precision treatment planning, it is likely that such cases will be invariably costly, and limited to the most complex and demanding cases.

The possible benefits of treatment planning in three dimensions with resulting optimized dose distributions can only be achieved if the delivery of such plans is likewise painstakingly performed. Improvements in immobilization will be required to reproduce the CT scan position on a daily basis on the treatment couch. Diagnostic quality films may be needed prior to each treatment for final alignment and positioning. Monitoring of patient position during therapy will be required in the most complex cases requiring absolute accuracy.

Despite the additional effort and complexity, precision radiation therapy is of interest, and is finding a place in radiation therapy, because it provides more accurate knowledge and control of the radiation delivered. Its foundation will be the volumetric anatomical information provided by computed tomography.

Acknowledgements. The author wishes to acknowledge the efforts of the members of the radiation therapy section of the Lawrence Berkeley Laboratory, especially Drs. SAMUEL PITLUCK, TODD RICHARDS and MARC KESSLER, in the development of computer programs which were used in the generation of the figures. The Heavy Ion Radiotherapy Project is supported by NCI 1P01CA19138.

References

Austin Seymour M et al. (1984) Assessment of liver radiation tolerance using dose volume histograms, Int J Rad Onc Bio Phys (abstract)

Battista J et al. (1980) Computed tomography for radiotherapy planning. Int J Rad Onc Bio Phys 6:99–108

Berry R et al. (1983) Computed tomography in therapy management: Tumors of the head and neck, In: Computed tomography in Radiation Therapy Ling, Rogers, and Morton eds. Raven Press, New York, p 89

Chen GTY, Singh RP, Lyman JT, Quivey JM, Castro JR (1979) Treatment planning for charged particle radiotherapy, Int J Rad Oncol Bio Phys 5:809–819

Chen GTY, Kessler MA, Saunders WM (1984a) Organ movement: Implications for CT based treatment planning, Med Phys 11:392 (abstract)

Chen G et al. (1984b) Dose volume histograms in the treatment planning evaluation of carcinoma of the pancreas, Proc 8th Int Conf on Computers in Radiotherapy, IEEE Computer Society Press, Silver Springs MD, ISBN 081860559-6 pp 264–268

Chin L et al. (1981) A computer-controlled radiation therapy machine for pelvic and para-aortic nodal areas, Int J Rad Onc Bio Phys 7:61–70

Cunningham JR (1983) Tissue Heterogeneity Characterization and Corrections, In: Advances in Radiation Therapy Treatment Planning, AAPM/AIP New York, pp 292–309

Cunningham JR, Ragan D, Van Dyke J eds (1984) Proc 8th Int Conf on Computers in Radiation Therapy IEEE Computer Society Press Silver Springs MD

Curran B, Sternick E (1984) The use of a display/array processor combination in radiation therapy treatment planning, In: Proc 8th Int Conf on Computers in Radiotherapy IEEE Computer Society Press, Silver Springs MD

Goitein M et al. (1979) The value of CT scanning in radiation therapy treatment planning: a prospective study, Int J Rad Oncol Bio Phys 5:1787–1798

Goitein M (1982a) Applications of computed tomography in radiotherapy treatment planning, In: Progress in Medical Radiation Physics, C. Orton, ed. Plenum New York, pp 195–287

Goitein M et al. (1982b) Curent and future developments in radiation therapy treatment planning. SPIE 318:359–364

Goitein M (1982c) Limitations of two dimensional treatment planning. Med Phys 9:580–586

Goitein et al. (1983) Multi-Dimensional treatment planning: I/II. Int J Rad Oncol Bio Phys 9:777–797

Hobday P, Hodson NJ, Husband J, Parker RP, MacDonald JS (1979) Radiol 133:477–82

Kijewski P (1984): private communication

Lichter A et al. (1983) An overview of clinical requirements and clinical utility of computed tomography based radiotherapy treatment planning. In: Computed Tomography in Radiation Therapy, C. Ling, C.C. Rogers and R.J. Marton, eds. Raven Press, New York, p 1–22

Ling CC, Rogers CC, Morton RJ eds (1983) Computed Tomography in Radiation Therapy, Raven Press, New York

Mah K, Henkelman M (1984) Time varying dose due to respiratory motion during radiation therapy of the thorax. In: Proc of 8th Int Conf on Computers in Radiotherapy, pp 294–298

Mayneord WV (1939) A dose contour projector and its application to three dimensional radiation distributions. Brit J Radiol 12:262–269

Purdy J (1983) Computer applications in Radiation Therapy Treatment Planning Radiation medicine, Vol 1, 161–173pp

Smith V et al. (1980) Development of a computed tomographic scanner for radiation therapy treatment planning. Radiology 136:489–493

Sontag M (1979) Photon beam dose calculations in regions of tissue heterogeneity using computed tomography. Ph.D. Thesis Univ of Toronto

Stewart JR et al. (1978) Computed tomography in Radiation Therapy, Int J Rad Onc Bio Phys vol 4 pp 313–324

Takizawa M et al. (1984) Automated design and cutting of compensating filters for precision radiotherapy using multi-CT image information. In: Proc 8th Int Conf on Computers in Radiotherapy, IEEE Computer Society Press Silver Springs MD, pp 452–455

Wong JW et al. (1984) The delta-volume method of three dimensional photon dose calculations. In: Proc 8th Int Conf Computers in Medicine IEEE Computer Society Press, Silver Springs MD

Wright A, Boyer AL (1983) Advances in Radiation Therapy Treatment Planning, Published by AAPM by AIP Medical physics monograph Nr 9

5.2 The Potential Application of Magnetic Resonance Imaging (MRI) in Radiation Oncology

Simon B. Sutcliffe, R. Mark Henkelman, and Peter Y. Poon

CONTENTS

1 Introduction

The clinical utility of imaging methods has generally focussed upon their diagnostic application. In addition to this role, imaging for the radiation oncologist provides a mechanism for definition of the target volume, routes of tumour spread and the diversity of tissue content within the target volume. Historically, the ready application of planar and three-dimensional imaging of tumour location and extent for radiation treatment planning, as exemplified by ultrasonography in the description of ocular tumours or the use of computed tomography for tumour imaging at various anatomical sites, stands as evidence of the importance of imaging to radiation oncology.

Imaging by nuclear magnetic resonance provides a new approach to descriptive anatomy, employing principles that, to a greater extent, reflect biological functions of tissue rather than the photon attenuations that characterize radiological im-

Simon B. Sutcliffe, M.D., Associate Professor
R. Mark Henkelman, Ph.D., Professor
Peter Y. Poon, M.D., Assistant Professor
500 Sherbourne Street
Toronto, Ontario M4X 1K9, Canada

ages. It is resonable to suppose, therefore, that magnetic resonance imaging (MRI) may provide information, either unique or complementary, to that currently available to the radiation oncologist. Relative to other imaging modalities, however, MRI is in an early stage of development and thus only preliminary statements of its potential application in oncology can be made. It must be recognised that the final role of MRI in oncological practice will become apparent following technological improvements in imaging and further clinical evaluation.

2 Principles of MRI

MRI measures signals from naturally-occurring, mobile protons in the human body that have been perturbed, by means of a radiofrequency pulse, from the equilibrium orientation that they adopt in a strong, externally applied, homogeneous magnetic field. The strength of the signal, and hence the contrast in the image, depends on: the density of protons within the imaging voxel; the relaxation time that it takes for them to return to equilibrium orientation after perturbation (T_1); the heterogeneity of the proton molecular environments which gives rise to a more rapid proton dephasing relaxation rate (T_2), and any movement, including flow, during the imaging time (Pykett et al. 1982). Different choices of the parameters defining the imaging sequence result in different functional dependencies of the image contrast on the various properties of the tissue. It is therefore necessary in MRI to ensure that an imaging pulse sequence is chosen which maximises the differential information required for the imaging task. Indiscriminate choices of pulse sequence can result in clinically important information being completely missed.

Spatial localisation of the signal is achieved by the application of appropriate magnetic field gradients during both the perturbation of the protons and the subsequent recording of the signal. MRI uses a computer system to record the signals and subsequently calculate the image. Initially, images were reconstructed by convolution back projection methods analogous to CT, but almost all clinical systems now use phase encoding methods which are unique to MRI. Most MR images use a two-dimensional Fourier transform algorithm with the data for multiple slices being acquired simultaneously (KAUFMAN et al. 1981). Direct 3-dimensional volume imaging can also be achieved.

Current state-of-the-art M.R.I. achieves spatial resolutions of about $1 \times 1 \times 5$ mm^3 in the head and $1 \times 2 \times 10$ mm^3 in the body. Greater resolution can be achieved over restricted regions using surface coils which have greater sensitivity. This ideal resolution is seldom achieved in clinical imaging where there is any degree of patient motion.

3 Freely Oriented Planes for 3-Dimensional Visualisation

Radiation therapy treatment planning is intrinsically a problem involving 3-dimensional geometry. Historically, this 3D nature has been ignored, initially because plans were constructed by hand on 2-dimensional paper. Even with computer techniques, plans have tended to remain 2D due to limited computational and memory computer resources and the use of 2-dimensional image display systems. Even CT. which is capable of obtaining 3D anatomical information, has been used most often in treatment planning as a single 2D transverse slice supplemented with crude assumptions about the cylindrical symmetry of the patient. The increasing availability of larger computer systems has resulted in some impressive and creative attempts to address computerised radiation treatment planning as the 3D problem that it really is (GOITEIN and ABRAMS 1983).

MRI readily contributes to a 3D understanding of the geometry of tumours and normal structures. Unlike CT, which is constrained by the mechanical rotation of the X-ray tube to imaging transverse slices of the patients, the image plane in MRI is electronically defined and can be arbitrarily oriented. Therefore, a diagnostic MR image is as likely to be in a sagittal or a coronal plane or, for that matter, in an arbitrary orientation as it is to be a transverse image. It must be stressed that these planes are not achieved by reformatting a series of transverse images as is done with CT data. Thus, MR is well suited to viewing patient anatomy from perspectives that are particularly appro-

priate for radiotherapy planning (i.e. perpendicular to or along the axis of the treatment beams). Furthermore, the ability to obtain 3D volume images encourages investigation of a complete 3D representation of the tumour and surrounding normal structures.

An example of the desirability of 3-dimensional radiation treatment planning is illustrated in Fig. 1, an MRI of a patient with an oesophageal tumor. Because of the close proximity of the oesophagus to the spinal cord, a structure of defined and limited radiation tolerance, and the change in cross-sectional anatomy at different levels in the thorax, beam localization in 2 dimensional planes is complex. MRI simplifies treatment planning, since it provides 3 dimensional information throughout the irradiation field.

A further example of a site requiring 3-dimensional information for radiation field planning is the posterior fossa and brain stem. In this situation, CT is limited in the definition of soft tissue tumour extent by the beam hardening artefact created by the presence of bone. MRI, however, is primarily sensitive to the soft tissues and provides excellent differentiation of the anatomy of the brain stem and cerebellum.

4 Differential Diagnosis

A common diagnostic problem in oncology is the evaluation of a space-occupying lesion. By virtue of the wide differences in relaxation times among different tissues, MRI provides good tissue contrast (KOENIG et al. 1984) permitting ready distinction of cystic and vascular lesions from solid tissue masses. This capability is of value, not only in discrimination within individual organs, but also in the evaluation of anatomical sites comprised of numerous tissue and vascular structures e.g. the mediastinum, the pulmonary hilum. While such distinction can be achieved with other imaging methods, in general there is a requirement for contrast enhancement to demonstrate vascular characteristics.

Based upon the observation that the T_1 relaxation time is generally longer in malignant tumours than in corresponding normal tissues, it was predicted that MRI might selectively distinguish malignant from benign masses (WEISMAN et al. 1972). However, this expectation has not yet been borne out in practice; and it is perhaps naive to presume that such distinctions could be made with current technology.

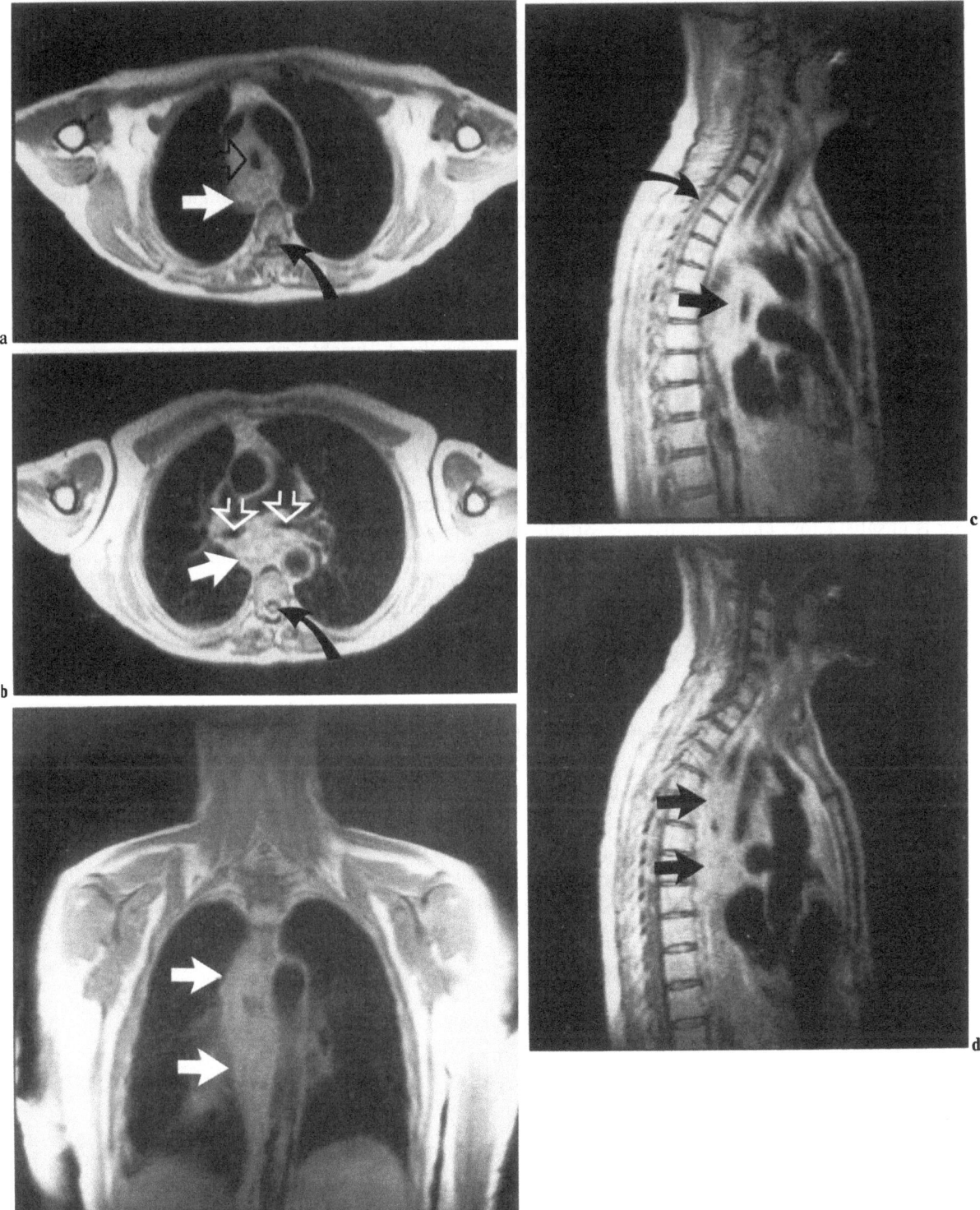

Fig. 1a–e. MRI of the thorax of a patient with proven carcinoma of esophagus. **a, b** Transverse sections; **c, d** sagittal sections; **e** coronal section. The tumor (*arrows*) is very extensive. It displaces the trachea (*open arrow*) and the main bronchi (*open arrow*) forward. Note its relation with the spinal cord (*curved arrow*) in the transverse and sagittal planes

5 Definition of the Target (Tumor) Volume and Description of Tissues

Radiation therapy is a localised therapeutic modality and to achieve a radiotherapeutic cure requires inclusion of the entire malignant process within the treatment volume. The target (tumor) volume therefore must include of the primary tumor, the direct routes of spread (contiguous invasion) and indirect routes of spread (lymphatic or vascular). Conventional imaging provides an anatomic or geographic representation of tumor volume – the physical tumor mass and its displacement or invasion of adjacent tissues. This geographic statement is also reproduced by MRI given its ability to provide good soft tissue contrast. An example of definition of anatomical extent is shown in Fig. 2, an MRI of the pelvis of a patient with a bladder tumour demonstrating tumor size, location and penetration. In this circumstance, radiological imaging is unsatisfactory and subjective assessment by examination under anaesthesia has conventionally provided the basis for assessment of tumour penetration.

Fig. 2a, b. MRI of pelvis showing a bladder carcinoma. **a** Transverse; **b** coronal. The large tumor (*arrow*) is well demonstrated. It extends into the perivesical fat (*curved arrow*). This was confirmed by examination under general anesthesia

Carcinoma of the prostate is another site where determination of tumor extent has defied reliable description by radiological imaging. As with bladder carcinoma, the generally available assessment of direct tumor penetration has been by the subjective approach of examination under anaesthesia. Although MRI has had limited success in the differential diagnosis of malignancy, it has provided a potential means of assessment of extracapsular penetration. Fig. 3a and b show NMR images of a clinically localised prostatic carcinoma and one assessed clinically to have invaded the capsule. The latter image demonstrates a breach in the normally visualised "bright" ring around the prostate, presumed to be the periprostatic venous plexus based on the similarity of its nuclear resonance characteristics with the corpora of the penis (POON et al. 1984). If this observation is borne out by further surgico-pathological studies, an objective measure of tumor penetration will be available with important attendant therapeutic implications.

A further example of tumor volume definition is shown in Fig. 4, an NMR image of a patient with bronchogenic carcinoma metastatic to mediastinal lymph nodes. In this instance, nodal metastasis was not apparent by mediastinoscopy, but was correctly identified at thoracotomy. The cited examples illustrate the potential for description of tumor spread by MRI, however the frequency and reliability of such observations require further study before general clinical utility can be determined.

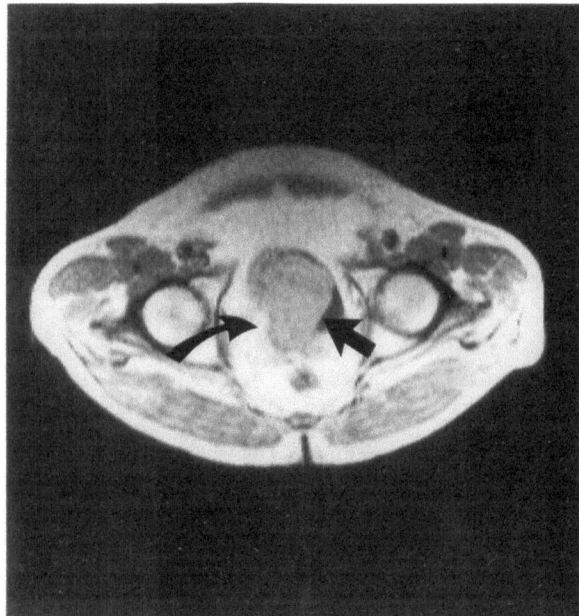
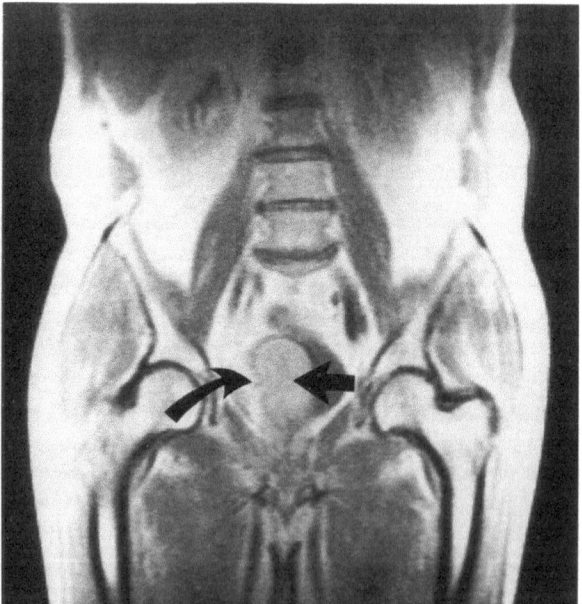

a   b

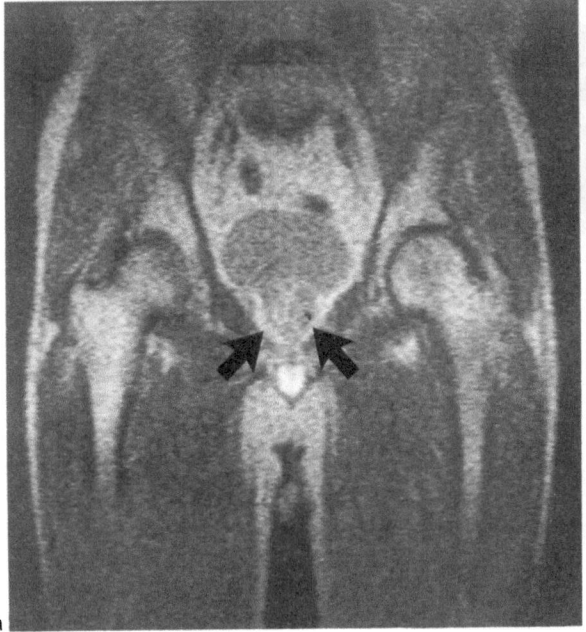
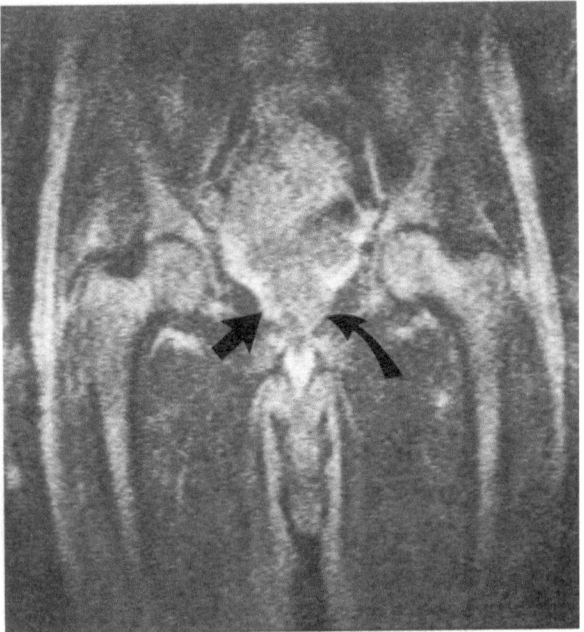

a   b

Fig. 3a, b. Coronal MRI of two patients both with carcinoma of prostate. **a** The periprostatic venous plexus (*arrows*) is intact inferring that the tumor is confined to the gland. **b** The periprostatic venous plexus (*arrow*) is deficient on the left (*curved arrow*) inferring that the tumor has extended beyond the capsule. The findings in both patients were confirmed by examination under general anesthesia

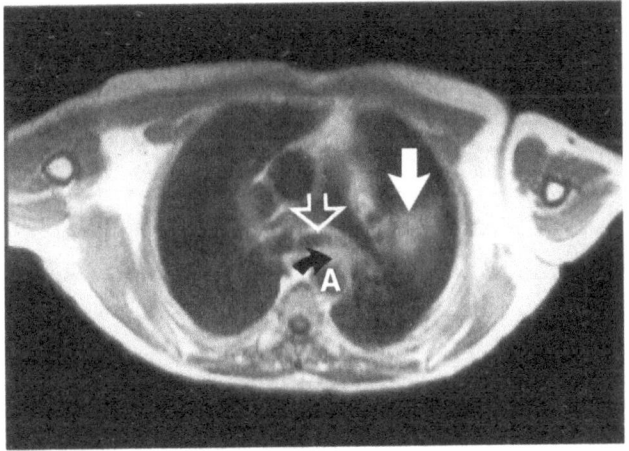

Fig. 4. MRI of thorax in a patient with bronchogenic carcinoma. The primary is in the left upper lobe together with consolidation (*arrow*). There are metastases to the subcarinal lymph nodes (*curved arrow*) between the left main stem bronchus (*open arrow*) and the aorta (*A*). The metastases were not detected at mediastinoscopy but were confirmed at thoracotomy

In addition to the demonstration of the anatomical relationship of tumor to adjacent structures, the significance of changes in signal intensity in contiguous "normal" tissues as an index of their functional state is an unexplored area. Consider the CT image of a patient with malignant intracranial disease (Fig. 5a). The tumor and the surrounding hypodense region are well characterised. The NMR image (Fig. 5b and c) also indicates the tumor, but shows an abnormality of surrounding tissue more extensive than the hypodensity revealed by CT, and interpreted as oedema. It is well recognised clinically that the extent of the malignant process exceeds that represented by radiological imaging. It is possible that the more extensive functional change distant from the primary tumor on MRI could correlate with a malignant process of diagnostically inapparent extent. If this were true, it would require a re-evaluation of the clinical concept of an appropriate "tumor mar-

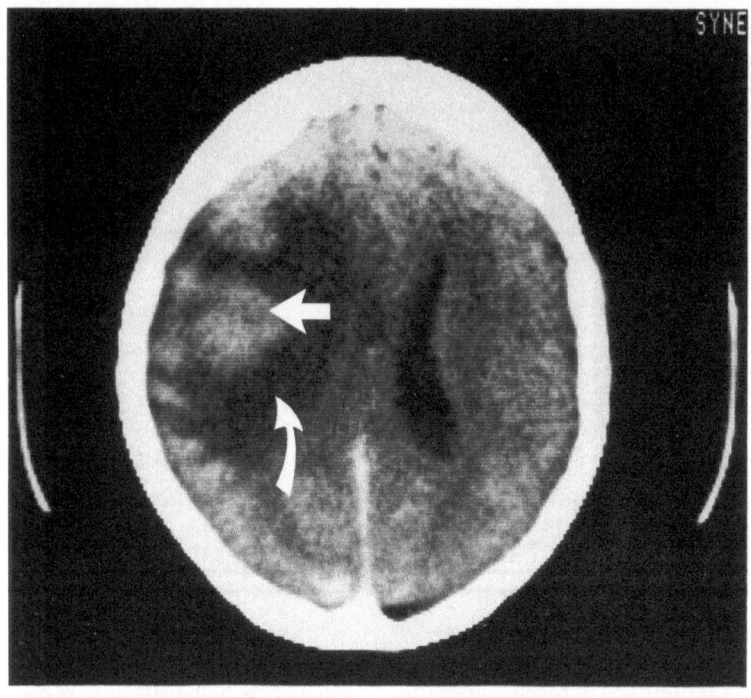

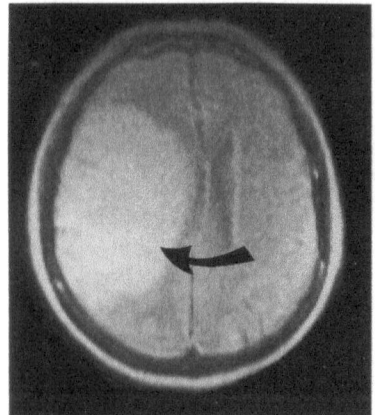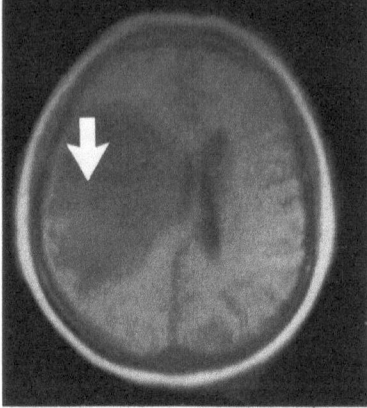

Fig. 5a–c. A patient with primary breast carcinoma. **a** CT examination of the brain after a bolus injection of contrast medium shows an enhanced metastasis (*arrow*) surrounded by a large amount of edema (*curved arrow*). **b** MRI obtained by spin-echo technique shows more mass effect than A (*curved arrow*). This is probably due to edema but additional contributing causes such as infiltrating tumor tissue cannot be excluded. The metastatic lesion is not clearly seen. **c** MRI obtained by inversion-recovery technique shows the metastasis (*arrow*) as well as the surrounding abnormality. Note the change of the edema from white to black between b and c

gin" for radiation therapy. Alternatively, the M.R.I. changes might reflect an increased sensitivity of this modality to detect intracranial oedema.

The principle of detecting functional tissue changes with M.R.I. can be extrapolated further. For example is it possible that MRI could define a malignant "field" change as is apparent with urothelial malignancies? Could more extensive metastases to bone marrow be demonstrated rather than the discrete lesions imaged radiologically in a situation where dissemination is the more likely clinical situation? The answers to these questions are unknown as yet, however, the capacity for functional as opposed to purely anatomical statements with MRI provides a dimension not served by radiological imaging, and a dimension amenable to assessment by quantitative MRI and appropriate clinical correlation.

6 Quantitative Data Concerning Tissue Heterogeneity

Besides providing 3-dimensional anatomical data for treatment planning, CT has provided quantitative estimates of the electron density distribution within the tissues, and hence the scattering cross sections presented to the therapy beam. Thus tissue inhomogeneity can be determined and incorporated into the development of algorithms used in computerised treatment planning programs.

The physical basis of signal intensity in MR images is completely different from that of X-ray imaging and bears no relationship to electron density. There is a complete lack of correlation between the MR intensities and the electron densities, nor would such a relationship be expected on theoretical grounds (HENKELMAN et al. 1984). This situation is further aggravated by the widely differing variety of imaging intensities with different MRI sequences. Thus, it will be impossible to use information from M.R. images to perform inhomogeneity dose corrections in the way that CT numbers have been used to infer electron densities using a bi-linear relationship as described by BATTISTA et al. (1980).

7 Correlation of Biological Activity with Magnetic Resonance Characteristics

The heterogeneity of response of local tumor to radiation therapy reflects a number of factors; one component of 'apparent' failure is that due to erroneous tumor localisation, whilst other factors describe genuine differences in biological behavior of the tumor and its response to irradiation.

The role of MRI in tumor localisation has been discussed in terms of anatomical description and functional changes in adjacent tissues.

It is premature to speculate on the capability of NMR to define biological correlates of malignancy e.g. mitotic activity or metastatic potential, particularly when these parameters are, as yet, described only in experimental settings without established clinical relevance. However, it is worth noting that NMR provides an in-vivo statement of both tumor extent and function, be this a description of the malignant cell population and/or its supporting stroma. In malignancies characterised by heterogeneity as a function of histological grade, e.g. soft tissue sarcomas, quantitative NMR may merit exploration as a means of objective assessment of grade, independent of the more subjective histological parameters.

8 Prediction of Local Tumor Control by Radiation

Hypoxic tumor cells are more radioresistant than fully oxygenated cells and therefore may be a dose-limiting factor in curative therapy. *A-priori* knowledge of the extent of hypoxia of a tumor could provide an indication of the need for more aggres-

sive therapy or for the use of radiation of high linear energy transfer.

Since molecular oxygen (O_2) is a paramagnetic contrast agent which reduces the T_1 relaxation time of tissue, it has been suggested that this effect could be used clinically to recognise hypoxic tumors (BYDDER GM 1981). However, to obtain measurable changes in T_1 in patients, very large changes in the concentration of O_2 are required, (of the order of 100 mm Hg). These are larger than the oxygen concentrations associated with radiobiological hypoxia, (i.e. 10 mm Hg). At present, therefore, although the MR imaging of hypoxia cannot be ruled out, it seems unlikely unless the sensitivity of detection is enhanced.

9 Assessment of Tumor Response and Normal Tissue Reactions

In many circumstances, complete sterilization of a tumor leaves residual anatomic distortions, or a mass, while on the other hand, residual viable tumor may be consistent with a normal clinical evaluation. The ability of NMR to provide both anatomic and functional information may be relevant in the assessment of local control of the tumor (KROEKER et al. 1984).

The late complications of radiation therapy in renewing tissues are thought to more reliably correlate with the integrity of the tissue stroma than with the acute effects in tissue epithelia. Serial information on functional properties of normal tissue within the irradiation field might form a basis for prediction of long term sequalae of treatment. Although definitive data are yet to be obtained, preliminary results suggest that MRI might give an early indication of radiation demyelination and radiation-induced pneumonitis. The early detection of changes in non-renewing tissues e.g. CNS, may indicate the future functioning potential of such tissues.

10 Conclusions

Any definitive statements concerning the role of NMR in radiation oncology are premature given the current technological limitations and the lack of appropriate clinical study to define its relevance.

There are, however, a number of areas of obvious interest – the diagnostic application based upon the soft tissue contrast properties, the ability to provide anatomic and functional statements of tumor and adjacent tissue with attendant implications for definition of tumor volume and the provision of freely-orientated planes. These benefits accrue without exposure to radiation and without evident risk. However, given the very low radiation exposures associated with radiological imaging, this benefit of NMR may be most apparent only in serial studies. It is not possible at present to indicate the unique contribution of MRI's capacity to influence radiation treatment planning. In most instances, the anatomic description of tumor extent by MRI has not exceeded that provided by other imaging modalities, although one notable exception may be in circumstances where bone artefact obscures the radiological image, e.g. the posterior fossa and brain stem. Other examples are cited in the text. The significance of change in signal intensity in tissues surrounding the tumor requires evaluation before any change in clinical judgment of appropriate tumor margin can be made.

Several experimental uses based upon the availability of *in-vivo* functional characterisation of tissue by NMR deserve exploration. These include the presence of hypoxia, biological tumor heterogeneity, assessment of tumor viability following therapy, and stromal effects potentially predictive of late effects of radiation.

Certain aspects of MRI are clearly inferior to the other imaging modalities, e.g. the failure to provide data analogous to the electron density measurements available from CT. Also the failure to image cortical bone resulting from the short T_2 relaxation time in the solid bone lattice removes the provision of bony landmarks for radiation therapy planning – a conventional method of field verification.

The evaluation of MRI will require that those properties unique to this modality be defined with appropriate technological improvements to establish quantification and economy of time and expense. The role that MRI subsequently assumes in radiation treatment planning will necessitate clinical evaluation against existing competitive methods and the demonstration that the benefits accruing from MRI translate into modifications of the treatment plans which result in improved clinical results.

Footnote. The images presented in this chapter have been produced using a prototype 0.15 Tesla Technicare Imager. A variety of different pulse sequences have been used, chosen to give maximum contrast of pathological structures.

Acknowledgement. The authors wish to acknowledge the receipt of Ministry of Health, Health Care Systems Research Grant D.M. 643 for development of M.R.I. at Ontario Cancer Institute/Princess Margaret Hospital.

References

Battista JJ et al. (1980) Computed Tomography for Radiotherapy Planning. Int J Radiat Oncol Biol Phys 6:99–107

Bydder GM (1981) NMR: Initial Clinical Results, In: Proceedings of an International Symposium on Nuclear Magnetic Resonance Imaging. Winston, Salem

Goitein M et al. (1983) Multi-Dimensional Treatment Planning: II Beam's View-Eye, Back Projection, and Projection through CT Sections. Int J Radiat Oncol Biol Phys 9, 6:789–797

Goitein M, Abrams M (1983) Multi-Dimensional Treatment Planning: I Delineation of Anatomy. Int J Radiat Oncol Biol Phys 9:777–787

Henkelman RM et al. (1984) Is Magnetic Resonance Imaging Useful for Radiation Therapy Planning, In: Proceedings of the Eighth International Conference on the Use of Computers in Radiation Therapy, pp 181–185, Toronto

Kaufman L, Crooks LE (1981) Hardware for NMR Imaging. In: Kaufman L, Crooks LE, Margulis AR (eds) Nuclear Magnetic Resonance Imaging in Medicine, Igaku-Shoin Ltd, Tokyo, Japan, pp 53–67

Koenig SH et al. (1984) Magnetic Field Dependence of $1/T_1$ of Protons in Tissue Investigative Radiology, 19:76–81

Kroeker RM et al. (1984) The Determination of tumour Recurrence After Radiotherapy with Relaxation Time Measurements. Soc. magnetic Resonance in Medicine. pp 439, New York

Poon PY et al. (1984) Magnetic Resonance Imaging of the Prostate, Radiology

Pykett IL et al. (1982) Principles of Nuclear Magnetic Resonance Imaging. Radiology 143:157–168

Weisman ID et al. (1972) Recognition of cancer in vivo by Nuclear Magnetic Resonance. Science 178:1288–1290

5.3 Applications of Positron Emission Tomography (PET) in Tumor Management

RANDALL A. HAWKINS and MICHAEL E. PHELPS

CONTENTS

1 Introduction

Positron emission tomography (PET), also referred to as positron computed tomography (PCT) provides cross sectional images of the body as do other axial tomographic techniques including x-ray computed tomography (x-ray CT) and nuclear magnetic resonance imaging (NMR) (also referred to as MRI, magnetic resonance imaging). Unlike x-ray CT images, which are anatomic representations of the attenuation characteristics of tissue, PET images reflect physiologic processes such as metabolism and blood flow (PHELPS et al. 1982 and PHELPS and MAZZIOTTA 1985). While most of the initial clinical experience with MRI has also resulted in primarily anatomic representations of pathology, the full potential of this technique, like PET, remains to be explored. Nevertheless, studies to date have already demonstrated the potential of PET to provide quantitative and pictorial physiologic descriptions of neoplasms that complement anatomic images obtained with other modalities. This information is particularly relevant to radiation therapy where varying levels of tissue oxygenation and blood flow can have significant therapeutic implications and to oncology in general

RANDALL A. HAWKINS, M.D., Ph.D.
MICHAEL E. PHELPS, Ph.D.
University of California
Los Angeles, CA 90024, USA

where metabolic parameters generated by PET studies can be significant both diagnostically and therapeutically.

Most of the initial PET tumor studies have concerned brain tumors, paralleling the neurologically oriented development of this imaging technique (PHELPS et al. 1982). While considerably progress in cardiac applications of PET have been made, the experience in other organ systems is limited. Therefore, this chapter will focus on brain tumors as a tumor paradigm, or model, while it must be remembered that the techniques described in the following pages are applicable in any region of the body.

A variety of clinically significant results are emerging from the initial PET tumor studies including the ability to distinguish between low grade astrocytomas and high grade astrocytomas (DI CHIRO et al. 1984), and to differentiate tumor recurrence from radiation necrosis (PATRONAS et al. 1982). These studies have also illustrated the efficacy of PET in differential diagnosis and monitoring therapy. Because extensive investigations in radiation biology have demonstrated a close relationship between physiologic parameters and tissue response to ionizing radiation (WITHERS and PETERS 1980), the clinical implementation of PET in radiation therapy should follow as a logical extension of those basic studies.

2 Methods

PET provides accurate measurements of the concentration of positron emitter labeled tracers in the organ or structure of interest as well as cross sectional and standard planar images of the distribution of the administered radioisotopes (PHELPS et al. 1982). Physiologic tracer kinetic models provide quantitative descriptions of the underlying physiologic processes in addition to the pictorial information available in the images themselves. The applications section below contains examples of tracer kinetic models specific for processes such

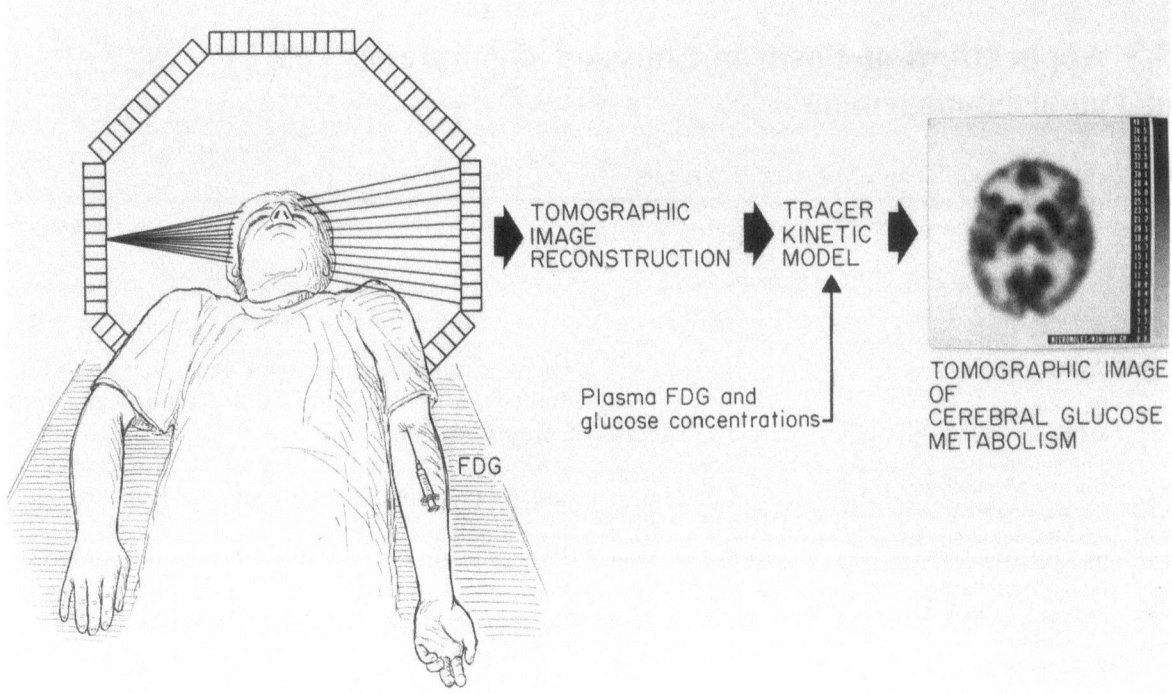

Fig. 1. PET studies. A PET study involves collecting projections of gamma ray emissions at many angles around the body illustrated by the bank of detectors surrounding the patient above. After the projection data is reconstructed into an image and the resultant image data is processed with an appropriate tracer kinetic model, a final tomographic image is produced which, in the above illustration, represents glucose metabolism. (From PHELPS et al. 1983)

as glucose and oxygen metabolism, blood flow, blood brain barrier diffusion and protein synthesis.

In addition to radiopharmaceuticals and tracer kinetic models, the third requirement for PET studies is the tomograph itself. While a full discussion of these tomographs is beyond the scope of this chapter, reviews of these devices are available in the literature (PHELPS et al. 1979a; TER-POGOSSIAN et al. 1981). PET, like x-ray CT and other forms of computed tomography, produces cross sectional images from projections of gamma ray emission from the body at many different angles. A superimposition of this angular data, after appropriate processing, produces the tomographic image. Pairs of detectors on opposite sides of the patient in a PET scanner are activated essentially simultaneously by two 511 KeV photons emitted 180 degrees apart that result from the emitted positron undergoing annihilation with an electron. Be-

cause many detectors are arranged circumferentially around the patient (Fig. 1), these "lines of coincidence" are entirely analogous to attenuation profiles generated in x-ray CT by circumferentially oriented x-ray tubes and detectors.

Early generation PET scanners produced a single image (slice) per scan while more modern units generate multiple slices per scan in addition to images of higher resolution than the earlier tomographs (PHELPS et al. 1979a; TER-POGOSSIAN et al. 1981; HOFFMAN et al. 1983).

Investigators have labeled a variety of compounds (over 200) with positron emitting isotopes (WELCH and TEWSON 1979; WOLF 1981). The short half lives (e.g., ranging from 2 minutes for ^{15}O to 109 minutes for ^{18}F) of most of these radioisotopes means that an on-site cyclotron is usually necessary for PET studies.

3 Applications

3.1 Glucose Metabolism

One of the most widely used and best validated approaches in PET is the F-18 deoxyglucose (FDG) method for measuring regional glucose metabolic rates. The method is an extension of the ^{14}C deoxyglucose autoradiographic model of

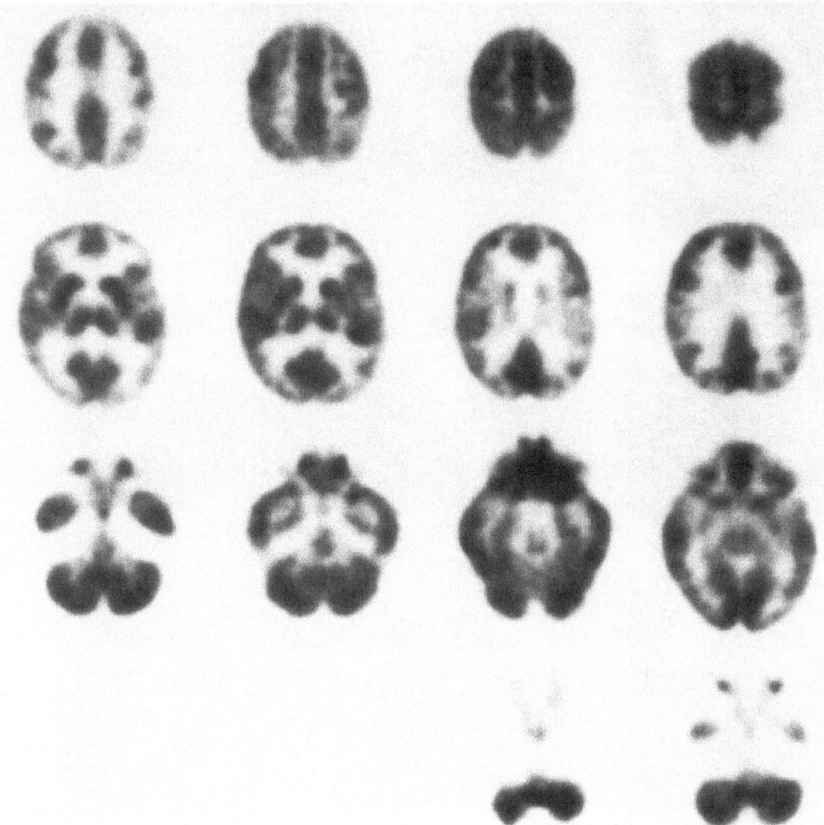

glucose metabolism developed by SOKOLOFF et al. (1977) and later extended to man (REIVICH et al. 1979; PHELPS et al. 1979b; HUANG et al. 1980). FDG is transported from the blood into the tissue space competitively with glucose. In the central nervous system, this transport occurs across the blood brain barrier (BBB) where FDG competes with glucose for facilitated carrier sites. Hexokinase catalyzes the phosphorylation of glucose and FDG to glucose-6-PO_4, and FDG-6-PO_4, respectively, in the cellular cytoplasm. Unlike glucose-6-PO_4, however, FDG-6-PO_4 is not a substrate for further metabolism, nor does it diffuse across cell membranes to any significant degree. It is therefore "metabolically trapped" in the tissue space. This facilitates imaging the tissue distribution of FDG with PET.

Based on the principles of competitive substrate kinetics, SOKOLOFF et al. (1977) developed a tracer kinetic model that provides estimates of the local glucose metabolic rate per unit volume of tissue. In the brain this is referred to as the cerebral metabolic rate of glucose, CMRGlc, in units of mg/min/100 g or μmol/min/100 g.

Fig. 2. Normal FDG study. Images from an FDG study in a normal subject. The images were obtained with a NeuroECAT tomograph at 8-mm intervals at planes parallel to the canthometal line with an in-plane system spatial resolution of 8.4 mm. The location of the tomographic planes can be superimposed on the rectilinear images on the lower right. Right is to the reader's right (this format is followed in all PET images in this chapter) and anterior is above. The darker areas of the image contain higher concentration of ^{18}F and have higher glucose metabolic rates. Normally, gray structure such as cortex, thalamus and basal ganglia have glucose metabolic rates several times higher than white matter. On the 3rd and 4th images on the second row, the basal ganglia and thalami are well seen. Visually, the ventricles are difficult to distinguish from white matter although numerical data resulting from region of interest analysis of the images may permit this distinction. (From PHELPS et al. 1982)

The following discussions of the FDG and other tracer kinetic approaches will focus upon cerebral applications. These methods may also be applied in other organ systems with appropriate modifications in parameters, normal values, etc., specific for other organ systems.

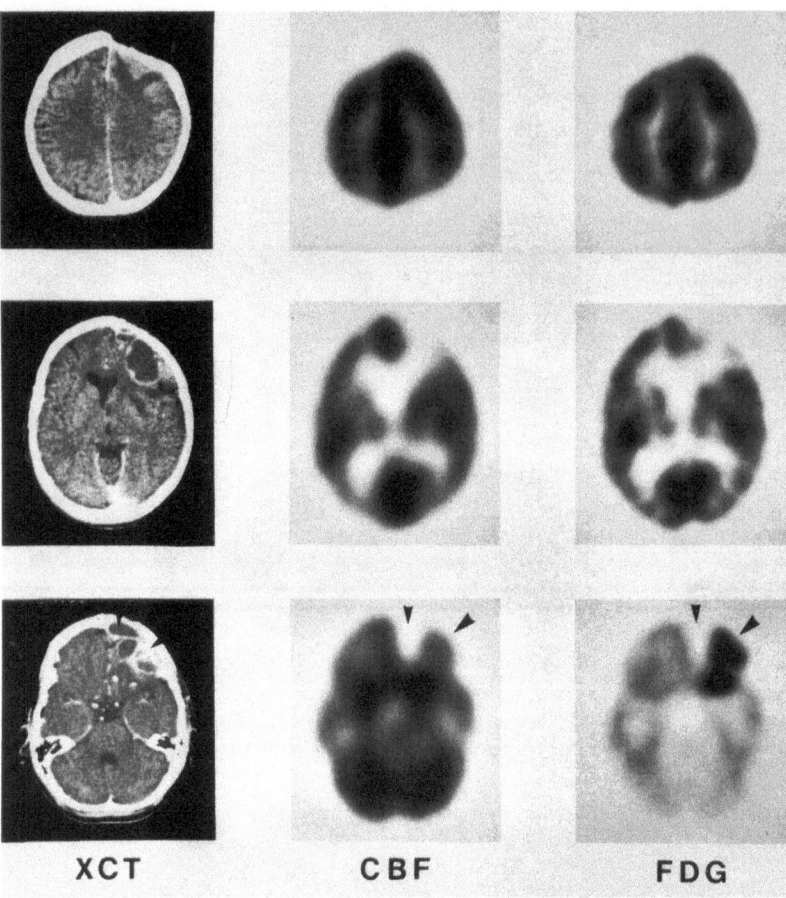

XCT   CBF   FDG

Fig. 3. Grade III astrocytoma. This patient underwent a craniotomy and 80% removal of a grade III astrocytoma is the right frontal area with subsequent radiation and chemotherapy. The figure contains contrast enhanced x-ray CT images (*left*), cerebral blood flow images obtained with $H_2^{15}O$ injected intravenously (*center*), and FDG images on the right. The image levels are near the vertex (*first row*), basal ganglia (*second row*), and inferior frontal/superior temporal levels (*third row*). The surgical defect is evident as a low density region with contrast enhancement on the superior and middle levels on the x-ray CT and as an area of decreased flow and glucose metabolism on the same levels on the CBF and FDG images. On the lowest level FDG image, there is an area of markedly increased glucose metabolism (*large arrowhead*), while flow in this region (*large arrowhead* on CBF images) is somewhat less than in contralateral tissue. The x-ray CT shows an area of contrast enhancement corresponding to this area (*large arrowhead*). The area of markedly decreased flow and glucose metabolism on this level (*small arrowheads* on CBF and FDG images) probably represents infarcted tissue, also suggested by a low density region on the x-ray CT study (*small arrowhead*). These findings are consistent with the presence of a viable high grade astrocytoma in the inferior right frontal region either as a recurrence or remaining after surgery, chemotherapy and radiation therapy. (From HAWKINS et al. 1985)

An FDG study requires the intravenous administration of FDG (usually 5–10 mCi intravenously) and the measurements of tissue ^{18}F activity (with region of interest analysis of the images) and the plasma concentration of FDG and glucose. Imaging is begun about 40 minutes after administration of the isotope and continued until the brain is adequately sampled. Scanning levels are parallel to the canthomental line and range from the cerebellum to the vertex; a complete set of images typically requires about a half-hour to obtain. The 40 minute delay between injection and scanning permits a near steady state tracer condition to be reached.

Figure 2 is a set of representative FDG images from a normal volunteer. With the FDG model incorporated on-line into the image display software package, regional, structure specific, values of glucose metabolism are immediately available for any brain region once it has been identified by the observer as a region of interest on a CRT (cathode ray tube image display) terminal. Several investigators have established normal values for

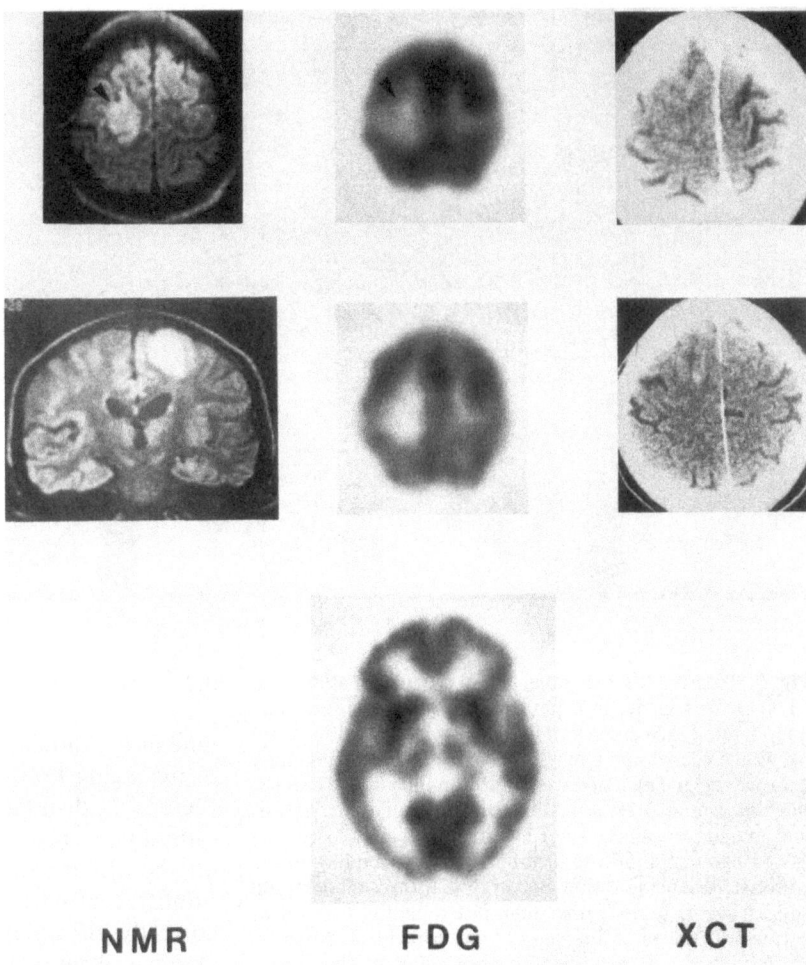

NMR **FDG** **XCT**

glucose metabolism regionally and globally in the brain (PHELPS et al. 1982; PHELPS and MAZZIOTTA 1985). The average global CMRGlc values in these FDG studies of approximately 5–6 mg/min/100 g agree well with earlier non-tomographic estimates of brain glucose metabolism.

3.1.1 Tumor Grade

The glycolytic rate is related to the degree of malignancy in a variety of tumors (WEBER 1977 and TIMPERLEY 1980). Additionally, even in the presence of adequate oxygen some tumors may preferentially metabolize glucose only through the glycolytic cycle rather than completing oxidative metabolism through the Krebs cycle. It therefore would be reasonable to expect that high grade gliomas could manifest greater levels of glycolysis than low grade gliomas, and this indeed appears to be the case. DI CHIRO et al. (1984) were the first to estab-

Fig. 4. Grade II astrocytoma. Preoperative NMR, FDG and x-ray CT images in a patient who presented with seizures. X-ray CT was the first study performed and was initially interpreted as normal although in retrospect minimal cortical effacement was noted on the vertex level corresponding to a region of decreased glucose metabolism (FDG) and high proton density (NMR) on the first row of images. The second row of images demonstrate a slightly lower level on the FDG and x-ray CT images and a coronal section on the NMR images. On the coronal NMR image the patient's left is to reader's right. The bottom FDG image demonstrates an essentially normal FDG pattern at the level of the basal ganglia. At craniotomy a grade II astrocytoma was found corresponding to the site of abnormalities on the FDG and NMR studies

lish this relationship in humans in vivo with FDG and PET. Reporting a series of over 100 consecutive gliomas, they found that the average glucose utilization rate in 38 patients with low grade astrocytomas (I and II) was 3.8 ± 1.8 (standard deviation) mg/min/100 g compared to values of 5.4 ± 2.7

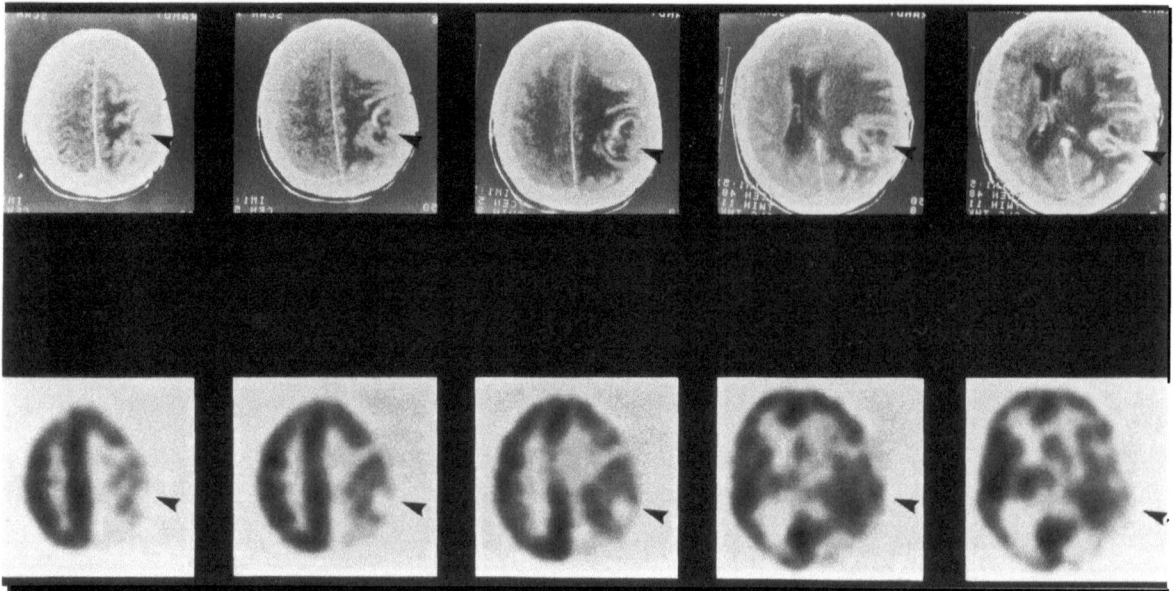

Fig. 5. Recurrent astrocytoma. X-ray CT images above and FDG images below in a patient who had previously had a moderate grade astrocytoma treated with radiation therapy. While edema and a mass effect as well as an irregularly contrast enhancing lesion were noted on the x-ray CT study, the differential diagnosis still included radiation necrosis and tumor recurrence. The FDG images below identify areas of significant glucose metabolism corresponding to the contrast enhancing lesion on x-ray CT (*arrowheads*) and suggest viable tumor rather than just radiation necrosis as a cause of the mass lesion. At a subsequent craniotomy, viable tumor was identified corresponding to the rim of metabolic activity noted on the FDG study. Also evident are regions of depressed metabolism surrounding the tumor on the FDG study, probably secondary to compression effects of edema

in 21 grade III patients and 7.3 ± 3.6 in 26 grade IV patients. They emphasize the appearance of a "hot spot" (Fig. 3) of increased FDG uptake reflecting a high regional CMRGlc value in high grade tumors.

Figure 4 is an example of a grade II astrocytoma evident as a focal depression of CMRGlc on the FDG study. Also included in the figure are the subject's NMR image showing a focal proton dense area and the x-ray CT study which revealed an almost normal appearance. In comparing the glycolytic rate in gliomas with contrast enhancement on x-ray CT in a group of 72 subjects PATRONAS et al. (1983) concluded that PET was more accurate than x-ray CT in the non invasive determination of histologic grade of gliomas.

3.1.2 Post-Radiotherapy Evaluation

One of the difficult clinical situations encountered in managing brain tumor patients after radiation therapy is distinguishing tumor recurrence from radiation necrosis. PATRONAS et al. (1982) reported on the differentiation of radiation necrosis from tumor recurrence using FDG (see Fig. 5). They correctly distinguished 3 recurrent grade II astrocytomas from 2 cases of radiation necrosis. The recurrent tumors all manifested increased glucose metabolism compared to surrounding normal brain tissue, while the 2 cases of radiation necrosis revealed regional hypometabolism. All cases were confired by biopsy or autopsy. The subjects had clinically deteriorated 24–52 months after irradiation and all had an increasing mass effect with contrast enhancement at the site of their original tumor.

3.2 Blood Flow and Oxygen Metabolism

Regional blood flow and oxygen metabolism are fundamental physiologic processes that, like glucose metabolism, can be quantified regionally and represented by cross sectional images with PET. Most methods currently in use for measuring these variables employ inhaled $^{15}O_2$ for measuring oxidative metabolism ($CMRO_2$ in the brain in units of μmol or ml of O_2/min/100 g) and injected $H_2{}^{15}O$ (or inhaled $C^{15}O_2$ which is converted to $H_2{}^{15}O$ by carbonic anhydrase in the lungs) for measuring blood flow. Either a bolus or continuous administration of these compounds generates, with the appropriate tracer kinetic model, measurements of the process of interest. Complete descriptions of the techniques are available in the literature (FRACKOWIAK et al. 1980; HUANG et al. 1983). The 2-minute half life of 0–15 mandates the presence of a cyclotron in the immediate vicinity of the tomograph. Normal values for cerebral blood flow and oxygen metabolism are also in the same range as those obtained by non-tomographic methods. When both flow and oxidative metabolism are measured, the oxygen extraction fraction (OEF) can be calculated. This term is the ratio of oxidative metabolism to the product of blood flow and arterial oxygen concentration and represents the fraction of oxygen delivered to the tissue that is subsequently extracted. The OEF is also sometimes referred to as the oxygen extraction ratio (OER), and should not be confused with the oxygen enhancement ratio (OER) well known in radiation biology and radiation therapy.

After observing that many tumors produced large amounts of lactic acid from glucose, WARBURG (1930) advanced the hypothesis that increased glycolysis in the presence of oxygen (aerobic glycolysis) was related to the malignant transformation of cells. In the over 50 years since that observation, many investigators have shown that the metabolic regulation of tumor cells is considerably more complex than WARBURG realized, although enhanced glycolysis has been demonstrated in many tumor systems, including human brain tumors as discussed above.

PET studies employing ^{15}O techniques for measuring blood flow and oxygen metabolism and FDG for glucose metabolism present an opportunity to examine the stoichiometric relationship of glycolysis to oxidative metabolism in human tumors in vivo. Studies in experimental brain tumors in rats have indicated that highly malignant tumors (glioblastoma, medulloblastoma, neuroblastoma, ependymoblastoma) tend to have uniformly low rates of oxygen consumption even though in their more differentiated forms they may have differing levels of oxygen usage (KIRSCH et al. 1977). Additionally, well differentiated astrocytomas appear to have uniformly low oxygen consumption rates as well (ALLEN 1972).

The first detailed PET study of brain tumors examining the glycolytic and oxidative metabolic interrelationship was performed by ITO et al. (1982). They examined 8 patients with primary and metastatic brain tumors and measured oxidative metabolism, blood flow and oxygen extraction fractions (OEF) with $C^{15}O_2$ by continuous inhalation. Using the x-ray CT scan as an anatomic template, they generated cross sectional profiles of OEF, blood flow and oxygen metabolism, and found that the tumors in their series had a generally lower OEF, oxygen metabolic rate and blood flow than in normal brain. The OEF is an indicator of ischemia; a high OEF implies oxygen delivery is inadequate to meet metabolic demands (ischemia), while a low OEF implies that the tissue is perfused by more oxygen than it needs. In normal subjects, oxygen extraction values in the brain are about 0.4 to 0.5. The finding of a low OEF in their tumors was somewhat surprising because of the significant number of hypoxic cells such tumors are believed to contain (WITHERS and PETERS 1980). They concluded that tumor cells may be employing aerobic or anaerobic glycolysis in preference to oxidative metabolism, which is consistent with the in vitro results mentioned above. However, they did not measure glucose metabolism.

In a follow-up study, RHODES et al. (1983), also from Hammersmith Hospital as were ITO et al., examined 7 patients with primary brain tumors with a similar methodology as that of ITO et al. but also measured glucose metabolism with FDG. Like ITO et al., RHODES et al. found a low $CMRO_2$ and OEF value in their tumors compared to contralateral cortical values. Glucose metabolic rates however, were comparable to contralateral cortical values. They also computed the "metabolic ratio" (MR) of the tumor and contralateral tissue, defined as the ratio of oxygen to glucose metabolic rates. The metabolic ratio is normally 0.67 ml of oxygen per milligram of glucose in normal brain, which is equivalent of 5.4 moles of oxygen per mole of glucose (SIESJO 1978). A low MR value is consistent with a higher glucose relative to oxygen utilization rate than normal (aerobic or anaerobic glycolysis) while a high value implies metabolism of alternative substrates to glucose. The MR value was significantly lower in tumors than in contralateral brain tissue.

Oxygen and glucose metabolism are normally closely linked in the brain. Glucose is the major metabolic substrate for cerebral metabolism (i.e., glucose normally provides over 90% of the brain's ATP) unlike the heart and other tissues which also metabolize fatty acids, lactate, amino acids, ketone bodies and other substrates. Therefore, the presence of a low MR value in this tumor series, associated with a a low OEF, implies a state of aerobic glycolysis existed in the tumors. It is important

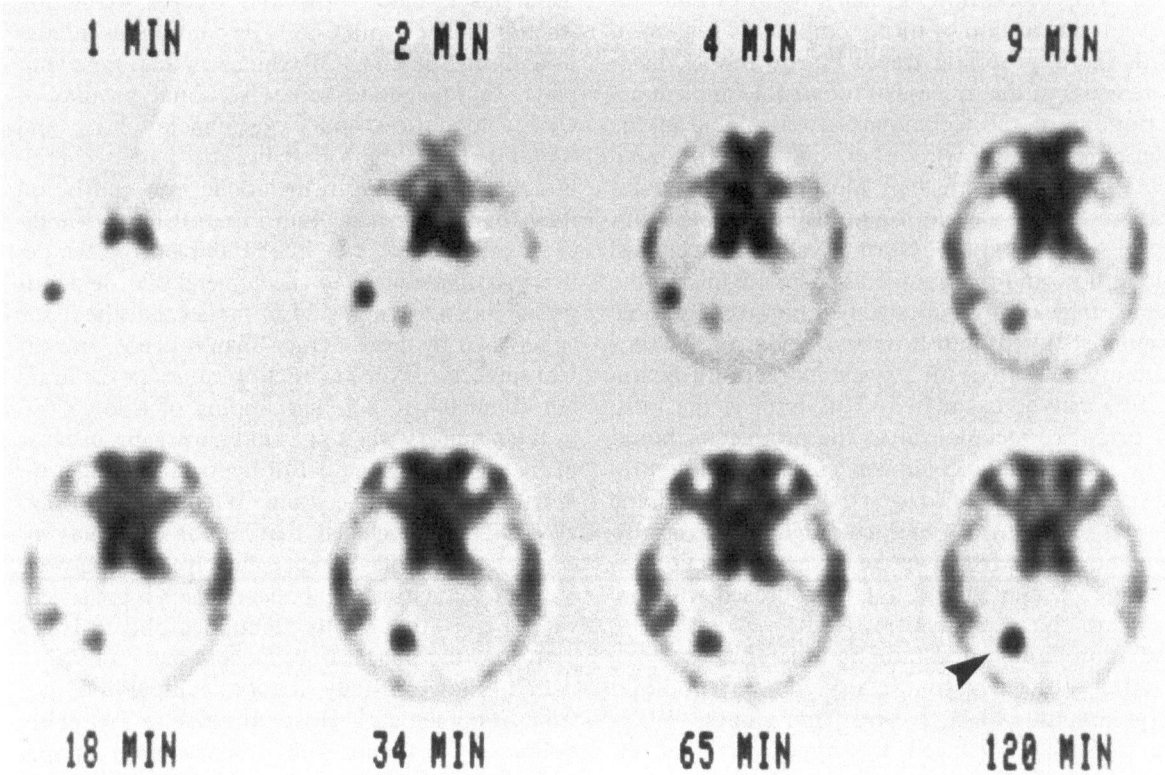

Fig. 6. Kinetic ^{68}Ga EDTA study. This patient had metastatic breast carcinoma to the left cerebellar hemisphere (*arrowhead* in 120-minute images). Images were acquired over progressively lengthening intervals (60 seconds to 10 minutes) for about 2 hours. In addition to activity in the tumor, all images show uptake in regions outside the blood brain barrier (scalp and soft tissues). Note that the uptake in the tumor compared with other areas becomes relatively more prominent with time. See text for further discussion. (From Hawkins et al. 1984)

to remember, however, that the absence of a significant degree of ischemia in tumor tissue in these series does not rule out the possibility of an associated hypoxic cell sub-population as the metabolic parameters derived with PET are reflective to average values of the entire cell population within the regions of interest (often the entire tumor mass or large subfractions of the tumor mass).

The above tumor studies with ^{15}O and FDG illustrate the potential of PET to physiologically characterize tumors before and after treatment and present an opportunity to examine issues such as in vivo radiosensitivity as a function of tissue oxygenation and blood flow.

3.3 Blood Brain Barrier

Functionally and structurally, the BBB is complex. Simplistically it may be regarded as a regulatory interface that excludes potentially neurotoxic materials from the brain and is composed primarily of endothelial cells in brain capillaries joined by tight junctions (Rapoport 1976). Increased BBB permeability is the presumed pathophysiological mechanism responsible for contrast enhancement on x-ray CT studies and for tracer uptake on planar nuclear medicine brain studies in brain tumors and other processes. These findings are consistent with the altered capillary characteristics of many brain tumors.

The first PET studies based on the altered BBB of tumors involved ^{68}Ga-EDTA for tumor localization. EDTA (ethelenediaminetetracetate) is an inert compound normally excluded from the brain by an intact BBB. Uptake in tumors is thus completely analogous to contrast enhancement on x-ray CT or traditional nuclear medicine images. In addition to anatomic localization of a barrier defect, however, PET can generate quantitative information about the degree of disruption of the BBB. Contrast enhancement on a x-ray CT study

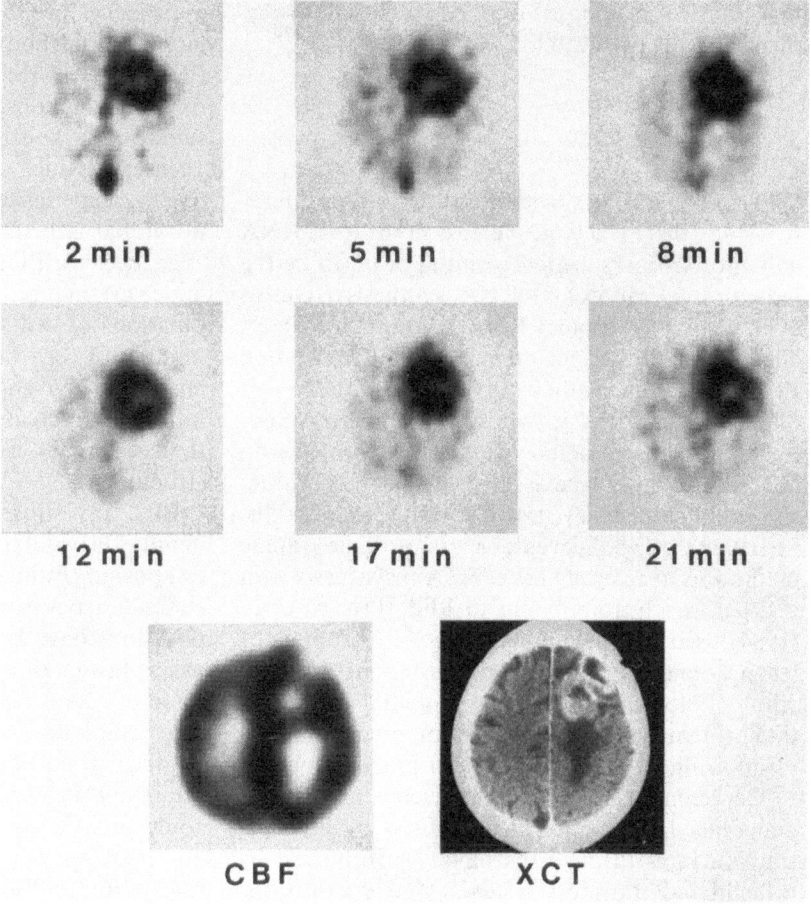

Fig. 7. Protein synthesis study. The top two row of images represent dynamic ^{11}C-leucine images obtained from 2 minutes to 21 minutes after intravenous injection of the tracer in this patient with a grade IV astrocytoma. A cerebral blood flow image obtained with H_2[15]O (*lower left*) and a contrast enhanced x-ray CT (*lower right*) are also included. Note that the ring of increased ^{11}C-leucine uptake corresponds to the high density rim of tumor tissue on the x-ray CT that also is characterized by high flow on the CBF study. A small region of infarcted tissue with surrounding contrast enhancement underlying a craniotomy defect in the skull on the x-ray CT corresponds to a region of decreased flow on the CBF study adjacent to the anterior/right surface of the tumor. Kinetic analysis of the leucine images, as discussed in the text, permits calculation of regional protein synthetic rates in tumor and normal tissue. This patient had also undergone radiofrequency hyperthermia with internal temperature monitoring of the tumor and normal brain tissue. There was no significant hyperthermic response in the tumor tissue, consistent with the high flow in the tumor noted in the CBF image

can signify variable degrees of BBB permeability (usually in a nonquantitative sense), as well as vascular effects. A variety of tracers have been used to investigate BBB permeability quantitatively in animal autoradiographic studies (BLASBERG et al. 1983). Permeability is usually measured in terms of a PS value (capillary permeability surface area product in units of ml/min/g) or a transfer constant (K_1) for a particular substance (such as EDTA) in the same units as PS values. HAWKINS et al. (1984) used ^{68}Ga EDTA with a two compartment tracer kinetic model to quantitate BBB permeability in human brain tumors. Fig. 6 is a set of representative images from that study. Quantification of changes in BBB permeability with this approach (i.e., after radiation therapy) could also have relevance in chemotherapy or combined chemotherapy and radiation therapy. Many current chemotherapeutic regimens are ineffective in CNS tumors, possibly because of limited access even through a damaged BBB. Coordinating chemotherapeutic and radiation therapy regimens with quantitative information about the BBB could

possibly help optimize clinical results. While other tracers can also be used to quantitate BBB permeability (LAMMERTSMA et al. 1984), all such approaches share the common goal of supplying a quantitative, as apposed to purely pictorial, assessment of BBB permeability.

3.4 Protein Synthesis

When a cell changes from a resting to a proliferative state, there is a large increase in the total RNA content. An early control point appears to be the induction of ribosomal RNA synthesis (KIRSCH et al. 1977). Ribosomal RNA accounts for about 40–50% of the weight of mammalian ribosomes. Because protein synthesis involves the attachment of messenger RNA to ribosomes and the subsequent linking of amino acids into a protein, an altered, probably increased rate of protein synthesis would seem likely in proliferating tumor cells. SMITH et al. (1980) developed an autoradiographic method for measuring brain protein synthesis with ^{14}C-leucine. Extrapolating to PET, PHELPS et al. (1984) used the metabolically active L isomers of leucine, phenylalanine and methionine labeled with ^{11}C to demonstrate the potential to quantitate protein synthesis as well as amino acid metabolism using an appropriate tracer kinetic model.

The essential L-amino acids leucine, methionine and phenylalanine are characterized by high extraction rates through the blood brain barrier by a facilitated transport system. After crossing the BBB, these amino acids may either be esterified to their corresponding tRNAs for incorporation into protein or become substrates for various metabolic pathways. If the labeled leucine is incorporated into proteins, the ^{11}C remains in the tissue and can be imaged with PET. Using a compartment model of transport, metabolism and incorporation into proteins, PHELPS et al. (1984) were able to calculate protein synthetic rates as well as the fractional distribution of leucine metabolism versus protein incorporation. Figure 7 illustrates the application of this technique in a patient with a grade IV astrocytoma. Other investigators have demonstrated the potential significance of amino acid PET studies in defining the extent of tumors (BERGSTROM et al. 1983).

4 Conclusions

The above overview demonstrates some of the potential applications of physiologic PET studies in tumor management. While the discussion has focused primarily on the brain, the tomographic imaging principles and many of the tracer kinetic approaches are applicable in tumors in other regions of the body. BEANEY et al. (1984) applied PET and ^{15}O techniques to measure blood flow, oxygen metabolism, and blood volume in breast tumors. They also demonstrated relatively low oxygen extraction values in breast tumors, paralleling the experience in the brain, again indicating no global ischemia in the regions studied. However, because PET produces estimates of physiologic variables on a per volume basis, small subpopulations of cells may be obscured by the larger number of cells with differing physiologic characteristics in a given volume. Improved scanner resolution will increase the reliability and accuracy of these estimates in smaller normal and abnormal structures.

PET investigations in tumors have focused mainly on validating the methods in tumors and establishing estimates of tumor flow and metabolic characteristics in vivo. Several clinically useful applications have laready emerged including noninvasive histologic grading of tumors and differentiation of tumor recurrence from radiation necrosis. The combined ^{15}O and FDG studies have demonstrated aspects of tumor biochemistry never before attainable in humans in vivo. These approaches could provide early detection of neoplastic lesions and more specific selection criteria for therapeutic interventions. Repeat studies allow one to follow and evaluate the course of therapy. Quantitative estimates of blood brain barrier permeability may, combined with flow and other techniques, permit quantification of tissue drug delivery as well as the development of optimal combined chemotherapy/radiation therapy regimens. Analogous applications in tumors in other body regions will also emerge. Additionally, other physiologic parameters of potential significance in tumors such as tissue pH can be evaluated with PET (ROTENBERG et al. 1984).

The major emphasis of PET to date has been on the study of disorders of the brain and heart, while future studies relating basic cancer studies in animals to in vivo studies in humans are of great potential value. Future investigations will define the full utility of these techniques in the dynamics of therapeutic interventions in tumor patients, including radiation therapy and chemotherapy.

References

Allen N (1972) Oxidative metabolism of brain tumors. Progr Exp Tumor Res 17:192–209

Beaney RP, Lammertsma AA, Jones T, McKenzie CG, Halnan KE (1984) Positron emission tomography for in vivo measurement of regional blood flow, oxygen utilization, and blood volume in patients with breast carcinoma. The Lancet, Jan. 21, 131–134

Bergstrom M, Collins VP, Ehrin E, Ericson K, Eriksson L, Greitz T, Halldin C, von Holst H, Langstrom B, Lilja A, Lundquist H, Nagren K (1983) Discrepancies in brain tumor extent as shown by computed tomography and positron emission tomography using [^{68}Ga]EDTA, [^{11}C]glucose, and [^{11}C]methionine. J Comput Assist Tomogr 7:1062–1066

Blasberg RG, Fenstermacher JD, Patlak CS (1983) Transport of α-aminobutyric acid across brain capillary and cellular membranes. J Cereb Blood Flow and Metabol 3:8–32

Di Chiro G, Brooks RA, Patronas NJ, Bairamian D, Kornblith PL, Smith BH, Mansi L, Barker J (1984) Issues in the in vivo measurement of glucose metabolism of human central nervous system tumors. Ann Neurol 15 (Suppl):S138–146

Frackowiak SJ, Lenzi GL, Jones T, Heather JD (1980) Quantificative measurement of regional cerebral blood flow and oxygen metabolism in man using ^{15}O and positron emission tomography: Theory, procedure and normal values. J Comput Tomogr 4:727–736

Hawkins RA, Phelps ME, Huang S-C, Wapenski JA, Grimm PD, Parker RG, Juillard G, Greenberg P (1984) A kinetic evaluation of blood brain barrier permeability in human brain tumors with [^{68}Ga]EDTA and positron computed tomography. J Cereb Blood Flow Metab 4:507–515

Hawkins RA, Phelps ME, Huang S-C, Wapenski JA, Silberman AW (1985) Quantitative estimations of blood brain barrier (BBB) permeability with Ga-68 EDTA and glucose metabolism with F-18 FDG in human brain tumors with PET. J Cereb Blood Flow Metab 5 (Suppl 1), S 583–584

Hoffman EJ, Ricci AR, van der Stee LMAM, Phelps ME (1983) ECAT III – Basic design considerations IEEE Trans Nucl Sci NS-30:729–733

Huang S-C, Phelps ME, Hoffman EJ, Sideris K, Selin CJ, Kuhl DE (1980) Noninvasive determination of local cerebral metabolic rate of glucose in man. Am J Physiol 238:E69–E82

Huang S-C, Carson RE, Hoffman EJ, Carson J, MacDonald N, Barrio JR, Phelps ME (1983) Quantitative measurement of local cerebral blood flow in humans by positron computed tomography and 150-water. J Cereb Blood Flow Metabol 3:141–153

Ito M, Lammertsma AA, Wise RJS, Bernardi S, Frackowiak RSJ, Heather JD, McKenzie CG, Thomas DGT, Jones T (1982) Measurement of regional cerebral blood flow and oxygen utilization in patients with cerebral tumors using ^{15}O and positron emission tomography: Analytical techniques and preliminary results. Neuroradiology 23:63–74

Kirsch WM, Tucker WS, Tabuchi K, Fink LM, Van Buskirk JJ, Low M (1977) The metabolism of the glioblastoma: Pathological correlates. Clin Neurosurg 25:310–325

Lammerstma AA, Brooks DJ, Frackowiak RSJ, Heather JD, Jones T (1984) A method to quantitate fractional extraction of rubidium-82 across the blood brain barrier using positron emission tomography. J Cereb Blood Flow Metab 4:523–534, 1984

Patronas NJ, Di Chiro G, Brooks RA, De La Paz RL, Kornblith PL, Smith BH, Rizzoli V, Kessler RM, Manning RG, Channing M, Wolf AP, O'Connor CM (1982) Work in Progress: [^{18}F]Fluorodeoxyglucose and positron emission tomography in the evaluation of radiation necrosis of the brain. Radiol 144:885–889

Patronas NJ, Brooks RA, De La Paz RL, Smith BH, Kornblith PL, Di Chiro G (1983) Glycolytic rate (PET) and contrast enhancement CT in human cerebral glomas. AJNR 4:533–535

Phelps ME, Hoffman EJ, Huang S-C (1979a) Single-slice versus multiple-slicepositron tomographs. J Nucl Med 20:800–802

Phelps ME, Huang S-C, Hoffman EJ, Selin C, Sokoloff L, Kuhl DE (1979b) Tomographic measurement of local cerebral glucose metabolic rate in humans with (F-18) 2-fluoro-2-deoxy-D-glucose: Validation of method. Ann Neurol 6:371–388

Phelps ME, Mazziotta JC, Huang S-C (1982) Study of cerebral function with positron computed tomography. J Cereb Blood Flow Metab 2:113–162

Phelps ME, Schelbert HR, Mazziotta JC (1983) Positron computed tomography for studies of myocardial and cerebral function. Ann Int. Med 98:339–359

Phelps ME, Barrio JR, Huang S-C, Keen RE, Chugani H, Mazziotta JC (1984) Criterial for the tracer kinetic measurement of cerebral protein synthesis in humans with positron emission tomography. Ann Neurol 15 (Suppl):S192–S202

Phelps ME, Mazziotta JC (1985) Positron emission tomography: human brain function and biochemistry. Science 228:799–809

Rapoport SI (1976) Blood brain barrier in physiology and medicine. Raven Press, New York

Reivich M, Kuhl DE, Wolf A, Greenberg J, Phelps ME, Ido T, Casella V, Fowler J, Hoffman E, Alavi, Som P, Sokoloff L (1979) The (^{18}F)-fluorodeoxyglucose method for the measurement of local cerebral glucose utilization in man. Circ Res 44:127–137

Rhodes CG, Wise RJS, Gibbs JM, Frackowiak RSJ, Hatazawa J, Palmer AJ, Thomas DGT, Jones T (1983) In vivo disturbance of the oxidative metabolism of glucose in human cerebral gliomas. Ann Neurol 14:614–626

Rottenberg DA, Ginos JZ, Kearfott KJ, Junck L, Bigner DD (1984) In vivo measurement of regional brain tissue pH using positron emission tomography. Ann Neurol 15 (Suppl):S98–S102

Siesjo BK (1978) Brain energy metabolism. John Wiley and Sons, Chichester, New York, Brisbane and Toronto

Smith CB, Davidsen L, Deibler G, Patlak C, Pettigrew K, Sokoloff L (1980) A method for the determination of local rates of protein synthesis in brain. Trans Am Soc Neurochem 11:94

Sokoloff L, Reivich M, Kennedy C, Des Rosiers MH, Patlak CS, Pettigrew KD, Sakurada O, Shinohara M (1977) The (^{14}C)-deoxyglucose method for the measurement of local cerebral glucose utilization: Theory, procedure and normal values in the conscious and anesthetized albino rat. J Neurochem 28:897–916

Ter-Pogossian MM, Mullani NA, Ficke DC, Markham J, Snyder DL (1981) Photon time-of-flight assisted positron emission tomography. J Comput Assist Tomogr 5:227–229

Timperley RW (1980) Glycolysis in neuroectodermal tumors. In: Thomas BT, Graham DI (eds) Brain tumors, scientific basis, clinical investigation and current therapy. Butterworth and Company, London, pp 145–167

Warburg O (1930) The metabolism of tumors. Arnold Constable, London, pp 75–327

Weber G (1977) Enzymology of cancer cells. N Engl J Med:486–493, 541–551

Welch MF, Tewson TJ (1979) Radiopharmaceuticals for neurological studies. In: Sorenson JA (ed) Radiopharmaceuticals II. Soc Nucl Med New York, pp 201–219

Withers HR, Peters LJ (1980) Biological aspects of radiation therapy. In: Fletcher GH (ed) Textbook of Radiotherapy, 3rd ed. Lea & Febiger, Philadelphia, pp 103–179

Wolf A (1981) Special characteristics and potential for radiopharmaceuticals for positron emission tomography. Semin Nucl Med 11:2–12

6 Modified Fractionation

6.1 Hyperfractionation

H. RODNEY WITHERS and JEAN-CLAUDE HORIOT

CONTENTS

1 Definitions

Clinical and experimental evidence suggests that, as an overall strategy, radiotherapy for most cancers should be given using the smallest practical dose per fraction and the shortest overall treatment duration. Any attempt to modify standard fractionation patterns to use smaller dose fractions and/or a shorter overall time will require more than 5 fractions per week. However, the fact that both strategies result in 2 or more treatments on some or every treatment day should not obscure the different biological reasons for adopting them. Shortening the overall treatment time (accelerated fractionation) aims to minimize the effect of regeneration of tumor clonogens during treatment while the use of small dose fractions (hyperfractionation) is aimed at exploiting differences in the radiobiology of the tumor and late responding normal tissues. Hyperfractionation is the use of dose fractions smaller than standard. Accelerated fractionation is a shortening of the overall duration of a fractionated dose regimen. (Hyperfractionated accelerated treatment involves both a reduced dose per fraction and a shorter overall time.)

Since radiotherapists use different fractionation schemes as standard practice, the relative terms are ambiguous. In this chapter, the smallest fraction size considered standard is 1.8 Gy: lower doses will be considered to constitute hyperfractionation regardless of the overall treatment duration. In a pure comparison of standard and hyperfractionated regimens the overall treatment duration should be the same in both arms, requiring the delivery of more than 5 fractions per week in the hyperfractionated treatment. Although it is not necessary that 2 or more fractions be given per day (e.g. by treating 7 days per week), hyperfractionated regimens have usually consisted of 10 fractions/week, each of 1.10–1.20 Gy given as two fractions per treatment day.

Other variations from standard fractionation may include an element of hyperfractionation. For example, in an accelerated regimen whose major purpose is to shorten overall treatment duration, doses per fraction less than 1.8 Gy may be given 2 or 3 times per day (HORIOT et al. 1985; WANG 1986). Such treatments should be described as accelerated hyperfractionation to distinguish them from pure hyperfractionation and from other approaches to shortening the overall treatment time in which standard doses per fraction may be used (e.g. when 5 fractions per week are intermittently supplemented by a concomitant boost). In practice, most hyperfractionated accelerated treatments must be given as a split course to avoid excessive acute reactions in normal tissues (e.g. HORIOT et al. 1985; WANG et al. 1985; WANG et al. 1986; WANG 1987), and when this is done, total doses need not be reduced below those given in standard regimens even though the overall treatment time can be reduced by up to 2 weeks.

In summary, hyperfractionation constitutes the use of dose fractions less than 1.8 Gy. In a strict comparison of its efficacy relative to a standard fractionation regimen, the overall treatment durations should be the same. It is undesirable to lengthen the treatment duration because such prolongation introduces the possibility of tumor "escape" through accelerated regeneration, or even through continued growth at its pre-radiation rate.

H. RODNEY WITHERS, M.D., D.Sc.
University of California
Los Angeles, CA 90024, USA

JEAN-CLAUDE HORIOT, M.D.
Centre Georges-Francois-Leclerc
Dijon, France

However, protraction may prove necessary in some hyperfractionated treatments because of a relative increase in acute toxicity when the total dose is increased sufficiently to produce late effects equivalent to those produced by a standard regimen (see later). Both hyperfractionation alone and accelerated treatment hold promise for an improved therapeutic outcome; and accelerated hyperfractionation, by combining the advantages of both, may be even better.

2 Biological Rationale for Hyperfractionation

A rationale for initially proposing hyperfractionation was that the redistribution to division cycle asynchrony that occurs in proliferating cells between successive dose fractions should provide a "self-sensitizing" effect among tumor cells not found in the non-proliferating "target" cells in critical late-responding normal tissues (WITHERS 1972, 1975). Such selective redistribution should contribute to a differential with standard fractionation, which should be increased further by hyperfractionation for two reasons: the number of fractionation intervals available for self-sensitization of proliferative tumor cells by redistribution is increased and, in addition, each small dose fraction is less "wasted" on cells in relatively radioresistant phases of the cycle, killing being confined more to the radiosensitive subpopulations. In this sense, redistribution is somewhat analogous to reoxygenation in which multiple fractionation intervals permit reoxygenation and small fractional doses kill large numbers of oxic cells without dose being "wasted" on hypoxic cells which can dominate the responses at high doses.

It is of interest that redistribution of surviving interphase cells into mitosis was a rationale put forward in 1914 by Schwarz for treating a young girl with histiocytic lymphoma with 6 fractions instead of one large single dose as was standard practice at that time. Although the concept was valid, the small percentage of cells in mitosis would not have been sufficient, of itself, to contribute greatly to a self-sensitizing effect on the cell population as a whole. We know now that interphase is composed of a variety of phases in which cells manifest differing radiosensitivities and that, in some phases, cells are nearly as radiosensitive as they are in mitosis. Thus, a greater proportion of the tumor cell population would be self-sensitized by redistribution than originally envisaged by Schwarz. It is also of historical interest that, in

irradiating the testis, REGAUD (1929) chose the only tissue in which redistribution appears to have a relatively easily detected sensitizing effect on the fractionation response (WITHERS 1974). (It can be detected in other tissues but in multifraction experiments is usually overshadowed by regeneration.) Regaud found that in a comparison with the skin of the scrotum, the germinative cells of the testis were relatively more sensitive to fractionated doses and suggested that tumors, being proliferative like the testis, may share a similarly more sensitive response.

By 1980, long after clinical trials of hyperfractionation had been initiated (ARCANGELI et al. 1979; BACKSTROM et al. 1973; DOUGLAS et al. 1982; HORIOT et al. 1982; JAMPOLIS et al. 1977; MEDINI et al. 1980; MEOZ et al. 1984; SHUKOVSKY et al. 1976), a second rationale for hyperfractionation became clear: those tissues which respond slowly to X-radiation show a *consistently* greater reduction in injury with decrease in dose per fraction than do acutely-responding tissues (BARENDSEN 1982; THAMES et al. 1982; WITHERS et al. 1982; WITHERS et al. 1983). Since most (although not all) tumors respond acutely to irradiation it is reasonable to assume that most of them will show a fractionation response similar to that of early responding normal tissues. The few appropriate studies on fractionation responses of tumors support this supposition (MACIEJEWSKI et al. 1986a, 1986b; MASON and WITHERS 1977).

The initial impetus for a comprehensive review in 1980 of the radiobiology of acutely- and late-responding tissues came from the realization that, during the preceding two decades, there had been a series of clinical catastrophies resulting from giving radiotherapy in a small number of large dose fractions (for refs. see THAMES et al. 1982 and WITHERS et al. 1983). Total doses in such hypofractionated regimens had been based on achieving the standard severity of acute response, or were determined using the NSD formula (ELLIS 1969), or one of its derivatives (SINGH 1978). The consistent finding was that if a small number of large dose fractions produced acute effects equivalent to those from a standard regimen, then late effects were more frequent and severe. A review of the radiobiology literature revealed a similar pattern (BARENDSEN 1982; THAMES et al. 1982; WITHERS et al. 1982a, 1982b; WITHERS et al. 1983). Tumor control rates were not easy to determine, but, at least, were not better with a small number of treatments (COX 1985). The obvious conclusion was that a therapeutically advantageous differential between late responses and tumor control had been achieved by decades of adjustment towards smaller dose fractions in clinical radiotherapy: this gain had been surrendered by a return to fewer, larger, fractions (usually for logistic and/or economic reasons). A reasonable extrapolation was that if standard fractionation is good, hyperfractionation should be better in that late responding tissues could be relatively spared by a further reduction in dose per fraction below 2 Gy with no loss in terms of tumor control rate, or better still, that for isoeffects in late responding tissues, tumor control could be increased, albeit with an increase in the severity of acute normal tissue responses.

A completely different goal of trials of hyperfractionation in Sweden was to circumvent the influence of hypoxic tumor cells on the outcome of radiotherapy. It was proposed that the influence of hypoxic cells could be minimized by exploiting a lower oxygen enhancement ratio and less capacity for sublethal injury in hypoxic cells at low doses (LITTBRAND et al. 1975; REVESZ et al. 1975).

3 Dose per Fraction

The fractionation responses of a wide range of tissues have been described in terms of isoeffect curves (Fig. 1). However, even now, responses of most early and late responding tissues are poorly quantified for doses per fraction less than 2 Gy (Fig. 2). Compared with acutely-responding nor-

mal and neoplastic tissues, late responding tissues should continue to "tolerate" a greater increase in total dose with reduction in dose per fraction below 2 Gy, as they do with reductions to 2 Gy from higher doses per fraction. However, for tissues other than lung and bone marrow, the existence and extent of this differential has not been established experimentally. Furthermore, even though clinical studies have begun, the isoeffectiveness for late sequelae of the doses used in standard and experimental regimens has not been established. Before the usefulness of hyperfractionated schemes can be assessed, it will be necessary to ensure that late sequelae are essentially equal to those from standard regimens.

In early pilot studies, isoeffective doses were based on acute mucosal reactions in the oro-pharynx (HORIOT et al. 1982; JAMPOLIS et al. 1977; SHUKOVSKY et al. 1976) resulting in a relative underdosage of late responding tissues. In the first randomized clinical trial in head and neck cancer (HORIOT et al. 1985) the daily dose in two fractions was 15% greater than the single daily dose (2 × 1.15 Gy compared with 1 × 2 Gy) with a comparable 15% increase in the total dose. Recently a daily dose 20% higher has been introduced into randomized RTOG studies. The continuing increase in total dose is being approached cautiously because the sequelae of concern develop slowly. It is not known whether a 20% increase in total dose will be too much, too little or just right for isoeffects in late responding tissues although it is

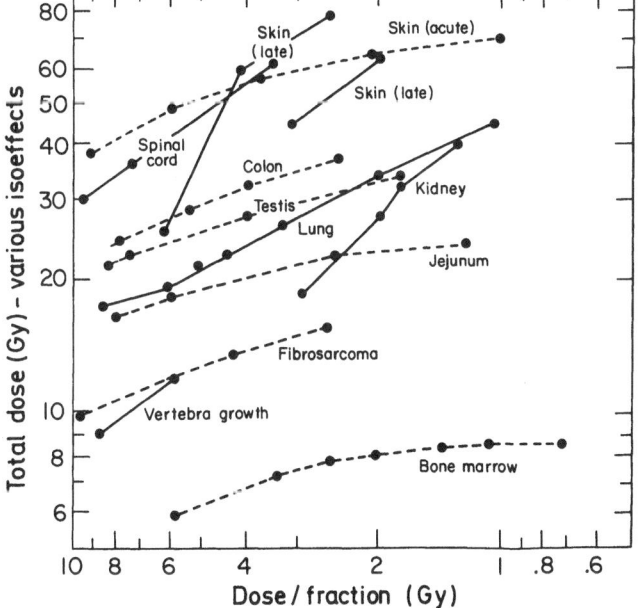

Fig. 1. Each (isoeffect) curve defines the change in the total multifraction dose required for a constant level of tissue injury as a function of size of dose per fraction. Dashed lines are for acutely-responding normal tissues and one tumor, solid lines for slowly-responding normal tissues. Note that the total dose for a late injury changes more with change in fraction size than it does for an acute response. (Reproduced from WITHERS 1985 with permission from LIPPINCOTT)

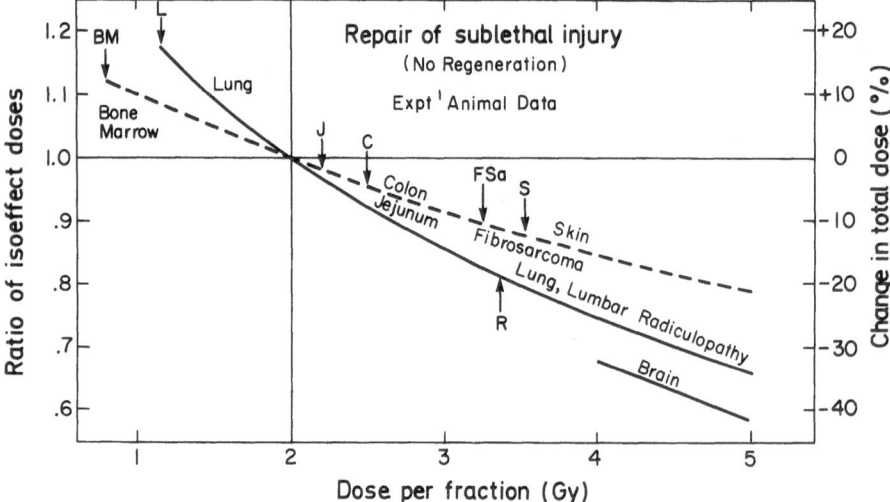

Fig. 2. Isoeffect curves relating total dose to fraction size for various endpoints in experimental animals, estimated using a linear quadratic dose response model. The total dose in 2 Gy fractions is that with which other total doses are compared. The arrows show, for the various effects, the lowest dose per fraction used in multifraction regimens. For most tissues the change in isoeffective dose with change in fraction size below 2 Gy is not defined by data. (Modified from Withers et al. 1983 b)

appreciated that, with such an increase, acute responses are more severe than in standard regimens (Parsons et al. 1986a, b). When the dose is increased by only 10–15%, acute sequelae are only slightly more severe than usual. In one pilot clinical study involving 139 patients (Loeffler 1983) the acute responses of the gastrointestinal tract were minimized by protracting abdominal irradiation for at least 8 weeks. In this circumstance, and using 2 doses per day ranging downwards from 1 Gy per fraction, the author estimated that the tolerance dose for late sequelae could be increased by 20–30%.

4 Fractionation Intervals

The rationale for hyperfractionation is that a differential can be expected between the responses of slowly-proliferating normal tissues and the majority of tumors, that is, those tumors showing an early response to irradiation. To obtain the maximum differential requires that the greater repair potential of slowly-responding tissues be fully exploited and that surviving tumor cells redistribute adequately within the division cycle between

dose fractions. Little is known about the redistribution kinetics of surviving tumor cells after one or more dose fractions but it seems likely that after doses of less than 1.80–2.0 Gy there would be some progression of survivors out of relatively radioresistant phases of the cycle within the time required for complete repair of sublethal injury in late responding tissues. It is the repair time in non-proliferating normal tissues which is the major factor determining the minimum acceptable fractionation interval.

Until recently, it was thought that an interval of 3 or 4 hours between dose fractions would be sufficient for complete repair of sublethal radiation damage. This estimate was based on the time to the first peak in recovery curves for cells in vitro and in acutely-responding tissues in vivo. It now seems likely that repair continues for longer than 3 or 4 hours in spinal cord (Ang et al. 1984), lung (Vegesna et al. 1985) and kidney (Withers and Mason 1986), the only three late responding tissues for which detailed data are available. In kidney, as in spinal cord, repair is more complete at 12 hours than at $4\frac{1}{2}$ hours (Fig. 3): in recent studies there was no evidence of a significant difference in survival from extending the fractionation interval from 12 to 24 hours. It generally becomes impractical to space daytime dose fractions longer than 6 to 8 hours, and even then it can be arduous for patients and staff.

A reasonable compromise between biological optimization and practical logistics is to require an interval of at least 6 hours between dose fractions on the same day, remembering that a longer interval may be slightly better. In a twice per day regimen this results in the other half of the frac-

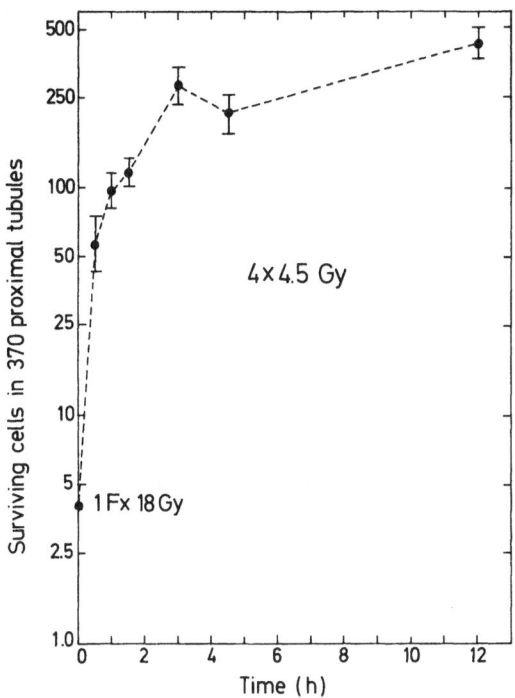

Fig. 3. Relative survival of renal tubule cells (WITHERS and MASON 1986) as a function of fractionation interval in a 4 fraction dose regimen. The 0 time point represents cell survival after a single dose of 18 Gy: other points are for survival after 18 Gy in 4 equal fractions separated by various intervals. Note that survival with 12 h fractionation intervals was higher than with 3 or $4^1/_2$ h intervals

tionation intervals being about 18 hours. A reasonable question is why treatments should not be given 7 days per week. There is unlikely to be any benefit from such measures because the 2 day gaps in treatment permit acutely-responding normal tissues to regenerate more quickly (ANG et al. 1985; VAN DER SCHUEREN et al. 1983) than they do if treated every day. Since acute normal tissue toxicity becomes the factor limiting the rate of hyperfractionated treatment, a 5 day per week regimen can probably be delivered in a shorter overall time than a 7 day per week scheme. (If the tumor were so rapidly growing that it outstripped normal tissue regeneration during treatment or during weekend breaks, then neither standard nor hyperfractionated treatment is appropriate and some form of accelerated treatment is logical.)

5 Field Reductions

Field reductions should be made at the same "biological" dose as in the standard regimen. For example, if 2 fractions of 1.2 Gy are substituted for 1 fraction of 2 Gy, field reduction should be made at doses 20% greater than in the standard treatment. However, relative isoeffective doses for 2 Gy and 1.2 Gy fractions have not been quantified sufficiently accurately for those late responding tissues such as spinal cord for which field reductions are critical (ANG et al. 1984). Accordingly, it is prudent at present to exclude the spinal cord from a hyperfractionated treatment volume at about the same dose as for a standard regimen e.g. at about 45–50 Gy. No cases of myelitis have been reported but total doses to spinal cord have not exceeded 50 Gy in any trials of hyperfractionation.

6 Clinical Studies

A variety of non-randomized and randomized trials have evaluated the feasibility and efficacy of hyperfractionation using two small (1.0–1.2 Gy) fractions per day. (A number of trials using 1.5–1.6 Gy/fraction given 2 or more times per day have been reported but will not be discussed here because their primary characteristic is acceleration, even though also hyperfractionated.) The consensus is that tumor control rates are at least as good, and probably better, than with standard regimens, that late sequelae are not worse, but that acute responses of normal tissues may be more severe. These are the results that would be predicted from prior radiobiological information.

A randomized prospective study by the European Organization for Research on Treatment of Cancer (EORTC) in patients with T2, T3, N_0, N_1 squamous carcinoma of the oropharynx (excluding base of tongue) was closed in 1985 (HORIOT et al. 1985). Dose regimens compared were 2 fractions of 1.15 Gy per day and daily doses of 2 Gy, carried to total doses of 80.5 Gy and 70 Gy, respectively. Preliminary analysis of results in 254 patients suggests that the acute mucosal reactions and late sequelae were similar while the actuarial local control rates at 36 months were 72% and 56% in the hyperfractionated and control arms, respectively. This difference has only an 85% probability of being true (not random chance). In those patients with Karnofsky indices of 90–100, there was a difference in local control at 3 years, 72% vs 42% which has more than a 95% probability of being true. Overall survival was slightly better (by 5%–10%) in the patients treated with the smaller dose fractions, but the difference is not significant.

At the Radiumhemmut, Stockholm, 168 patients with bladder cancer were treated in a randomized trial with either 64 Gy in 32 fractions, 5 fractions per week, or 84 Gy in 84 fractions, 15 fractions per week with 3 fractions being given on each of 5 weekdays with a daytime fractionation interval of 4 hours (Littbrand et al. 1975; Edsmyr et al. 1985). In both regimens, a break of 2 weeks was introduced after the first half. The overall treatment time was essentially equal for both groups. At the time of last report on this trial (Edsmyr 1985) the minimum follow up time was 5 years and the results show that hyperfractionation yielded a local control rate at 6 months of 65%, significantly ($p < 0.001$) better than 36% for patients treated with 2 Gy fractions. Overall survival at 5 years also improved from 22% to 34% ($p = 0.01$), the improvement being in the more advanced cases, especially those with T3 tumors. Acute toxicity was apparently circumvented by the 2 week break in both regimens. There was a higher incidence of major late complications in the hyperfractionated regimen (12% vs 5%) but, after allowing for the better survival of patients, the difference was not significant. A criticism of this trial has been that 84 Gy in 1 Gy fractions may be a higher biological dose to late responding tissues than 64 Gy in 2 Gy fractions. For the 2 regimens to be iso-effective in terms of late responses, the alpha/beta ratio for the most relevant tissues (those responsible for peritoneal adhesions, fistulae and strictures of bowel wall) would have to be 2.2 Gy. However, even if the dose in the hyperfractionated regimen was too high, the lesser increase in complications than in local tumor control suggests that the use of small doses per fraction may offer a therapeutic advantage.

A number of randomized studies by the Radiotherapy Oncology Group (RTOG) using 1.2 Gy fractions twice daily are still in a dose escalation phase. However, Marcial et al. (1986) report that in initial studies in head and neck cancers, local control rates were comparable even when the total dose in the hyperfractionated series was lower, instead of higher than in the conventional regimen. Another interesting conclusion from their studies was that when daytime fractionation intervals were longer than 4 hours, the late sequelae were less severe than when the intervals were 4 hours or less. This clinical observation supports the notion that repair of sublethal injury requires longer than 4 hours for completion in late-responding tissues.

A continuing non-randomized study showing encouraging results has been reported by Parsons and co-workers (1984; 1986a, 1986b). They conclude that hyperfractionation offers some therapeutic advantage in advanced head and neck malignancies. They have reported on 132 patients with 136 tumors treated by radiotherapy alone who received a range of total doses, but usually between 74.4 and 79.2 Gy in 1.2 Gy fractions given twice daily. Nineteen patients received a supplemental dose of 10–15 Gy from a radium implant. Doses were given twice per day, 5 days per week, the daytime fractionation interval being 4–6 hours. The tumors treated were selected, in that early lesions were treated with standard therapy, the worst cases being entered into the experimental study. Standard treatment was 1.8 Gy/day, requiring up to 1.5–2 weeks longer than the experimental series. Thus, in that center, the twice per day treatment represents accelerated hyperfractionation.

In patients with greater than 2 years follow-up, local control after doses of 74.4 Gy or more was generally better, and never worse than in patients treated once daily with a standard regimen. In T2 lesions of tonsillar fossa and supraglottic larynx the results were similar, 14/17 (82%) local control in hyperfractionated series and 49/61 (80%) with standard therapy. In T2–3 carcinomas of hypopharynx 7/10 (70%) were controlled in the twice per day regimen compared with 17/32 (53%) in the control series. The generally better results with T3 lesions are shown in Table 1 (Parsons et al. 1986b). There was no therapeutic gain detected in 12 patients treated for T4 oropharyngeal lesions, 4/12 (33%) achieving local control compared with 7/25 (28%) in comparable patients treated once daily. In a separate group of 8 patients with 2 years follow-up after preoperative hyperfractionated irradiation (50.4 to 60 Gy) and surgical resection, 4/5 with T3 disease and 2/3 with T4 lesions had local control: this is thought to be somewhat better than expected with standard therapy. When the planned treatment was given (radiotherapy or radiotherapy plus surgery) metas-

Table 1. Comparison of once-a-day and twice-a-day irradiation T3. (From Parsons 1986)

Site	Continuous course once-a-day	twice-a-day
Tonsillar region	17/26 (65%)	13/16 (81%)
Base of tongue	14/18 (78%)	7/7 (100%)
Supraglottic larynx	3/5 (60%)	7/11 (64%)
True vocal cord	7/13 (54%)	7/10 (70%)

U.F., 3/78–4/81; analysis 4/86

tases in neck nodes were usually controlled. Acute mucosal reactions were more severe than with the standard regimen, about 20% of the patients developing significant problems, 11% requiring nasogastric feeding. Seven of 132 (5%) of patients treated with radiotherapy alone developed severe late sequelae (3 with cartilage necrosis, 1 with bone necrosis, 1 esophageal stricture and 2 requiring a permanent tube for gastric feeding). An additional 4 (5%) patients had moderately severe late sequelae and 15 (10%) had mild (transient) late sequelae, mainly soft tissue necrosis. Elective surgical dissection of neck nodes in 33 patients was associated with no greater problems than after standard therapy: 7 developed wound complications. In general, the late sequelae were less than would be anticipated after standard therapy for these advanced stages of disease.

In another pilot study from the Radiumhemmut (BACKSTROM et al. 1973), 17 patients with cancer of gingiva or tongue were treated with 3 fractions of 1.0 Gy per day, 8 to a total dose of 42 Gy prior to planned surgery, and 9 to 84 Gy as primary treatment. Five of the second group were subsequently subjected to surgery. Local control rate was about 75%, normal tissue sequelae were minimal and surgery presented no problems.

7 Summary

Total doses in hyperfractionated regimens will vary with size of dose per fraction but should result in late sequelae equivalent to those from standard therapy. If isoeffects are produced in late responding tissues, there is reason to anticipate improved tumor control rate, and more severe acute normal tissue toxicity. (If tumor control rates are satisfactory, hyperfractionation could be used to deliver slightly lower total doses with the aim of decreasing late sequelae.) Present evidence is that when 1 fraction of 2 Gy is replaced by 2 fractions per day, the total dose in the hyperfractionated arm can be safely increased by 15%: the amount by which it should be increased may be greater, but needs further investigation. Fractionation intervals should not be less than 6 hours if the full differential in repair between late responding normal tissues and the tumor is to be exploited. Clinical trials of hyperfractionation suggest an advantage to using small doses per fraction. Since tumor regeneration during treatment appears to be a significant cause of failure (MACIEJEWSKI et al. 1986b; TROTT and KUMMERMEHR 1985), innova-

tive methods for shortening the overall treatment duration (PETERS and ANG 1987) in association with hyperfractionation are likely to hold further promise for improvements in radiotherapy.

Acknowledgements. This investigation was supported by PHS grant numbers CA-31612 and CA-29644 awarded by the National Cancer Institute, DHHS.

References

Ang KK, van der Kogel AJ, van Dam J, van der Schueren E (1984) The kinetics of repair of sublethal damage in the rat cervical spinal cord during fractionated irradiation. Radiother Oncol 1:247–253

Ang KK, Xu F-X, Vanuytsel L, van der Schueren E (1985) Repopulation kinetics in irradiated mouse lip mucosa: The relative importance of treatment protraction and time distribution of irradiations. Radiat Res 101:162–169

Arcangeli G, Mauro F, Morelli D, Nervi C (1979) Multiple daily fractionation in radiotherapy: Biological rationale and preliminary clinical experiences. Europ J Cancer 15:1077–1083

Backstrom A, Jakobsson DA, Littbrand B, Wersall J (1973) Fractionation scheme with low individual doses in irradiation of carcinomas of the mouth. Acta Radiol Ther Phys Biol 12:401–406

Barendsen GW (1982) Dose fractionation, dose rate and isoeffect relationships for normal tissue responses. Int J Radiat Oncol Biol Phys 8:1981–1997

Cox JD (1985) Large dose fractionation (hypofractionation). Cancer 55:2105–2111

Douglas B, Worth A (1982) Superfractionation in glioblastoma multiforme: Results of a phase II study. Int J Radiat Oncol Biol Phys 8:1787–1794

Edsmyr F, Andersson L, Esposti PL, Littbrand B, Nilsson B (1985) Irradiation therapy with multiple small fractions per day in urinary bladder cancer. Radiother Oncol 4:197–203

Ellis F (1969) Dose, time and fractionation: A clinical hypothesis. Clin Radiol 20:1–7

Horiot JC, Nabid A, Chapman G (1982) Clinical experience with multiple daily fractionation in the radiotherapy of head and neck carcinoma. Cancer Bulletin 34:230–233

Horiot JC, van den Bogaert W, de Pauw M, van Glabbeke M, Gonzales DG, van der Schueren E (1985) EORTC prospective trials of altered fractionation using multiple fractions per day (MFD). Proceedings 16th Int. Congress of Radiology, Honolulu, Hawaii, 1985, p 95

Horiot JC, Chaplain G, van der Schueren E et al. (1985) European Organization for Research and Treatment on Cancer (EORTC) Cooperative Group of Radiotherapy: Protocol 22581 "A phase III study of accelerated fractionation in the radiotherapy of advanced head and neck carcinoma"

Jampolis S, Pepard G, Horiot JC, Bolla M, LeDorze C (1977) Preliminary results using twice a day fractionation in the radiotherapeutic management of advanced cancers of the head and neck. Am J Roentgenol 129:1091–1093

Littbrand B, Edsmyr F, Revesz L (1975) A low dose fractionation scheme for the radiotherapy of the carcinoma of the bladder. Experimental and preliminary results. Bull Cancer 62:241

Loeffler RK (1983) Improved tolerance with two radiation fractions per day for treatment of abdominal and pelvic malignancies. Am J Clin Oncol (CCT) 6:619–627

Maciejewski B, Taylor JMG, Withers HR (1986a) Alpha/beta value and the importance of size of dose per fraction for late complications in the supraglottic larynx. Radiother Oncol 4:323–326

Maciejewski B, Withers HR, Taylor JMG, Hliniak A (1986b) Dose fractionation and regeneration in radiotherapy for cancer of the oral cavity and oropharynx. Part 1. Tumor dose-response and repopulation. Int J Radiat Oncol Biol Phys (submitted)

Mason KA, Withers HR (1977) RBE of neutrons generated by 50 MeV deuterons on beryllium for control of artificial pulmonary metastases of a mouse fibrosarcoma. Br J Radiol 50:652–657

Medini E, Rao Y, Kim T, James TK, Levitt SH (1980) Radiation therapy for advanced head and neck squamous cell carcinoma using twice-a-day fractionation. Radiology 134:531–532

Meoz RT, Fletcher GH, Peters LJ, Barkley HT, Thames HD (1984) Twice-daily fractionation schemes for advanced head and neck cancer. Int J Radiat Oncol Biol Phys 10:831–836

Parsons JT, Cassisi NJ, Million RR (1984) Results of twice-a-day irradiation of squamous cell carcinomas of the head and neck. Int J Radiat Oncol Biol Phys 10:2041–2051

Parsons JT, Million RR (1986a) Radiation therapy with multiple fractions per day in the treatment of head and neck cancer. In: Jacobs C (ed) Head and Neck Oncology. Martinus Nijhoff, The Hague (in press)

Parsons JT, Mendenhall W, Cassisi J, Million RR (1986b) Accelerated hyperfractionation for head and neck cancer. Int J Radiat Oncol Biol Phys (in press)

Peters LJ, Ang KK (1987) Accelerated fractionation. In: Withers HR, Peters LJ (eds) Innovations in Radiation Oncology. Springer-Verlag, Heidelberg

Regaud C (1929) Radium therapy of cancer at the Radium Institute of Paris. Technique, biological principles and results. Am J Roentgenol Rad Therapy 21:1–24

Revesz L, Littbrand B, Midander J, Scott OCA (1975) Oxygen effects in the shoulder region of cell survival curves. In: Alper T (ed) Proceedings 6th LH Gray Conference. John Wiley and Sons Ltd, London/New York, p 141

Schwarz G (1914) Dauerbestrahlung mit täglichen kleinen Dosen. Münchener Med Wochenschr 61:1733–1735

Shukovsky L, Fletcher GH, Montague ED, Withers HR (1976) Experience with twice-daily fractionation in clinical radiotherapy. Am J Roentgenol 126:155–162

Singh K (1978) Two regimes with the same TDF but differing morbidity used in the treatment of stage III carcinoma of the cervix. Br J Radiol 51:357–362

Thames HD, Withers HR, Peters LJ, Fletcher GH (1982) Changes in early and late radiation responses with altered dose fractionation: Implications for dose-survival relationships. Int J Radiat Oncol Biol Phys 8:219–226

Trott K, Kummermehr J (1985) What is known about tumor proliferation rates to choose between accelerated fractionation or hyperfractionation? Radiother Oncol 3:1–9

van der Schueren E, van den Bogaret W, Ang KK (1983) Radiotherapy with multiple fractions per day. In: Steel GG, Adams GE, Peckham MJ (eds) The Biological Basis of Radiotherapy. Elsevier Science Publishers, Amsterdam, p 195

Vegesna V, Withers HR, Thames HD (1985) Multifraction radiation response of mouse lung. Int J Radiat Biol 47:413–422

Wang CC, Blitzer PH, Suit H (1985) Twice-a-day radiation therapy for cancer of the head and neck. Cancer 55:2100–2104

Wang CC, Suit HD, Blitzer PH (1986) Twice-a-day radiation therapy for supraglottic carcinoma. Int J Radiat Oncol Biol Phys 12:3–7

Wang CC (1987) Accelerated fractionation. In: Withers HR, Peters LJ (eds) Innovations in Radiation Oncology. Springer-Verlag, Heidelberg

Withers HR (1972) Cell renewal concepts and the radiation response. In: Vaeth JM (ed) Frontiers of Radiation Therapy and Oncology, vol 6. Karger, Basel, p 93

Withers HR (1975) Cell cycle redistribution as a factor in multifraction irradiation. Radiology 114:199–202

Withers HR, Hunter N, Barkley HT, Reid BO (1974) Radiation survival and regeneration characteristics of spermatogenic stem cells of mouse testis. Radiat Res 57:88–103

Withers HR, Thames HD Jr, Peters LJ (1982a) Differences in the fractionation response of acute and late responding tissues, In: Karcher KH, Kogelnik HD, Reinartz G (eds) Progress in Radio-Oncology II. Raven Press, New York, p 287

Withers HR, Thames HD Jr, Peters LJ (1982b) Biological bases for high RBE values for late effects of neutron irradiation. Int J Radiat Oncol Biol Phys 8:2071–2076

Withers HR, Thames HD, Peters LJ, Fletcher GH (1983a) Normal tissue radioresistance in clinical radiotherapy. In: Fletcher GH, Nervi C, Withers HR (eds) Biological Bases and Clinical Implications of Tumor Radioresistance. Masson, New York, p 139

Withers HR, Thames HD, Peters LJ (1983b) A new isoeffect curve for change in dose per fraction. Radiother Oncol 2:187–192

Withers HR (1985) Biologic basis for altered fractionation schemes. Cancer 55:2086–2095

Withers HR, Mason KA, Thames HD (1986) Late radiation response of kidney assayed by tubule cell survival. Br J Radiol 59:587–595

6.2 Accelerated Fractionation

Lester J. Peters and K. Kian Ang

CONTENTS

1 Background

Accelerated fractionation is defined as reducing the overall duration of a radiotherapy regimen without a significant change in the size of dose per fraction or total dose. This is achieved by giving two or more fractions on some or all of the treatment days.

The rationale for attempting to improve the therapeutic ratio by accelerated fractionation is based primarily on the premise that shortening the overall time of radiotherapy reduces the opportunity for tumor cells to regenerate during treatment and, therefore, increases the probability of tumor control for a given dose level. By giving more than one dose fraction per day, the size of dose per fraction can be kept constant or even slightly reduced. Since the probability of late normal tissue injury is much more dependent on size of dose per fraction than on overall treatment time (Thames et al. 1983), an improvement in the therapeutic ratio between tumor control and late complications may therefore be expected with accelerated fractionation. For this to be true, however,

This investigation was supported in part by grants CA06294 and CA16672 awarded by the National Cancer Institute, U.S. Department of Health and Human Services

Lester J. Peters, M.D.
K. Kian Ang, M.D.
The University of Texas M.D. Anderson Hospital and Tumor Institute
Houston, TX 77030, USA

when two or more fractions are given on the same day, the treatments must be spaced sufficiently to allow repair processes to approach completion. Experimental data relating to the kinetics of repair in normal tissues are sparse, but suggest that repair proceeds more slowly in late responding normal tissues such as spinal cord (Ang et al. 1984) and kidney (Withers chapter on "Hyperfractionation" this volume) than in acutely responding tissues such as the bone marrow, jejunum and colon (Thames et al. 1984). In the late responding tissues, the half-time for repair was on the order of 1.5 hours. Thus, to prevent significant cumulative interaction of sublethal radiation injury, treatments delivered on the same day should be separated by at least six hours.

Since most human tumors are relatively slow growing with respect to the duration of a conventional course of radiotherapy, it is not immediately apparent why overall treatment time should influence tumor control probability to any appreciable extent. However, the growth rate of an untreated tumor gives little or no indication of the regenerative capability of the clonogenic cells within the tumor, and this determines the total number of cells that must be sterilized during a fractionated course of treatment to effect cure. For example, if two tumors of the same physical size differed in regenerative capability such that the number of clonogenic doublings during treatment differed by a factor of 3, it would be the same radiobiologically as if one tumor were 8 times larger than the other but with equal regenerative capability.

The potential importance of tumor clonogen regeneration in determining the outcome of radiotherapy can be derived from two different types of clinical observation.

1) Time to recurrence data suggest that tumor clonogens surviving radiation proliferate much more rapidly than might be expected from pretreatment volume doubling times. Analysis of recurrences of squamous cell carcinomas of various head and neck sites (Fletcher 1980; Pene and Fletcher 1976) shows that approximately three

quarters are manifest within the first year of treatment and over 90% within 2 years. These recurrences have occurred in populations of patients where the majority have been cured, implying that most of the recurrences must have arisen from one or a very few surviving clonogenic cells. Since approximately 30 volume doublings are required for a single malignant cell to proliferate to a clinically manifest recurrence, these data demonstrate that the cells surviving a course of radiation have significant regenerative potential.

2) Retrospective studies of large numbers of patients with all stages of carcinoma of the upper respiratory and digestive tracts have shown that introduction of a $2–2^1/_2$ week break in treatment (split-course) without changing the total dose or number of dose fractions has resulted in inferior tumor control rates than those achieved with a continuous course of irradiation (Parsons et al. 1984; Vikram et al. 1985). A corollary of these data is the observation of Holsti (1984) that in a split-course regimen the total dose must be escalated by about 10% to compensate for a treatment interruption of 2 to 3 weeks.

It may be argued that tumor regeneration rates determined from time to recurrence and split-course data are not representative of the situation during a continuous course of radiotherapy because of the division delay induced by treatment. Recently Kummermehr (1985) has quantitated the extent of regeneration in several murine tumors during the first and second weeks of continuous fractionated irradiation. While the exact patterns differed between histologic types, all tumors showed significant regenerative potential. For example, in a squamous cell carcinoma treated with 12 fractions over 2 weeks, half of the total dose delivered was required to offset tumor regeneration during the treatment. Clinically, because of the interrelationship between fraction size (and number) and overall time, this question can be addressed only indirectly. Nonetheless, in an analysis of time dose factors relating to control of squamous cell carcinoma of the larynx, Maciejewski et al. (1983) concluded that tumor control depended strongly on overall time, especially between weeks 4 and 7, where each 4 days of prolongation required an extra 200 cGy to compensate for tumor repopulation.

The capacity for rapid regeneration in certain human tumors is consistent with the rather limited data available on their detailed proliferation kinetics. For example, the median potential doubling time of 198 human squamous cell carcinomas re-

ported by Sasaki et al. (1980) was only 4.1 days. In reviewing the literature and their own data, Trott and Kummermehr (1985) concluded that squamous cell carcinomas of the head and neck region and of the uterine cervix, poorly differentiated bladder cancers, and colorectal adenocarcinomas are most capable of a rapid regenerative response (i.e., potential doubling time of 3–4 days) and suggested an advantage of treating these tumors with accelerated fractionation.

The limitation of accelerated fractionation is the severity of acute reactions in rapidly proliferating normal tissues and the consequential late sequelae of such reactions. By consequential late sequelae, we refer to late normal tissue injury, e.g., scarring, persistent ulceration, exposed bone, fistulae, etc., that results from severe acute reaction or complications thereof, rather than from direct radiation injury of late reacting normal tissues. The distinction is important, since the probability of direct late radiation injury is relatively insensitive to overall time of treatment, whereas consequential late sequelae are clearly a function of the severity of the acute reaction which is strongly time dependent. Thus, attempts to give high doses in very short overall times to patients with head and neck cancer (Peracchia and Salti 1981) have been attended by unacceptable rates of *both* acute reactions and consequential late sequelae. Another serious problem associated with the use of very intensive treatment regimens is that of hemorrhage following ultra-rapid tumor lysis which can sometimes be fatal (Van den Bogaert et al. 1982).

Because of severe acute reactions, the use of pure accelerated fractionation in the treatment of head and neck tumors is generally not feasible, and one must either introduce a split in the treatment regimen or reduce the total dose to make the treatment tolerable. If the total dose is reduced, it must be assumed that the dose saved through restricting tumor regeneration to a shorter treatment time exceeds that by which the total dose is reduced. Clearly, without a detailed knowledge of the proliferation kinetics and radiation dose response for individual tumors such a conclusion cannot be made and the rationale of accelerated fractionation regimens with reduced total doses is therefore suspect. On the other hand, introduction of a split course in treatment defeats the purpose of accelerated fractionation if the overall duration of treatment, including the split, is not less than that of a conventional regimen. Experiments conducted in our own laboratory assessing curability of a murine fibrosarcoma (FSa) when treated with

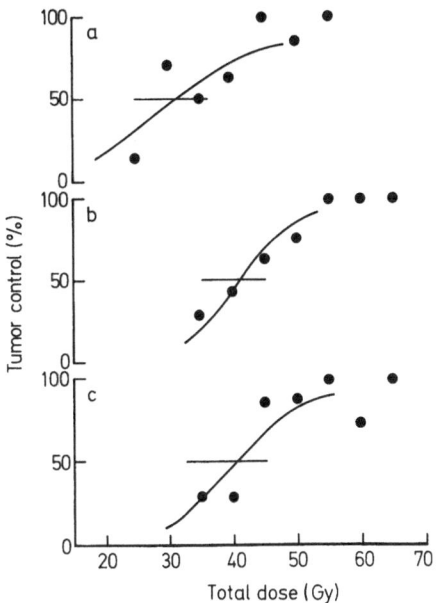

Fig. 1 a–c. Local cure probability of a 5 mm fibrosarcoma (FSa) as a function of total dose and fractionation schedule. **a** Accelerated fractionation: 10 fractions given in 3 days (TCD$_{50}$: 31.5 Gy). **b** Daily fractions: 10 fractions given in 11 days (TCD$_{50}$: 41 Gy). **c** Split course acclerated fractionation: 2 treatment courses, each consisting of 5 fractions administered in $1^1/_2$ days, separated by a rest period of 8 days (TCD$_{50}$: 40.4 Gy)

conventional schedule, accelerated fractionation, or a split course regimen have demonstrated this point (Fig. 1). In some cases, a measure of acceleration can be achieved even with a split course, but it is usually modest.

A variant treatment strategy, the so called "concomitant boost" technique can help to overcome the limitation of acute reactions (KNEE et al. 1985). With this technique the boost is delivered as a second daily dose during the basic course of treatment rather than sequentially as in a conventional schedule, thereby reducing the volume of tissue treated at accelerated rate. The concomitant boost affords a modest degree of treatment acceleration, usually by no more than 2 weeks, but since the total dose does not have to be reduced with this strategy it may have the best radiobiologic rationale.

2 Clinical Experience

Several clinical studies have been reported using fractionation schedules that have features of accelerated fractionation although relatively few conform to the strict definition. The clinical experience is summarized in Table 1, and is elaborated in the following sections. These are grouped according to tumor site/type and presented in the chronological order of the first trial reported for that site.

2.1 Brain Tumors

The concept of treatment acceleration was first applied by SIMPSON and PLATTS (1976) for the management of patients with glioblastoma multiforme. Two subgroups of patients received a dose of 40 Gy in 21 fractions delivered in either 1 week or 3 weeks. There was no difference in survival between the groups, probably reflecting the low biological dose given. Since the total dose is significantly reduced, the schedule used in their study cannot be considered as a prototype accelerated fractionation.

The randomized malignant glioma study of the EORTC (European Organization for Research on Treatment of Cancer) Radiotherapy Group comes closest to meeting the criteria of accelerated fractionation (VAN DER SCHUEREN et al. 1985). In this trial a dose of 60 Gy was given in 2 treatment courses, each consisting of 30 Gy delivered in 15 fractions and spread over 5 days (3 fx/day). In order to avoid excessive acute skin reaction a rest period of 2 weeks was inserted between the 2 treatment courses resulting in an overall treatment time of 4 weeks. This regimen was well tolerated by the patients, but no survival benefit for accelerated fractionation over conventional fractionated treatment (60 Gy/30 fx/6 weeks) was observed. These results suggest that conventional therapy is too far from the threshold of cure for most patients with glioblastoma multiforme for any modest improvement in therapeutic efficacy to be resolved.

2.2 Burkitt's Lymphoma

The early results of a pilot study on Burkitt's lymphomas (NORIN and ONYANGO 1977) showed improvement in complete tumor regression rate when an average dose of 29 Gy was given in approximately 2 weeks overall time as opposed to approximately 31 Gy administered in 3 weeks. Although these data support the concept of accelerated fractionation, the total dose administered and the fractionation schedules used varied considerably from one patient to another, and only response rates, not tumor control rates, are available. Hence, it

Table 1. Clinical studies with features of accelerated fractionation

Tumor site	Type of study	No. of patients	Dose/fx (Gy)	No. fx/ day	Total dose (Gy)	Time (wks)	Split (wks)	Results	Authors
Brain (Gliomas)	R	47	1.9	3	40	1	–	No improvement in survival	Simpson and Platts 1976
			1.9	1	40	3	–		
	R	160	2	3	60	4	2	No difference in median survival time (48 vs 47 wks)	Van der Schueren et al. 1985
			2	1	60	6	–		
Burkitt's	P	34	1–1.25	3	25–31	2	–	Complete tumor regression: 74%	Norin and Onyango 1977
Breast (Inflammatory)	P	31	1.25	2	71	5.5	–	Local control rate: 77%	Barker et al. 1980
Advanced head and neck (Various sites)	P	22	2	3	48–54	1.5	–	Complete response at 8 months: 68%	Peracchia and Salti 1981
Head and neck (various stages)	P	59	1.75–2.3	3	50–55	2	–	Complete response within 3 months: 86% 3-yrs survival: 44%	Svoboda 1984
Neck nodes	P	35	1.5–2	3	60	2.5	–	Complete response at 12 months: 42%	Arcangeli et al. 1984
Advanced head and neck (Various sites)	R	208	1.6	3	67.2–72	6–7	3–4	No difference in 2-yr actuarial local control rate (32% for both arms)	Horiot et al. 1985
			2	1	70	7	–		
Head and neck (Various stages)	P C	321 303	1.6 1.8	2 1	64–67.2 65	6 7.2	2 –	Highly significant improvement in 3-year actuarial local control rate (68% vs 46%)	Wang et al. 1985
Advanced head and neck	P	53	1.2–2	2	70–74	6	–	2-yr actuarial local control rate: 65%	Knee et al. 1985
Melanoma (Brain metastases)	P	20 23	3–3.75 1.9–2.4	2 2	30–37.5 37.5–48	1 2	– –	Median survival time: 50 wks Median survival time: 28 wks	Choi et al. 1985

P, Pilot; C, Control; R, Randomized

is difficult to draw firm conclusions regarding the efficacy of these regimens.

2.3 Breast Cancer

The results of a pilot study assessing the efficacy of accelerated fractionation in the treatment of inflammatory breast cancer (Barker et al. 1980), one of the rapidly progressing human tumors, are rather impressive. Using twice daily fractionation a total dose of about 71 Gy could be administered in $5^1/_2$ weeks. The local-regional control rate, with a minimum follow-up of 2 years in patients treated with accelerated fractionation was significantly improved over that of an historical control group treated with conventional schedule (77% versus 62%). No increase in undue late effects was observed.

2.4 Head and Neck Cancer

The feasibility and efficacy of accelerated fractionation have extensively been investigated in cancers of the upper respiratory and digestive tracts (see Table 1). The overall treatment time was drastically reduced in 3 pilot studies. Svoboda (1984) reported his experience in 59 patients treated to doses of 50 to 55 Gy given in fractions of 1.75 to 2.3 Gy, 3 times a day over 10 to 16 days. Acute reactions were tolerable when small treatment volumes were used. However, the acute mucosal reactions became limiting when larger volumes were irradiated, so it was necessary to limit the dose per fraction to 1.75 Gy (RESOULY and SVOBODA 1982). The local control rate was good, but 6 patients developed severe late reactions such as laryngeal or esophageal stenosis, or cartilage necrosis, without tumor recurrence (SVOBODA 1984). By contrast, PERRACHIA and SALTI (1981) reported serious complications (necrosis, fistula) in 12 of 22 patients with head and neck cancers given thrice daily fractions of 2 Gy (4 hrs interval) to total doses of 48–56 Gy over about $1^1/_2$ weeks. ARCANGELI et al. (1984) reported on a series of patients with neck node metastases from head and neck cancer treated with accelerated fractionation and found that reduction of overall time resulted in a higher complete response rate at 12 months after therapy (42% versus 20% achieved with conventional treatment). The late effects of treatment were not mentioned.

Two other studies have employed "split course accelerated fractionation." In the randomized study of the Radiotherapy Cooperative Group of the EORTC (VAN DEN BOGAERT et al. 1982), patients in the experimental arm received 3 fractions of 1.6 Gy on each treatment day to a dose of 48 Gy in 2 weeks. Due to severe mucosal reactions, treatment was interrupted at this point, but generally could be resumed after a rest period of 3 to 4 weeks again with 1.6 Gy × 3 each day to total doses of 67.2 to 72 Gy in 6 to 7 weeks. Thus, on the average the overall time of this regimen is only a few days shorter than that of the conventional schedule used in the control arm of the trial (70 Gy in 35 fractions over 7 weeks), and cannot be considered as accelerated fractionation by our definition. The preliminary results of this trial showed no advantage of the split-course regimen over conventional treatment (VAN DEN BOGAERT et al. 1985). Acute toxicity was worse in the experimental arm, but no increase in late normal tissue reactions have been observed to this point. In the pilot study of WANG et al. (1985), 2 fractions of 1.6 Gy, separated by a 4 hr interval, were given on each treatment day to a dose of 38.4 Gy over 12 days. After giving a 2-week break for symptoms of acute mucosal reaction to subside, therapy was resumed for an additional 8 to 9 days to total doses of 64–67.2 Gy. Comparing the data of the study group to those of historical control patients treated with conventional fractionation (64–65 Gy given in fractions of 1.8 Gy over $7^1/_2$ weeks) it was found that $1^1/_2$ weeks acceleration of treatment resulted in a significant improvement in the local tumor control rate. No increase in late complications was observed during the 4-year follow-up period. (See Chapter 6.3 for more details).

Finally, the experience of concomitant boost technique for the management of advanced head and neck cancers was reported by KNEE et al. (1985). In this pilot study all patients received basic daily treatment of 1.8 to 2 Gy to a total dose of approximately 55 Gy. The boost was delivered as a second daily treatment, 1.2 to 1.5 Gy, 2–3 times a weeks for 3–5 weeks. Thus, a total tumor dose of approximately 72 Gy was delivered in about 6 weeks without a treatment break. The acute reactions were rather severe, but treatment could be completed in 50 of 53 patients without interruption. For the entire group of patients with a median follow-up of 31 months, the actuarial 2-year probability of local-regional disease control was 65% and of survival 55%. Fourteen patients sustained moderate to severe late complications, 7 of which were associated with neck dissection following radiotherapy.

2.5 Melanoma

CHOI et al. (1985) reported on a series of patients with brain metastases from malignant melanoma treated with accelerated fractionation. These patients received either 30–37.5 Gy in 10 fractions over 1 week or 37.5–48 Gy in 20 fractions over 2 weeks. In both schedules, 2 treatments were delivered per day separated by at least a 6 hour interval. The results showed that patients who had intracranial metastases only at the time of treatment (i.e., no visceral disease) survived longer when treated with the more accelerated 1 week schedule (median survival time: 50 vs 28 weeks). Besides the difference in overall time, there was also a difference in the size of dose per fraction used in the 2 treatment schemes. However, in this analysis, fraction size was not found to be a significant factor in modifying tumor effect.

3 Summary and Perspective

The potential benefit of using accelerated fractionation regimens in the treatment outcome of various human tumors has been investigated in several centers during the past decade. Although diverse treatment schemes have been tested in different groups of patients, the available clinical data summarized in this chapter allow the tentative conclusion that accelerated fractionation, when used appropriately, does offer the prospect of an improvement in therapeutic ratio between tumor control and late complications in certain groups of patients. As can be observed from Table 1, the majority of the experience has been acquired from treatment of cancers of the upper respiratory and digestive tracts. Therefore, we have attempted to analyze this material in more detail in order to identify features that would be useful in refining the radiotherapy schedule.

Data on head and neck cancers show that acute mucosal reactions limit the rate by which treatment can be accelerated, particularly when large volumes of mucous membranes are irradiated. The results of Peracchia and Salti (1981) and Svoboda (1984), for example, demonstrate that it is virtually impossible to deliver a total dose of more than 48–50 Gy when the overall time is limited to 2 weeks. This observation has been substantiated by the EORTC study (Van den Bogaert et al. 1982) in which severe mucosal reactions, occurring after a dose of 48 Gy given in 2 weeks, necessitated a 3–4 week treatment break. As noted above, the preliminary data of this randomized study (Horiot et al. 1985) showed that a split course regimen of this type, delivering a total dose of approximately 70 Gy in $6^1/_2$ to 7 weeks did not lead to a significant improvement in treatment outcome over a conventional schedule. This indicates that treatment strategies in which a reduced total dose is delivered in a very short overall time, e.g., 48–50 Gy in 2 weeks, as used in a few centers, are unlikely to be beneficial since they correspond to only the first part of the split course schedule employed in the EORTC trial.

The results of Wang et al. (1985) and Knee et al. (1985), on the otherhand, demonstrate that it is feasible to reduce the treatment time by 1.2–2 weeks without diminishing the total dose. By using either two fractions a day (BID) schedule with a short break (2 weeks) or the concomitant boost technique without interruption, they were able to administer a dose of 64–74 Gy in 6 weeks. These strategies appear promising. A high local control rate has been achieved apparently without increasing the incidence of late complications.

Based on the clinical experience acquired thus far, two studies aiming at further refinement of scheduling of accelerated fractionation have recently been initiated. Horiot (personal communication, 1986) has shown, in a pilot study, that it was feasible to administer a dose of 70–72 Gy in 5 weeks by introducing a gap of approximately 2 weeks after 24–33.6 Gy was delivered in 5–8 days

(3 fractions of 1.6 Gy per day). The efficacy of this schedule is currently being tested against that of conventional fractionation by the EORTC Radiotherapy Cooperative Group in advanced head and neck cancer patients. At the U.T.M.D. Anderson Hospital we are conducting a Phase II randomized trial assessing the optimal timing of delivery of the concomitant boost. Patients with squamous cell carcinoma of the oropharynx or nasopharynx receive a basic course of 54 Gy given in 30 exposures over 6 weeks (1.8 Gy per fraction). At the outset, they are randomly assigned to receive one of three concomitant boost schedules (10–12 fractions of 1.5 Gy). In each arm, all patients receive a total dose of 69–72 Gy, only the timing of administering the second daily exposure differs between the 3 study arms. Each of the schedules to be tested has potential advantages and disadvantages. In the first arm the boost will be given twice-a-week during the basic treatment. Delivering the boost twice a week reduces the maximum dose received during any one week to 12 Gy, and therefore may be the best tolerated. However, it is logistically the most difficult, and increases the risk of technical error. It has no specific radiobiological rationale beyond reducing the overall time of treatment. In the second arm the boost is given every day, 5 times a week during the first $2–2^1/_2$ weeks of the basic course. Delivering the boost at the beginning of the course of treatment allows a greater proportion of the total tumor dose to be delivered before a tumor regenerative response is triggered (Barendsen and Broerse 1970). An early boost also results in a more rapid tumor volume reduction, and as demonstrated in the pilot study (Knee et al. 1985) will in nearly all cases arrest the growth of tumors that progress under therapy at 9–10 Gy per week. This schedule should increase the probability of complete tumor regression at the end of treatment, which, with conventional treatment, has been associated with improved tumor control (Barkley and Fletcher 1977). The major disadvantage of this technique is that the risk of treatment interruption is greatest since a large dose is received by the stem cells of the mucous membranes before a regenerative response has been triggered. Another theoretical disadvantage is that the boost will be delivered at least in part before reoxygenation by volume regression has had a chance to take place. However, this is not a major concern, since functional reoxygenation has been demonstrated experimentally within hours of radiation exposure without any volume changes (Howes 1969; Thomlinson 1970;

van Putten and Kallman 1968). In the third arm, the boost is given every day, 5 times a week during the last $2-2^{1}/_{2}$ weeks of the basic treatment. Delivering the boost during the last part of the basic treatment has the greatest probability of ensuring that the full dose is given without interruption, even though an exacerbation of the acute reaction may be predicted following completion of therapy. However, the regenerative response of rapidly proliferating normal tissues has been shown to increase during fractionated irradiation (Withers and Mason 1974; Denekamp 1973; Ang et al. 1985), and this will act to offset the toxicity of this schedule. Delivering the boost towards the end of the basic course may be beneficial in terms of reoxygenation, but is less likely to achieve a complete tumor regression by the completion of therapy. Another possible disadvantage is that of stimulating a regenerative response in the tumor analogous to that in normal rapidly proliferating tissues before the boost is given.

From first principles, it is readily apparent that patients whose tumors have rapid regenerative potential are the ones that should preferably be treated with accelerated fractionation. However, detailed knowledge of the proliferation kinetics of individual tumors is necessary to select such patients on a rational basis. For example, although cytokinetic studies (Sasaki et al. 1980; Trott and Kummermehr 1985) have shown that squamous cell carcinomas of the head and neck region as a group have a high regenerative potential (short potential doubling time), the proliferation kinetics of individual tumors may differ considerably. Up to the present time, it has been difficult to measure the cytokinetic parameters of human tumors, but the development of new techniques of cell labeling with monoclonal antibodies to halogenated analogs of deoxyuridine now makes individual patient measurements feasible (Begg et al. 1985). This technique has been adopted in our Institution so that it is possible to estimate the potential doubling time of human tumors using a single preradiotherapy biopsy sample labeled in vitro. If this parameters represents the true regenerative response of the tumor during fractionated treatment, it should soon be possible to select patients who would benefit most from accelerated fractionation on individual basis.

Note Added in Proof:

Since submission of this chapter, preliminary data from a new trial of accelerated fractionation in the treatment of bronchial, esophageal and head and neck cancers have been reported (Saunders and Dische, 1986). These data are included in our most recent review of the rationale and results of different strategies for delivery of accelerated fractionation (Peters et al. 1987).

Peters LJ, Ang KK, Thames HD Jr (1987) Accelerated fractionation in the treatment of head and neck cancer: A critical comparison of different strategies. Acta Radiol Oncol (in press)

Saunders MI, Dische S (1986) Radiotherapy employing three fractions in each day over a continuous period of 12 days. Br J Radiol 59:523–525

References

Ang KK, van der Kogel AJ, Van Dam J, van der Schueren E (1984) The kinetics of repair of sublethal damage in the rat cervical spinal cord during fractionated irradiations, Radiotherapy & Oncology 1:247–253

Ang KK, Xu F-X, Vanuytsel L, van der Schueren E (1985) Repopulation kinetics in irradiated mouse lip mucosa: The relative importance of treatment protraction and time distribution of irradiations, Rad Res 101:162–169

Arcangeli G, Nervi C, Cividalli A, Mauro F, Pardini MC (1984) Clinical implication of the radiobiological data in multiple fractions per day (MFD) radiotherapy. In: Proceedings of Varian's Fourth European Clinac Users Meeting, (Malta, May 25–26, 1984), Varian, Zug, Switzerland, pp 36–43

Barendsen GW, Broerse JJ (1970) Experimental radiotherapy of rat rhabdomyosarcoma with 15 MeV neutrons and 300 KV x-rays. II. Effect of fractionated treatments applied five times a week for several weeks, Europ J Cancer 6:89–109

Barker JL, Montague ED, Peters LJ (1980) Clinical experience with irradiation of inflammatory carcinoma of the breast with and without elective chemotherapy. Cancer 45:625–629

Barkley HT Jr, Fletcher GH (1977) The significance of residual disease after external irradiation and squamous cell carcinoma of the oropharynx, Radiology 124:493–495

Begg AC, McNally NJ, Shrieve DC, Karcher H (1985) A method to measure the duration of DNA synthesis and the potential doubling time for a single sample. Cytometry 6:620–626

Choi KN, Withers HR, Rotman M (1985) Metastatic melanoma in brain: Rapid treatment of large dose fractions. Cancer 56:10–15

Denekamp J (1973) Changes in the rate of repopulation during multifractionation irradiation of mouse skin. Br J Radiol 46:381–387

Fletcher GH (1980) Textbook of Radiotherapy, 3rd Edition, Lea & Febiger, Philadelphia, pp 330–363

Holsti L (1984) An introduction to unconventional fractionation. Clinical experiences and future indications. In: Proceedings of Varian's Fourth European Clinac Users Meeting, (Malta, May 25–26, 1984), Varian, Zug, Switzerland, pp 51–56

Horiot JC, Van den Bogaert WV, De Pauw M, Glabbeke

MV, Gonzalez DG, Van der Schueren E (1985) EORTC prospective trials of altered fractionation using multiple fractions per day (MFD). In: Proceedings of the XVI International Congress of Radiology (Hawaii, July 8–12, 1985), pp 95–98

Howes AE (1969) An estimation of changes in the proportions and absolute numbers of hypoxic cells after irradiation of transplanted C3H mouse mammary tumors. Br J Radiol 42:441–447

Knee R, Fields RS, Peters LJ (1985) Concomitant boost radiotherapy for advanced squamous cell carcinoma of the head and neck, Radiotherapy & Oncology 4:1–7

Kummermehr J (1985) Regeneration in tumors (Abstract #Fd-4), In: Abstracts of Papers for the Thirty-Third Annual Meeting of the Radiation Research Society, Los Angeles, California, May 5–9

Maciejewski B, Preuss-Bayer G, Trott K (1983) The influence of the number of fractions and of overall treatment time on local control and late complication rate in squamous cell carcinoma of the larynx. Int J Radiat Oncol Biol Phys 9:321–328

Norin T, Onyango J (1977) Radiotherapy in Burkitt's lymphoma: Conventional or superfractionated regime – early results. Int J Radiat Oncol Biol Phys 2:399–406

Parsons JT, Cassisi NJ, Million RR (1984) Results of twice-a-day irradiation of squamous cell carcinomas of the head and neck. Int J Radiat Oncol Biol Phys 10:2041–2051

Pene F, Fletcher GH (1976) Results in irradiation in the in situ carcinomas of the vocal cords. Cancer 37:2586–2590

Peracchia G, Salti C (1981) Radiotherapy with thrice-a-day fractionation in a short overall time. Int J Radiat Oncol Biol Phys 7:99–104

Resouly A, Svoboda VHJ (1982) Management of advanced head and neck squamous carcinoma by multiple daily sessions of radiotherapy and surgery. In: Karcher KH, Kogelnik HD, Reinartz G (eds) Progress in Radio-Oncology, II, Raven Press, New York, pp 339–347

Sasaki T, Sato Y, Sakka M (1980) Cell population kinetics of human solid tumors. A statistical analysis in various histological types, GANN 71:520–529

Simpson WJ, Platts ME (1976) Fractionation study in the treatment of glioblastoma multiforme. Int J Radiat Oncol Biol Phys 1:639–644

Svoboda VHJ (1984) Accelerated fractionation: The Portsmouth experience 1972–1984. In: Proceedings of Varian's Fourth European Clinac Users Meeting, (Malta, May 25–26, 1984), Varian, Zug, Switzerland, pp 70–75

Thames HD Jr, Peters LJ, Withers HR, Fletcher GH (1983) Accelerated fractionation vs hyperfractionation: Rationales for several treatments per day. Int J Radiat Oncol Biol Phys 9:127–138

Thames HD, Withers HR, Peters LJ (1984) Tissue repair capacity and repair kinetics deduced from multifractionated or continuous irradiation regimens with incomplete repair. Brit J Cancer 49 (Suppl. VI) 263–269

Thomlinson RH (1970) Reoxygenation as a function of tumor size and histopathological type. In: Bond VP, Suit HD, Marcial V (eds) Conference on Time and Dose Relationships in Radiation Biology as Applied to Radiotherapy, Clearinghouse Federal Scientific Technical Information, Brookhaven National Laboratory Report BNL 50203 (C-57), Springfield, Virginia, pp 242–247

Trott K-R, Kummermehr J (1985) What is known about tumor proliferation rates to choose between accelerated fractionation or hyperfractionation? Radiotherapy & Oncology 3:1–9

Van den Bogaert W, van der Schueren E, Horiot JC, Chaplain G, Arcangeli G, Gonzalez D, Svoboda V (1982) The feasibility of high-dose multiple daily fractionation and its combination with anoxic cell sensitizers in the treatment of head and neck cancer. A pilot study of the Radiotherapy Group of the EORTC. Int J Radiat Oncol Biol Phys 8:1649–1655

Van den Bogaert W, van der Schueren E, Tongelen CV, Horiot JC, Chaplain G, Arcangeli G, Gonzalez D, Svoboda V (1985) Late results of multiple fractions per day (MFD) with misonidazole in advanced cancer of the head and neck. A pilot study of the EORTC radiotherapy group. Radiotherapy & Oncology 3:139–144

Van der Schueren E, Ang KK, Horiot JC, Gonzalez DG, Glabbeke MV, De Pauw M (1985) Concentrated radiotherapy schedules: role of repair and repopulation. In: Proceedings of the XVI International Congress of Radiology (Hawaii, July 8–12, 1985), pp 99–103

Van Putten LM, Kallman RF (1968) Oxygenation status of transplantable tumor during fractionated radiotherapy JNCI 40:41–451

Vikram B, Mishra UB, Strong EW, Manolatos S (1985) Patterns of failure in carcinoma of the nasopharynx. I. Failure at the primary site. Int J Radiat Oncol Biol Phys 11:1455–1459

Wang CC, Blitzer PH, Suit H (1985) Twice-a-day radiation therapy for cancer of the head and neck. Cancer 55:2100–2104

Withers HR, Mason K (1974) The kinetics of recovery in irradiated colonic mucosa of the mouse. Cancer 34:896–903

6.3 Accelerated Hyperfractionation

C.C. WANG

CONTENTS

1 Introduction

Radiation therapy given in multiple daily fractions has drawn great interest in the management of malignant disease. Many schemes have been developed with various fraction sizes, number of daily fractions and duration of treatment course (BACKSTROM et al. 1973; JAMPOLIS et al. 1977; MEDINI et al. 1980; MILLION et al. 1985; PERACCHIA et al. 1981). Two commonly used multi-fraction-per-day (MFD) programs have emerged, including: 1) accelerated fractionation with similar fraction size and total dose as conventional once-a-day radiation therapy but significantly shorter treatment time, 2) hyperfractionation in which a large number of treatments are given as multiple smaller-sized fractions daily with a similar or higher total dose and the same overall treatment time in order to minimize tumor regeneration and the latter is thought to beneficially spare late normal tissue effects of radiation therapy.

2 Accelerated Hyperfractionation Program

Radiation therapy given twice-a-day (b.i.d.) with fraction size of slightly less (10%) than the once-a-day program has been carried out at the Massa-

C.C. WANG, M.D.
Harvard Medical School, Boston, MA 02114, USA

chusetts General Hospital for the past five years for treatment of advanced squamous cell carcinoma of the head and neck area, esophagus, lung, cervix and a few undifferentiated carcinomas of the thyroid, inflammatory carcinomas of the breast, and others. This paper is a report of our experience with b.i.d. radiation therapy for treatment of carcinoma of the head and neck from October 1979 through April 1984, and specifically for two anatomic sites, oropharynx and supraglottis. Some results have been published elsewhere. (WANG 1985; WANG et al. 1985; WANG et al. 1986.)

The b.i.d. program consists of 1.6 Gy per fraction, two fractions per day with a minimum of 4 hours between fractions, for 12 days, 5 days a week. All fields were treated per session with megavoltage radiations. After 38.4 Gy the patients were given a rest period of approximately two weeks and then resumed treatment using a shrinking field technique. Initially one fraction of 1.8 Gy per day was given up to 65 Gy. This is designated as the b.i.d.-q.d. regimen. Since August, 1982, the patients resumed a twice-a-day daily regimen after the two-week break, receiving 1.6 Gy per fraction for 8 additional days, resulting in a total dose of 64 Gy in 6 weeks. In some instances, an additional b.i.d. dose was directed to the primary site through markedly reduced portals as a final boost for a grand total of 67.2 Gy. This is designated as the b.i.d.-b.i.d. program. The spinal cord dose was excluded after the first $2^1/_2$ weeks, receiving 38.4 Gy in 24 fractions.

3 Techniques of B.I.D. Radiation Therapy

In order to avoid excessive amounts of acute and late effects of radiation therapy, careful treatment techniques must be meticulously observed. Because of the high propensity for regional lymph node metastases for most of the advanced head and neck carcinomas, the treatment portal for the initial 38.4 Gy must be large to include the primary

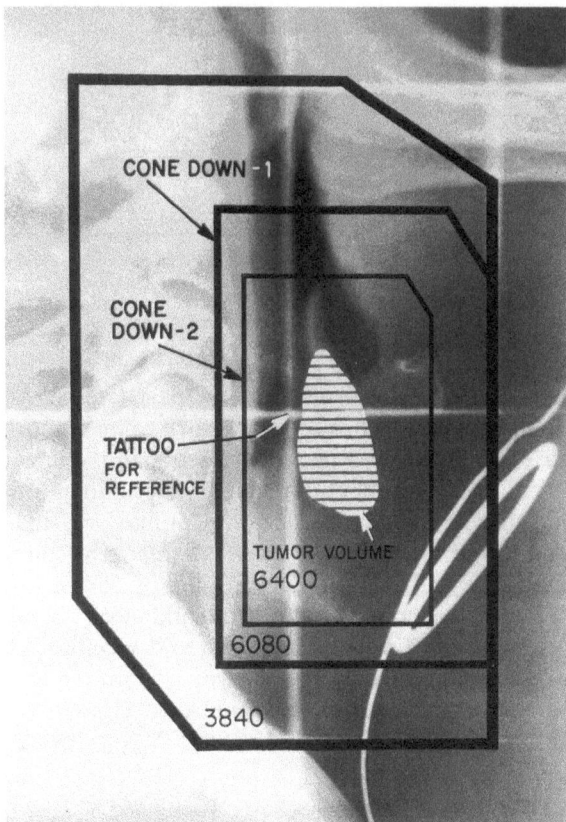

Fig. 1. Diagram showing shrinking field technique for placement of various portals vs dose for treatment of supraglottic carcinoma

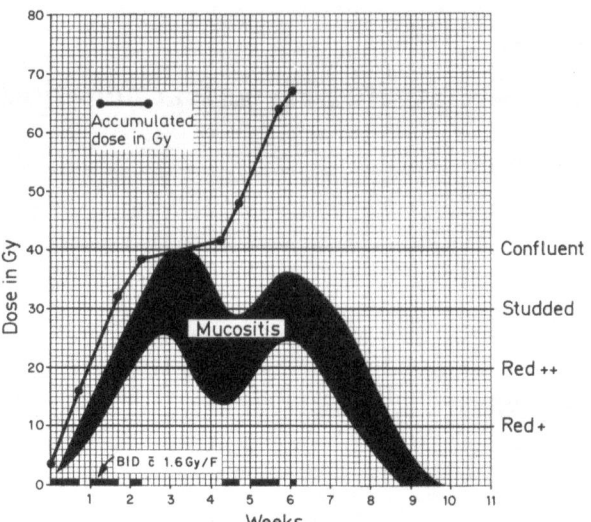

Fig. 2. Diagram showing composite biphasic mucositis of the oropharynx during b.i.d. radiation therapy course versud dose and time. Extent of mucosal reaction shown on right of graph divided into four categories

lesions and their first echelon lymphatic drainage areas. When the patients resume the latter portion of the program the radiation therapy fields are reduced to spare the spinal cord, but encompass the primary lesions and the regional nodes up to a grand total of 64 to 67.2 Gy. Any bulky posterior cervical nodes which cannot be included in the reduced portals are irradiated with low energy electrons. Figure 1 illustrates the important concept of a shrinking field for treatment of supraglottic carcinoma.

4 Acute and Late Effects on Normal Tissues After Twice-Daily Radiation Therapy

Acute effects after b.i.d. radiation therapy consist mostly of severe sore throat and development of patchy to confluent radiation mucositis. The reactions vary in degree and extent in various anatomic sites and with portal size and irradiated volume, as well as the physical condition of the patient. In general, the mucosal reaction follows a rather regular pattern of development: it occurs rapidly reaching a peak of studded and/or confluent mucositis 2.5 to 3 weeks after commencement of therapy. It then decrease rather rapidly during the two-week break. After the patient resumes b.i.d. radiation therapy, a similar mucositis may be reactivated, but to a lesser extent toward the completion of the entire course of radiation therapy. With the aid of topical and systemic analgesics, the symptoms of biphasic peak mucosal reactions generally are well-tolerated. Very few patients require hospitalization because of severe dehydration during the course of irradiation. Figure 2 relates the development and subsidence of radiation mucositis of the oropharynx and larynx to radiation dose and time.

The late effects are insignifint. Thus far, the patients followed for as long as 48 months after b.i.d. radiation therapy show no undue skin and subcutaneous fibrosis at the irradiated site nor increased incidence of mucosal ulceration or osteoradionecrosis. No patient after the b.i.d. program as outlined has developed radiation myelitis. The few patients who underwent salvage surgery to the primary site and/or neck for recurrent or persistent disease did not experience unusual postoperative complications.

5 Results of Treatment

In order to assess the efficacy of the twice daily radiation therapy program (including the b.i.d.-q.d. and b.i.d.-b.i.d. regimens), we retrospectively analyzed a comparison group of patients with oropharyngeal and supraglottic carcinomas treated by conventional once daily radiation from 1975 through 1979 in the same department with 1.8 Gy per fraction, one fraction per day, 5 days a week continuously for a total of 65 Gy in 7 weeks. An additional 5 Gy in two days was given as a boost to the bulky disease if needed. Using a computer (DEC/VAX Digital Equipment Corp., Marlborough, MA), standard life tables were obtained for both groups, and various risk factors affecting local control such as T and N stages, sex, etc. were analyzed and compared. The statistical differences were calculated by Mantel-Haenzel statistic. A p value of less than 0.05 was considered statistically significant (Cox 1972; LEW et al. 1983; MANTELL 1966; PETO et al. 1977).

5.1 Carcinoma of the Oropharynx

A total of 99 patients with oropharyngeal cancer were entered into the b.i.d. fractionation program and 134 patients into the conventional once daily radiation therapy (q.d.) program. As shown in Table 1, the 36 month actuarial local control was higher for the b.i.d. groups except in the early stages of the disease (T1–2 and N0).

5.2 Carcinoma of Supraglottic Larynx

A total of 106 patients with supraglottic carcinoma were entered into the b.i.d. fractionation program and 79 into the conventional once daily (q.d.) program. Results of these treatment schedules are shown in Table 2 and show b.i.d. to be superior to q.d., although the difference was not significant if patients characterized by negative nodes were considered as a group.

5.3 Comparison of B.I.D.-Q.D. and B.I.D.-B.I.D. Schedules

In the beginning of the program, the twice daily radiation therapy program consisted of twice daily radiation therapy for 12 days to deliver 38.4 Gy tumor dose. After a two-week break, treatment was resumed with 1.8 Gy per fraction once daily for a total of 64–67.2 Gy (designated as b.i.d.-q.d. schedule). After August 1982, patients resumed radiation therapy after a two-week break with a twice daily schedule of 1.6 Gy per fraction for a

Table 1. Oropharyngeal carcinoma (faucial tonsil and base of tongue). 36 Month actuarial local control rates

	B.I.D. Total cases/ # At risk	NED %	Q.D. Total cases/ at risk	NED %	P value
T1–4	99/16	58	134/51	45	0.0074
T1–2	35/7	77	57/33	73	0.15
T3–4	64/9	48	77/18	25	0.0024
N0	44/6	48	49/27	66	0.33
N1–3	55/10	67	85/24	33	0.0001

Table 2. Supraglottic carcinoma. 36 Month actuarial local control rates

	B.I.D. Total cases/ # At risk	NED %	Q.D. Total cases/ At risk	NED %	P value
T1–4	106/12	76	79/32	50	0.0017
T1–2	49/4	88	44/23	63	0.029
T3–4	57/8	66	35/9	33	0.0037
N0	72/8	76	51/28	62	0.25
N1–3	34/4	76	28/4	28	0.0001

Analyzed June 1984

Table 3. Oropharyngeal carcinoma treated by two B.I.D. schedules. 36 Month actuarial local control rates

	Schedule I Total cases/ # At risk	NED %	Schedule II Total cases/ # At risk	NED %	P value
T1–4	53/18	52	46/5	89	0.008
T1–2	13/7	77	22/2	95	0.80
T3–4	40/11	43	24/3	83	0.02
N0	24/22	42	19/0	84	0.11
N1–3	29/11	60	27/5	91	0.05

N.B. Schedule I 1.6 Gy/f × 2/d × 12 days 2-week break
                        1.8 GY/f/d × 15 = 65 Gy (b.i.d.-q.d.)
         Schedule II 1.6 Gy/f × 2/d × 12 days 2-week break
                         1.6 Gy/f × 2/d × 8 days = 64 Gy
                         (b.i.d.-b.i.d.)

Analyzed 2/27/85

similar total dose (designated as b.i.d.-b.i.d. schedule). Thus the double b.i.d. schedule was 10 days shorter than the b.i.d.-q.d. program.

53 patients with oropharyngeal carcinoma were treated with b.i.d.-q.d. schedule, and 46 patients with b.i.d.-b.i.d. program. As shown in Table 3, the 36 months actuarial local control rates were better in the b.i.d.-b.i.d. series except that in the

earlier stage lesions the differences were smaller and the follow-up times too short to ensure statistical significance.

6 Discussion

Although the patients under study were not randomized and the number was small, the findings seem to indicate significant improvement in local control over the results achieved by once-a-day radiation therapy in the years immediately prior to the b.i.d. program in our institution. A comparison of Tables 1 and 3 shows that there was an improvement in local tumor control rate as a result of the change from q.d. to b.i.d.-q.d. schedules. The impressive improvement in results is most apparent from a comparison of the b.i.d.-b.i.d. results with those from the b.i.d.-q.d. schedule (Table 3) or with the old q.d. results (Table 4). The improvement is particularly evident in patients with T3–4 lesions. Although the rates of improvement for the T1–2 lesions have not generally reached a statistical level, the high successful results for the representative lesions, i.e. supraglottic and faucial tonsil, suggest a trend toward significant improvement; a sufficient number of patients has not yet been entered into the program.

The reason for improvement in local tumor control has been discussed in detail in previous communications (WANG et al. 1986) and is thought to be due mainly to shortening of the total treatment course. The entire duration of the b.i.d.-b.i.d. program, including the rest period of two weeks, is 1.4 weeks shorter than the continuous q.d. program using 1.8 Gy per fraction.

The two-week rest period after 38.4 Gy is necessary because mucosal radiation reactions would be too severe without it. The break in treatment is not thought to be detrimental to the therapeutic ratio because, although some tumor cell repopulation may occur it is likely to be exceeded by the regeneration in the normal epithelium, a prerequisite to delivering the second phase of the treatment. The reduction in dose per fraction to 1.6 Gy (vs 1.8 Gy) favors an improvement in the therapeutic ratio but is probably too small a change to be a significant factor in the improved differential response between tumor and late responding normal tissues.

The question of whether an accelerated treatment given in the same overall time as the b.i.d.-b.i.d. but using larger doses per fraction in a once-a-day radiation program, e.g. 2.3 Gy per fraction

Table 4. Oropharyngeal carcinoma treated by Q.D. and B.I.D.-B.I.D. schedules. 36 Month actuarial local control rates

	Q.D. #/At risk	B.I.D.-B.I.D. #/At risk	P value
T1–4	134/51 (45%)	46/5 (89%)	0.00045
T1–2	57/33 (73%)	22/2 (95%)	0.11
T3–4	77/18 (25%)	24/3 (83%)	0.00033
N0	49/27 (66%)	19/0 (84%)	0.45
N1–3	85/24 (33%)	27/5 (91%)	0.000056

for 28 fractions in $5^1/_2$ weeks or 3.2 Gy per fraction for 20 fractions in $5^1/_2$ weeks, would result in similar improvement in local control remains speculative. However, a continuous once-a-day treatment of 2.3 Gy per fraction would produce too severe an acute mucosal reaction and 3.2 Gy per fraction regimen would lead to more severe late sequelae even if the acute reaction were to prove tolerable (WITHERS 1985). The split of 2 weeks in the b.i.d. regimens described here permits more rapid regeneration of mucosa than would occur with a continuous regimen (ANG et al. 1984) and the slightly lower dose per fraction together with the same total dose ensures that late sequelae will not be worsened. No increase in late radiation reactions of normal tissues has been noted in patients surviving four or more years. Likewise, salvage surgery, such as total laryngectomy for radiation therapy failure and/or radical neck dissection for residual nodes has been readily feasible with acceptable complications.

Because of the improved results thus far achieved at this and other sites in the head and neck area, all patients, except those with T1 lesions, are currently treated by the twice-a-day radiation therapy program at Massachusetts General Hospital.

References

Ang KK, Landuyt W, Rijnders A, van der Schueren E (1984) Differences in repopulation kinetics in mouse skin during split course multiple fractions per day (MFD) or daily fractionated irradiations. Int J Radiat Oncol Biol Phys 10:95–99

Backstrom A, Jackobsson PA, Littbrand B, Wersall J (1973) Fractionation scheme with low individual doses in irradiation of carcinoma of the mouth. Acta Radiol Ther Phys Biol 12:401–406

Cox DR (1972) Regression models and life-tables. J of Royal Stat Assn B 34:187–220

Jampolis S, Pipard G, Horiot J-C, Bolla M, LeDorze C

(1977) Preliminary results using twice-a-day fractionation in the radiotherapeutic management of advanced cancers of the head and neck. Am J Roentgenol 129:1091–1093

Lew DA, Day CL, Harrist TJ, Wood CWC, Mihm MC (1983) Multivariate Analysis. JAMA 249 (5):641–643

Mantell N (1966) Evaluation of survival data and two new rank order statistics arising in its consideration. Cancer Chemotherapy Reports 50:163

Medini E, Rao Y, Kim T, Jones TK, Levitt SH (1980) Radiation therapy for advanced head and neck squamous cell carcinoma using twice-a-day fractionation. Radiology 134:531–532

Million RR, Parsons JT, Cassisi NJ (1985) Twice-a-day Irradiation Technique for squamous cell carcinoma of the head and neck. Cancer 55:2096–2099

Peracchia G, Salti C (1981) Radiotherapy with twice-a-day fractionation in a short overall time: Clinicl experiences. Int J Radiat Oncol Biol Phys 7:99–104

Peto R, Pike MC, Armitage P et al. (1977) Design and analysis of randomized clinical trials requiring prolonged observation of each patient. II Analysis and examples. Brit J Cancer 35:1–39

Thames HD, Peters LJ, Withers HR, Fletcher GH (1983) Accelerated fractionation vs hyperfractionation: rationales for several treatments per day. Int J Radiat Oncol Biol Phys 9:127–138

Wang CC (1985) Improved local control for advanced oropharyngeal carcinoma following twice daily radiation therapy. Am J Clin Oncol 8:512–516

Wang CC, Blitzer PH, Suit HD (1985) Twice-a-day radiation therapy for cancer of the head and neck. Cancer 55:2100–2104

Wang CC, Suit HD, Blitzer PH (1986) Twice-a-day radiation therapy for supraglottic carcinoma. Int J Radiat Oncol Biol Phys 12:3–7

Withers HR (Personal communication October 1985)

7 Drugs and Radiation

7.1 Sensitizers in Radiotherapy

J. Martin Brown

CONTENTS

1 Introduction

The fact that radiotherapy is not 100% successful in controlling local disease means that there is a basis for improving the cure rate of cancer using physical or chemical modifiers of the radiation response of normal or malignant tissues. The goal for the use of sensitizers is to increase the sensitivity of tumor cells to a greater extent than those of the normal tissues which are irradiated along with the tumor. A number of diverse approaches to achieve this goal have emerged from laboratory studies. Some have been tested clinically, while others are still in the development stages. This chapter will review the more promising of these

J. Martin Brown, Ph.D., Professor
Stanford University Medical Center
Stanford, CA 94305, USA

approaches, with the emphasis where possible on their clinical use.

How much impact on local control could we expect from the use of a sensitizer combined with radiotherapy? It would be of little use, for example, to use a sensitizer which produced a sensitizer enhancement ratio (SER) of 1.5 to the tumor – in effect giving 50% more dose to the tumor cells – if a 50% increase in radiation dose to that particular tumor would produce little or no change in local control. Thus it is vital to have some idea of the dose response curve of the particular tumor under study.

Williams et al. (1984) have reviewed the available data on the dose response relationship for human tumors and have concluded that, despite the fact that the available clinical data are, for the most part, individually unsatisfactory (because they are retrospective and involve small numbers of patients), the data as a whole show that relatively small changes in x-ray dose to the tumor can produce improvements in local control. A dose increment of less than 12% was required to increase local control from 40% to 60% in more than half of the studies. Thus it is reasonable to conclude from these data that dose increments of the order of 10% to 30% (SERs of 1.1 to 1.3) would produce measurable improvements in local control. It should be noted however that the majority of the studies in the literature are for carcinomas for the head and neck (but including one or two studies of cervix, bladder and breast) so that this figure may not apply to all tumors.

2 Hypoxic Cell Radiosensitizers

2.1 Is Hypoxia Important in Clinical Radiotherapy?

Since the early 1920s it has been known that tissues irradiated in the absence of oxygen are 2.5 to 3.0 times more resistant to the damaging effects of ionizing radiation than in the presence of oxygen.

The possibility that this might present a problem in radiotherapy was soon appreciated (CRABTREE and CRAMER 1933), but it was not until the pioneering work of Gray and colleagues (GRAY et al. 1953; THOMLINSON and GRAY 1955) that this problem was considered to involve serious limitations in the cure rates in radiotherapy. THOMLINSON and GRAY (1955) showed that the histological structure of human bronchogenic carcinoma fitted a model in which necrosis occurred as a result of the utilization of oxygen through respiring tumor tissue. Specifically, they showed that the distance from the blood vessel in the normal tissue stroma to necrosis in the tumor was typically 100 to 150 μm. They suggested that viable hypoxic tumor cells might be present in a thin rim around the necrotic areas, that is, at a distance of 100 to 150 μm from the blood vessels. This is the classic model of hypoxia in tumors. These hypoxic cells have been termed "chronically hypoxic cells" to distinguish them from cells made hypoxic ("acutely hypoxic cells") by a mechanism involving the temporary occlusion of a blood vessel or a momentary slowing of bloodflow in such a vessel (BROWN 1979; SUTHERLAND and FRANKO 1980).

However likely these models are, they do not prove the presence of viable, radiobiologically resistant hypoxic cells in tumors. However, the presence of such cells can be demonstrated by a variety of methods involving the radiosensitivity of tumors or their cells. Such methods have shown that hypoxic cells are a common feature of solid tumors in rodents and provide no evidence that hypoxic cells should not also be present in human tumors (MOULDER and ROCKWELL 1984).

However, the question to be addressed is not only whether human tumors contain hypoxic cells, but whether these cells are a significant problem in conventional radiotherapy. There is now considerable evidence to suggest that, at least for some human tumors, hypoxia limits the cure rate of these tumors to conventional daily fractionated irradiation. Some of this evidence comes from clinical trials using hyperbaric oxygen (HBO) with radiotherapy. Table 1 shows the results of one such trial, a cooperative study done by the British Medical Research Council (MRC), in which stage III carcinoma of the cervix was treated using conventional fractionated radiotherapy with or without hyperbaric oxygen. It can be seen that treatment of tumors with HBO increased the local control rate and five-year survival of the patients – dramatically so for the six fraction treatments, but also for the conventional daily treatments. These

Table 1. MRC hyperbaric oxygen trial-carcinoma of the cervix uteri, stage III. (Data extracted from WATSON et al. 1978)

	HBO (%)	Air (%)	Comments
5-yr Survival			
6 Fr. Portsmouth (37 pts)	42	17	In air results
6 Fr. Oxford (23 pts)	46	8	were poor
25 Fr. Glasgow (127 pts)	50	37	Combined
30 Fr. Mt. Vernon (56 pts)	39	28	$P < 0.05$
Local Control 5 yr			
Glasgow	87	60	Highly signifi-
Mt. Vernon	76	50	cant differences
Severe Morbidity			
Bowel	12	4	

results show that hypoxic cells are present and limit the control rate of these tumors even in conventional daily fractionation.

Other evidence that hypoxic cells limit the local control rate in human tumors comes from the data of Bush and colleagues (BUSH et al. 1978) on the role of anemia and pretreatment blood transfusion on the cure rate of carcinoma of the cervix. They found that patients with stages 2B and 3 disease and hemoglobin levels during treatment of less than 12 g% had a significantly higher pelvic recurrence rate and a lower cure rate than patients whose hemoglobin levels were 12 g% or more. When they corrected the anemia by blood transfusions prior to radiotherapy, the rate of pelvic recurrence decreased, demonstrating radiosensitization.

A particularly interesting result, combining blood transfusion with HBO, has been reported by DISCHE et al. 1983. Anemic patients with carcinoma of the cervix who were transfused prior to radiotherapy showed poorer local tumor control when treated conventionally, but very good local control when treated with HBO. This identifies a subgroup of patients with this disease where tumor hypoxia is clearly implicated as a significant cause of failure in radiotherapy.

Although these data show that the radioresistance of hypoxic cells is likely to be a problem for some human tumors, it is quite likely that they may not be a problem in others. For example, hyperbaric oxygen trials of carcinoma of the bladder have not shown improved tumor response to conventional radiotherapy given with HBO (CADE et al. 1978). This may be the result of rapid reoxy-

Table 2. Hypoxic cell sensitizers-randomized controlled trials employing misonidazole. (From DISCHE 1984)

Site	Significant benefit	Margin in favor	No difference	Margin against	Significant adverse effect	Indeter-minate	Total
Head and neck	4	0	7			1	12
Bladder		1	3				4
Bronchus		1	5	1			7
Cervix			2				2
Glioblastoma	1		6				7
Esophagus			1				1
Total	5	2	24	1	0	1	33

genation of the tumor cells between fractions, or may be a reflection of a shallow dose response curve of tumor control versus radiation dose for this particular neoplasm. Despite this caveat, it is clear that any method of overcoming the radioresistance of hypoxic cells in tumors could produce a worthwhile gain in the overall cure rate of subgroups of cancer patients.

2.2 Expectations and Reality of Hypoxic Cell Radiosensitizers in the Clinic

2.2.1 Clinical Results

Although we have seen that hyperbaric oxygen can increase local control rates for some tumors, it is too complex, time consuming and difficult for standard clinical practice. Other ways of overcoming, at least in part, the problem of hypoxic cells, such as the use of neutrons or other high LET particles, are also likely to be inappropriate for routine clinical practice, in this case because of cost. It is easy to understand, therefore, that there was considerable excitement during the mid-1970s when specific radiosensitizers of hypoxic cells, notably metronidazole (MET) and misonidazole (MISO) were shown to be able to radiosensitize hypoxic cells both in vitro and in mouse tumors in vivo. These compounds, particularly MISO, rapidly went into clinical studies, and expectations were high. DISCHE (1983) has estimated that there have been over 100 clinical trials of MISO with more than 5000 patients entered on a worldwide basis since the first patient was treated in November, 1974. What has been achieved by all of these trials?

Table 2 shows a listing of the results of 33 randomized, controlled clinical studies of MISO listed by type of cancer. It is clear from this compilation

that the majority of studies have shown no benefit in the addition of MISO to radiotherapy. Only in the case of tumors of the head and neck is there any suggestion that MISO may have had a noticeable effect on the tumor response. However even for these tumors, significant improvements in local control have yet to be reported.[1] This lack of a demonstrable change in local tumor control has led to widespread disappointment in the use of radiosensitizers in the clinic. For example, researchers closely associated with the introduction of radiosensitizers into clinical use have expressed pessimism:

"...most of the Phase III trials with misonidazole have failed to show the expected gains of 20 to 40% in either survival or tumor response" (URTASUN et al. 1984). And also

"We can contrast this dismal failure of result with the great success of misonidazole in improving tumor control in practically every animal tumor system which is used in the laboratory" (DISCHE 1983).

These sentiments illustrate what would appear to be a growing feeling of many clinicians and biologists: radiosensitizers have simply not produced the hoped for benefit in radiotherapy, and thus hypoxic cells are probably not a significant limitation to local control of human tumors.

2.2.2 What Should We Expect from Misonidazole?

Do the above statements reflect a reasonable conclusion? To answer this, we must examine closely the doses of sensitizers which have been given to

---

[1] This situation has now changed. J. OVERGAARD (personal communication) has found a statistically significant improvement in local control and survival in patients with carcinoma of the pharynx treated with misonidazole in the large, randomized DAHANCA study.

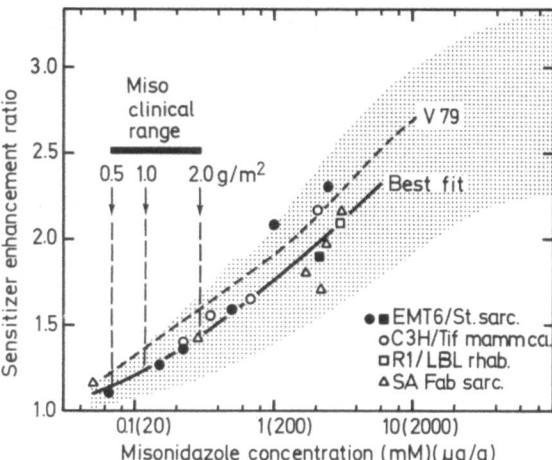

Fig. 1. Sensitizer enhancement ratios determined from large single x-ray doses as a function of measured tumor levels of MISO. The shaded area shows the range of the in vitro data from the literature with one of these sets of data (marked V79) shown. The solid line marked "Best Fit" is the author's best fit (by eye) of the published data points for the animal tumors. The range of tumor concentrations for the clinical range of MISO doses is shown. See Brown (1984) for the references for the data on which this curve is based. (From Brown (1984) with permission)

patients and ask what effect, based on laboratory studies, we would have expected from these doses. Fig. 1 shows the published data on tumor sensitization versus MISO concentration obtained from experiments in vivo and the range of a data obtained from mammalian cells in vitro (the shaded area). Also shown in this diagram is the range of tumor concentrations obtained from the doses of MISO given clinically. This range of tumor concentrations arises because of the different ways in which misonidazole can be combined with a fractionated regimen. Neurotoxicity limits the total dose of misonidazole which can be delivered to approximately 12 g/m^2 (Dische et al. 1978). Thus if MISO is given with each dose in a daily conventional fractionated regimen only approximately 0.5 g/m^2 can be given with each radiation dose. This would produce an expected sensitizer enhancement ratio (SER of the hypoxic cells) of only 1.15. On the other hand, if the radiation dose is given as 6 large fractions, then a MISO dose of 2 g/m^2 can be given with each dose. This would produce an expected SER of approximately 1.45.

For a variety of reasons both practical and theoretical it is likely that if sensitizers are to be effective, they will be have to be given for the most part in combination with conventional daily fractionation. Thus the most important part of the clinical

range of MISO concentration shown in Fig. 1 is the lower part in which individual MISO doses of 0.5 g/m^2 have been delivered. As noted above, this produces an expected SER of 1.15 for the hypoxic cells, equivalent to a dose increment of 15%. However, this is not the dose increment to be expected for the whole tumor for the fractionated regimen. This value would apply if all the tumor cells were hypoxic and the radiation dose was delivered in one large fraction. This is not the case, and it is known that tumor cells reoxygenate between fractions, a phenomenon which considerably lessens the impact of the hypoxic cells on the tumor population (Denekamp 1983). Thus this 15% dose increment predicted for 0.5 g/m^2 has to be *reduced* to allow for reoxygenation between doses. By how much must it be reduced? Examination of animal data for sensitizers given with single and fractionated doses suggests that for individual dose fractions of 2–4 Gy a factor of roughly 5–10 must be used (Hill 1986), thereby reducing the dose increment from 15% to 1.5–3%. Since we saw earlier that a dose increment of at least 10% would be required to see a significant improvement in local control, this value is clearly below that necessary to produce significant sensitization. In addition to this, many of the clinical trials so far conducted with MISO have suffered from serious limitations of design or heterogeneity of tumor populations (Maor and Peters 1984).

Thus, the conclusion is inescapable that the doses of MISO achieved in the clinical trials performed to date were too low to expect a detectable increase in local tumor control except for tumors with little or no reoxygenation. Only with a new sensitizer giving much higher dose increments could be expect to see a clinically useful increase in local control rates of those tumors for which hypoxia is a limiting factor.

2.2.3 Is There Sensitization at Low Radiation Doses Per Fraction?

The above analysis of the amount of radiosensitization to be expected as a function of MISO concentration (e.g., Fig. 1) is based on data obtained at high radiation doses. Recently it has been suggested, however, that at lower, clinically relevant radiation doses, the SER values for MISO are considerably less than at high radiation doses because (it is claimed) MISO does not sensitize at doses within the initial slope (α component) of the radiation survival curve (Palcic et al. 1984). If this were

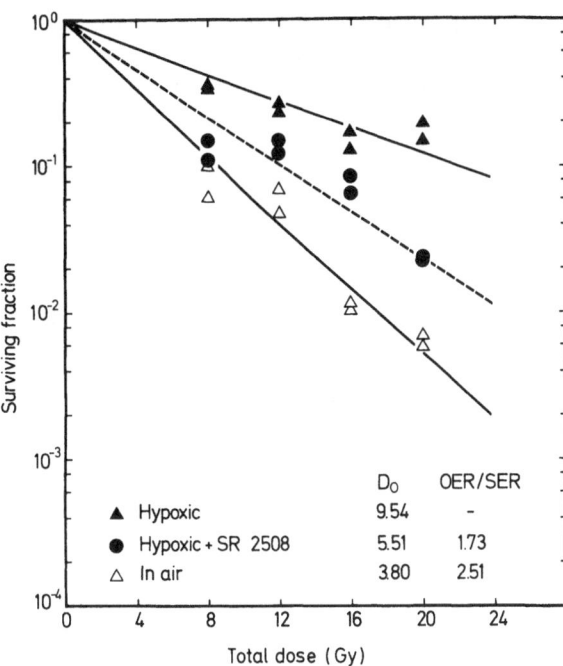

Fig. 2. Multifraction survival curve of RIF-1 tumors irradiated with 2 Gy/fraction 2 times/day (12 h fraction interval). The tumors were either clamped 2 min prior to each radiation dose to render them hypoxic, or left untouched ("In air"). SR 2508 (1000 mg/kg) was injected 45 min prior to each radiation dose. Each point represents a separate survival determination on a single tumor. All the data were obtained in one experiment. (From BROWN and YU (Int. J. Radiat. Oncol. Biol. Phys. *10*:1207–1212, 1984) with permission)

mice received a single injection of SR 2508 (1000 mg/kg) or saline 45 min prior to the irradiation. Also included were unclamped tumors irradiated under the same conditions without sensitizer. The tumors were removed after varying numbers of fractions, single cell suspensions made and plated as described previously (TWENTYMAN et al. 1980) and multifraction survival curves plotted. Fig. 2 shows the results of one such experiment. It is clear that there is significant radiosensitization by SR 2508 of the hypoxic cells at 2 Gy per fraction. The pooled results of six similar experiments gave an SER of 1.73 ± 0.25 (95% confidence limits) for radiation doses of 1–4 Gy/fraction. This enhancement ratio is very close to that predicted by the best fit line in Fig. 1 obtained from large single dose experiments at the measured tumor concentration of 1.7 mM.

These data together with those of others (GRDINA et al. 1984), show that there is substantial enhancement of the radiation response of hypoxic cells at low doses per fraction of radiation. Thus, little or no radiosensitization at low radiation doses appears not to be the explanation of the lack of clinical benefit of MISO. The data suggest, therefore, that a more efficient sensitizer than MISO, or one that is less toxic, could lead to significant radiosensitization of those human tumors for which hypoxia is a problem.

2.3 Radiosensitizers Superior to Misonidazole

2.3.1 General Considerations

We have seen from the preceding discussion that although the clinical studies with MISO have not led to improved local control of tumors with radiotherapy, this fact cannot be used to conclude that hypoxic cells are not a problem in conventional fractionated radiotherapy. If hypoxic cells are a significant contributor to tumor radioresistance, the doses of MISO used with conventional therapy have been too low to achieve radiosensitization likely to be detactable in a trial. This is the rationale for the need for improved radiosensitizers, and several laboratories have expended considerable effort in this direction.

In several ways the search for an improved hypoxic cell radiosensitizer is easier than, for example, searching for a better alkylating agent. First, the ultimate goal is clear: to achieve an SER comparable to that produced by oxygen (i.e. 2.5 to 3.0) at a drug dose that can be given with each radia-

the case, there would be less radiosensitization at doses of 2 Gy/fraction than predicted from the high dose studies, since the radiation response of most mammalian cells is dominated by the α component at these dose levels. This would significantly lessen the benefit that radiosensitizers could play in conventional radiotherapy, and could well account for the negative results seen in the clinic.

This possible explanation of the lack of positive results of the clinical trials is more important than the one proposed above based on inadequate radiosensitizer concentrations, since it would render fruitless attempts to make better radiosensitizers of the MISO class.

We have performed a series of experiments to examine this question in some detail. RIF-1 tumors were implanted subcutaneously in syngeneic C3H mice and irradiated with small doses per fraction of 1–4 Gy with varying numbers of fractions up to a maximum total dose of 20 Gy. During irradiation the tumors were clamped so as to render them fully hypoxic for each dose, and the

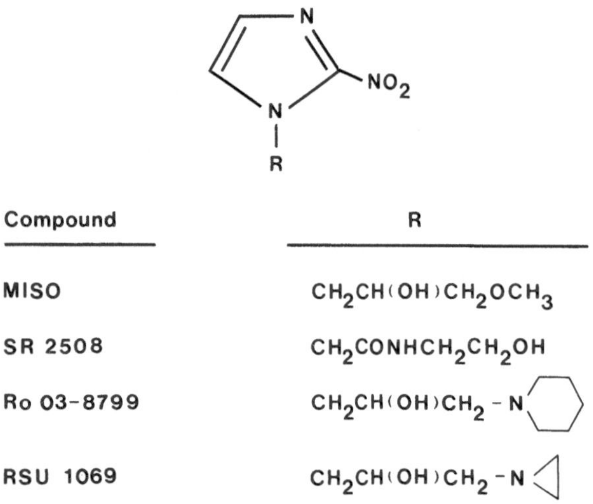

Compound	R
MISO	$CH_2CH(OH)CH_2OCH_3$
SR 2508	$CH_2CONHCH_2CH_2OH$
Ro 03-8799	$CH_2CH(OH)CH_2-N\bigcirc$
RSU 1069	$CH_2CH(OH)CH_2-N\triangleleft$

Fig. 3. The structure of MISO and three new analogs which promise to be superior radiosensitizers in the clinic

tion treatment. This may not be attainable: but if we can use a drug with each radiation dose for which the SER is 2.0 or greater, this would almost certainly be sufficient to test the hypothesis that hypoxia limits tumor control.

A second way in which drug development is easier is that radiosensitization of hypoxic cells occurs at a physico-chemical level and consequently is, for the most part, independent of cellular biochemistry. Thus radiosensitization is similar for mouse and human cells, and a drug concentration in a mouse tumor which gives a certain radiosensitization is likely to give a similar radiosensitization in a human tumor.

Finally, because they act at the physico-chemical level, it is only the drug concentration in the tumor at the time of irradiation that determines the extent of radiosensitization. Systemic toxicity, however, is governed by overall tissue exposure, or area under the curve (AUC) of drug concentration versus time.

These factors have been used to develop and to evaluate new hypoxic cell radiosensitizers for clinical application. We will review here three of the most promising of these drugs. The structures of these drugs together with that of MISO are shown in Fig. 3.

2.3.2 SR 2508

The dose-limiting toxicity of MISO is neuropathy, both peripheral and central. It follows therefore that a possible way to reduce, or eliminate this is to exclude the drug from neural tissues without

affecting its distribution in the tumor. Brown and colleagues (BROWN and WORKMAN 1980; BROWN and LEE 1980) showed that such selective exclusion from neural tissues compared to tumors could be achieved with nitroimidazole analogs of MISO with similar electron-affinities but reduced lipophilicities. BROWN and LEE (1980) further showed that although adequate tumor levels could be obtained for drugs of low lipophilicities, radiosensitization was considerably reduced at very low lipophilicity. Subsequent in vivo and in vitro studies identified the drug SR 2508, with an octanol : water partition coefficient of 0.046 (cf MISO, 0.43), as the optimum compound in the series (BROWN et al. 1981). Although nitroimidazoles with partition coefficients less than this were less toxic to mice (and progressively more excluded from neural tissues), their radiosensitizing effectiveness both in vivo and in vitro fell off even faster as a result of a progressive inability to cross the cell membrane and enter the cell (BROWN et al. 1983). SR 2508 was shown both from in vitro and in vivo studies to have the same radiosensitizing efficiency as MISO (BROWN et al. 1981).

Preclinical toxicology studies with SR 2508 in dogs showed that peripheral neuropathy would be the dose-limiting toxicity and suggested that a total dose 6 times higher than MISO would be achievable in multidose studies (BROWN 1984). In addition to this factor of lower toxicity, WHITE et al. (1980) showed that for equal i.v. injected doses, tumor concentrations of SR 2508 at least 2 times higher than those of MISO were achieved in spontaneous tumors of the dog. Thus, it was a reasonable prediction that tumor concentrations of SR 2508 at least 10 times higher than those of MISO would be achievable in the clinic (BROWN 1984).

Phase I trials of SR 2508 have now been completed and have confirmed its lower toxicity than MISO and the fact that peripheral neurotoxicity (with no indication of central neurotoxicity) is the dose-limiting toxicity. However, the factor of 6 predicted from the preclinical studies with dogs was not achieved: the highest non-toxic dose was approximately 36 g/m^2 when given over 6 weeks (N. Coleman, written communication, March, 1985). This is 3 times more than achievable with MISO, and with the approximately two-fold higher tumor concentrations following an i.v. injection (also confirmed in preliminary studies with patients), means that tumor concentrations of SR 2508 5–6 times higher than those obtained with MISO should be achievable clinically.

Phase II/III studies with SR 2508 are now beginning in the U.S. (through the Radiation Therapy Oncology Group) with head and neck cancer, and with cancers of the prostate and bladder. A total dose of 36 g/m² is planned giving the drug 3 times per week (2 g/m² × 18), with the radiotherapy 4–5×/week (N. Coleman, written communication). An SER of approximately 1.6 is to be expected with each of the sensitizer doses (Fig. 1).

2.3.3 Ro 03-8799

SMITHEN et al. (1980) reported the results of their in vitro testing of a large number of (2-nitro-1-imidazolyl) alkanolamines, the majority of which were propanolamines. The reason for the focus on this class of agents were data which showed that the presence of a basic function in the side chain (such as a morpholine, piperidine or pyrrolidine group) capable of being ionized at physiological pH, can lead to an improvement in the radiosensitizing efficiency by approximately an order of magnitude. The authors chose six compounds for further evaluation based on the ratio of drug concentration to produce a given level of radiosensitization versus that to produced a specified level of cytotoxicity in air.

In vivo testing of one of the most promising of these compounds, Ro-03-8799, has been performed using regrowth delay of a transplanted mouse fibrosarcoma as the endpoint (WILLIAMS et al. 1982). On the basis of injected dose it was not found to be superior to MISO. However, when expressed in terms of tumor concentration it was shown to be up to four times more potent than MISO, but only at high doses. At clinically realistic dose levels no significant advantage over MISO was found. Constant infusion or multiple injections of drug to prolong plasma and tumor levels did not improve radiosensitization (HILL et al. 1983). On the basis of promising toxicity testing with rats and monkeys, plus the fact that Ro-03-8799 was shown to be at least as efficient a radiosensitizer in mouse tumors as MISO (WILLIAMS et al. 1982), clinical phase I testing was begun in 1981 (DISCHE et al. 1982).

Toxicity testing of Ro-03-8799 in humans has now been performed (SAUNDERS et al. 1984). A dose of 750 mg/m² appears to be the maximum tolerated single dose, particularly in daily administration, but it should be possible to deliver this at least 20 times. Central neuropathy (not liver damage as predicted by the monkey testing) is the dose-limiting toxicity. Apart from this slightly lower toxicity than MISO (total dose 15 g/m² compared to 12 g/m² for MISO) the principal advantage of the drug which has emerged from clinical testing is the high initial tumor concentration. This is a result of the i.v. injection of a highly polar drug (95% protonated) plus the fact that the tumor is at a lower pH than plasma and concentrates this basic drug. The extent to which Ro-03-8799 is superior to MISO is in some doubt, but it should be of the same order as SR 2508 (i.e. equivalent to tumor concentrations approximately 5 fold greater than MISO) (DISCHE et al. 1986).

2.3.4 RSU 1069

The third new drug of promise, RSU 1069, has been developed by Adams and colleagues (ADAMS et al. 1984). Its promise lies in the fact that it is the first compound which clearly shows superior radiosensitization to MISO in vivo. This appears to be the result of the alkylating aziridine ring on the side chain (Fig. 3). RSU is now in phase I clinical trials, and initial results show that toxicities other than neurotoxicity are likely to be dose limiting. It also appears that this particular drug may be too toxic to be tested further, but there are additional compounds in this alkylating series which appear to be equally efficient as radiosensitizers in vivo but which are significantly less toxic (Adams, G.E., personal communication).

2.3.5 Combining Sensitizers with Glutathione Depletion

Figure 4 shows in diagrammatic form the most widely held hypothesis for the mechanism of sensitization of hypoxic cells by electron-affinic radiosensitizers, including oxygen. It is basically the "oxygen fixation" hypothesis of ALPER (1956) and HOWARD-FLANDERS (1960), later extended by WILLSON and EMMERSON (1970) and by CHAPMAN et al. (1973) to include the mechanism of sensitization by electron-affinic chemicals. In essence the model proposes a competition between reducing species, particularly non-protein sulfhydryls, and oxidizing species (oxygen or electron-affinic sensitizers), for interaction with the free radicals formed in the DNA target molecule. The reaction with sulfhydryls (SH) produces hydrogen donation to the free radical, thereby returning it to its undam-

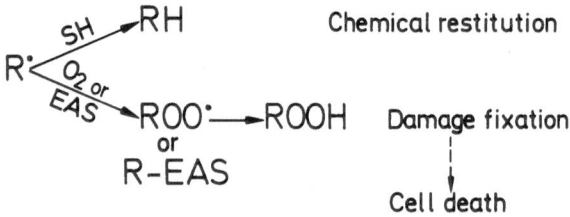

Fig. 4. The "oxygen-fixation" hyotheses for the mechanism of action of oxygen and electron-affinic sensitizers (EAS). R˙ represents the target (DNA) free radical which has arisen from direct or indirect radiation damage to the DNA of the cell, and -SH represents nonprotein sulfhydryl compounds in the cell

aged form. This is "chemical restitution" and would not lead to any cell killing. On the other hand, reaction with an oxidizing species would "fix" (or make permanent) the damage leading to the possibility of cell death.

In terms of this model, the development of improved radiosensitizers can be seen as a method of increasing the amount, or the efficiency, of electron-affinic sensitizers (EAS), thereby "weighting" the competitive reaction towards the damage fixation arm. Viewed in these terms, however, an alternative strategy would also seem feasible; that of reducing the endogenous levels of competing non-protein sulfhydryls. Of these non-protein sulfhydryls, the tripeptide glutathione (GSH) is the most important (MEISTER 1983).

Several depletors of non-protein sulfhydryls have been used to sensitize hypoxic cells, including N-ethylmaleamide (NEM) (BRIDGES 1969) and diamide (HARRIS 1979). However, these have also affected protein sulfhydryls and have been too toxic to be used in vivo. More recently, BUMP et al. (1982) have shown that the agent diethylmaleate (DEM) is a more specific depletor of GSH, and can be given to mice in concentrations sufficient to deplete GSH levels. They showed, moreover, that GSH depletion could increase the radiosensitizing efficiency of MISO both in vitro and in vivo. Fig. 5 shows their data for CHO cells in vitro.

An even more promising drug for clinical use is the specific inhibitor of γ-glutamyl cysteine synthetase, buthionine-SR-sulfoximine (BSO) developed by GRIFFITH and MEISTER (1979). HODGKISS and MIDDLETON (1983) showed that V79 cells treated with BSO so as to partially deplete their GSH levels were more sensitive to MISO radiosensitization, and BROWN (1984) and YU and BROWN (1984) have demonstrated similar effects with mouse tumors in vivo with combinations of DEM and BSO sufficient to deplete GSH levels to less than 10% of normal. However, although BSO is a drug of very low toxicity in the mouse, and repeated daily injections can be given which deplete GSH levels without toxicity (YU and BROWN 1984), the same is not true of DEM. Thus, it is unrealistic to assume that tumor GSH levels as low as 10% of controls (obtainable with DEM + BSO) will be achievable in patients each day throughout a course of radiotherapy. It is more realistic to expect that tumor levels of GSH will be obtained which are 20–50% of controls. Such levels are achievable on a daily basis in mice with non-toxic levels of BSO alone (MINCHINGTON et al. 1984; YU and BROWN 1984). Although it has yet

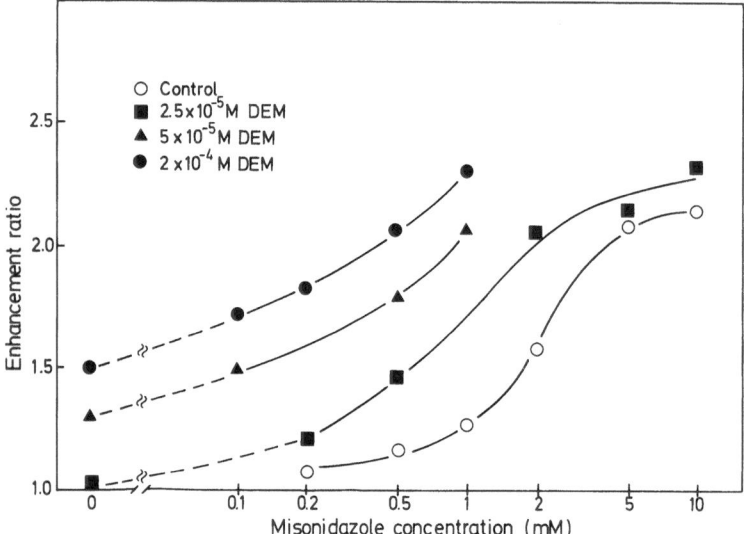

Fig. 5. Effect of glutathione depletion by diethylmaleate (DEM) on ability of MISO to radiosensitize hypoxic Chinese hamster ovary (CHO) cells. The CHO cells were incubated for 1 hr at 25° C under hypoxic conditions prior to irradiation with the various DEM concentrations with various concentrations of MISO. Glutathione levels for the above curves were (from right to left): 100%, 35%, 20%, and 5% of control values. (From BUMP et al. (1982) with permission)

to be demonstrated that depletion of GSH by BSO to these moderate levels will produce a significant increase in the efficiency of either of the two radiosensitizers likely to be used clinically – SR 2508 and Ro 03 8799 –, we might expect an increased sensitizer efficiency in the range of 2–5 using DEM and MISO as the model (Fig. 5).

This would be a significant gain *provided* there was not an increase (or, at least, a comparable increase) in the toxicity of the radiosensitizers. Although animal experiments with daily BSO and MISO doses have shown little or no increase in the toxicity of MISO (YU and BROWN 1984) this does not guarantee no enhanced toxicity in the patient since there is reason to suspect that even chronic toxicity studies in the mouse are not predictive of clinical neuropathy (COLEMAN et al. 1984). Nonetheless, this is a promising approach, and preclinical toxicology testing of BSO is presently being performed by the U.S. National Cancer Institute (T. Strike, personal communication, 1985).

3 Halogenated Pyrimidine Analogs

3.1 Experimental Studies

The halogenated thymidine analogs 5-bromodeoxyuridine (BUdR) and 5-iododeoxuridine (IUdR) have long been known to be radiosensitizers of bacterial and mammalian cells in vitro (DJORDJEVIC and SZYBALSKI 1960; GREER 1960). Unlike the nitroimidazole radiosensitizers, which act essentially instantaneously once they enter the cell, the halogenated pyrimidine analogs require extended contact with the cells prior to irradiation because of the requirement for their incorporation into the DNA (which occurs only in those cells undergoing DNA synthesis). Although the precise mechanism for radiosensitization is not known, it is clear that incorporation into the DNA is required (ERICKSON and SZYBALSKI 1963). The basis for a differential radiosensitization of malignant cells compared to normal cells is a more rapid proliferation rate of the tumor cells compared to the dose-limiting normal cells adjacent to the tumor. It is reasonable to suppose that such situations would occur for tumors in the brain, liver and lung, or indeed in any tissue the dose to which is limited by late, rather than early, effects.

The principal effect of incorporation of the pyrimide analogs is on the slope of the radiation survival curve, although a reduction in the

shoulder (or extrapolation number, n) has also been reported, particularly for the higher drug concentrations (ERICKSON and SZYBALSKI 1963; MOHLER and ELKIND 1963). Although careful studies at low radiation doses have yet to be performed, there is no suggestion in the data obtained to date that the extent of radiosensitization would be reduced at low doses: indeed if n were reduced, the sensitizer enhancement ratio would be greater at low radiation doses than at high doses. Greater radiosensitization would also be expected for fractionated than for single doses providing the pyrimidine analog were infused throughout the course of therapy (BROWN and ELLIS 1969). This would be particularly true if any recruitment of non-proliferating clonogenic cells or acceleration of proliferation occurred during the treatment regime.

Following these in vitro studies several authors attempted to radiosensitize tumors in vivo. SUIT et al. (1970) found a significant enhancement of the radiosensitivity of a transplanted mammary tumor in mice following multiple injections of IUdR (which in themselves were not cytotoxic to the tumors cells). This radiosensitization occurred for tumors irradiated under hypoxic conditions or with the animals breathing hyperbaric oxygen. In early experiments of our own (BROWN et al. 1971), the radiosensitizer bromodeoxycytidine BCdR (which is rapidly deaminated in plasma to BUdR) was infused intra-arterially in mice during a multifraction course of 10 daily radiation doses. We found an enhanced tumor response (SER = 1.3) for the multifraction regime with no significant radiosensitization of the skin over the mouse foot: i.e. a therapeutic gain comparing this tumor with the skin as the normal tissue. We were also able to demonstrate radiosensitization of the glioma SK-26 implanted in the mouse brain with continuous intra-carotid artery infusion of BCdR during fractionated radiotherapy (GOFFINET et al. 1972).

At that time it was believed that the rapid dehalogenation of the pyrimidine analogs by the kidney in rodents and man (KRISS and REVESZ 1962; KRISS et al. 1963) necessitated the use of intra-arterial infusion in order to deliver the drug to the tumor before it could pass through the liver. Consequently the two early clinical trials both used intra-arterial infusions (BAGSHAW et al. 1967; HOSHINO and SANO 1969). However, in some more recent experiments we found that radiosensitization of the EMT-6 mouse tumor by intravenously infused BUdR was not affected by blocking dehalogenation by the liver, and that the only advantage (though this can be considerable) of intra-

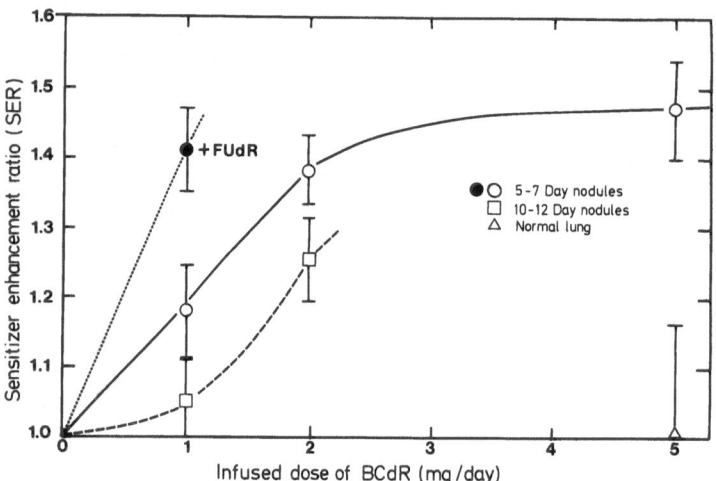

Fig. 6. Sensitizer enhancement ratios obtained from full radiation survival curves of EMT6 tumor cells growing as pulmonary nodules in Balb/c mice. The mice were infused for 2 days prior to irradiation of the cells with various doses of BCdR or with saline. The tumor cells were either in exponential growth in the lungs (5–7 days old nodules) or had experienced a slowing of growth (10–12 day old nodules). In one group FUdR (0.5 μg/day) was added to the BCdR infusion. Radiosensitization of normal lung was assayed by determining the effect of BCdR infusion on the $LD_{50/160}$ of thorax-irradiated mice. (Data from BROWN 1975, 1977)

arterial infusion is the higher local concentrations achievable (GOFFINET and BROWN 1977). A second stimulus to the clinical use of intravenous rather than intra-arterial pyrimidine analogs was the findings that the pharmacokinetics of thymidine (ENSMINGER and FRIE 1978) and the halogenated thymidine analog FUdR (COLLINS et al. 1980) showed a non-linear profile of drug concentration at higher intravenous infusion rates. This demonstrated that the metabolic pathways for these drugs could be saturated, thereby allowing higher blood levels to be obtained during infusion.

Nonetheless, intra-arterial infusion has the major advantage of delivering high local drug concentrations to the tumor and the high rate of uptake on the first pass means greater radiosensitization is achieved in the infused tissue compared to tissue supplied by the systemic circulation. This was clearly seen in the normal tissues sensitized by carotid artery infusion in the clinical studies of BAGSHAW et al. (1967). However, there is one situation in which the equivalent of intra-arterial infusion should be achievable with intravenous infusion. This is the case of pulmonary metastases which, according to the elegant studies of MILNE et al. (1969), have a blood supply from the pulmonary system. Thus the first capillary bed reached by drugs infused intravenously is that of the lungs and any pulmonary metastases.

We have attempted to exploit this situation by infusing BCdR intravenously into mice bearing lung metastases and assaying the response of the tumor cells by irradiating in vitro known dilutions of the disaggregated lung containing the nodules following 2 days of infusion (BROWN 1975, 1977). Survival curves of the tumor cells can be obtained

in this way with no influence of the lung cells on the plating efficiency of the tumor cells (BROWN 1977). Fig. 6 shows a summary of the data. All the infusions produced dose-modifying radiosensitization (no change in the extrapolation number) so the SER was independent of dose. The effect of the highest infused dose (5 mg/kg/day) on the radiosensitivity of normal lung parenchyma was tested by determining the LD_{50} of thorax-irradiated (non tumor-bearing) mice at 160 days after irradiation. The values obtained (with 95% confidence intervals) were 13.5 (12.2–15.0) Gy and 13.6 (12.0–15.4) Gy in saline infused and BCdR infused mice respectively. In other words, there was no significant radiosensitization of the normal tissue. This would therefore appear to offer the possibility of clinical exploitation.

3.2 Clinical Studies

Based on the early experimental studies, two clinical trials were conducted during the mid-1960's combining conventional radiotherapy with selective intra-arterial infusion of BUdR. In a non-randomized study of primary brain tumors HOSHINO and SATO (1969) reported an apparent improvement in survival compared to historical controls in approximately 200 patients with brain tumors, of whom half had high-grade gliomas. They reported little local or systemic toxicity, suggesting a therapeutic gain.

On the other hand, in a smaller but randomized prospective clinical trial of patients with advanced head and neck cancer BAGSHAW et al. (1967) reported no benefit of comparing intra-arterial BUdR and concomitant irradiation with radiation alone. However, they did find a marked increase in the reactions of the normal tissue (buccal mucosa and tongue) in the side infused with BUdR. This necessitated a reduction in the total dose delivered. In retrospect it is clear that this is not the ideal site for BUdR studies: not only is the buccal mucosa a normal tissue with a relatively rapid proliferation rate, it is also likely that it will accelerate its proliferation rate during a course of therapy (DENEKAMP 1973). However, this negative result discouraged further clinical use of pyrimidine analog radiosensitizers for approximately 15 years.

Quite recently renewed clinical interest in pyrimidine analogs has developed. At the U.S. National Cancer Institute a phase I/II study of intermittent intravenous BUdR and concomitant conventional fractionated radiation is underway for patients with glioblastoma multiforme (KINSELLA et al. 1984). The rationale for selective tumor radiosensitization is the expectation that the proliferation rate of the glioblastoma cells will be substantially greater than that of the dose limiting normal cells in the surrounding brain. The intermittent infusion rate (12 hours/day for 14 days and repeated with a 10–14 day interruption between the two infusion periods) was chosen to limit systemic toxicity. Bone marrow suppression, especially thrombocytopenia was the primary dose-limiting toxicity, and the maximum tolerable dose of BUdR was found to be 650–700 mg/m^2/12 hrs when given over 14 days. A secondary but significant toxicity of dry desquamation and scaling of palms and soles has also been seen. This is probably the result of photosensitization by BUdR, and may be preventable by using IUdR rather than BUdR as the sensitizer (MITCHELL et al. 1984).

The authors of this clinical study have been able to demonstrate that the blood levels of the infused BUdR are sufficient to produce substantial radiosensitization of proliferating cells in the patients. This was done by comparing the radiation survival curves of bone marrow colony-forming units taken from the patients before and after the 14 days of infusion (MITCHELL et al. 1983). Sensitizer enhancement ratios, calculated by dividing the pretreatment D_0 by the post-treatment D_0 ranged from 1.0 to 2.2, with a trend of increasing radiosensitization with increasing BUdR dose (Fig. 7). Although it is unlikely that such large SER's will be obtained for the glioblastoma cells, such data promise a real therapeutic gain for this procedure.

A similar study is also currently underway at the University of California at San Francisco (T.

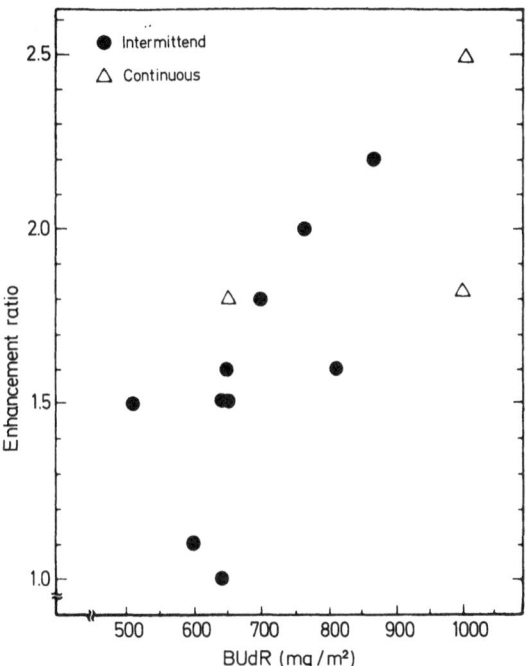

Fig. 7. Radiation enhancement ratios of human bone marrow CFUC (D_0 preinfusion/D_0 postinfusion) as a function of BUdR infused dose. Ten patients received a 2 week infusion of BUdR as an intermittent infusion (12 hours/day) while 3 patients (triangles) received a continuous (24 hours/day) two week infusion. (From KINSELLA et al. 1984 (Int. J. Radiat. Oncol. Biol. Phys. *10*:1399–1406) with permission)

Phillips, personal communication). In this trial a 24 hour continuous infusion for 4 days followed by a 3 day break and then repetition of the cycle until toxicity ensues is being used. As in the National Cancer Institute study, bone marrow suppression and skin toxicity are dose-limiting.

3.3 Future Prospects

It seems reasonable to conclude from the experimental and clinical studies conducted so far that the clinical possibilities of pyrimidine analog infusion to enhance conventional radiotherapy have not been fully explored. There seems to be no reason why therapeutic gains in a number of sites will not be realizable. In particular i.v. infusion with localized or whole lung irradiation for pulmonary metastases would seem to be worthwhile. In addition, technical developments in infusion pumps, an HPLC assay for BUdR levels (RUSSO et al. 1984) and the development of monoclonal antibodies to identify cells with incorporated BUdR and IUdR (MORSTYN et al. 1983), will simplify future trials as well as allowing greater sophistication in patient monitoring than previously.

Nonetheless, selective radiosensitization with the pyrimidine analogs used to date relies entirely on a greater proliferation rate of tumor cells than the cells of the surrounding dose-limiting normal tissue. Although these compounds may therefore be of potential use wherever late effects limit the radiation dose, it would obviously be of great help to find an additional method of selective incorporation into the tumor cells.

A possible approach to obtaining selective radiosensitization without relying on differential proliferation rates has recently been suggested by Perez et al. (1984). These investigations have used 5-chlorodeoxycytine (CldC) with tetrahydrouridine (H_4U), the latter to prevent plasma deamination by cytidine deaminase to chlorodeoxyuridine before DNA incorporation. They propose that the CldC will then be incorporated into DNA in the following manner: $CldC \xrightarrow{1} CldCMP \xrightarrow{2} CldUMP \xrightarrow{3} CldUTP \xrightarrow{4} DNA$ (with the enzymes as follows: 1-deoxycytidine kinase, 2-deoxycytidylate deaminase, 3-thymidylate kinase and 4-DNA polymerase). They suggest that all of these enzymes are elevated in many malignant tumors, especially deoxycytidylate deaminase which is reported to be elevated 20 to 80-fold over that of equivalent normal tissues (Giusti et al. 1970). In their experimental studies Perez et al. (1984) have found significant enhancement of the radiosensitivity of HEp-2 cells in vitro with CldC + H_4U particularly when combined with inhibitors of the *de novo* pathway of pyrimidine biosynthesis.

However, in experiments of our own (Russell et al. 1986), we have not been able to demonstrate any significant advantage of CldC over BUdR in sensitizing the RIF-1 tumor in vivo to radiation following a 72 hour infusion period of the two drugs at equitoxic levels. Nonetheless, this approach, based on potential differences in enzyme levels between normal and tumor cells is worthy of further exploration, and could add significantly to the potential use of these drugs in clinical radiotherapy.

4 Inhibitors of Potentially Lethal Damage Repair

4.1 Introduction

Potential lethal damage (PLD) was first discovered and defined by Phillips and Tolmach (1966). They found that the survival of cells could be either increased or decreased by changing the postirradiation conditions of the cells. Repair of PLDR is said to occur when the postirradiation conditions are such that damage that would normally have been lethal to the cell is repaired. Inhibition of protein synthesis in HeLa cells by cycloheximide was the first condition noted to induce PLDR (Phillips and Tolmach 1966). Other conditions reported to facilitate PLDR in cells in vitro include exposure to low temperature (Whitmore et al. 1970), incubation in balanced salt solution (Belli and Shelton 1969), and culture in a density-inhibited (plateau-phase) state after irradiation prior to subculture at low density (Little 1969; Hahn and Little 1972). All of these conditions are associated with a slowing down or inhibition of the normal progression of cells through their life cycle.

Because tumors are known to contain a large proportion of nondividing or slowly dividing cells, it has been suggested that plateau-phase cultures may be an appropriate in vitro model for the tumors with respect to response to radiation damage (Hahn and Little 1972). PLDR was first clearly demonstrated in tumors by Little et al. 1973 and Hahn et al. 1974. They showed that in the EMT6 and NCTC tumors, cell survival increased when excision of the tumors was delayed up to 24 hours after radiation. Subsequently, other authors have demonstrated a similar phenomenon of PLDR in some, but not all, animal tumors (Shipley et al. 1975; Rasey and Nelson 1981, 1983; McNally and DeRonde 1980) and in human tumors in nude mice (Guichard et al. 1984). Although it remains to be demonstrated that PLDR occurs in tumors in humans following irradiation, there is no reason to suppose that it does not.

Evidence for the possible importance of PLDR in affecting the response of human tumors is the reported correlation between the radiocurability of human tumors and the ability of cell lines derived from these tumors to undergo PLDR (Weichselbaum et al. 1980; Guichard et al. 1984). These authors found that in density-inhibited stationary phase (plateau) cultures, the extent of PLDR was greatest in radioincurable tumors (osteosarcoma, melanoma, glioblastoma) and least in radiocurable tumors (neuroblastoma, breast carcinoma). Weichselbaum and Little (1982) have also shown that this difference is seen with low dose per fraction daily irradiations. They measured PLDR after fractionated radiation in plateau-phase cultures of two human cell lines derived from tumors of different radiocurabilities (melanoma and breast). Although the radiation-survival parameters of these cells in exponential growth were similar, the PLDR after fractionated treatment of the plateau cultures with four doses of 125 to 175 rads conferred significant radioresistance on the melanoma cells but not on the breast cancer cells, giving a slope of the multifraction cell survival curve (D_0) almost five times greater for the melanoma than for the breast cells.

Caution has to be exercised in extrapolating these results to the clinical situation however. First, it is possible that differences in radiocurability between tumor types *may* be related to differences in PLDR as determined in vitro, but this does not mean that the radiosensitivity of the tumors of individual patients will be predictable from PLDR measurements. In this regard, WEICHSELBAUM et al. (1984) has failed to find a correlation between the PLDR of early passage cells in vitro and the radiation response of the head and neck cancers from which the cell lines were derived. Second, it is not clear that PLDR measured in vitro in density inhibited cultures is the same as, or correlates with, that measured in vivo by delaying removal of the tumor before assaying for surviving fraction. For example, RASEY and NELSON (1983) found that RIF-1 tumor cells exhibited a large degree of PLDR in vitro, but little or none in vivo.

Nonetheless, these problems could be the result of our as yet crude methods of measuring potentially lethal damage and its repair in vitro, and particularly in vivo. There is no doubt that repair of radiation damage in mammalian cells is extensive and is probably the most important factor governing tumor cell survival during fractionated radiotherapy. It therefore remains a viable (and testable) hypothesis that failure to cure some human tumors by radiotherapy is a result of their repair of PLD, and inhibitors of such repair may be able to preferentially sensitize these resistant tumors.

4.2 Inhibition of PLDR as a Clinical Strategy

The rationale for inhibition of PLDR as a clinical strategy has to be based on a differential response of normal and malignant tissue. However, it does not depend on the assumption that normal cells do not repair PLDR – this would be an unreasonable assumption, and has in any case been contradicted, at least in vitro, by studies of normal human fibroblasts (MINARIK et al. 1985). Nor does it depend on the assumption tumor cells exhibit

greater repair of PLDR than normal cells. Its rationale is based on the assumption that in tumors and normal tissues alike there will be a range of PLDR, and that there will be circumstances – for example, with a radioresistant tumor in a radiosensitive normal tissue – in which inhibition of repair of PLDR will radiosensitize the tumor to a greater extent than the surrounding dose-limiting normal tissue.

4.3 Compounds That Inhibit PLDR

Although as yet unproven, a reasonable working hypothesis is that PLDR results from molecular processes involved in the repair of DNA damage postirradiation. This is supported by the findings that fibroblasts taken from patients suffering from the autosomal recessive disease, ataxia telangiectasia, which show a defect in the repair of γ-irradiation-induced DNA damage (PATERSON et al. 1976), also exhibit deficient recovery from PLD produced by ionizing radiation (WEICHSELBAUM et al. 1978). There has also been shown to be an excellent correlation between the time course of PLDR and both the rejoining of chromosome breaks (CORNFORTH and BEDFORD 1983), and the repair of DNA strand breaks (VAN ANKEREN and WHEELER 1984).

Based on the above findings, it would be predicted that agents which interfere with DNA synthesis and/or DNA repair would also interfere with PLDR. This has been found to be the case with such agents as actinomycin-D (DRITSCHILO et al. 1979), β-arabinofuranosyladenine (β-ara A) (ILIAKIS 1980), cordycepin (NAKATSUGAWA and SUGAHARA 1980), and other purine nucleoside analogs (NAKATSUGAWA et al. 1982a). However, inhibition of DNA synthesis *per se* does not prevent PLDR, as is indicated by the fact that concentrations of the drug aphidicolin sufficient to completely inhibit DNA synthesis by specifically inhibiting DNA polymerase α, are ineffective at reducing PLDR in the same cell line (ILIAKIS et al. 1982).

Two other classes of agents reported to inhibit PLDR, at least in some systems, are (a) the methylxanthine caffeine, an inhibitor of post-replication repair (NAKATSUGAWA and SUGAHARA 1980), and (b) such energy depletors as 2'-deoxy-d-glucose, which has been reported to inhibit PLDR in yeast (JAIN et al. 1977), and lonidamine, which has been shown to inhibit PLDR at nontoxic concentrations in CHO HA-1 cells (HAHN et al. 1984).

The close involvement of DNA repair with PLDR suggested by the above studies indicates that other inhibitors of DNA repair may be effective in inhibiting PLDR, and it has been shown recently that inhibitors of the chromosomal enzyme poly(ADP-ribose) polymerase are capable of inhibiting PLDR in cells in vitro (BEN-HUR et al. 1984; BROWN et al. 1984).

An unexpected finding – first noted in vivo and then in vitro – is the fact that the hypoxic cell radiosensitizers MISO and SR 2508 also inhibit repair of PLD (BROWN et al. 1984; GUICHARD et al. 1979; GUICHARD and MALAISE 1983; SAKAMOTO and ARITAKE 1981). This is an interesting phenomenon and is far from being understood. However, it would appear from the results of Guichard and colleague that the radiosensitizing effect of these drugs, at least for some tumors, may be a combination of hypoxic cell radiosensitization and PLDR inhibition. Moreover, they noted full PLDR inhibition at the relatively low dose of 100 mg/kg, which would produce tumor concentrations achievable in humans in the forthcoming trials with SR 2508.

Apart from these investigations with MISO and SR 2508, the only other in vivo studies with PLDR inhibitors have been with the purine nucleoside analogs, which reportedly enhanced the effects of radiation on the EMT6 and RIF-1 tumors in mice (NAKATSUGAWA et al. 1982b). However, although these studies have shown that the compounds are effective when given after irradiation, it is not clear that their mechanism of action was through inhibition of PLDR. Further work is urgently needed on the in vivo effects of these inhibitors, on both a variety of tumors and normal tissues. Clearly this is a promising field for future clinical application and is – like the field of hypoxic cell radiosensitizers – an excellent area for collaboration between biologists, chemists and, ultimately, clinicians.

5 Summary

The principle that radiation sensitizers can be used to differentially affect the radiosensitivity of normal versus malignant tissues in animals is established. This chapter reviews the experimental and clinical data and future prospects for three classes of radiosensitizers: hypoxic cell radiosensitizers, halogenated pyrimidine analogs and inhibitors of potentially lethal damage repair (PLDR).

The most effective of these sensitizers, at least with single large doses of radiation, are hypoxic cell radiosensitizers. These have been developed and improved in the laboratory and the most widely used drug, misonidazole (MISO), has undergone extensive clinical trials with radiation. However, despite some suggestive improvements in several of the trials with head and neck tumors, there have been no significant increases in local control using this drug. This has led some to conclude that hypoxic cells might not be important in clinical radiotherapy and hence that radiosensitizers may not have a role in the clinic. However, it can be demonstrated that little or no radiosensitization would be *expected* at the clinically achievable dose levels of MISO. Thus, a major effort has been underway to develop more efficient, less toxic radiosensitizers of hypoxic cells. Several of these are now available for clinical trials and phase I testing has already shown them to be significantly superior to MISO. Nonetheless, further improvements in the design of hypoxic cell sensitizers are necessary before a drug is available which can radiosensitize the hypoxic cells in the tumor to the maximum extent possible. One method for improving these new drugs still further is the commitant use of the sensitizer with a depletor of intracellular glutathione, a tripeptide which makes up more than 95% of the non-protein sulfhydryls in the cell. Gluthathione competes with the exogenous sensitizer, so that its depletion enhances the effectiveness of the sensitizer. Buthionine sulfoximine (BSO) appears to be a powerful and non-toxic agent for achieving glutathione depletion in vivo.

The halogenated pyrimidine analogs bromodeoxyuridine (BUdR) and iododeoxyuridine (IUdR) have been known since 1960 to be radiosensitizers if incorporated into DNA. Animal experiments have shown that they are capable of producing differential radiosensitization of tumors compared to normal tissues if infused either intra-arterially, or intravenously, before single doses or during a course of fractionated radiation. Despite this early promise, interest waned in the use of these compounds principally because of the perceived need to deliver them intra-arterially and because the one early randomized clinical trial (on head and neck cancers) reported no benefit. This Stanford study, however, did note a marked enhancement of normal tissue reactions, and it is now clear that this site is not suitable for pyrimidine analog sensitizers since these agents depend on a much slower rate of normal tissue proliferation than that of the tumor (a condition which does not hold in this site). However, interest has recently been rekindled and studies are presently underway of BUdR (and IUdR) infused intravenously with concomitant conventional radiotherapy of glioblastomas. Substantial radiosensitization in proliferating bone marrow cells has been demonstrated in patients, proving that the systemic drug levels are high enough to achieve a therapeutic gain. Further studies in other sites, particularly with pulmonary metastases, would seem warranted.

Finally, the phenomenon of repair of potentially lethal damage (PLD) after radiation is discussed. There is evidence that this could contribute to the radioresistance of human tumors. Based on this, a rationale can be developed for the use of an inhibitor of PLDR combined with radiotherapy of a radioresistant tumor surrounded by a relatively radiosensitive normal tissue (assuming the sensitivity of the latter is a result of lower PLDR than for the tumor). Several classes of inhibitors of PLDR are known; most either interfere with DNA synthesis or with its repair. It also appears that (for entirely unknown reasons) the hypoxic cell radiosensitizers misonidazole and SR 2508 are capable of inhibiting PLDR after radiation both in vivo and in vitro. In addition to this class, several purine nucleoside analogs have also been used in vivo and enhance the effect of radiation and some chemotherapeutic drugs on mouse tumors. More work and more drug development is probably required before the most effective clinical trials of these agents can be mounted. Nonetheless, they represent a very promising class of potentially selective tumor radiosensitizing agents.

References

Adams GE, Ahmed I, Sheldon PW, Stratford IJ (1984) Radiation sensitization and chemopotentiation: RSU 1069, a compound more efficient than misonidazole in vitro and in vito. Br J Cancer 49:571–577

Alper T (1956) The modification of damage caused by primary ionization of biological targets. Radiat Res 5:573–586

Bagshaw MA, Doggett RLS, Smith KC, Kaplan HS, Nelsen TS (1967) Intra-arterial 5-bromodeoxyuridine and X-ray therapy. Radiology 99:886–894

Belli JA, Shelton M (1969) Potentially lethal radiation damage: repair by mammalian cells in culture. Science 165:490–492

Ben-Hur E, Utsumi H, Elkind MM (1984) Inhibitors of poly (ADP-ribose) synthesis enhance X-ray killing of log-phase Chinese hamster cells. Radiat Res 97:546–555

Bridges BA (1969) Sensitization of organisms to radiation by sulphydryl-binding agents. In: Advances in Radiation Biology, vol 3. Academic Press, New York, pp 123–187

Brown DM, Dionet C, Brown JM (1984) Inhibition of X-ray-induced potentially lethal damage (PLD) repair in aerobic plateau-phase Chinese hamster cells by misonidazole. Radiat Res 97:162–170

Brown DM, Evans JW, Brown JM (1984) The influence of inhibitors of poly (ADP-ribose) polymerase on X-ray-induced potentially lethal damage repair. Br J Cancer 49, Suppl VI:49–53

Brown DM, Gonzales-Mendez R, Brown JM (1983) Factors influencing intracellular uptake and radiosensitization by 2-nitroimidazoles in vitro. Radiat Res 93:492–505

Brown JM (1975) Exploitation of kinetic differences between normal and malignant cells. Radiology 114:189–197

Brown JM (1977) Effects of radiation and chemotherapeutic agents on the incidence and treatment of blood-borne metastases. Gann Monograph on Cancer Research 20:207–225

Brown JM (1979) Evidence for acutely hypoxic cells in mouse tumours, and a possible mechanism of reoxygenation. Br J Radiol 52:650–656

Brown JM (1984) Clinical trials of radiosensitizers: What should we expect? Int J Radiat Oncol Biol Phys 10:425–429

Brown JM (1984) Radiosensitizers and radioprotectors: Current status, and future prospects. In: Broerse JJ, Barendsen GW, Kal HB, Van der Kogel AJ (eds) Proceedings of 7th International Congress of Radiation Research Reviews and Summaries, pp 281–289. Martinus Nijhoff, Amsterdam

Brown JM, Ellis F (1969) Use of pyrimidine analogues in radiotherapy (letter to editor). Br J Radiol 42:155–157

Brown JM, Goffinet DR, Cleaver JE, Kallman RF (1971) Preferential radiosensitization of mouse sarcoma relative to normal skin by chronic intra-arterial infusion of halogenated pyrimidine analogs. J Nat Cancer Inst 47:75–89

Brown JM, Lee WW (1980) Pharmacokinetic considerations in radiosensitizer development. In: Brady LW (ed) Radiation Sensitizers: Their Use in the Clinical Management of Cancer. Masson: New York, pp 2–13

Brown JM, Workman P (1980) Partition coefficient as a guide to the development of radiosensitizers which are less toxic than misonidazole. Radiat Res 82:171–190

Brown JM, Yu NY, Brown DM, Lee WW (1981) SR-2508: A 2-nitroimidazole amide which should be superior to misonidazole as a radiosensitizer for clinical use. Int J Radiat Oncol Biol Phys 7:695–703

Bump EA, Yu NY, Brown JM (1982) Radiosensitization of hypoxic tumor cells by depletion of intracellular glutathione. Science 217:544–545

Bush RS, Jenkin RDT, Allt WEC, Beale FA, Bean H, Dembo AJ, Pringle JF (1978) Definitive evidence for hypoxic cells influencing cure in cancer therapy. Br J Cancer 37, Suppl III:302–306

Cade IS, McEwen JB, Dische S, Saunders MI, Watson ER, Halnan KE, Wiernik G, Perrins DJD, Sutherland I (1978) Hyperbaric oxygen and radiotherapy: a Medical Research Council trial in carcinoma of the bladder. Br J Radiol 51:876–878

Chapman JD, Reuvers AP, Borsa J, Greenstock CL (1973) Chemical radioprotection and radiosensitization of mammalian cells growing in vitro. Radiat Res 56:291–306

Coleman CN, Hirst VK, Brown DM, Halsey J (1984) The effect of vitamin B$_6$ on the neurotoxicity and pharmacology of desmethylmisonidazole and misonidazole: Clinical and laboratory studies. Int J Radiat Oncol Biol Phys 10:1381–1386

Collins JM, Dedrick RL, King FG, Speyer JL, Myers CD (1980) Non-linear pharmacokinetic models for 5-fluorouracil in man: Intravenous and intraperitoneal routes. Clin Pharmac Ther 28:235–246

Cornforth MN, Bedford JS (1983) X-ray induced breakage and rejoining of human interphase chromosomes. Science 222:1141–1143

Crabtree HG, Cramer W (1933) The action of radium on cancer cells II Some factors determining the susceptibility of cancer cells to radium. Proc Roy Soc B 113:238–250

Denekamp J (1973) Changes in the rate of repopulation during multi-fraction irradiation of mouse skin. Br J Radiol 46:381–387

Denekamp J (1983) Does physiological hypoxia matter in cancer therapy? In: Steel GG, Adams GE, Peckham MJ (eds) The Biological Basis of Radiotherapy. Elsevier: Amsterdam, pp 139–155

Dische S (1983) Clinical trials with hypoxic cell sensitizers – the European experience. In: Mirand EA, Hutchinson WB, Mihich E (eds) Proceedings of the 13th International Cancer Congress, Part D: Research and Treatment. Alan R Liss Inc: New York, pp 293–303

Dische S (1984) Randomized controlled clinical trials of the chemical sensitizer for hypoxic cells – misonidazole. Radiosensitization Newsletter 3:No 4,5

Dische S, Anderson PJ, Sealy R, Watson ER (1983) Carcinoma of the cervix – anaemia, radiotherapy and hyperbaric oxygen. Br J Radiol 56:251–255

Dische S, Saunders MI, Anderson P, Stratford MRL, Minchington AI (1982) Clinical experience with nitroimidazoles as radiosensitizers. Int J Radiat Oncol Biol Phys 8:335–338

Dische S, Saunders MI, Anderson P, Urtasun RC, Karcher KH, Kogelnik HD, Bleehen N, Phillips TL, Wasserman TH (1978) Neurotoxicity of misonidazole – pooling of data from 5 centers. Br J Radiol 51:1023–1024

Dische S, Saunders MI, Dunphy EP, Bennet MH, des Rochers C, Stratford MRL, Minchington A (1986) Concentrations achieved in human tumors after administration of misonidazole, SR 2508 and Ro 03-8799. Int J Radiat Oncol Biol Phys 12:1109–1111

Djordjevic B, Szybalski W (1960) Genetics of human cell lines III Incorporation of 5-bromo and 5-iododeoxyuridine into the deoxyribonucleic acid of human cells and its effect of radiation sensitivity. J Exp Med 112:509–531

Dritschilo A, Piro A, Belli JA (1979) Interaction between radiation of drug damage in mammalian cells III The effect of Adriamycin and actinomycin-D on the repair of potentially lethal radiation damage. Int J Radiat Biol 35:549–560

Ensminger WD, Frie E (1978) High-dose intravenous and hepatic artery infusions of thymidine. Clin Pharmac Ther 24:610–615

Erickson RL, Szybalski W (1963) Molecular radiobiology of human cell lines V Comparative radiosensitizing properties of 5-halodeoxycytidines and 5-halodeoxyuridines. Radiat Res 20:252–262

Giusti G, Mangoni C, De Petrocellis B, Scarano E (1970) Deoxycytidine deaminase in normal and neoplastic human tissues. Enzym Biol Clin 11:375–383

Goffinet DR, Brown JM (1977) Comparison of intravenous and intra-arterial pyrimidine infusion as a means of radiosensitizing tumors in vivo. Radiology 124:819–822

Goffinet DR, Brown JM, Bagshaw MA, Kaplan HS (1972) Prolonged carotid arterial radiosensitizer infusion and radiation therapy of mouse gliomas. Am J Roentgenol 114:7–15

Guichard M, Weichselbaum RR, Little JB, Malaise EP (1984) Potentially lethal damage repair as a possible determinant of human tumor radiosensitivity. Radiother and Oncol 1:263–269

Gray LH, Conger AD, Ebert M, Hornsey S, Scott OCA (1953) The concentration of oxygen dissolved in tissues at the time of irradiation as a factor in radiotherapy. Br J Radiol 26:638–648

Grdina DJ, Thames HD, Milas L (1984) Tumor sensitizing effect by misonidazole in a clinically relevant radiation dose range. Int J Radiat Oncol Biol Phys 10:379–385

Greer S (1960) Studies on ultraviolet irradiation of Escherichia coli containing 5-bromouracil in its DNA. J Gen Micro 22:618–634, 1960

Griffith OW, Meister A (1979) Potent and specific inhibition of glutathione synthesis by buthionine sulfoximine (S-n-Butylhomocysteine Sulphoximine). J Biol Chem 254:7558–7560

Guichard M, de Langen-Omri F, Malaise E-P (1979) Influence of misonidazole on the radiosensitivity of a human melanoma in nude mice: Time-dependent increase in surviving fraction. Int J Radiat Oncol Biol Phys 5:487–489

Guichard M, Malaise EP (1983) Radiosensitizing effects of misonidazole and SR 2508 on a human melanoma transplanted in nude mice: Influence on repair of potentially lethal damage. Int J Radiat Oncol Biol Phys 8:465–468

Hahn GM, Little JB (1972) Plateau-phase cultures of mammalian cells: An in vitro model for human cancer. Curr Top Radiat Res Q 8:39–83

Hahn GM, Rockwell S, Kallman RF, Gordon LF, Frindel E (1974) Repair of potentially lethal damage in vivo in solid tumor cells after x-irradiation. Cancer Res 34:352–354

Hahn GM, Van Kersen I, Silvestrini B (1984) Inhibition of recovery from potentially lethal damage by lonidamine. Br J Cancer 50:657–660

Harris JN (1979) Mammalian cell studies with diamide. Pharmac Ther 1:375–384

Hill SA, Fowler JF, Minchinton AI, Stratford MRL, Denekamp J (1983) Radiosensitization of a mouse tumour by Ro 03-8799: Acute and protracted administration. Int J Radiat Biol 44:143–150

Hill RP (1986) Sensitizers and radiation dose fractionation: Results and interpretation. Int J Radiat Oncol Biol Phys 12:1049–1054

Hodgkiss RJ, Middleton RW (1983) Enhancement of misonidazole radiosensitization by an inhibitor of glutathione biosynthesis. Int J Radiat Oncol Biol Phys 43:179–183

Hoshino T, Sano K (1969) Radiosensitization of malignant brain tumors with bromouridine (thymidine analog). ACTA Radiol Ther Phys Biol 8:15–26

Howard-Flanders P (1960) Effect of oxygen on the radiosensitivity of bacteriophage in the presence of sulphydryl compounds. Nature 186:485–487

Iliakis G (1980) Effects of β-arabinofuranosyladenine on the growth and repair of potentially lethal damage in Ehrlich ascites tumor cells. Radiat Res 83:537–552

Iliakis G, Nusse M, Bryant P (1982) Effects of aphidicolin on cell proliferation, repair of potentially lethal damage and repair of DNA strand breaks in Ehrlich ascites tumor cells exposed to x-rays. Int J Radiat Biol 42:417–434

Jain VK, Holtz GW, Pohlit W, Purohit SC (1977) Inhibition of unscheduled DNA synthesis and repair of potentially lethal x-ray damage by 2'-deoxy-D-glucose in yeast. Int J Radiat Biol 32:175–180

Kinsella TJ, Russo A, Mitchell JB, Rowland J, Jenkins J, Schwade J, Myers CE, Collins JM, Speyer P, Kornblith P, Smith B, Kufta C, Glatstein E (1984) A phase I study of intermittent intravenous BUdR with conventional irradiation. Int J Radiat Oncol Biol Phys 10:69–76

Kriss JP, Maruyama Y, Tung LA, Bond SB, Revesz L (1963) The fate of 5-bromodeoxyuridine, 5-bromodeoxycytidine, and 5-iododeoxycytidine in man. Cancer Res 23:260–268

Kriss JP, Revesz L (1962) The distribution and fate of bromodeoxyuridine in the mouse and the rat. Cancer Res 22:254–265

Little JB (1969) Repair of sublethal and potentially lethal radiation damage in plateau phase cultures in human cells. Nature 224:804–806

Little JB, Hahn GM, Frindel E, Tubiana M (1973) Repair of potentially lethal damage in vitro and in vivo. Radiology 106:689–694

Maor MH, Peters LJ (1984) Selection of appropriate studies for Phase III trials of radiosensitizers. Int J Radiat Oncol Biol Phys 9:271

McNally NJ, DeRonde J (1980) Radiobiological studies with tumours in situ compared with cell survival. Br J Cancer 41 (suppl 4):259–265

Meister A (1983) Selective modification of glutathione metabolism. Science 220:472–477

Milne ENC, Noonan CD, Margulis AR, Stoughton JA (1969) Vascular supply of pulmonary metastases: Experimental study in rats. Invest Radiol 4:215–229

Minarik L, Marchese M, Zaider M, Hall EJ (1985) Potential lethal damage repair and survival in human AG1522 fibroblasts in plateau phase under acute- and low-dose-rate ^{137}Cs irradiation. Endocuriether/Hypertherm Oncol 1:5–8

Minchington AI, Rojas A, Smith KA, Soranson JA, Shrieve DC, Jones NR, Bremner JC (1984) Glutathione depletion in tissues after administration of buthionine sulphoximine. Int J Radiat Oncol Biol Phys 10:1261–1264

Mitchell JB, Kinselly TJ, Russo A, McPherson S, Rowland J, Kornblith P, Glatstein E (1983) Radiosensitization of hematopoietic precursor cells (CFUc) in glioblastoma patients receiving intermittent intravenous infusions of bromodeoxyuridine (BUdR). Int J Radiat Oncol Biol Phys 9:457–463

Mitchell JB, Morstyn G, Russo A, Kinsella TJ, Fornace A, McPherson S, Glatstein E (1984) Differing sensitivity to fluorescent light in Chinese hamster cells containing equally incorporated quantities of BUdR versus IUdR. Int J Radiat Oncol Biol Phys 10:1447–1451

Mohler WC, Elkind MM (1963) Radiation response of mammalian cells grown in culture III Modification of X-ray survival of Chinese hamster cells by 5-bromodeoxyuridine. Exp Cell Res 30:481–491

Morstyn G, Hsu S-M, Kinsella T, Gratzner H, Russo A, Mitchell JB (1983) Bromodeoxyuridine in tumors and chromosomes detected with a monoclonal antibody. J Clin Invest 72:1844–1850

Moulder JE, Rockwell S (1984) Hypoxic fractions of solid tumors: Experimental techniques, methods of analysis, and a survey of existing data. Int J Radiat Oncol Biol Phys 10:695–712

Nakatsugawa S, Kumar A, Ono K, Nishidai T, Yukawa Y, Takahashi M, Abe M, Sugahara T (1982b) Increased

tumor curability by radiotherapy combined with PLDR inhibitors in murine cancer. In: Prospective methods of radiation therapy in developing countries. IAEA-TEC-DOC 266. International Atomic Energy Agency, Vienna, pp 77–86

Nakatsugawa S, Sugahara T (1980) Inhibition of x-ray-induced potentially lethal damage (PLD) repair by cordycepin (3'-deoxyadenosine) and enhancement of its action by 2'-deoxycoformycin in Chinese hamster hai cells in the stationary phase in vivo. Radiat Res 84:265–275

Nakatsugawa S, Sugahara T, Kumar A (1982a) Purine nucleoside analogues inhibit the repair of radiation-induced potentially lethal damage in mammalian cells in culture. Int J Radiat Biol 41:343–346

Palcic B, Faddegon B, Skarsgard LD (1984) The effect of misonidazole as a hypoxic radiosensitizer at low dose. Radiat Res 100:340–347

Paterson MC, Smith BP, Lohman PHM, Anderson AK, Fishman L (1976) Defective excision repair of x-ray-damaged DNA in human (ataxia telangiectasia) fibroblasts. Nature 260:444–447

Perez LM, Mekras JA, Briggle TV, Greer S (1984) Marked radiosensitization of cells in culture to X ray by 5-chlorodeoxycytidine coadministered with tetrahydrouridine, and inhibitors of pyrimidine biosynthesis. Int J Radiat Oncol Biol Phys 10:1453–1458

Phillips RA, Tolmach LJ (1966) Repair of potentially lethal damage in X-irradiated HeLa cells. Radiat Res 29:414–432

Rasey JS, Nelson NJ (1981) Repair of potentially lethal damage following irradiation with x-rays or cyclotron neutrons: Response of the EMT-6/UW tumor system treated under various growth conditions in vitro and in vivo. Radiat Res 85:69–84

Rasey JS, Nelson NJ (1983) Discrepancies between patterns of potentially lethal damage repair in the RIF-1 tumor system in vitro and in vivo. Radiat Res 93:157–174

Russell KJ, Rice GC, Brown JM (1986) In vitro and in vivo radiation sensitization by the halogenated pyrimidine 5-chloro-2'-deoxycytidine. Cancer Res 46:2883–2887

Russo A, Gianni L, Kinsella TJ, Klecker RW, Jenkins J, Rowland J, Glatstein E, Mitchell JB, Collins J, Myers CE (1984) A pharmacologic evaluation of intravenous delivery of BUdR to patients with brain tumors. Cancer Res 44:1702–1705

Sakamoto K, Aritake S (1981) Effects of misonidazole on tumur cell radiation sensitivity and potentially lethal damage repair in vivo and in vitro,. Eur J Cancer Clin Oncol 17:825–830

Saunders MI, Anderson PJ, Bennett MH, Dische S, Minchinton A, Stratford MRL, Tothill M (1984) The clinical testing of Ro 03-8799 – Pharmacokinetics, toxicology, tissue and tumor concentrations. Int J Radiat Oncol Biol Phys 10:1759–1763

Shipley WU, Stanley JA, Courtenay WD, Field SB (1975) Repair of radiation damage in Lewis lung carcinoma cells following in situ treatments with fast neutrons and x-rays. Cancer Res 35:932–938

Smithen CE, Clarke ED, Dale JA, Jacobs RS, Wardman P, Watts ME, Woodcock M (1980) Novel (nitro-1-imidazolyl)-alkanolamines as potential radiosensitizers with improved therapeutic properties. In: Brady LW (ed) Radiation sensitizers: Their use in the clinical management of cancer. Masson: New York, pp 22–32

Suit HD, Hewitt R, Urano M (1970) Effect of radiation

sensitizing agents in radiation therapy of mouse mammary carcinoma. Radiol 94:185–195

Sutherland RM, Franko AJ (1980) On the nature of the radiobiologically hypoxic fraction in tumors. Int J Radiat Oncol Biol Phys 6:117–120

Thomlinson RH, Gray LH (1955) The histological structure of some human lung cancers and the possible implications for radiotherapy. Br J Cancer 9:539–549

Twentyman PR, Brown JM, Gray JW, Franko AJ, Scoles MA, Kallman RF (1980) A new mouse tumor model system (RIF-1) for comparison of end-point studies. J Nat Cancer Inst 64:595–604

Urtasun RC, Coleman CN, Wasserman TH, Phillips TL (1984) Clinical trials with hypoxic cell sensitizers: Time to retrench or time to push forward? Int J Radiat Oncol Biol Phys 10:1691–1696

van Ankeren SC, Wheeler KT (1984) Relationship between the repair of radiation-induced DNA damage and recovery from potentially lethal damage in 9L rat brain tumor cells. Cancer Res 44:1091–1097

Watson ER Halnan KE, Dische S, Saunders MI, Cade IS, McEwen JB, Wiernik G, Perrins DJD, Sutherland I (1978) Hyperbaric oxygen and radiotherapy: a Medical Research Council trial in carcinoma of the cervix. Br J Radiol 51:879–887

Weichselbaum RR, Dahlberg W, Little JB, Ervin TJ, Miller D, Hellman S, Rheinwald JG (1984) Cellular X-ray repair parameters of early passage squamous cell carcinoma lines derived from patients with known responses to radiotherapy. Br J Cancer 49:595–601

Weichselbaum RR, Little JB (1982) The differential response of human tumours to fractionated radiation may be due to a post-radiation repair process. Br J Cancer 46:532–537

Weichselbaum RR, Nove J, Little JB (1978) Deficient recovery from potentially lethal radiation damage in ataxia telangiectasia and xeroderma pigmentosum. Nature 271:261–262

Weichselbaum RR, Nove J, Little JB (1980) Radiation response of human tumor cells in vitro. In: Meyn RE, Withers HR (eds) Radiation Biology in Cancer Research. Raven Press, New York, pp 345–351

White RAS, Workman P, Brown JM (1980) The pharmacokinetics, tumor and neural tissue penetrating properties in the dog of SR-2508 and SR-2555 – hydrophilic radiosensitizers potentially less toxic than misonidazole. Radiat Res 84:542–561

Whitmore GF, Gulyas S, Kotalik J (1970) Recovery from radiation damage in mammalian cells. In: Bond VP, Suit HD, Marcial V (eds) Time and dose relationships in radiation biology as applied to radiotherapy. Brookhaven National Laboratory, Upton, New York, pp 41–46

Williams MV, Denekamp J, Fowler JF (1984) Dose-response relationships for human tumors: Implications for clinical trials of dose modifying agents. Int J Radiat Oncol Biol Phys 10:1703–1707

Williams MV, Denekamp J, Minchinton AI, Stratford MRL (1982) In vivo assessment of basic 2-nitroimidazole radiosensitizers. Br J Cancer 46:127–137

Willson RL, Emmerson PT (1970) Reaction of triacetone-N-oxyl with radiation-induced radicals from DNA and from deoxyribonucleotides in aqueous solution. In: Moroson HL, Quintiliani M (eds) Radiation Protection and Sensitization. Taylor and Francis Ltd: London, pp 72–79

Yu NY, Brown JM (1984) Depletion of glutathione in vivo as a method of improving the therapeutic ratio of misonidazole and SR 2508. Int J Radiat Oncol Biol Phys 10:1265–1269

7.2 Optimizing Combinations of Drugs and Radiation. The Interdigitated Alternating Regimen

Maurice Tubiana, Rodrigo Arriagada, and Jean-Marc Cosset

CONTENTS

Numerous reviews have been devoted to considering the combination of radiotherapy (RT) and chemotherapy (CT) (Bleehen 1981; Vaeth 1979; Peckham and Collis 1981; Tubiana 1981; Rubin 1984) and they have underlined the importance of the relative timing of the administration of the drugs and the radiation. The time interval and sequence between the delivery of CT and RT exerts an influence on both the tolerance of normal tissues and the probability of local control of the tumor.

The combination of the two modalities, RT and CT, has two aims. The first is to increase the probability of control of the primary tumor. This requires either the potentiation of one of the two modalities by the other or the addition of their effect on tumor cells without a concomitant increase in the toxic effects on critical normal tissues. Local failure to control primary tumors is still the cause of a large proportion of cancer deaths (Suit 1982). A small increase in the effectiveness of local treatment may markedly improve long term survival (Suit 1982), in particular because it may decrease the incidence of distant metastases (Anderson and Dische 1981).

The second aim of this combination is spatial cooperation, RT being used for the control of the primary tumor and/or of sanctuary sites and CT for the control of disseminated disease. In various types of cancer, adjuvant chemotherapy is capable of destroying small occult neoplastic deposits and to maximize this beneficial effect, its scheduling should not be altered.

In these two strategies, radiotherapy and chemotherapy should be given up to full dose for maximum efficacy. The main risk is an increase in the number and severity of the early and late side effects.

In order to circumvent this problem, two possibilities are being explored: 1) the use of drugs without serious toxic effects on those critical tissues which are included in the irradiated volume; 2) the avoidance of concomitant administration and the introduction of a sufficiently long time gap between the completion of one modality and initiation of the other. However, in such sequential treatment, delaying chemotherapy until after the completion of radiotherapy, or suspending chemotherapy while giving radiotherapy, may allow any occult metastases to increase in size. A similar delay in initiation of radiotherapy is also detrimental, as drugs are often not as effective in treating bulky tumors. Moreover, during chemotherapy the cells in the primary tumor which are resistant to the cytotoxic drugs may disseminate and initiate chemoresistant metastases.

The purpose of this paper is to examine the various types of scheduling which have been employed and to report the results which have been obtained in the Institut Gustave-Roussy with a new scheme of alternating treatment.

1 Concomitant Administration

The main advantage is the delivery, without undue delay, of the two modalities. The major risk is cumulative toxicity on normal tissue. A therapeutic gain is only obtained when the increase in the effect on neoplastic tissues outweighs that observed on normal tissues. The potentiation of the effect on normal tissues (Peckham and Collis 1981; Tubiana 1981; Rubin 1984) should therefore be less than the increase in the probability of tumor control.

Maurice Tubiana, M.D.
Rodrigo Arriagada, M.D.
Jean-Marc Cosset, M.D.
Institute Gustave-Roussy
F-94800 Villejuif

Drug administration or irradiation induces some synchronization of the viable tumor cells (ROCKWELL et al. 1978; DEMEESTERE et al. 1980). However, in human tumors, the therapeutic effectiveness of such a kinetically-based approach has never been found to be superior to conventional scheduling. This is true in both combination treatments (TUBIANA et al. 1975; COSTANZI et al. 1976; CAMPLEJOHN 1980; NIAS 1980) and in the few attempts in which vaious associations between CT and RT were studied (FAZEKAS et al. 1980). Even when preliminary results appeared promising (PRICE et al. 1978; PRICE and HILL 1980), later, more rigorous trials did not support a role for this type of approach (TANNOCK et al. 1982; STELL et al. 1983). For example, in the EORTC LR$_2$ lymphoma trial, a chemotherapy regimen aiming at so-called synchronization and another regimen delivering the same drugs without such a preconceived idea obtained identical relapse-free survivals and total survivals (BURGERS et al. 1985).

Another theoretic advantage of concomitant administration is to exploit the increase in chemosensitivity due to tumor cell recruitment triggered by the first sessions of RT or CT administration (ROCKWELL et al. 1978; DEMEESTERE et al. 1980; MALAISE and TUBIANA 1966; BARENDSEN and BROERSE 1969; HERMENS and BARENDSEN 1978; POTMESIL and GOLDFEDER 1980; DENEKAMP and THOMLINSON 1971; GRISWOLD et al. 1970; STEPHENS and STEEL 1980). However, during a course of RT, an increase in labeling index (LI) is observed in only a small proportion of tumors (COURDI et al. 1980), whereas an acceleration of the proliferation rate occurs in a large number of normal tissues such as bone marrow stem cells, intestinal epithelium, epidermis and several others (POTTEN and HENDRY 1983). From this, one should expect a negative therapeutic gain; this is what has been observed. For example, in head and neck tumor trials, when RT and CT were administered concomitantly, mucosal reactions have been much more severe (CACHIN et al. 1977; FU et al. 1979) than in sequential administration (PECKHAM and COLLIS 1981; MARCIAL et al. 1980). Concomitant administration resulted in a reduction of the normal tissue tolerance and therefore the radiation dose had to be reduced (CACHIN et al. 1977). Of the numerous controlled trials comparing RT alone, and RT with concomitant CT, all (CACHIN et al. 1977; FU et al. 1979) but one (SHANTA and KRISHNAMURTHI 1980) failed to reveal any improvement in survival.

Similar disappointing results were also observed in concomitant treatment of tumors which are both chemosensitive and radiosensitive such as small cell lung cancer. A randomized study testing concomitant administration showed an improvement in the complete response rate, in the median survival and in the 2-year actuarial survival, but these effects were counterbalanced by an increased toxicity (BUNN et al. 1983; MORSTYN et al. 1984).

The increase in the toxic effect on normal tissues can still be observed following moderate doses of RT and low doses of CT. For example, the incidence of radiation pneumonitis was higher than 50% in patients with unresectable lung cancer treated by 40 Gy in 10 fractions, in two split-courses, plus concomitant doxorubicin 10 mg/m^2 (LAGRANGE et al. personal communication). Thus, only a few groups still explore this regimen on selected groups of patients in phase II trials.

2 Sequential Administration

The main advantage of sequential administration is avoidance of interaction between the two modalities and reduction of cumulative effects as long as the time interval between the delivery of the two modalities is sufficient.

Several sets of experimental and clinical data show the importance of timing with respect to early or late complications (PECKHAM and COLLIS 1981; TUBIANA 1981; RUBIN 1984). For example, in a report by ARISTIZABAL et al. (1977), four out of six patients receiving concurrent radiation and cyclophosphamide and adriamycin had cutaneous complications, whereas none of 14 patients receiving a drug radiation-drug sequence at 7–10 day intervals had untoward reactions.

In fact, in sequential administration, toxic effects are much lower and immediate reactions are generally not much greater than after one modality alone (PECKHAM and COLLIS 1981). A sequential scheme of administration was successful in treating several types of cancer such as malignant lymphoma, Ewing sarcoma, medulloblastoma rhabdomyosarcoma, nephroblastoma, small-cell carcinoma of the lung (PECKHAM and COLLIS 1981; TUBIANA 1981; RUBIN 1984), and early stages of non-Hodgkin lymphoma (CARDE et al. 1984; BONADONNA et al. 1984). However, often the gain is relatively small and can be demonstrated only by comparison with a control arm in a randomized trial.

Table 1. Incidence of recurrence in an irradiated territory in patients treated by radiotherapy alone or combination of radiotherapy and chemotherapy.

In H_1 EORTC trial (1964–1970), patients with CS I+II Hodgkin's disease were randomized between mantle field irradiation, or mantle field irradiation plus a weekly injection of Velban for two years.

In H_2 trial, patients received a subtotal radiotherapy (mantle + spleen + para-aortic region) with or without Velban or Verban + Procarbazine.

In H_5 trial (1975–1982), patients with poor prognostic indicators were randomized between total nodal irradiation or 3 MOPP, mantle field 3 MOPP [40]

		Patient at risk	Relapse in an irradiated territory (%)
H_1	Mantle field	177	16 ± 3
	Mantle field + VLB	171	6 ± 2
H_2	Mantle field +	202	9 ± 2
	para aortic id. + VLB $\pm$ PCZ	98	4 ± 2
H_5	TNI	152	7 ± 2
	MOPP + RT + MOPP	144	2 ± 1

Logrank test: $p = 0.017$

In Hodgkin's disease (TUBIANA et al. 1984), the incidence of local recurrence in irradiated territory was about halved (Table 1) using either monochemotherapy with vinblastine or combination chemotherapy with MOPP. This showed that previous irradiation with a dose of 40 Gy did not interfere with the drug availability in the tumor. However, even for this chemosensitive type of tumor, the effect of drugs is relatively limited. Thus, it is not surprising that, for other less chemosensitive tumor types, the incidence of local control is not significantly improved (BARKER et al. 1980). This is particularly the case for head and neck tumors (FAZEKAS et al. 1980; TANNOCK et al. 1982; MARCIAL et al. 1980; GLICK et al. 1980; GLICK and TAYLOR 1981; MEAD and JACOBS 1982; VOGL et al. 1982). For this tumor, none of the randomized trials shows any improvement in control of primary tumor from adding chemotherapy to radiotherapy (STELL et al. 1983; CACHIN et al. 1977; STEFANI et al. 1971; PETROVICH et al. 1981).

Let us discuss, as an example, small-cell carcinoma of the lung. In a retrospective survey by Cox et al. (1979), the median dose required to produce control of the thoracic tumor was claimed to be less with the combined modality treatment than with radiation alone; this result suggested a cumulative effect of the two treatment modalities on the primary tumor. However, the aim should be

a significant increase in the incidence of local control and not the delivery of a smaller radiation dose. SALAZAR and CREECH (1980) reviewed the published data and showed that, from this point of view, the improvement, if any, is small (recurrence in the tumor was observed in 33% of 446 patients receiving radiation alone, versus 28% of the 1.047 patients treated with an association of RT and CT). At the Institut Gustave-Roussy, when patients in a combined modality regimen received 45 Gy, the incidence of local recurrence at 2 years remained too high (approximately 40% of the patients); however it was reduced to 20% when the dose was increased to 55 Gy (LE CHEVALIER et al. 1982; ARRIAGADA et al., 1985).

In non-Hodgkin lymphoma of unfavorable histology, local failures were also observed when the radiation dose was too low (30 Gy) and the dose had to be maintained at the level given when RT was used alone (45 Gy) in order to fully profit from the association with CT (COSSET et al. 1985). Thus, it may be that in combined modality treatments, the radiation dose should not be reduced significantly. The same is true for CT; in combined regimens the CT must be as intense as when used alone. This is illustrated by the data of the EORTC non-Hodgkin lymphoma trial (LR_2) in which the survival rate was not improved in clinical stage I and II when relatively low dose CVP was added to RT (CARDE et al. 1984).

If both CT and RT have to be given in full doses, the main disadvantage becomes the long protraction of the treatment. The chronology of this administration has been long debated (BLEEHEN 1981). The advantage of using radiation therapy first is that it directs effective therapy to the primary site. However, this delays the employment of CT, and thus may permit further growth of untreated occult metastases. For example, if the tumor's doubling time is equal to one month, which is a realistic figure for rapidly growing tumors such as NHL or small-cell carcinoma of the lung (CHARBIT et al. 1971; STEEL 1977), a delay of two months would allow the metastases to become four times larger (Fig. 1). This is why CT is usually given first; however, RT cannot be delayed too long for two reasons: i) cytotoxic drugs are generally less effective on bulky tumors; ii) under chemotherapy, the clones of cells resistant to the cytotoxic drugs administered will expand (SCHABEL et al. 1980), and may disseminate and initiate chemoresistant metastases. Therefore, RT is usually carried out after two to four cycles of chemotherapy.

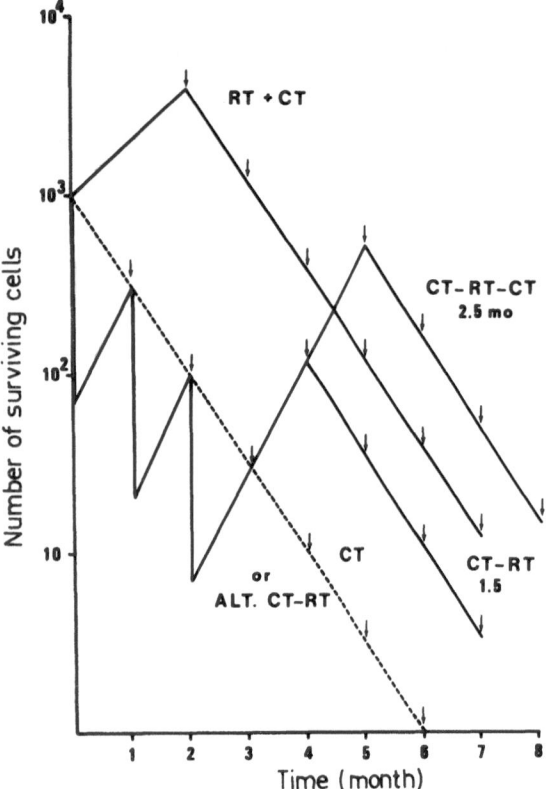

Fig. 1. Time course changes of the volume of occult metastases located outside of the irradiated field. The doubling time is taken equal to 1 month before treatment and 0.5 month during repopulation between cycles of chemotherapy. Four options are considered: 1. Radiotherapy first, chemotherapy is initiated after a two-month delay ($RT + CT$). 2. Chemotherapy is initiated first and then interrupted for 2.5 months during the course of radiotherapy ($CT - RT - CT$). 3. Chemotherapy first, thereafter an interruption of 1.5 month is introduced for radiotherapy. 4. Undisturbed course of chemotherapy or alternating chemotherapy and radiotherapy. Each arrow indicates a chemotherapy cycle. The proportion of surviving clonogenic cells after each chemotherapy course is taken equal to 7%

After such CT the tumor cells which are still viable undergo an acceleration of their proliferation rate (TUBIANA 1982). A number of studies have well documented repopulation in rodent (ROCKWELL et al. 1978; DEMEESTERE et al. 1980; MALAISE and TUBIANA 1966; BARENDSEN and BROERSE 1969; HERMENS and BARENDSEN 1978; DENEKAMP and THOMLINSON 1971; TUBIANA 1982; TUBIANA and MALAISE 1976) and human tumors (VAN PEPERZEEL 1972; MALAISE and CHARBIT 1972). Malaise and Tubiana discovered in 1966 that mouse fibrosarcoma tumors regrew earlier after irradiation than would have been expected if the surviving cells maintained the doubling time

of the original tumor. In 1968–1970, BARENDSEN and BROERSE (1969), and HERMENS and BARENDSEN (1978) demonstrated in an irradiated rhabdomyosarcoma that the viable clonogenic cells had a doubling time only one-third of that of unirradiated tumors. GRISWOLD et al. (1970) found in 1970 a similar acceleration of the proliferation rate of clonogenic cells of a plasmocytoma after administration of a cytotoxic drug. ROCKWELL et al. (1978) and DEMEESTERE et al. (1980) showed that the clonogenic tumor cell recruitment occurs within one day. Several other investigators have since confirmed the occurrence of a phase of rapid repopulation in treated experimental tumors (TUBIANA 1982).

In patients, a rapid regrowth of cutaneous (RAMBERT et al. 1968) or pulmonary metastases (VAN PEPERZEEL 1972; MALAISE et al. 1972) has been observed. The acceleration can be characterized by the ratio of the doubling time before treatment to that during the repopulation phase. In 31 human metastases in which it was measured, the value of this ratio ranged from 2.5 to 5 (MALAISE et al. 1972).

Thus, if the pretreatment tumor doubling time, as in the previous example, is taken to be one month, after a few cycles of CT one can presume a doubling time equal to 10–15 days. Taking 0.5 months as a conservative estimate, after the two-month interruption caused by the radiotherapy course, the occult metastases located outside the irradiated volume are sixteen times larger (Fig. 1). As the size is a very critical parameter, this may significantly reduce the effectiveness of adjuvant CT. For example, we have been able to show, using a simulation model of tumor growth (GUIGUET 1982; KOSCIELNY et al. 1984) that the occult metastases of breast cancer, which are controlled by adjuvant chemotherapy, do not contain more than one million cells. Multiplying by 2 or 4 the average size of the occult metastases would considerably lower the effectiveness of adjuvant CT (TUBIANA 1982; GUIGUET 1982).

Hence, with both types of chronology, the long duration of the radiotherapy causes an interruption of the chemotherapy, which allows a critical growth of occult metastases. This is one of the reasons for which several medical oncologists are reluctant to consider the use of combined treatment despite the obvious advantages. To take again the example of small cell carcinoma of the lung, despite the high local recurrence rate in patients treated by CT alone and the decreased incidence in patients treated by sufficient doses of ionizing radiation (BLEEHEN et al. 1983; BYHARDT and COX 1983), several authors criticize the use of RT (COHEN 1983). They argue that association between RT and CT alters both schedule and dosage of CT. However, in spite of the high rate of responses to CT the percentage of complete remissions is moderate: 30–50% (AISNER et al. 1983; IHDE and BUNN 1982) and the percentage of long term survivors remains very low: 8–12%; only patients evidencing complete response have the potential to be long-term survivors (MORSTYN et al. 1984; HANSEN et al. 1980). All these factors call for a role of combined RT and CT but the question is still what is the best timing of this combination.

At Villejuif, from the onset, we recognized the importance of combining RT and CT, which are agents without cross resistance and, if well chosen, with minimal cross toxicity (TUBIANA 1981). On the other hand, our aim was to avoid disturbance of the scheduling of cytotoxic drug administration which, we feel, is of paramount importance. Our first attempt was to irradiate only after completion of the CT course; this is what we called iceberg RT, which appears to be useful in the treatment of disseminated lymphoma (AMIEL et al. 1971). However, this sequencing between CT and RT can only be used in advanced and very chemosensitive tumors and therefore had only limited application. Along these lines, our second attempt was to deliver a small radiation dose at the end of each cycle of CT (AMIEL et al. 1980; ARRIAGADA et al. 1981). However, the therapeutic results of this type of combination were poor, and the toxicity was far from negligible. This is why, in 1980, we proposed another type of association which alternated CT and RT (TUBIANA 1981; TUBIANA et al. 1982).

3 The Interdigitated Alternating Regimen

This new scheme alternates multiple short courses of RT with CT. The rationale of the proposed timing is the following: 1) CT should be initiated immediately after the histological diagnosis has been made and staging investigations completed; 2) CT should be administered regularly every month during the whole induction treatment; 3) RT should be given early in the schedule to the maximal dose tolerated and should not interrupt the CT, so reducing the risk of resistant cells developing; 4) a seven-day interval between CT and RT was introduced in order to avoid the increased

toxicity associated with concurrent therapy (PEARSON and STEEL 1984).

As, in two weeks, it is hazardous to deliver more than 20–25 Gy, the radiotherapy course should be carried out as a split course: for example, twice 25 Gy in two weeks, separated by a time interval of about three weeks.

Such an alternating interdigitated protocol avoids concomitant administration of drugs and radiation and does not alter the rhythm of chemotherapy. It has been used at Villejuif in four feasibility trials in order to assess both the tolerance of normal tissues and the effects on the tumor.

For small cell carcinoma of the lung, two subsequent pilot studies were conducted. The preliminary results of the first pilot study (LE CHEVALIER et al. 1982; ARRIAGADA et al. 1985) were encouraging in terms of tolerance and relapse free survival (23% at 4 years). In 1981, we started the second pilot study introducing two modifications to the first study: 1) Methotrexate was replaced by CDDP in order to decrease hematological toxicity, and 2) the total dose of thoracic RT was increased from 45 to 55 Gy. It seemed to us important to reach the tolerance dose, unknown for this kind of combination, in an attempt to optimize the results. The second protocol can be summarized as follows: six cycles of induction CT were given according to the schedule: Doxorubicin 40 mg/m², d1, VP 16213 75 mg/m² d1–3, Cyclophosphamide 300 mg/m² d3–6, CDDP 100 mg/m² d2. Radiotherapy was initially delivered in 2 courses of 20 Gy given in 8 fractions over 14 days; the target volume included all the initially visible tumor (with a 1.5 cm margin of normal lung tissue) as well as the mediastinum and both hilar and supraclavicular regions. A third course of RT was given using two lateral fields, sparing the spinal cord and delivering 15 Gy in 6 fractions over 10 days. Prophylactic cranial irradiation – PCI – (30 Gy in 10 fractions over 14 days) was given during the first course of thoracic RT. The schedule of the alternating protocol can be summarized as follows: CT --- CT – RT 20 Gy — RT 20 Gy — CT — RT 15 Gy — CT --- CT, where (—) represents a gap of 1 week.

The actuarial local control and the relapse free survival for the 28 patients treated in the first alternating regimen and the 45 patients treated in the second protocol are given in Fig. 2. The detailed results have been recently reported (ARRIAGADA et al. 1985; ARRIAGADA et al. 1985; ARRIAGADA et al. 1987) and we shall only briefly comment upon them in these pages. It is as yet too early

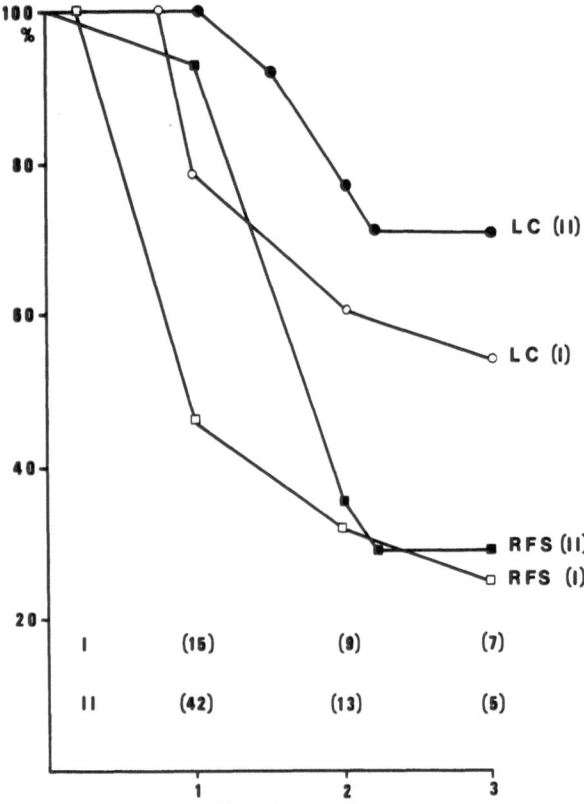

Fig. 2. Results obtained in small cell lung cancer treated by two protocols of an interdigitated alternating regimen: 28 patients in the first protocol (*I*) delivering 45 Gy to the mediastinum and 45 patients in the second protocol (*II*) delivering 55 Gy to the mediastinum. LC: local control for complete responders. *RFS* relapse free survival for all patients in each protocol

to compare the two subgroups of patients or to assess the long-term results; nevertheless, several conclusions can be made.

Both protocols obtained a rate of complete response higher than 85% (evaluated by chest X ray and fiberoptic bronchoscopy). The incidence of local recurrence at 2 years is low (37.5% in the first protocol, 20% in the second). The 3 year RFS (25% and 28% respectively) is remarkably high. It is comparable to that reported by others (MORSTYN G. et al. 1984; GRECO and OLDHAM 1982; FELD et al. 1984) for the subset of complete responder patients who represent a selected group of the population. It is noteworthy that the marked increase in the probability of local control comparing the second with the first protocol did not result in a concomitant increase in either relapse free survival or total survival. This suggests that the relatively large tumors which were not previously controlled and which are now controlled

had already metastasized and these occult metastases are too large to be eradicated by current CT regimens. No death due to early toxicity was observed among the 45 patients of the second protocol.

The late toxicity can be evaluated on the 73 patients included in both protocols for whom the follow-up ranges from 2 to 4.5 years. An asymptomatic radiation fibrosis was detected by chest X-ray in 75% of patients treated with the first protocol and 51% of the patients treated with the second one. Symptomatic pneumonitis with cough and shortness of the breath was observed in 7% of the patients. In 8% of the patients, alteration of the ECG necessitated cessation of adriamycin. A late bone marrow hypoplasia was observed in 11% of the patients of the first protocol (among them, one grade 5 toxicity) and 6% of the second. A grade 2 pericarditis was noticed in one patient. In two patients, neurologic symptoms were found, though these were probably due to cranial irradiation. It can be concluded that the late toxicity is acceptable and that no untoward late complication was observed.

In non-Hodgkin lymphoma of unfavorable histologic types, the protocol is similar (COSSET et al. 1985). It consists of eight monthly courses of CT alternating with two or three RT courses, which do not alter the scheduling of CT. Chemotherapy consisted of eight monthly courses of CHVP, according to previous EORTC LR_2 trial:

Doxorubicin	50 mg/m²	day 1
VM 26 (Teniposide)	60 mg/m²	day 1
Cyclophosphamide	300 mg/m²	day 3 and 4
Prednisone	40 mg	day 3 *to* 7

At least two RT courses were alternated with CT courses: between CT courses 2 and 3, and 3 and 4. Each RT course delivered 15 Gy in six fractions over ten days. The irradiated volumes were usually the initially-involved areas and the adjacent lymph node groups. A third irradiation course was optional, and only given in the case of residual disease after one or two RT courses (between CT courses 4 and 5). This third irradiation sequence delivered 15 Gy, with the same fractionation, in as small a volume as possible. The time intervals between CT and RT or RT and CT were to be no shorter than eight days and no longer than ten days.

Thirty four patients have been included in this protocol. The 4-year TS is approximately 65% (Fig. 3). Seven relapses were observed; 2 were local within the irradiated volumes, 4 outside the irradiated areas; 1 patient experienced simultaneously a local and a systemic relapse. The analysis of our data shows the influence of the dose on the incidence of local recurrence: 2 local recurrences out of 9 patients treated with only two courses of 15 Gy (according to a first version of the protocol), versus one local recurrence out of the 15 patients who received 3 courses of 15 Gy; moreover this relapsing patient presented at the same time a widespread extra nodal dissemination. Thus, even when chemotherapy is combined with RT, a dose of at least 45 Gy appears to be required to obtain a local control of the bulky lesions. Of the 4 relapses which occurred outside the irradiated volume, two were in lymph nodes located on the other side of the diaphragm; one was located in the brain, and the last one was a gastric relapse. Rather than extending the irradiation volumes, these data suggest the usefulness of a more extensive work-up and of an intensification of the chemotherapy regimen. Hematological, systemic and digestive tolerances were good. No increase in late toxicity was detected and no severe untoward reaction occurred. As expected, these observations suggest that the 8–10 day gap between drug and radiation helps to avoid the enhanced toxicity of normal tissues associated with the concomitant schedules. We are investigating whether a systematic use of three courses of irradiation (15 Gy each), combined with a more aggressive chemotherapy regimen, can further improve the therapeutic results.

Thirty-six patients with stage III cancer of the uterine cervix were treated with an alternating scheme of Rt and chemotherapy which included CDDP. No increase in early or late side effects was noted: It was not possible to demonstrate a therapeutic gain for this series compared to previous experience with RT alone, but it is probable that a moderate dose of CDDP as single agent therapy is not effective enough in squamous cell carcinoma. In the inflammatory breast cancer study, with the present follow-up no improvement in relapse-free survival or total survival has been noted. However, the immediate skin tolerance is excellent in spite of the use of a 5 drug chemotherapy (5-Fluoracil, Doxorubicin, Cyclophosphamide, Vincristine, Methotrexate).

4 Discussion

The alternating treatment schedule which is proposed interdigitates radiotherapy and chemotherapy. Its aim is to reconcile the needs for early and sequential administration of both agents.

This scheme has several advantages. Alternating two different treatment modalities with minimal cross toxicity gives more time for recovery of critical normal tissue for each modality. The critical tissues generally are different for radiotherapy and chemotherapy. For radiotherapy the limiting factor is late effects on connective tissue surrounding the tumor whereas for most combination chemotherapy regimens, bone marrow failure is the main complication. Thus, in this integrated scheme, radiotherapy must be planned in order to avoid irradiation of bone marrow as much as possible.

In fact, in patients treated with this alternating scheme, early tolerance is as good as that following sequential administration. Theoretically, late toxicity should also not be greater than following sequential administration since radiation and drugs cause late effects by different mechanisms (RUBIN 1984). Currently, in our series of patients, late toxicity appears acceptable; however, the number of patients with a follow-up longer than two years after completion of treatment is still relatively small.

The main advantage of this scheme is that it avoids a long gap in the CT delivery and shortens the time interval between the various agents which act on the tumor. We have previously shown, using a simulation model (GUIGUET et al. 1982), that in occult metastases which are controlled by adjuvant combination chemotherapy, for example in the study of BONADONNA et al. (1977), the number of cells is about one million. Let us assume that the proportion of clonogenic cells is one per thousand. Thus, in order to achieve sterilization, the six cycles of combination chemotherapy should reduce the proportion of viable clonogenic cells to less than 10^{-3}. This corresponds to a proportion of surviving cells equal to 30% one month after each CT course, at the time at which a new CT cycle is initiated (Fig. 1). If we assume a doubling time of 0.5 month (as discussed above), this means that the proportion of viable clonogenic cells at the completion of the CT course was about 7%. If in a sequential chemotherapy radiotherapy regimen the CT is interrupted for two months, this interruption therefore annihilates the therapeutic effect of one or two cycles of CT. In the alternating regimen, the efficacy of CT is not reduced as its rhythm is not altered.

With regard to the primary tumor, if irradiation starts ten days after completion of CT, the proportion of surviving cells at this time is about 10%. Thus, with 3 courses of CT intercalated between RT courses and six given with the conventional

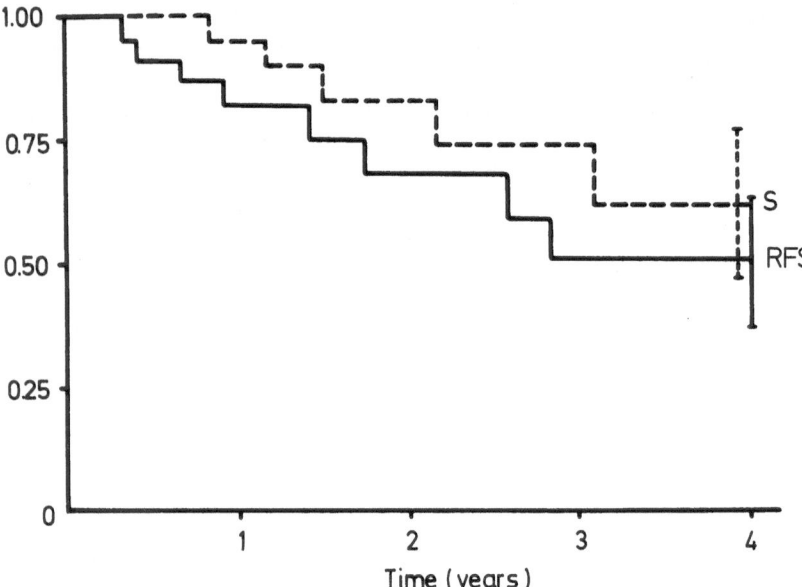

Fig. 3. Total survival and relapse-free survival in 24 patients with clinical stage II NHL of diffuse histological pattern treated at Villejuif with an alternating combination of radiotherapy and chemotherapy. (From Cosset et al. 1985; results updated in April 1985)

scheme the reduction in the proportion of viable cells resulting from CT will be about 10^{-4}, equivalent to that obtained with about 25 Gy.

Besides this advantage from the point of view of growth kinetics, the alternating regimen has the theoretic addition of preventing the proliferation of drug-resistant cells. Spontaneous mutation of single drug resistant cells is relatively frequent (SCHABEL et al. 1980). In addition to selection of drug resistant cells which were initially present, mutation to drug resistance may occur during treatment. It is commonly observed, both in man and rodent, that initially drug sensitive tumors become progressively less responsive and ultimately fail to respond during continuous treatment (SCHABEL et al. 1980).

The main aim of combination chemotherapy is to avoid the consequences of the presence of drug resistant cells. However, resistance to as many as six separate drugs has been shown to occur in treatment of human or experimental tumors. When many drugs are used in combination, the individual drug doses must be reduced in order to avoid cumulative toxicity, and some of the drugs are only toxic to vital normal cells without contributing to tumor cell kill. Thus, the addition of irradiation is advantageous as there is no cross resistance between ionizing radiation and drugs.

The mathematical model constructed by GOLDIE and COLDMAN (1979) and GOLDIE et al. (1982) shows that when both CT and RT are to be administered, it is preferable to deliver both of them as early as possible. The essential features of this

model are that mutations to resistance arise spontaneously and with a measurable frequency independent of treatment. When two agents are used, a delay in the administration of one of them increases the probability of development of a resistant tumor cell line. If it is assumed that the development of a doubly-resistant tumor cell line results in the incurability of the tumor, alternating the treatment regimen at every cycle markedly increases the effectiveness of the strategy. Although this model was built for predicting the effects of combining various cytotoxic drugs, its conclusion remains valid with respect to an association between RT and CT, and it suggests that each modality should be given as early as readily achievable.

These theoretic considerations and the promising clinical results are corroborated by an interesting series of experiments reported by LOONEY et al. (1983), and LOONEY et al. (1981, 1983). These authors studied a rat hepatoma for which no cure was achieved with either radiotherapy or chemotherapy given alone. They obtained a tumor cure rate of 60% when 3 series of combined radiation (15 Gy) and cyclophosphamide (150 mg/kg) were given sequentially and the time between modalities was held constant at 7 days. The time interval between the 2 modalities and between successive sequences was relatively critical. For example, a time interval of 7 days between radiation and cyclophosphamide was the most effective in controlling tumor growth with least acute host toxicity. The cure rate was reduced to 10% when the time between the first sequence of cyclophosphamide and radiation and the following sequence was increased from 7 to 25 days. The existence of an optimum delay between the two modalities has probably two explanations: i) the sensitivity of a tumor to either RT or CT is enhanced at the time of repopulation; ii) if the time interval between successive sequences is too long, an increase in the number of clonogenic viable cells due to repopulation lowers the cure probability.

The delay that we have chosen (7–10 days) which is optimal for the experimental tumor studies by LOONEY et al. (1983a, 1983b) might not be the optimal one in patients. However, a shorter delay might enhance the toxic effect on normal tissues (Conference on Combined Modalities..., 1979; PECKHAM and COLLIS 1981; TUBIANA 1981; RUBIN 1984). Moreover, studies carried out in human tumors show that repopulation is certainly ongoing at that time (TUBIANA 1982; TUBIANA et al. 1985). Nevertheless, from the point of view of reduction of the cumulative effect on normal tissue and therefore of the therapeutic efficacy, a slightly longer delay might be preferable. Without perturbation of the CT scheduling, a slight increase of the delay between the two modalities might be achieved by shortening the duration of each of the RT courses. Studies with multifraction irradiation in patients suggest that 18.75 Gy should be delivered in five days (three fractions daily of 1.25 Gy during five consecutive days). LOONEY et al. (1985) have shown in the rat hepatoma that multiple fractions daily given intermittently and alternated with cyclophosphamide resulted in a cure rate of 50% with 6,000 rad compared to 11,250 rad given as daily radiation; the use of multiple fractions daily and cyclophosphamide also eliminated the risk of metastatic dissemination. MITCHELL et al. (1984) have shown that small cell lung cancer cell lines are characterized by small survival curve shoulders. Thus, these cells would not be expected to repair sublethal damage as readily as normal lung. This finding would imply that the use of multiple daily fractions may be appropriate in the treatment of small cell lung cancer.

In conclusion, the preliminary clinical data obtained with this alternating schedule of CT and RT which have been previously reported (ARRIAGADA et al. 1985; COSSET et al. 1985; TUBIANA et al. 1985) and which are updated in the present paper, are promising. They are supported by experimental data and theoretic considerations. The scheme deserves to be further investigated, since combination of CT and RT constitutes one of the solid approaches for further progress in cancer treatment.

It is more convenient for both the radiotherapist and the chemotherapist to carry out this part of the treatment with the conventional and familiar schedule. However, when both modalities are combined, this usual schedule is probably not the optimal one. Our data show that other types of sequencing are well tolerated and might be more effective. This integration requires an organizational pattern in which radiotherapist and medical oncologist work closely together. This cooperation has several other advantages for the patients and for the institution.

References

Aisner J, Alberto P, Bitran J, Comis R, Daniels J, Hansen H, Ikegami H, Smyth J (1983) role of chemotherapy in small cell lung cancer: a consensus report of the International Association for the Study of Lung Cancer Workshop. Cancer Treat Rep 67:37–43

Amiel JL, Cosset JM, Arriagada R, Droz JP, Tursz Th, Ben Ayed F (1980) Les chimiothérapies et les radiothérapies imbriquées. Application aux métastases pulmonaires multiples des cylindromes. Nouv Presse Med 9:2545–2547

Amiel JL, Mathé G, Tubiana M, Schlumberger JR, Rouessé J, Pouillart P (1971) Traitement des maladies de Hodgkin stades III et IV par la séquence chimiothérapie, radiothérapie, chimiothérapie. Bull Cancer (Paris) 58:191–202

Anderson P, Dische S (1981) Local tumor control and the subsequent incidence of distant metastatic disease. Int J Radiat Oncol Biol Phys 7:1645–1648

Aristizabal SA, Miller RC, Schlichtemeier AL, Jones SE, Boone MLM (1977) Adriamycin-irradiation cutaneous complications. Int J Radiat Oncol Biol Phys 2:325–331

Arriagada R, Le Chevalier T, Baldeyrou P et al. (1985) Alternating radiotherapy and chemotherapy (Doxorubicin, Etoposide, Cyclophosphamide, CDDP) in small cell lung cancer limited disease. Cancer Treat Symp 2:115–117

Arriagada R, Le Chevalier T, Baldeyrou P et al. (1985) Alternating radiotherapy and chemotherapy schedules in small cell lung cancer, limited disease. Int J Rad Oncol Biol Phys 11:1461–1467

Arriagada R, Le Chevalier T, Ruffié P et al. (1987) Optimizing combinations of alternating radiotherapy and chemotherapy in limited small cell lung cancer. In: Karcher KH, Kogelnik HD, Szepesi T, eds. Progress in Radio-Oncology III. Vienna: ICRO 226–230

Arriagada R, Le Chevalier T, Sillet-Bach I (1981) Association de chimiothérapie et de radiothérapie séquentielles dans le traitement des carcinomes épidermoïdes bronchiques inopérables. Bull Cancer (Paris) 68:163–165

Barendsen GW, Broerse JJ (1969) Experimental radiotherapy of a rat rhabdomyosarcoma with 15 MeV neutrons and 300 kV X-Rays. I: Effects of single exposures. Eur J Cancer 5:373–391

Barker JL, Montague ED, Peters LJ (1980) Clinical experience with irradiation of inflammatory carcinoma of the breast with and without elective chemotherapy. Cancer 45:625–629

Bleehen NM (1981) Combined drug-radiation treatment: indications and clinical problems. Bull Cancer (Paris) 68:127–131

Bleehen NM, Bunn PA, Cox JD et al. (1983) Role of radiation therapy in small cell anaplastic carcinoma of the lung. Cancer Treat Rep 67:11–19

Bonadonna G, Bajetta E, Lattuada A, Buzzoni R, Valagussa P, Rilke F, Banfi A (1984) CVP versus VACOP chemotherapy sequentially combined with irradiation in stage II diffuse non Hodgkin's lymphoma. In: Adjuvant Therapy of Cancer IV. Grune and Stratton Inc. 661–667

Bonadonna G, Zucali R, Delene M, Valagussa P (1977) Combined chemotherapy (MOPP or ABVD) radiotherapy approach in advanced Hodgkin's disease. Cancer Treat Rep 61:769–777

Bunn P, Cohen M, Lichter A et al. (1983) Randomized trial of chemotherapy versus chemotherapy plus radiotherapy in limited stage small cell lung cancer. Proc Amer Soc Clin Oncol 2:200

Byhardt RW, Cox JD (1983) Is chest radiotherapy necessary in any or all patients with small cell carcinoma of the lung. Cancer Treat Rep 67:209–215

Cachin Y, Jortay A, Sancho H et al. (1977) Preliminary results of a randomized EORTC study comparing radiotherapy and concomitant Bleomycine to radiotherapy alone in epidermoid carcinomas of the oropharynx. Eur J Cancer 13:1389–1395

Camplejohn RS (1980) A critical review of the use of Vincristine (VCR) as a tumor cell synchronizing agent in cancer therapy. Cell Tissue Kinet 13:27–335

Carde P, Burgers JMV, Van Glabbeke M et al. (1984) Combined radiotherapy-chemotherapy for early stages non-Hodgkin's lymphoma. The 1975–1980 EORTC controlled lymphoma trial. Radiotherapy and Oncology 2:301–312

Charbit A, Malaise EP, Tubiana M (1971) Relation between the pathological nature and the growth rate of human tumors. Eur J Cancer 7:307–315

Cohen MH (1983) Is thoracic radiation therapy necessary for patients with limited-stage small cell lung cancer? No. Cancer Treat Rep 67:217–221

Conference on Combined Modalities Chemotherapy-Radiotherapy. Int J Radiat Oncol Biol Phys 5 (Nos 8 and 9):1139–1723

Cosset JM, Ozanne F, Henry-Amar M et al. (1985) An alternating chemotherapy and radiotherapy combination for non-Hodgkin's lymphomas of unfavourable histologies: preliminary results. Radiotherapy and Oncology 3:133–138

Costanzi JJ, Loukas D, Gagliano RG, Griffiths C, Barranco S (1976) Intravenous bleomycin infusion as a potential synchronizing agent in human disseminated malignancies; a preliminary report. Cancer 38:1503–1506

Courdi A, Tubiana M, Chavaudra N, Malaise EP, Le Fur R (1980) Changes in labeling indices of human tumors after irradiation. Int J Radiat Oncol Biol Phys 6:1639–1644

Cox JD, Byhardt R, Komaki R, Wilson JF, Libnoch JA, Hansen R (1979) Interaction of thoracic irradiation and chemotherapy on local control and survival in small cell carcinoma of the lung. Cancer Treat Rep 63:1251–1255

Demeestere M, Rockwell S, Valleron AJ, Frindel E, Tubiana M (1980) Cell proliferation in EMT6 tumors treated with single doses of X-rays or hydroxyurea. II: Computer simulations. Cell Tissue Kinet 13:309–317

Denekamp J, Thomlinson RH (1971) The cell proliferation kinetics of four experimental tumors after acute X-irradiation. Cancer Res 31:1279–1284

Fazekas JT, Sommer C, Kramer S (1980) Adjuvant intravenous methotrexate or definitive radiotherapy alone for advanced squamous cancers of the oral cavity, oropharynx, supraglottic larynx or hypopharynx. Int J Radiat Oncol Biol Phys 6:533–541

Feld R, Evans WK, Deboer G (1984) Combined modality induction therapy without maintenance chemotherapy for small cell carcinoma of the lung. J Clin Oncol 2:294–304

Fu KK, Silverberg IJ, Phillips TL, Friedman MA (1979) Combined radiotherapy and multidrug chemotherapy for advanced head and neck cancer: results of Radiation Therapy Oncology Group pilot study. Cancer Treat Rep 63:351–358

Glick JH, Marcial V, Richter M, Velez-Garcia E (1980) The adjuvant treatment of inoperable stage III and IV epidermoid carcinoma of the head and neck with platinum and bleomycin infusions prior to definitive radiotherapy: an RTOG pilot study. Cancer 46:1919–1926

Glick JH, Taylor SG (1981) Integration of chemotherapy into a combined modality treatment plan for head and neck cancer: a review. Int J Radiat Oncol Biol Phys 7:229–242

Goldie JH, Coldman AJ (1979) A mathematic model for relating the drug sensitivity of tumors to their spontaneous mutation rate. Cancer Treat Rep 63:1727–1733

Goldie JH, Coldman AJ, Gudauskas GA (1982) Rationale for the use of alternating non-cross-resistant chemotherapy. Cancer Treat Rep 66:439–449

Greco FA, Oldham RK (1982) Combined therapy in limited stage small cell bronchial carcinoma. In: Williams CJ, Whitehouse JMA, ed. Recent Advanced in Clinical Oncology I. Edinburgh: Churchill Livingstone 325–339

Griswold DP, Simpson-Herren L, Schabel FM (1970) Altered sensitivity of a hamster plasmacytoma to cytosine arabinoside. Cancer Chemother Rep (Part 1) 54:337–346

Guiguet M, Tubiana M, Valleron AJ (1982) Distribution des tailles des métastases à la détection et traitement adjuvant. Approche biomathématique. Comptes Rendus Acad Sciences (Paris) 294:15–18

Hansen M, Hansen HH, Dombernowsky P (1980) Long term survival in small cell carcinoma of the lung. JAMA 144:247–250

Hermens AF, Barendsen GW (1978) The proliferative status and clonogenic capacity of tumor cells in a transplantable rhabdomyosarcoma of the rat before and after irradiation with 800 rad of X-rays. Cell Tissue Kinet 11:83–100

Ihde DC, Bunn PA (1982) Chemotherapy of small cell bronchogenic carcinoma. In: Williams CJ, Whitehouse JMA, ed. Recent Advances in Clinical Oncology I. Edinburgh: Churchill Livingstone 305–323

Koscielny S, Tubiana M, Le MG, Valleron AJ, Mouriesse H, Contesso G, Sarrazin D (1984) Breast cancer: relationship between the size of the primary tumor and the probability of metastatic dissemination. Brit J Cancer 49:709–715

Lagrange JL, Verschoore J, Boubil JL et al. Synchronous chemotherapy and radiotherapy in lung cancer. (personal communication)

Le Chevalier T, Arriagada R, Pico JL et al. (1982) Chimiothérapie et radiothérapie séquentielles dans les carcinomes anaplasiques à petites cellules. Résultats préliminaires. Bull Cancer (Paris) 69:98–101

Looney WB, Hopkins HA, Carter WH (1984) Solid tumor models for the assessment of different treatment modalities. XXII. The alternate utilization of radiotherapy and chemotherapy. Cancer 54:416–425

Looney WB, Hopkins HA, Carter WH (1985) Solid tumor models for the assessment of different treatment modalities. XXIII. A new approach to the more effective utilization of radiotherapy alternated with chemotherapy. Int J Rad Oncol Biol Phys 11:2105–2117

Looney WB, Hopkins HA, Kovacs CJ et al. (1983) Single and combined (radiation-cyclophosphamide) modality therapy in experimental solid tumors. Adv Radiation Biology 10:305–403

Looney WB, Hopkins HA, Longerbeam MB, Carter WH Jr (1983) Solid tumor models for the assessment of different treatment modalities: XX. Comparison of effects of daily versus hyperfractionated, split course radiation schedules with and without cyclophosphamide on median survival, metastatic dissemination, tumor cure and growth rates. Cancer Res 43:60–67

Looney WB, Ritenour ER, Hopkins HA (1981) Solid tumor models for the assessment of different treatment modalities: XVI. Sequential combined modality (cyclophosphamide-radiation) therapy. Cancer 47:860–869

Malaise EP, Charbit A, Chavaudra N, Combes PF, Douchez J, Tubiana M (1972) Change in volume of irradiated human metastases. Investigation of repair of sublethal damage and tumor repopulation. Brit J Cancer 26:43–52

Malaise E, Tubiana M (1966) Croissance des cellules d'un fibrosarcome expérimental irradié chez la souris C 3H. CR Acad Sciences 263D:292–295

Marcial VA, Velez-Garcia E, Figueroa-Valles NR, Cintron J, Vallecillo LA (1980) Multidrug chemotherapy (vincristine-bleomycin-methotrexate) followed by radiotherapy in inoperable carcinomas of the head and neck: preliminary report of a pilot study of the Radiation Therapy Group. Int J Radiat Oncol Biol Phys 6:717–722

Mead GM, Jacobs C (1982) Changing role of chemotherapy in treatment of head and neck cancer. Am J Med 73:582–595

Mitchell JB (1984) Radiobiology of lung cancer. Workshop on radiotherapy for lung cancer (IASLC). Cambridge, England, June 26–30

Morstyn G, Ihde DC, Lichter AS et al. (1984) Small cell lung cancer 1973–1983: Early progress and recent obstacles. Int J Radiat Oncol Biol Phys 10:515–539

Nias AHN, Camplejohn RS (1981) Minimal criteria for synchronization in clinical trials. Cell Tissue Kinet 14:337–339

Pearson AE, Steel GG (1984) Chemotherapy in combination with pelvic irradiation: a time-dependence study in mice. Radiotherapy and Oncology 2:49–55

Peckham MJ, Collis CH (1981) Clinical objectives and normal tissue responses in combined chemotherapy and radiotherapy. Bull Cancer (Paris) 68:132–141

Petrovich Z, Block J, Kuisk H et al. (1981) A randomized comparison of radiotherapy with a radiotherapy-chemotherapy combination in stage IV carcinoma of the head and neck. Cancer 47:2259–2264

Potmesil M, Goldfeder A (1980) Cell kinetics of irradiated experimental tumors: cell transition from the non-proliferating to the proliferating pool. Cell Tissue Kinet 13:563–570

Potten CS, Hendry JH (1983) Cytotoxic Insult to Tissue. Effects on Cell Lineages. Londres: Churchill Livingstone 421

Price LA, Hill BT (1980) Safe and effective combination chemotherapy for squamous cell carcinomas of the head and neck. J Laryngol Otol 94:89–90

Price LA, Hill BT, Calvert AH et al. (1978) Improved results in combination chemotherapy of head and neck cancer using a kinetically-based approach: a randomized study with and without adriamycin. Oncology 35:26–28

Rambert P, Malaise E, Laugier A, Schlienger M, Tubiana M (1968) Données sur la vitesse de croissance de tumeurs humaines. Bull Cancer (Paris) 55:323–342

Rockwell S, Frindel E, Valleron AJ, Tubiana M (1978) Cell proliferation in EMT6 tumors treated with single doses of X-rays or hydroxyurea. I: Experimental results. Cell Tissue Kinet 11:279–289

Rubin P (1984) Late effects of chemotherapy and radiation therapy. A new hypothesis. Int J Radiat Oncol Biol Phys 10:5–34

Salazar OM, Creech RH (1980) The stage of the art towards defining the role of radiation therapy in the management of small cell bronchogenic carcinoma. Int J Radiat Oncol Biol Phys 6:1103–1117

Schabel FM, Skipper HE, Trader MW, Laster WR, Corbett TH, Griswold DP (1980) Concept for controlling drug resistant tumor cells. In: Mouridsen HT, Palshof T, ed. Breast Cancer, Experimental and Clinical Aspects. Oxford: Pergamon Press, 199–211

Shanta V, Krishnamurthi S (1980) Combined bleomycin and radiotherapy in oral cancer. Clin Radiol 31:617–620

Somers R, Burgers JMV, Qasim M, van Glabbeke M, Duez N, Hayat M. (1987) EORTC trial non-Hodgkin Lymphomas. Eur. J. Cancer 23:283–293

Steel GG (1977) Growth Kinetics of Tumours. Cell Population Kinetics in Relation to the Growth and Treatment of Cancer. Oxford: Clarendon Press

Stefani S, Eells RW, Abbate J (1971) Hydroxyurea and radiotherapy in head and neck cancer. Radiology 101:391–396

Stell PM, Dalby JE, Strickland P, Fraser JG, Bradley PJ, Flood RM (1983) Sequential chemotherapy and radiotherapy in advanced head and neck cancer. Clinical Radiology 34:463–467

Stephens TC, Steel GG (1980) Regeneration of tumors after cytotoxic treatment. In: Meyn and Withers, ed. Radiation Biology in Cancer Research. New York, Raven Press, 385

Suit H (1982) Potential for improving survival rates for the cancer patient by increasing the efficacy of treatment of the primary lesion. Cancer 50:1227–1234

Tannock I, Sutherland D, Osoba D (1982) Failure of short-course multiple drug chemotherapy to benefit patient with recurrent metastatic head and neck cancer. Cancer 49:1358–1361

Tubiana M (1981) Les associations radiothérapie-chimiothérapie. Bull Cancer (Paris) 68:109–115

Tubiana M (1982) Cell kinetics and radiation oncology. Int J Radiat Oncol Biol Phys 8:1471–1489

Tubiana M, Arriagada R, Cosset JM (1982) New types of fractionation for optimization of combinations of radiotherapy and chemotherapy. In: Karcher et al. ed. Progress in Radio-Oncology II. New York: Raven Press 387–391

Tubiana M, Arriagada R, Cosset JM (1985) Sequencing of drugs and radiation. The integrated alternating regimen. Cancer 55:2131–2139

Tubiana M, Frindel E, Vassort F (1975) Critical survey of experimental data on in vivo synchronization by hydroxyurea. In: Grundmann E, Gross R, ed. Recent Results in Cancer Research, vol. 62. Berlin New York: Springer Verlag, 187–205

Tubiana M, Henry Amar M, Hayat M et al. (1984) The EORTC treatment of early stages of Hodgkin's disease: the role of radiotherapy. Int J Radiat Oncol Biol Phys 10:197–210

Tubiana M, Malaise E (1976) Comparison of cell prolifera-
tion kinetics in human and experimental tumors: response to irradiation. Cancer Treat Rep 60:1887–1895

Vaeth JM (1979) Combined Effects of Chemotherapy and Radiotherapy on Normal Tissue Tolerance. Frontiers of Radiation Therapy and Oncology, vol. 13. Basel, New York: S Karger, 251

Van Peperzeel HA (1972) Effects of single doses of radiation on lung metastases in man and experimental animals. Eur J Cancer 8:665

Vogl SE, Lerner H, Kaplan BH et al. (1982) Failure of effective initial chemotherapy to modify the course of stage IV (MO) squamous cancer of the head and neck. Cancer 50:840–844

8 Neutrons

8.1 Fast Neutron Therapy: Problems and Promise

MOSHE H. MAOR

CONTENTS

1 Introduction

It took only six years from the discovery of the neutron and the production of fast neutron beams with cyclotrons for Dr. Robert Stone to start his pioneering work on human cancer. At that time (1938), there was no theoretical indication that neutron therapy might be more effective in controlling human cancer than conventional x-ray therapy. Thus, neutrons were empirically tested, just as x-rays had been shortly after their discovery in 1895. Stone and his colleagues knew that neutrons had a higher relative biologic effectiveness (RBE) compared to x-rays and used a ratio of 2.5 for their dose estimation. This factor was derived from single-fraction experiments on human skin. The fact that the RBE increases with fractionated small-dose irradiation was not known then. This led to a significant overdosage in many patients treated in this first trial with neutrons with consequent severe late normal tissue injury. In summarizing his experience with neutrons, STONE (1948), concluded that "neutron therapy as administered by us resulted in such bad delayed se-

MOSHE H. MAOR, M.D., Associate Professor
The University of Texas M.D. Anderson Hospital
and Tumor Institute
Houston, TX 77030, USA

quelae in proportion to a few good results that it should not be continued." Since a sound biologic rationale for neutron therapy was lacking, this unfavorable experience was enough to discourage further attempts at neutron therapy for 25 years.

The rebirth of neutron therapy was fathered by Gray in the late fifties at the Hammersmith Hospital, London. Radiobiologic considerations led Gray to believe that neutron therapy should be more effective than photons in controlling human tumors. They were based on two discoveries: 1) neutrons are less dependent on oxygen as a radiosensitizer; and 2) human cancer contains anoxic cells. These foci of anoxia were believed to be the reason for radioresistance in human tumors that remain uncontrolled with conventional photon therapy. Later discoveries such as the diminished capability of tumor cells to repair injury inflicted by neutrons and a lesser variation in sensitivity in the various phases of the cell cycle have made the rationale for neutron therapy even more attractive (RAJU 1980). The modern clinical experience with neutrons started in 1966 at the Hammersmith Hospital with the support of the Medical Research Council. In the United States the second era of neutron therapy began in 1972 at M.D. Anderson Hospital and Tumor Institute employing the Texas A & M Variable Energy Cyclotron. Since then other institutions have acquired the capability of neutron therapy in the United States, Europe, and Japan. Approximately 9,000 patients were treated with neutrons to date and they form the basis of our current assessment of neutron therapy reported here.

2 Clinical Experience With Fast Neutron Therapy

2.1 High-Grade Gliomas

Based on tumor-related considerations, high-grade gliomas should be ideally suited for neutron therapy: they rarely metastatize, and patients invariably die of progressive local disease. Moreover, identification of necrosis is a sine qua non for the histological diagnosis of glioblastoma multiforme. It was conjectured that conventional radiation therapy fails due to the survival of hypoxic clonogenic tumor cells. Pilot studies with neutron therapy reported from Seattle (LARAMORE et al. 1978) were encouraging. Although there was no improvement in survival for patients treated with neutrons, they did not seem to die of progressive tumor. Autopsies on 15 patients treated with neutrons showed no evidence of gross tumor progression in 14 cases despite their poor survival. Death occurred as a result of diffuse degeneration and demyelination of the white matter. This experience led to Radiation Therapy Oncology Group (RTOG) randomized study in which the whole brain was given x-ray therapy to a dose of 50 Gy in 2 Gy fractions. An additional boost of 15 Gy with photons, or an RBE-adjusted neutron dose, was given to the tumor volume according to randomization. With 83 patients in each arm, there was no difference in survival and this remained the case when data were analyzed separately for grade III or grade IV astrocytoma (GRIFFIN et al. 1983). Autopsies were performed in 24 cases, 12 in each arm. In nine out of 12 patients treated with neutrons, no mass effect or an infiltrating tumor could be identified. There was significant necrosis at the primary tumor site. In contrast, all autopsy patients treated with photons revealed an infiltrating viable tumor mass. Similar results in a randomized trial were reported from England (CATTERALL et al. 1980). There were 33 patients treated with photons and 30 were treated with neutrons. Five patients treated with neutrons showed symptoms of dementia without signs of tumor recurrence. Autopsy studies showed that local tumor control was achieved in most neutron-treated patients but at the expense of a fatal gliosis.

The question of whether an optimal dose of neutrons exists, a dose which would give maximal tumor control or palliation with minimal late changes was addressed by a subsequent RTOG study. Patients were treated with whole-brain irradiation with photons, 45 Gy in 30 equal fractions over 6 weeks. The patients received a concomitant boost dose with neutrons to the tumor-bearing area twice per week using six different total neutron doses ranging from 3.6 to 6.0 Gy. There was no significant survival benefit for any of the dose levels (LARAMORE, oral communication, 1984). There was no difference in survival between patients treated with the lower three doses, as compared to patients treated with the higher three doses. The number of autopsies was too low to make a meaningful comparison. However, tumor progression was found in almost all cases.

In summary, the results of fast neutron therapy treatment for high-grade gliomas are disappointing: in no instance was tumor control reported without a fatal complication. With photon therapy, to trade off tumor recurrence for a complication in the brain prolong survival since the time to a complication is, on the average, 18 months (SHELINE 1980). However, the complications encountered with neutron irradiation administered to patients with brain tumors occurred much earlier; on the average, even before the median time for tumor recurrence. One is therefore forced to conclude that the vulnerability of the central nervous system to injury by fast neutron therapy precludes its effective use in the treatment of malignant gliomas.

2.2 Squamous Cancer of the Upper Aerodigestive Tract

The main cause of death in patients with advanced head and neck cancer is failure to control the primary or regional tumor. Hence, it is likely that an improvement in local control will favorably influence survival. It is now 10 years since the reports on the randomized trial on head and neck cancer from Hammersmith were published (CATTERALL et al. 1975, 1977). In this study, 70 patients were treated with neutrons and 63 with photons. Complete regression of the tumor was achieved in 77% of the neutron series and 43% of the photon series. Only one tumor recurred in the patients treated with neutrons compared with 15 recurrences in patients treated with photons. The ultimate local control was 76% for neutrons and 19% for photons but survival was only slightly better in the neutron series. This impressive achievement in local control was recently corroborated by a RTOG trial comparing neutrons with photons (GRIFFIN et al. 1984b) in a small group of patients. Both these trials are open to criticism because of the poor control rates achieved in patients treated with conventional radiation. This, in turn, may have resulted, at least in part, from the design of both studies, which allowed treatment of patients in the control arm by outside institutions.

Other attempts to emulate the good results from Hammersmith in larger phase III protocols were not successful. In a randomized trial in Edinburgh,

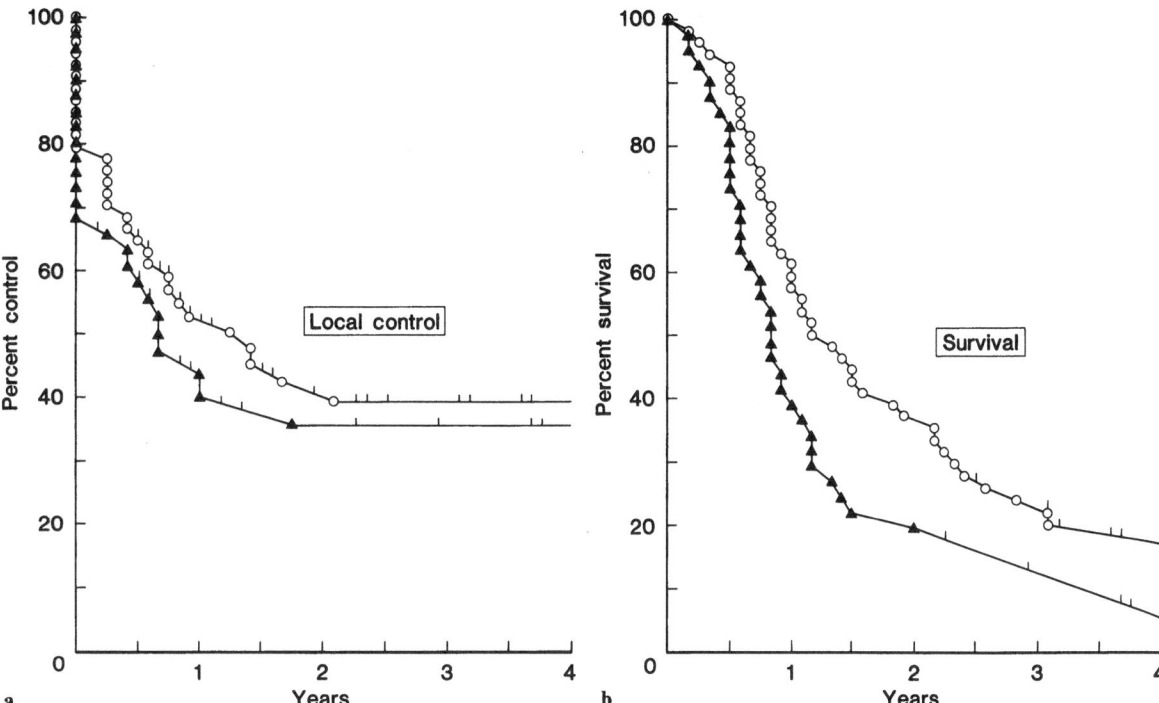

Fig. 1a, b. Local control and survival in patients with advanced head and neck cancer treated at M.D. Anderson Hospital. ○ Mixed beam (54 pts.); △ conventional treatment (41 pts)

64 patients were treated with neutrons and 66 with photons (ARNOTT and DUNCAN 1984a). Serious morbidity in both arms was about the same, hence the biologic doses administered in each arm were similar. Complete regression and permanent local control were no different in the two arms. Survival was better in patients treated with photons at $P = 0.064$. No analysis of the causes of death is given in this paper. In the United States, studies with neutrons alone became unpopular in the 1970's because all investigators reported high rates of complications with neutrons alone in head and neck cancer. Thus a mixed schedule of neutrons and photons was selected as the investigative arm to be tested against conventional irradiation with photons alone in a randomized phase III trial. Five institutions participated in this RTOG study (76–10): University of Washington (Seattle), Great Lakes Neutron Therapy Association (GLANTA), Cleveland, Naval Research Laboratories (NRL), Washington, D.C., Texas A&M Variable Energy Cyclotron (TAMVEC) – The University of Texas M.D. Anderson Hospital (UT MDAH) Houston and Fermi Laboratories, Batavia, Illinois. The re-

sults of treating 306 patients were analyzed. Actuarial local control and survival showed no difference between the two arms. The rate of complications was the same (GRIFFIN et al. 1984a). An interesting result in this study was that when clearance of metastatic neck nodes was analyzed separately, there was a significant difference favoring mixed beam treatment over photons, 69% vs. 55%, ($P = 0.024$). The improved control in the nodes was not associated with better overall local control or survival. A separate analysis of the patients treated at The University of Texas M.D. Anderson Hospital (UT MDAH) and Tumor Institute at Houston-TAMVEC showed a higher clearance rate for mixed beam and a better local control and survival in the first 2 years (Fig. 1A, 1B). After 2 years these differences equalled out (MAOR et al. 1983). The superiority of mixed-beam irradiation for nodal neck disease was confirmed in these patients by a further analysis (HUSSEY et al. 1983). For N_3 neck disease, the failure rate with mixed beam was 26.3% compared to 50% with photons.

2.3 Salivary Gland Tumors

The largest experience in the treatment of this tumor with neutrons has been gained at Hammersmith Hospital, London (CATTERALL 1981). Forty

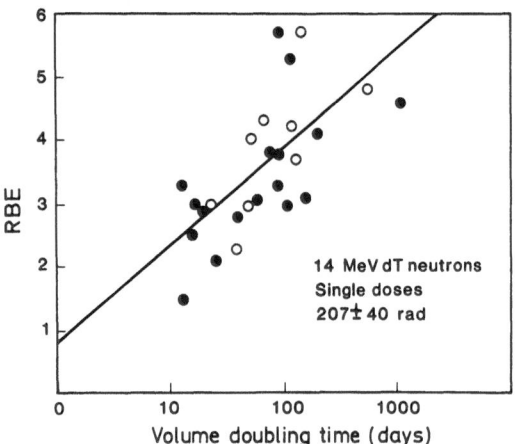

Fig. 2. RBE η/γ vs. volume doubling time in human lung metastases. (From BATTERMANN et al. 1981)

patients with different histologies were treated: 18 adenoid cystic, 7 mucoepidermoid, 6 adenocarcinoma, 5 anaplastic, and 4 malignant mixed. Fourteen of the patients were treated for cancer recurrence after surgery. All patients had complete regression of the tumor and 34/40 (85%) patients had long term local-regional control of their tumor. Of the six recurrences, three were marginal recurrences outside the irradiated field and the other three followed an inadequate dose. A local control rate of 72% (18/25) in patients with salivary gland tumors of various histologies was reported from the Fermilab facility (KURUP et al. 1984). Because this tumor is relatively rare, a randomized trial of the RTOG is accruing patients very slowly, and although the trend is in favor of fast neutron therapy, no statistical significance has yet been demonstrated. By analogy with the high RBE values for slowly-growing tumors (Fig. 2), the favorable clinical results with neutrons for salivary gland tumors may be related to the long doubling time of some lower grade tumors in this site. Of interest is the measurement of 5.7

for RBE η/γ in adenoid cystic carcinoma metastatic to the lung (BATTERMANN et al. 1981).

2.4 Lung Cancer

Experience to date with fast neutron therapy for non-oat cell lung cancer has not been encouraging. Two comparative trials have recently been reported.

In the Heidelberg study (SCHNABEL et al. 1984), patients with squamous cell carcinoma of the lung were assigned to either neutrons or photons, depending on the availability of the DT generator. Fifty-nine patients were treated with neutrons and 79 with ^{60}Co. The doses selected were 18 Gy for neutrons and 54 Gy for photons. All treatments were given in 20 fractions over 5 weeks. The overall response rates were 75% and 77% for neutrons and photons, respectively, with similar incidences of radiologically complete response. Lung fibrosis was the same in both arms. One year survival and median survival were also similar in both arms. The authors concluded that fast neutron therapy offered no advantage in the treatment of squamous cancer of the lung and discontinued this study.

In the United States a RTOG trial (79-07) included patients with squamous, adeno, and large cell carcinomas who were randomized between three treatments: photons only, mixed schedule of neutrons and photons, and neutrons only. The results were recently analyzed (LARAMORE et al. 1986). Dose selection, number of patients, and results are shown in Table 1. Three patients treated with neutrons and one patient treated with mixed beam developed myelitis. Thus, the American experience confirms the conclusions from Heidelberg. Better local control with a combination of neutrons and photons compared to photons was reported from East Germany (EICHORN et al. 1980); however, the survival was poorer in the mixed beam-treated arm.

Table 1. Comparison of treatment modalities for non-oat cell cancer of the lung (RTOG 79-07)

Treatment	No. of patients	Complete response (%)	Partial response (%)	Overall response (%)	Median survival (mo)	No. of complications
Photons	38	44	15	59	8.4	2
Neutrons	30	24	31	55	7.1	10
Mixed beam	36	29	24	53	7.0	4

2.5 Esophageal Cancer

A RTOG phase I study of neutron therapy in squamous carcinoma of the esophagus was reported (LARAMORE et al. 1983). Thirty patients were treated with a mixed schedule of neutrons and photons and nine with neutrons. The median survivals were 10.9 and 9 months for mixed irradiation and neutrons, respectively. There was a high rate of severe or fatal complications. The results were considered so poor in terms of local control and complications that no phase II–III study was designed.

The experience in Chiba-shi, Japan was much more favorable (TSUNEMOTO et al. 1982). At 1 year, the survival of patients treated with neutrons or with photons was the same at 35%. Later, however, the survival curves separated. At 5 years, survival rates were 20% and 10.5% for neutrons and photons respectively, but because of the small number of patients, this finding was not statistically significant.

2.6 Pancreatic and Stomach Cancer

Since neutron therapy was effective in the treatment of salivary gland tumors, it was hoped that it might also be effective in other carcinomas of exocrine glands such as the pancreas. The widest experience to date has been gained at Fermilab (KAUL et al. 1981). Thirty-one patients with primary pancreatic adenocarcinomas with no evidence of distant metastases were treated. Most patients received a dose of 19.5 Gy in 13 fractions in 6 weeks. Median survival was 9 months. Eleven patients developed complications, two of which were fatal. At the NRL facility in Washington, the median survival of 20 patients with pancreatic cancer was only 6 months (SMITH et al. 1981). Two randomized trials to evaluate neutrons and mixed neutrons and photons compared to conventional radiation was initiated in february 1980 by RTOG. Although only 46 patients were evaluable, the survival in the neutron arms was shorter and the complication rate was higher. Based on physical considerations, the pancreas is an unfavorable site for neutron therapy. Its close anatomical relations with the small bowel, stomach, kidneys, and spinal cord demands a high precision beam as well as optimal tumor localization and treatment planning. All these features were lacking in patients treated with neutrons. The high rate of metastasis and the difficulty in evaluating the local outcome compound the problem of assessing the real value of neutrons in this disease. For these reasons, pancreatic cancer has a low priority for future investigations with neutron therapy.

Stomach cancer, another major tumor site in the upper abdomen, has similar unfavorable features for neutron therapy. The experience on patients with stomach cancer treated at Hammersmith was reported in 1976 (KINGSLEY et al. 1976). Autopsy showed microscopic tumor in all but one case examined. No survival data were given.

2.7 Uterine Cervix Cancer

Relatively few studies have been carried out using fast neutron therapy for cervical cancer, no doubt because only fixed, mostly horizontal neutron beams have been available until recently. Furthermore, neutrons have an inferior depth dose when compared to high energy photons; this is especially unfortunate in cervical cancer since the external diameters at this level are greatest. A horizontal beam requires that patients be treated in an upright position for the anterior and posterior positions, which not only increases the A–P dimension of the patient but also the volume of normal bowel irradiated. To minimize the unfavorable physical characteristics of the neutron beam, a mixed beam schedule of neutrons and energetic photons was chosen in studies conducted in the United States and Japan. Preliminary results of a randomized trial were reported from UT MDAH (MORALES et al. 1981). In this study, 75 patients with locally advanced cancer of the uterine cervix were treated by either 1) a combination of 50 MeV neutrons and 25 MeV photons, or 2) 25 MeV photons. In both arms of the study, an intracavitary radium system was allowed, when appropriate, after 5 weeks of external radiation. At the time of analysis, there was no difference between the mixed beam and photon groups with regard to local tumor control, frequency of major complications, or patient survival. The patients treated at UT MDAH were part of a national cooperative clinical trial conducted under the RTOG with the participation of Catholic University, Brussels, Belgium. The cooperative study was closed in May 1984 and the data were recently analyzed (MAOR et al. 1987). Of 156 cases randomized, 146 are evaluable for analysis. Eighty patients were treated with mixed beam and 66 with photons. The actuarial survival in two arms are approximately the same (Fig. 3). However, there were 15 cases (19%)

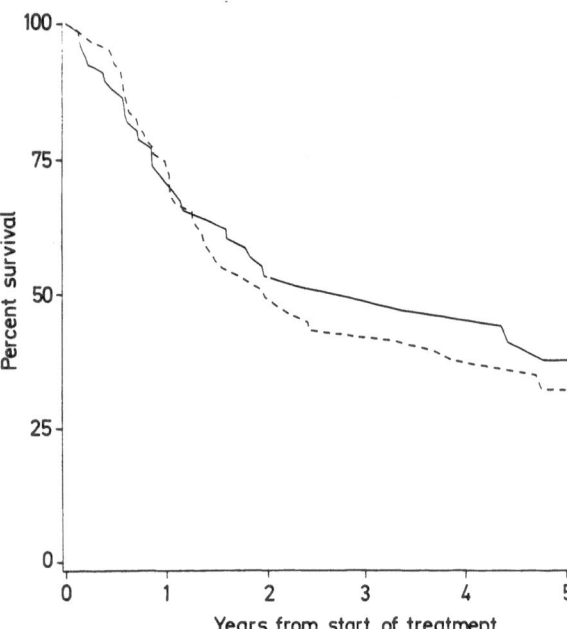

Fig. 3. Survival in patients with advanced cervical cancer treated by mixed beam or photons (RTOG 76-08). —— Photons; ――― mixed beam

Table 2. Fast neutron therapy for rectal and bladder cancers in Amsterdam

	Rectum	Bladder
No. of patients	25	22
Local control	13	10
Complications	16	7
2-year survival	4	5
Survival at analysis	0	1

of severe late bowel or bladder injury in the mixed-beam arm as compared to seven (11%) in the photon arm.

At the National Institute of Radiological Sciences (NIRS) in Chiba, Japan, a similar trials was conducted on 98 patients with advanced cervical cancer randomized between mixed-beam irradiation and photons (MORITA et al. 1985). Local control rates were 73% and 66% for mixed beam and photons, respectively. Complications were higher with mixed beam irradiation.

Although the results with neutron therapy in cervical cancer to date have been disappointing, it is difficult to evaluate the biological potential of the modality in view of the technical limitations noted above.

2.8 Rectal and Bladder Cancer

Both tumors share biologic similarities other than their location in the pelvis. Local tumor control with conventional radiation therapy is low. Surgery with or without radiation achieves a better local control rate but at a high price in function. A significant experience in the treatment of these tumors with neutrons was gained in Amsterdam (BATTERMANN 1982). Patients were treated using a DT generator, with a depth dose similar to a ^{60}Co machine. The results of this experience are summarized in Table 2. Local tumor control was achieved in approximately half the patients and confirmed by autopsy in many. However, the rate of complications was very high and contributed significantly to the patients' demise. A change in technique to a 6-portal arrangement seemed at first to decrease the complication rate, but with further follow-up, the complication rate was still high (ARNOTT and DUNCAN 1984b).

In a pilot study of the RTOG, mixed-beam irradiation was given to 29 patients with advanced cancer of the bladder (LARAMORE et al. 1984). Seventeen of the patients had stage D_1 disease. Local clearance was achieved in 21/29 (72%) of the patients, but of the 21 patients 10 relapsed later in the bladder for an ultimate local control rate of 38%. A small group of patients had preoperative irradiation with mixed beam dose equivalent to 50 Gy photons in 5 weeks followed by cystectomy in 4–6 weeks. Negative specimens were obtained in 7/12 (58%) of the patients. This rate of downstaging is superior to the rate obtained with preoperative photons.

2.9 Prostate Cancer

The results of a RTOG phase trial comparing conventional and neutron irradiation on locally advanced prostate cancer were recently made available (LARAMORE et al. 1985a). Patients with stages C and D_1 disease were treated with megavoltage photons to 70 Gy with a field reduction to the gross tumor at 50 Gy or with a combination of high-energy photons and neutrons in a mixed-beam schedule to the same equivalent dose, and using the same techniques. A total of 91 patients were analyzed, 55 treated with mixed beam, and 36 with photons. The randomization was unbalanced by design to include more patients in the mixed-beam arm. Patient and tumor characteris-

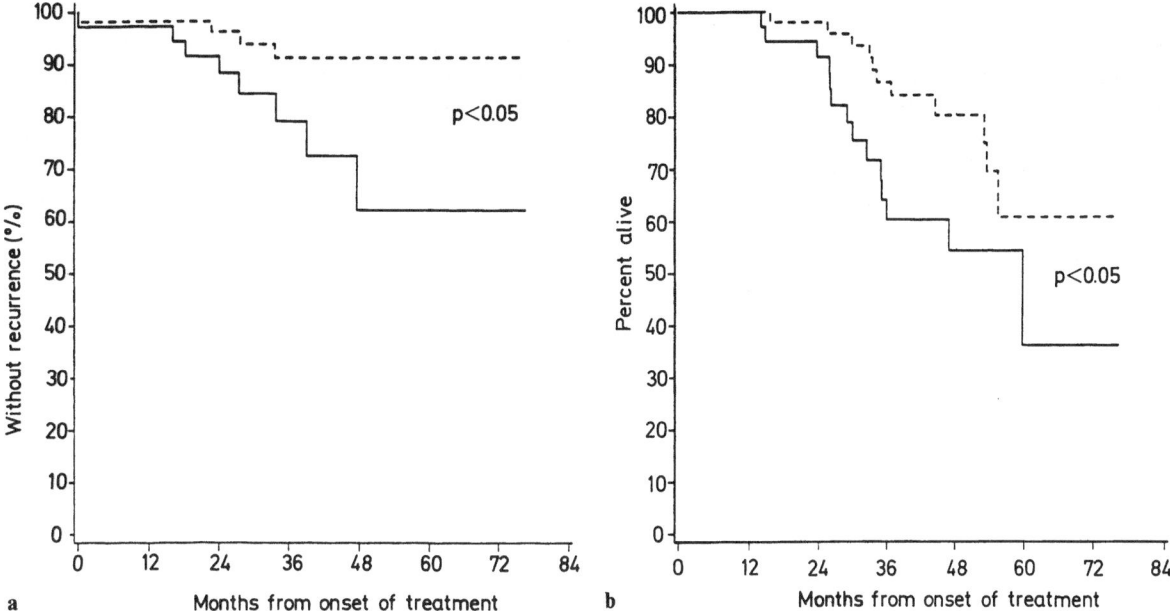

Fig. 4a, b. Local control and survival in prostate cancer treated with mixed beam or photons (RTOG 77-04). —— Photons; ——— mixed beam

tics were balanced in the two treatment arms except for gland size, which was larger in the patients treated with photons. Actuarial analysis of the time to local failure is shown in Fig. 4A. At 5 years, the actuarial failure rate was 7% for the mixed-beam group compared to 38% for the photon group. The actuarial survival of the patients treated with mixed beam was also significantly longer, compared to patients treated with photons (Fig. 4B). The incidence of severe complications was comparable in the two treatment groups, for the mixed beam – 9% and for photons – 7%.

Localized prostatic cancer has anatomical and biologic features that separates it from other pelvic tumors and makes it more suitable for neutron therapy. The major problem with neutron therapy to most tumor sites in the abdomen and pelvis is the morbidity associated with the unavoidable bowel irradiation. The prostate, on the other hand, is located very low in the pelvis and is extraperitoneal permitting irradiation of only a limited volume of the bowel. Also, prostate cancer is usually more slowly growing than other tumors in the pelvis which may be associated with a higher RBE η/γ for this tumor.

Though promising, the results of the RTOG phase III trial need to be confirmed in a larger study which should include stratification by histologic grade. This important prognostic characteristic was not available in approximately half the patients in the RTOG trial.

2.10 Sarcomas of the Soft Tissues and Bone

Conservative surgery for the gross tumor combined with radiation therapy for subclinical cancer foci achieves a high rate of local control in soft tissue sarcoma. However, conventional radiation for inoperable tumors is much less effective (SLATER et al. 1986).

The largest experience with fast neutron therapy comes from Essen, West Germany (SCHMITT and SCHNABEL 1984). Fifty-eight patients were treated with neutrons alone or with a neutron boost following photons to a wider volume. Long term local tumor control was achieved in half of these patients. For patients treated with neutrons alone, the complication rate was 28.6% but for patients treated with a neutron boost, with a shorter follow-up time, the complication rate was only 5%. The change in technique did not affect the local control rate. Results at other institutions in Europy vary. For local control, the range is between 18 and 75% and for complications, the range is between 18% and 44% (WAMBERSIE et al. 1984). This wide range of results is probably due to differences in tumor size and grade among the institutions. Experience in the United States is also favorable (SALINAS et al. 1980; COHEN et al. 1984). It is generally agreed that a control rate of 50% can be achieved with a reasonable rate of complications. This treatment allows the patient to retain a functioning limb and avoid amputation. The option of radical salvage surgery is not lost and can be offered to patients with treatment failure or with a devastating complication. Soft tissue sarcomas are uncommon tumors displaying a wide range of prognostic heterogeneity. Thus the prospects of establishing the superiority of neutrons over photons in a randomized trial treating only those tumors which are inoperable are poor. It is the consensus, however, that neutrons offer a therapeutic advantage.

Limited experience exists in the treatment of osteosarcoma with neutrons. At NIRS, 36 patients were treated with neutrons and compared with 17 patients treated with photons (TSUNEMOTO et al. 1982). All patients received chemotherapy prior to and after irradiation. Survival rate at 2 years was 75% for neutrons and 29% for photons. At 5 years the survival rates were 63% and 18% for neutrons and photons, respectively. Biopsies and surgical specimens were evaluated for tumor response. No viable tumor cells were demonstrated in 66% of the specimens obtained from patients treated with neutrons, as compared with 41% of those who received photons. There was no difference in the late tissue reactions between the two treatments.

The incidence of chondrosarcoma is lower than osteosarcoma and experience in its treatment is more limited. On the other hand, chondrosarcoma is an appropriate tumor for neutron therapy because it is often well differentiated with a low potential for distant metastases and a relatively low growth rate. Furthermore, chondrosarcoma occurs mainly in adults and problems associated with neutron irradiation in children can be avoided. Favorable results were reported from the Fermilab facility (Cohen et al. 1984). Sixteen patients were treated and 9 (56%) were controlled.

3 Conclusions

Before 1984, neutron therapy was delivered with inferior equipment characterized by poor depth dose, fixed beams and low output. Nevertheless, neutron therapy has yielded promising results in a number of tumor sites: salivary glands, prostate, soft tissue and bone sarcoma, and metastatic neck nodes. New and better facilities dedicated to patient care have been installed during the last few years in the United States and abroad. It is envisaged that results with neutron therapy will improve with the superior neutron delivery systems in the same way that the introduction of ^{60}Co and more energetic photons improved the results that could be achieved with orthovoltage equipment.

While further randomized clinical trials must be carried out to establish the value of fast neutron therapy, it is important not to exclude from further consideration tumors in sites where previous studies have yielded a null result since it is conceivable that the random allocation of a heterogeneous series of patients to receive fast neutron or conventional therapy could mask the advantage of neutrons for subsets of patients who could benefit from this modality. For this reason, a major effort is currently being directed to the development of predictive assays able to identify individual tumors that will be more sensitive to neutrons than to photons. The treatment of only these patients would improve the overall results in disease categories that hitherto yielded negative results for neutrons with randomized trials.

Acknowledgement. This work was supported in part by Grants CA06294 and CA16672 from the National Cancer Institute, Department of Health and Human Services, U.S.A.

References

Arnott SJ, Duncan W (1984a) An interim assessment of the experience of fast neutron therapy in patients with head and neck cancer in Edinburgh. J Eur Radiother 5:138–141

Arnott SJ, Duncan W (1984b) Workshop on Progress in High LET Radiation Therapy. Munich, Sept. 22, 1984

Battermann JJ, Breur K, Hart GAM, Van Peperzeel HA (1981) Observations on pulmonary metastases in patients after single doses and multiple fractions of fast neutrons and cobalt-60 gamma rays. Eur J Cancer 17(5):539–548

Battermann JJ (1982) Results of d + T fast neutron irradiation on advanced tumors of bladder and rectum. Int J Radiat Oncol Biol Phys 8:2159–2164

Catterall M, Sutherland I, Bewley DK (1975) First results of a randomized clinical trial of fast neutrons compared with X or gamma rays in treatment of advanced tumors of the head and neck. Br Med J 2(5972):653–656

Catterall M, Bewley DK, Sutherland I (1977) Second report on results of a randomised clinical trial of fast neutrons compared with X or gamma rays in treatment of advanced tumors of head and neck. Br Med J 1(6077):1642

Catterall M, Bloom HJ, Ash DV, Walsh L, Richardson A, Uttley D, Gowing NF, Lewis P, Chaucer B (1980)

Fast neutrons compared with megavoltage x-rays in the treatment of patients with supratentorial glioblastoma: A controlled pilot study. Int J Radiat Oncol Biol Phys 6(3):261–266

Catterall M (1981) The treatment of malignant salivary gland tumors with fast neutrons. Int J Radiat Oncol Biol Phys 7(12):1737–1738

Cohen L, Hendrickson F, Mansell J, Kurup PD, Awschalom M, Rosenberg I, TenHaken RK (1984) Response of sarcomas of bone and of soft tissue to neutron beam therapy. Int J Radiat Oncol Biol Phys 10:821–824

Eichhorn HJ, Lessel A, Dalluge KH (1980) Five years of clinical experience of radiotherapy using a combination of neutrons and photons. In: Karcher KH, Kogelnik HD, Meyer HJ (eds) Progress in Radio-Oncology, Thieme-Stratton Inc., New York, p 168

Griffin TW, Davis R, Laramore G, Hendrickson F, Rodriguez-Antunez A, Hussey D, Nelson J (1983) Fast neutron radiation therapy for glioblastoma multiforme. Results of an RTOG study. Am J Clin Oncol 6(6):661–667

Griffin TW, Davis R, Laramore GE, Maor MH, Hendrickson FR, Rodriguez-Antunez A, Davis L (1984a) Mixed beam radiation therapy for unresectable squamous cell carcinomas of the head and neck: The results of a randomized RTOG study. Int J Radiat Oncol Biol Phys 10:2211–2215

Griffin TW, Davis R, Hendrickson FR, Maor MH, Laramore GE (1984b) Fast neutron radiation therapy for unresectable squamous cell carcinomas of the head and neck: The results of a randomized RTOG study. Int J Radiat Oncol Biol Phys 10:2217–2221

Hussey DH, Maor MH, Fletcher GH (1983) A detailed analysis of the MDAH-TAMVEC neutron therapy trials for head and neck cancer. In: The 13th International Cancer Congress, Part D. Research and Treatment, Alan R. Liss Inc, New York, pp 267–277

Kaul R, Cohen L, Hendrickson F, Awschalom M, Hrejsa AF, Rosenberg I (1981) Pancreatic carcinomas: Results with fast neutron therapy. Int J Radiat Oncol Biol Phys 7(2):173–178

Kingsley D, Gad A, Catterall M (1976) Adenocarcinoma of the stomach: Radiological and pathological correlation of effects of treatment with fast neutrons. Gut 17(8):624–632

Kurup PD, Mansell J, TenHaken RK, Hendrickson FR, Cohen L, Awschalom M, Rosenberg I (1984) Response of epidermoid and non-epidermoid cancers of the head and neck to fast neutron irradiation: The Fermilab experience. Int J Radiat Oncol Biol Phys 10:473–479

Laramore GE, Griffin TW, Gerdes AJ, Parker RG (1978) Fast neutron and mixed (neutron/photon) beam teletherapy for grades III and IV astrocytomas. Cancer 42(1):96–103

Laramore GE, Davis RB, Olson MH, Cohen L, Raghaven V, Griffin TW, Rogers CC, Al-Abdulla AS, Gahbauer RA, Davis LW (1983) RTOG phase I study on fast neutron teletherapy for squamous cell carcinoma of the esophagus. Int J Radiat Oncol Biol Phys 9(4):465–473

Laramore GE, Davis RB, Hussey DH, Griffin TW, Maor MH, Hendrickson FR, Davis LW, Dupre E (1984) Radiation therapy oncology group phase I–II study on fast neutron teletherapy for carcinoma of the bladder. Cancer 54:432–439

Laramore GE, Krall JM, Thomas FJ, Griffin TW, Maor MH, Hendrickson FR (1985) Fast neutron radiotherapy for advanced carcinomas of the prostate: Results of an RTOG randomized clinical trial. Int J Radiat Oncol Biol Phys 11:1621–1627

Laramore GE, Bauer M, Griffin TW, Thomas FJ, Hendrickson FR, Maor MH, Griffin BR, Saxton JP (1986) Fast neutron and mixed beam radiotherapy for inoperable non-small cell carcinoma of the lung: Results of an RTOG randomized study. Am J Clin Oncol 79:233–243

Maor MH, Hussey DH, Barkley HT Jr, Peters LJ (1983) Neutron therapy for head and neck cancer: II. Further follow-up on the M.D. Anderson TAMVEC random trial. Int J Radiat Oncol Biol Phys 9:1261–1265

Maor MH, Gillespie BW, Peters LJ, Wambersie A, Griffin TW, Thomas FJ, Conner N, Gardner P (1987) Neutron therapy in cervical cancer: Results of a phase III RTOG study. Int J Radiol Oncol Biol Phys (in press)

Morales P, Hussey DH, Maor MH, Hamberger AD, Fletcher GH, Wharton JT (1981) Preliminary report of the M.D. Anderson Hospital randomized trial of neutron and photon irradiation for locally advanced carcinoma of the uterine cervix. Int J Radiat Oncol Biol Phys 7(11):1533–1540

Morita S, Arai T, Nakano T, Ishikawa T, Tsunemoto H, Fukuhisa K, Kasamatsu T (1985) Clinical experience of fast neutron therapy for carcinoma of the uterine cervix. Int J Radiat Oncol Biol Phys 11:1439–1445

Raju MR (1980) Biological Effects of High-LET Radiations. In: Heavy Particle Radiotherapy, Academic Press, New York, pp 39–77

Salinas R, Hussey DH, Fletcher GH, Lindberg RD, Martin RG, Peters LJ, Sinkovics JG (1980) Experience with fast neutron therapy for locally advanced sarcomas. Int J Radiat Oncol Biol Phys 6(3):267–272

Schmitt G, Schnabel K (1984) Neutron irradiation of soft tissue sarcomas in Essen and Heidelberg. An evaluation of the treatment period 1978–1982. J Eur Radiother 5(3):150–152

Schnabel K, Berberich W, Vogt-Moykopf J, Abel U (1984) Fast neutron therapy of squamous cell carcinoma of the lung. J Eur Radiother 5(3):147–149

Sheline GE (1980) Irradiation injury of the human brain: A review of clinical experience. In: Gilbert HA, Kagan AR (eds) Radiation Damage to the Nervous System, A Delayed Therapeutic Hazard, Raven Press, New York, pp 39–58

Slater JD, McNeese MD, Peters LJ (1986) Radiation therapy for unresectable soft tissue sarcomas. Int J Radiat Oncol Biol Phys 12:1729–1734

Smith FP, Schein PS, Wooley PV, Rogers C, Macdonald JS, Ornitz R (1981) Fast neutron irradiation for locally advanced pancreatic cancer. Int J Radiat Oncol Biol Phys 7(11):1527–1531

Stone RS (1948) Neutron therapy and specific ionization. Am J Roentgen and Radium Therapy 59(6):771–785

Tsunemoto H, Arai T, Morita S, Ishikawa T, Aoki Y, Takada N, Kamata S (1982) Japanese experience with clinical trials of fast neutrons. Int J Radiat Oncol Biol Phys 8:2169–2172

Wambersie A, Battermann JJ, Breteau N (1984) Survey of the clinical results of neutrontherapy. J Eur Radiother 5(3):120–131

9 Adjunctive Therapies

9.1 Externally Induced Hyperthermia

Frederic A. Gibbs, Jr.

CONTENTS

1 Introduction

Hyperthermia continues to be the subject of numerous clinical trials and intensive multidisciplinary investigations in biology, physics and engineering laboratories. Progress has been steady but painstaking since investigators are continually challenged by the complex problems of determining how to combine hyperthermia with the already effective modalities of X-radiation and chemotherapy and whether treatment has been improved by the addition of heat. Perhaps even more challenging is the task of safely and effectively heating anatomic regions of clinical importance. The purpose of this chapter is to summarize the present art and science of externally or non-invasively induced hyperthermia; reasonable restrictions on its length do not permit an exhaustive discussion of the relevant subject material. It is assumed that the reader is familiar with some of the basic principles of the developing field of hyperthermia (see STEWART and GIBBS 1984 for review).

2 Heating Methods

All of the non-invasive heating techniques have relative advantages and disadvantages; none has

FREDERIC A. GIBBS, Jr., M.D., Associate Professor
University of Utah Medical Center
Salt Lake City, UT 84132, USA

universal applicability to all anatomic sites and clinical circumstances. Uniform tumor heating without excessive normal tissue heating is not yet a common-place occurrence with any technique except in relatively small superficial subcutaneous sites. The following is a brief discussion of the fundamental difficulties associated with the various techniques.

Non-invasive heating may be accomplished by electromagnetic (EM) or mechanical means, the latter being practically restricted to ultrasound (US).

Electromagnetic Techniques. The EM techniques may be categorized as capacitive, inductive, or radiative.

Capacitive heating is most simply exemplified by two metal plates, connected to a radiofrequency (RF) generator (usually 13.56 or 27.12 mHz), which are placed on opposite sides of the tissue to be heated (A, Fig. 1). An alternating current passes between the plates with resulting heating of the interposed tissue. Heating is most intense in the high resistence fat planes lying perpendicular to the direction of the current. Differential fat heating may be ten-fold or more greater than that of underlying muscle equivalent tissue and, even with surface cooling, pain and fat necrosis often prevent effective tumor heating. Precautions must be taken to avoid excessive heating near the edges of the plates where the current density tends to be greatest. The electric field lines also diverge or balloon-out between the plates resulting in decreased power density in a larger central volume. Plate diameters approximately equal to the separation between the plates must be used to counteract this latter effect. Since heating patterns may reflect uncertain low-resistance current paths through complex tissue planes, attempted targeting of volumes to be heated at depth may be rather imprecise. Also, regions where current paths may be constrained into a small cross-sectional area (such as the retropharynx between the spine and pharyngeal air column in heating across the neck) may be subjected to excessive heating.

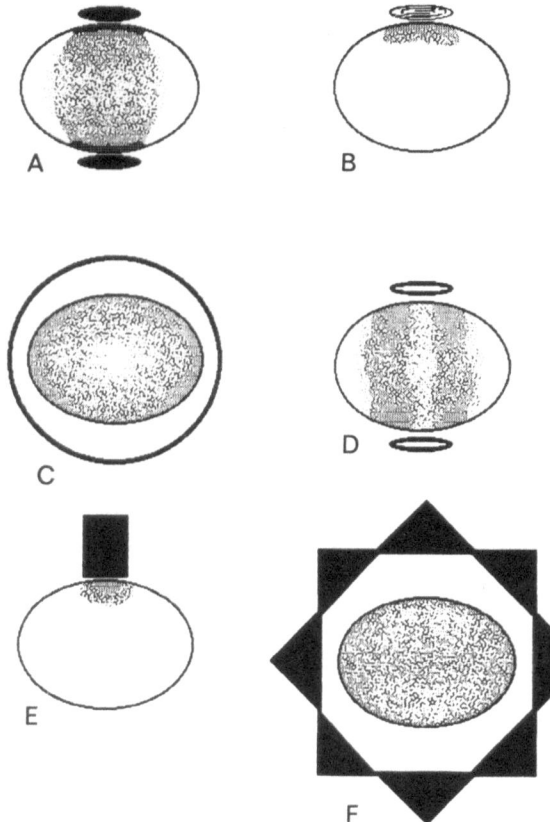

Fig. 1. Visual representations of the approximate cross-sectional heating patterns (in a schematic human torso) associated with various external EM heating methods (also schematically represented). The regions of darkest stippling represent the regions of greatest power density. *A* capacitive coupling (note dark bands representing subcutaneous fat heating); *B* "pancake coil"; *C* concentric coil (Magnetrode®); *D* transaxial coils (depicted pattern is variable and highly dependent on geometry and tissue properties); *E* radiative (single waveguide applicator); *F* radiative (annular array applicator)

Inductive heating is produced by an appositional RF current loop (e.g. a "pancoke coil", B, Fig. 1) when its electromagnetic field lines traverse the tissue to be heated. However, the field intensity decreases rapidly with distance from the coil and effective heating to more than a few centimeters in depth is unusual. In order to heat more effectively at depth using inductive principles it is necessary to avoid fieldline divergence at depth and also avoid regions where intense electric fields cross subcutaneous fat planes. One approach is to surround the patient's torso or limb with a concentric coil (CC) made from an impedance matched cylindrical sheet of metal carrying an RF current. A device utilizing this principle has been manufactured for experimental hyperthermia (Magne-

trode®, Henry Medical Electronics) and used rather extensively. Although this method of heating produces a relatively uniform axial magnetic field within the encompassed body segment, it does not produce uniform power deposition. Heat is produced by the electrical currents generated in the tissue by the alternating magnetic field. The physical laws describing this phenomenon state that the power deposited at any point is directly proportional to the square of the distance of that point from the center of the heated object and relatively independent of the position of the object within the surrounding RF current loop. Therefore, the cross-sectional power density or rate of temperature rise in a cylindrical tissue equivalent phantom is paraboloidal with the greatest heating occurring near the surface and none at the center (PALIWAL et al. 1982) as illustrated in C, Fig. 1.

Other inductive approaches of interest are the coaxially oriented helical coil (RUGGERA and KANTOR 1984) and a transaxially oriented pair of coils (OLESON et al. 1984) positioned on opposing sides of the heated subject. The helical coil differs from the previously discussed CC in that the electric field, which now is oriented parallel to the axis of the coil and the patient's body, is responsible for the heating. This method appears promising but has not been tested clinically and requires further development (the anticipated heating pattern will probably resemble F, Fig. 1). The transaxial coils (TC) would be theoretically expected to have a power null like the CC only oriented perpendicularly to the body axis. The anticipated heating pattern of the TC is illustrated in D, Fig. 1. However, its heating characteristics are complicated and highly dependent on coil and phantom geometry and tissue properties. The potential advantage of the TC over the CC is that the field theoretically could be positioned so that the regions of ineffective heating would be least likely to be located within the tumor volume.

Radiative heating, the last classification of the EM techniques, is usually referred to as microwave heating. However, since the microwave frequency range is generally considered to be above 300 mHz and the same technological approaches can be used at lower frequencies, the more descriptive generic term is better. The basic limitation with this technique is poor penetration with effective heating to more than a few centimeters being unusual (E, Fig. 1). Lower frequencies offer slightly better penetration but in order to affect a substantial improvement in penetration, frequencies below 50 mHz are needed which require much larger applicators, which are clinically cumbersome and heat a proportionately larger total volume. Though the depth of heating from a single radiative aperture is not very great, it is possible to use an array of such apertures to improve penetration. If a cylindrical arrangement of apertures is powered by a single generator so that a common wavefront is generated with the electric field parallel to the axis of the cylinder, it is possible to achieve much better heating than would be expected from mere plane wave penetration (TURNER 1984) as illustrated by F, Fig. 1. By changing the relative field strengths and phasing, it is possible to "steer" the heating pattern to a limited extent. Such a device has been designed and manufactured for experimental use (Annular Phased Array System [AA], BSD Medical Corp.), although the phase-control capability of the presently available system is not well developed and has been essentially clinically unutilized.

A disadvantage of any of the preceeding low frequency EM techniques is that they are essentially "regional" methods which heat broad areas of both tumor and normal tissue unselectively. If any preferential tumor heating occurs, it is due to a difference in blood flow between the tumor and surrounding normal tissue resulting in a relatively diminished capacity of the tumor to cool itself. The occurrence of such preferential tumor heating is often but not invariably seen in humans but is not quantitatively predictable.

3 Ultrasound Techniques

US is more penetrating than radiative EM techniques and it is also more directional, coherent and focusable, thus permitting more selective heating of tumor masses. Fixed-focus acoustic lenses can be used to produce a small, well-defined region of heating, or such a focal region may be rapidly and repetitively scanned under computerized control through or around a tumor volume to produce controlled heating of slightly larger more irregularly shaped masses (LELE 1983). The size of tumor which can be heated is limited by the scanning time and the fact that the "window" of body surface through which the beam passes must remain substantially larger than the focal region in order to prevent excessive superficial heating. Alternatively, a fixed array of US transducers can be focused on a tumor bearing region (FESSENDEN 1984a). Unfortunately, the problems with US are as numerous as its advantages. It is reflected by

tissue-air interfaces resulting in potential hot-spots on the near side of air containing structures and lack of heating beyond the interface. It is heavily absorbed by bone which can result in pronounced periosteal heating and associated pain unless the angle of incidence of the acoustic beam is sufficiently acute to result in reflection off the bone surface. Therefore, US would be of no use for deep heating in the chest and must be used with great caution and selectivity in the head and neck region around the upper aerodigestive tract and mandible. Applications in the abdomen and pelvis are frequently limited by air containing bowel or by bony obstacles or juxtaposition of the volume to be heated to large bones.

A technical problem associated with both US and EM methods, aside from achieving deep heating, is the difficulty of producing uniform temperature elevations over sizeable surface areas for large superficial lesions such as locally recurrent breast carcinoma. Radiative EM applicators typically produce a power distribution which tapers to zero near the edges of the applicator. In order to heat a large area, multiple adjacent applicators are needed with appropriate precautions to provide uniform power output from each applicator or independent temperature dependent feedback control for each applicator. Alternatively, a single applicator may be rapidly mechanically scanned over the area to be heated. Similar techniques employing multiple transducers or mechanical scanning are also necessary to heat a large area with US.

4 Thermometry and Thermal Dosimetry

The effect of hyperthermia on cell killing in vitro (with the attendant implications for both tumor cure and potential normal tissue complications) doubles with every one degree rise in temperature above 42–43° C, if the treatment time is held constant. Therefore, the importance of temperature monitoring and a concept of thermal dose should be intuitively clear. There are three fundamental problems in thermal dosimetry: 1) Clinically practical thermometers providing accurate temperature measurement are necessary. 2) Temperatures should be known throughout the tumor and surrounding normal tissue. 3) A means of incorporating temperature and time into a measurement of thermal dose is needed.

The availability of suitable thermometers is no longer a significant problem. Electromagnetically noninteractive high resistance lead thermisters or fiber-optic probes with accuracies of $\pm 0.2°$ C in EM fields are now manufactured by several companies. Additional improvements in such hardware is ongoing, including multi-sensor probes. It was previously thought that temperature measurement in EM fields was a major problem; one that could be avoided by using US heating. With further study it has become apparent that previously unsuspected sources of potential thermometry artifacts are present with US as well (FESSENDEN et al. 1984b).

Small needle thermisters or thermocouples pose no problem for routine clinical studies using US though "smearing" of temperatures by heat conduction in the needle shaft can cause errors in regions of high thermal gradients. Difficulties arise when plastic tubes are used to encapsulate flexible multi-sensor probes since most plastics have a coefficient of acoustic absorption greater than that of tissue and will differentially heat, causing artifactually high temperature readings. When the probe diameter approximates the US wavelength in tissue (e.g. 0.8 mm at 2 mHz) artifactually high measurements can also occur due to heating by friction between the tissue and probe ("viscous effect").

No matter how accurate the measurement at a single tissue point, the problem of knowing the temperature at other points remains. The fact that it is possible to observe temperature gradients in tissue as high as 7° C/cm (due to differences in local blood flow) even with the fairly uniform regional power density produced with the AA (GIBBS et al. 1985) gives one some perspective on the difficulties of measuring and predicting the temperature throughout a tumor mass. Multi-sensor probes are a step in the right direction. Fiber-optic probes having four sensing points are commercially available (VAGUINE et al. 1984; Luxtron, Mountain View, CA.). However, spacing of the sensors at 1–1.5 cm intervals (and sometimes closer) is necessary to accurately document thermal gradients commonly encountered in clinical practice (GIBBS et al. 1985). The technique of "thermal mapping" (TM) has been a useful solution to this problem under conditions near thermal equilibrium. This technique uses a moving single-sensor probe inside a small implanted catheter to scan the temperatures of the tissue through which the catheter passes. Apparatus has been developed to move several probes at once by a computer controlled steppermotor and display the temperature-distance plots from each catheter automatically on a video monitor (GIBBS 1983). It is prob-

able that a hybrid probe employing four or more sensing points and short distance TM capability to fill the information gap between the sensing points will be the best practical clinical thermometry probe in the oming decade.

Even with multiple TM probes inserted through a tumor bearing region, not all of the points throughout the tumor can be measured. The ideal thermometry device would determine temperatures in 3 dimensions non-invasively. Unfortunately, there does not appear to be a physical basis on which to design a practically useable non-invasive thermometry system in the foreseeable future (CETAS 1984). Another approach which seems more promising is the use of numerical modeling techniques based on projections of heat conduction and convection in tissue (ROEMER and CETAS 1984). Because of the uncertainties of local blood flow it is improbable that such techniques will be able to predict thermal distributions without invasive thermometry but they may well be capable of providing sufficiently accurate predictions of the temperatures throughout a large volume based on TM measurements at specific points.

A number of considerations make it extremely desirable to have a method of calculating a thermal dose based on both time and temperature that could be represented as iso-thermal-dose distributions analogous to those used in radiation therapy. It is rare that tumors can be heated to uniform temperatures maintained for fixed periods of time, and practical constraints often restrict the temperatures that can be achieved. In addition, extensive temperature measurements over the course of a treatment, such as are obtained with TM, produce a volume of data that is nearly incomprehensible (without substantial study) to an observer wishing to understand what was achieved in a given treatment. The use of on-line "thermal-dose-mapping" would provide a solution to some of these problems as well as enable the treating physician to continue a temperature restricted treatment for sufficient duration to achieve a desired minimum dose distribution across the tumor volume. The use of the following formula relating temperature and time has been proposed by a number of investigators (FIELD and MORRIS 1983; SAPARETO and DEWEY 1984).

$$\text{Thermal Dose} = \int_{\text{Beginning}}^{\text{End of treatment}} F(T)\,dt$$

where T = temp. (°C); t = time (min)

and where

$$F(T) = R(T_{Trans} - T) = 1 \quad \text{for} \quad T = T_{Trans}$$

and

$$R \text{ is a constant } \geq 0.17 \text{ and } \leq 0.25 \quad \text{for} \quad T < T_{Trans}$$
$$= 0.5 \qquad\qquad\qquad \text{for} \quad T > T_{Trans}$$

In uncomplicated terms, this equation describes the observed effect that the rate of heat induced cell killing in vitro increases by 4 to 6 fold with every 1° C rise up to a critical transition temperature (T_{Trans}). Above T_{Trans} the rate increases by only a factor of 2 with each 1° C rise. The transition is thought to occur at 42.5 to 43° C but its exact value and the value of R in the $< T_{Trans}$ range remain uncertain and could conceivably vary with tissue and cell type. The thermal dose is expressed in units of equivalent heating time at T_{Trans}. There are many dose modifying factors such as pre-heating ("step-up" heating), post-heating ("step-down" heating), rate of heating, "thermotolerance", tissue pH and nutritional status, physiologic effects such as blood flow modification by heating, and the interactions of heat with X-radiation and/or chemotherapy that modulate the treatment outcome (PEREZ and SAPARETO 1984). The existence of such dose modifying factors and the slight uncertainties regarding the values of T_{Trans} and R do not diminish the importance and utility of the clinical application of the preceding thermal dose formula, although it is important that a hyperthermia treatment be conducted so as to standardize as many of these potential variables as possible.

The ultimate accuracy with which tumor and normal tissue temperatures will have to be known in routine clinical applications cannot be presently determined. The answer will depend on the efficacy and therapeutic index of the treatment. If the range between substantial therapeutic benefit and the onset of complications is wide, then the accuracy with which the treatment must be documented will be less stringent. The most prudent path to follow at present is to obtain the best achievable documentation.

5 Clinical Efficacy

5.1 Local Superficial Heating

Hyperthermia has been used in a number of clinical trials employing radiation alone, hyperthermia alone and a combination of both for treatment

Table 1. Response of matched superficial tumors. (From STEWART 1984)

Authors	No. of tumors	Tumors with a complete response[a] (%)	
		Radiation alone	Radiation and heat
OVERGAARD 1983 (review)	186	31	74
KIM et al. 1982[b]	99	46	70
ARCANGELI et al. 1983	123	39	76
SCOTT et al. 1984[c]	62	39	83

[a] Radiation dose same in each arm, [b] Randomized trial, [c] Results at 6 mos

of superficial tumor nodules (generally cutaneous, subcutaneous or lymphatic metastases). MEYER (1984) summarized the results of this experience. From eight reported series using hyperthermia alone in a total of 131 cases, 15% had complete responses (CR's) and 32% partial responses (PR's) with little variation in response rate between the individual series. Table 1 (from STEWART 1984) summarizes the data from a number of series using radiation alone or combined with hyperthermia. These treatments were accomplished with superficial external heating techniques employing radiative or inductive EM methods or unfocused US. The treatment sequence (i.e. heat before or after X-ray), temperatures achieved, heating duration, accuracy and uniformity of heating and radiation dose all varied. In all series the X-ray dose was purposely chosen to be subcurative so that the additional value of hyperthermia could be convincingly demonstrated. Given the variability of the treatment parameters, the consistency of the results is truly remarkable. Nearly every series has shown roughly a doubling of CR's with the addition of hyperthermia. In addition, there does not appear to have been any significant correlation between histology and the degree of improved response. Though these results are exciting, one must bear in mind that the duration of observation was often short, due to the fact that most of the patients had metastatic disease and often died within months of treatment. The results of a pioneering study on pet animals (DEWHIRST and SIM 1984) serve to emphasize that response durability is a more elusive goal than CR and that both are related to the adequacy of tumor heating. Their results are summarized in Fig. 2. The defined variables are the Thermal Relative Response (TRR =

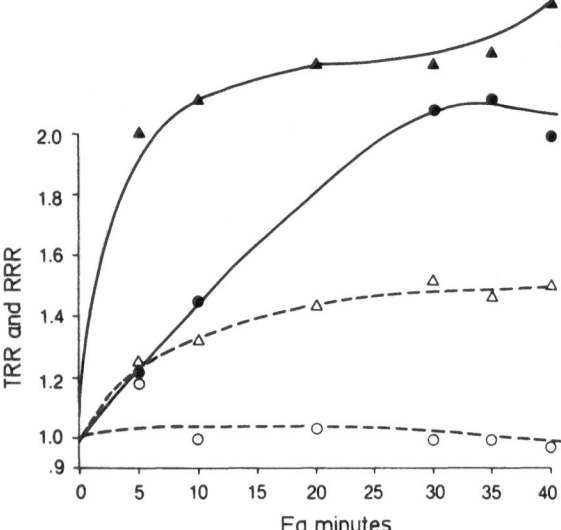

Fig. 2. The influence of inadequately heated regions of spontaneous tumors arising in pet animals on the tumor response relative to radiation therapy (XRT) alone. △ (TRR), enhancement in CR rate for heat + XRT versus XRT alone; ○ (RRR), enhancement in duration of response. Solid symbols (▲, ●), all monitored tumor points were heated in excess of the indicated thermal dose (in units of equivalent minutes at 43° C). Open Symbols (△, ○), only some of the monitored tumor points were heated in excess of the indicated dose. (Reprinted by permission from Dewhirst and Sim 1984)

the ratio of the probabilities of obtaining a CR with heat + X-ray versus X-ray alone) and the Relative Relapse Rate (RRR, an index of the relative differences in response duration). Both indices were constructed so that a value greater than 1 indicates benefit from X-ray plus heat relative to X-ray alone. The target "dose" for these studies was 44° C for 30 min during 4 treatments but not all points in all tumors during all 4 sessions achieved temperatures that high. The abscissa of Fig. 2 represents equivalent minutes of heating at 43° C (Eq43) using the previously stated thermal dose formula (with the transition temperature taken as 43° C and R = 0.25 for $T < T_{Trans}$). The minimum thermal dose for the entire course of treatments was determined but the value stated on the abscissa is a per-treatment average. The solid lines denote circumstances where all of the measured tumor points exceeded the indicated thermal dose and the dotted lines represent data from tumors where only some of the measured points exceeded the stated thermal dose. It can be seen that when only some of the tumor points were heated above the index dose there was a dose response with respect to TRR (CR rate) but no benefit as measured by RRR (response duration).

Similarly, when all of the measured tumor points were heated to the indicated thermal doses, the TRR doubled at very low doses and then increased only slowly at higher doses. However, the RRR did not reach similar levels of benefit until all of the measured tumor points exceeded a thermal dose of 30 Eq43 (i.e. treatments equivalent to 30 min at 43° C). By implication, one may state that if the human data were able to be followed long enough, some patients would relapse and that only those who were treated within the heating parameters indicated in the work of Dewhirst and Sim (1984) would show improvement in freedom from relapse over that expected with radiation alone. However, if tolerance doses of conventionally fractionated X-radiation that might more effectively control the possibly better perfused and oxygenated tumor periphery were to be employed in both the human and pet animal studies there might not be such a clear relationship between minimum thermal dose and local tumor control. Furthermore, though cold spots may be disadvantageous, it has not been proven that higher central tumor temperatures are without therapeutic benefit. In other words, will a tumor heated to a minimum of 15 Eq43 at the periphery but higher doses in its center have the same or a better chance of cure than a tumor heated uniformly to 15 Eq43? In future studies, if documentation with thermal dose mapping is adequate, important questions such as these will be answered.

5.2 Deep Heating

Most of the reported progress with non-invasive deep heating has been with regional heating techniques in trials primarily directed at determining tolerance, toxicity and heating characterictics in patients with advanced cancer who either failed customary treatments or were considered essentially untreatable by conventional means. Because these studies were uncontrolled and the hyperthermia was added to already generally effective treatment, it is not possible to draw any strong conclusions as to its therapeutic impact. However, a good deal has been learned about the heating characteristics and acute side effects of several of the available devices, particularly the CC and the AA.

The AA has been used experimentally at the University of Utah since 1980 and the results of a pilot series of 46 patients with abdominal tumors have been reported (Sapozink et al. 1984) as has a comparative study of the CC (at LDS Hospital,

Salt Lake City) and the AA in the same patients (GIBBS 1984 and SAPOZINK et al. 1985). TM was done to document tumor and normal tissue temperatures at multiple points and at radial depths of up to 12 cm in both of these studies. Of the initial 46 patients treated with the AA, 22 completed sufficient treatment with extensive thermometry to qualify for detailed analysis. Half had upper abdominal masses and half lower abdominal or pelvic tumors. Nine pelvic and 5 abdominal tumors achieved temperatures of 43° C or greater and 2 others, which were regulated at 42–43° C as an early precaution against unexpected complications, were considered likely to have achieved >43° C if they had not been restricted. However, without using significant sedation or increased analgesia it was possible in the overall series of treatments to achieve ≥41° C at only 75% of the pelvic and 63% of the abdominal monitored tumor points. For 43° C the proportions were 29 and 22% respectively. The mean time it was possible to hold temperatures at 43° C was only 14 min of the intended 30 min in the pelvis and 12 min in the abdomen. In the pelvis the treatments were most often restricted in temperature or duration by pelvic or lower extremity pain and in the abdomen they were most often restricted by systemic heating ≥40° C, tachycardia >150 beats/min and general anxiety. The treatments were noted to be generally stressful and uncomfortable but no significant treatment related complications were reported and it was proposed that increased thermal doses might be achieved in future studies with cautious increases in sedation and accrual of less critically ill patients, with more potentially curable disease, who could better tolerate the stress of the treatment.

In the comparative study it was found that the AA was clearly superior to the CC in the pelvis but that both devices had separate limitations in the upper abdomen that required further study. Neither device has been studied sufficiently in the thorax. In all circumstances where radial catheters were placed through normal tissue and tumor the CC was found to produce decreasing temperatures with depth unless a poorly perfused tumor interface was penetrated in which case abrupt temperature rises were observed followed by a furthur decline with increasing depth. In general, the AA produced a progressive rise in temperature with depth in the same temperature monitoring catheters. This rise was attributed to an increase with depth in the relative number of less well perfused intratumor points monitored. These characteristics

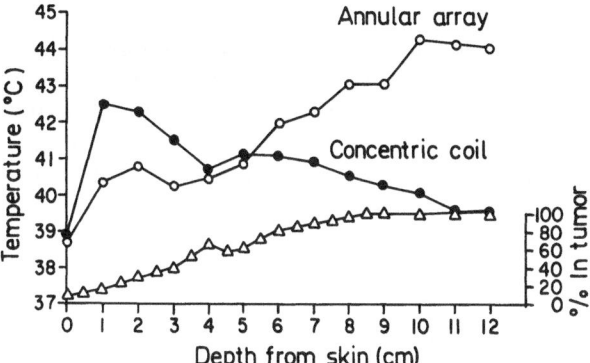

Fig. 3. Maximum temperatures (means of measurements from 14 radial percutaneously placed thermometry catheters in 13 patients) achieved at various depths in patients with advanced abdominal/pelvic tumors heated with the CC (●) and the AA (o). The same patients and identical catheter sites were compared during sequential treatments with the two devices. The percentage of monitored points that were in tumor tissue (△) increases with depth and is indicated by the ordinate scale on the right. (Reprinted by permission from GIBBS 1984)

are shown in Fig. 3. The central location of pelvic tumors and an invariably power–limiting complaint of sacrococcygeal pain appeared to be the reasons for the failure of the CC to heat tumors in this region. Despite its better penetration, the AA was often limited by systemic heating in the upper abdomen such that its performance was not substantially better than the CC in the patients studied.

Though studies such as these have pointed out a problem with treatment-limiting systemic heating with the AA, recent evidence has established that a significant part of this systemic heating is due to resonance coupling of the patient's entire body with the EM field, and not merely blood-flow redistribution of the regional power load. Furthermore, it is possible to manipulate this EM field so as to significantly decrease power deposition in the patient's upper torso and legs (Paul Turner, BSD Medical, Salt Lake City, UT, unpublished results, 1986).

The University of Utah experience has been further updated with two subsequent reports. The first of these (SAPOZINK et al. 1986a) is a multivariate analysis of 43 patients with advanced pelvic tumors treated with the AA in which it was shown that both concurrent radiation dose and number of satisfactory heat treatments were statistically significant independent correlates of tumor response and that survival of responders was better than that of nonresponders. The second (SAPO-

ZINK et al. 1986b), describes the results of 28 patients treated for upper abdominal tumors. A similar multivariate analysis did not suggest a benefit from hyperthermia and the authors felt that the temperatures obtained were generally too low and treatments too short to expect significant radiosensitizing or heat-only effects but that the heating technique might be useful in combination with chemotherapy due to the lower temperatures required for hyperthermic chemosensitization with certain drugs.

In a much larger but less well documented study, STORM et al. (1985) reviewed 1170 patients treated with the CC. Hyperthermia was given adjunctively with radiation therapy or chemotherapy in 85%. The overall complete, partial, and minimal regression rates were 9, 18, and 10% respectively with median response durations of 7, 4, and 3 months. There were 142 patients treated with heat alone of which 23% regressed. The authors felt that there were demonstrable benefits from the hyperthermia treatments. However, though most of these patients were heavily pretreated and had failed various treatments, it is possible that the response rates noted could be explained mostly on the basis of the use of the conventional modalities of treatment alone. The relationship of response to treatment temperature was assessed and there appeared to be no significant correlation unless the highest measured tumor temperatures that could be maintained throughout treatment (30–60 min) were in excess of 45° C, in which case 28/41 (68%) showed regression as compared to 195/444 (44%) when temperatures were below 45° C. Tumor temperature measurements were performed in only half the patients and more than one position was sampled in only 16%. Because of the tendency of the CC to heat best in superficial locations and the probability that those superficial locations were also the points that were sampled, it is extremely likely that there were substantial portions of most of the heated tumors where temperatures were well below those reported. One would predict from in vivo studies (GIBBS 1981) and the work of DEWHIRST and SIM (1984) that the response would be most likely to correlate with the adequacy of heating in the least effectively heated portion of the tumor. The lack of apparent correlation of response with temperature except in the few cases where values exceeding 45° C were reached, may be explained by the reasonable assumption that only in this latter group were substantial parts of the tumors likely to have been heated to effective temperatures.

Despite the problem of subcutaneous fat heating with capacitive heating methods, Japanese investigators have reported apparently successful heating of deep seated abdominal tumors using this technology with an experimental device employing cooling of the skin contact paddles (HIRAOKA et al. 1984; KATO et al. 1985). Tumor center temperatures were maintained at or above 42° C in 75% (99/133) of treatments. Though thick fat layers did diminish the likelihood of successful tumor heating, there were no serious subcutaneous burns and the treatments were reported as well tolerated. Despite the sophisticated clinical engineering of their apparatus it does not appear to employ any fundamentally new ideas in heating technology. It is possible that this approach has been prematurely discarded without adequate evaluation. Additional ongoing studies will be needed to determine the relative merits of all such present and future heating techniques.

6 Normal Tissue Consequences

The possibility of enhanced normal tissue radiation injury as a result of adding hyperthermia to radiation therapy is one of the major subjects of in vivo laboratory investigations. There is now a substantial body of laboratory data indicating that all normal tissues from laboratory animals studied thus far, including skin, connective tissue, cartilage and small intestine, exhibit thermal sensitization of both acute and chronic radiation reactions (HUME 1985). Whether tumors are relatively more responsive than normal tissues to adjunctive hyperthermia and what conditions of administration will lead to optimization of any relatively tumor specific effect, it is still not possible to say with confience. A problem in common with other radiobiological research is that most of the preclinical models tested have dealt with rapidly growing transplantable tumor models (that do not necessarily accurately model the physiology or growth kinetics of large spontaneous human tumors) treated with large radiation doses per fraction (that do not mimic clinical conditions and constraints). Although the issue of potential normal tissue injury has not been settled, it is clear that the risks are real and should not be underestimated.

In contrast to the preclinical results, enhanced clinical radiation toxicity with adjuvant hyperthermia has been mimimal thus far. Most investigators have reported only occasional mild burns due to inadequate temperature control and no greater acute or late normal tissue response than that expected with radiation therapy alone. However, the nature of the heating methods employed and the geometry of most of the lesions treated would tend to concentrate the power deposition in the region of the tumor with relative sparing of surrounding tissues. Furthermore, the skin, the most obvious indicator of potentially enhanced reactions, was frequently cooled. When skin cooling has not been used, increased skin reactions have been described (MARMOR and HAHN 1980; ARCANGELLI et al. 1983 and 1984). Data from the previously mentioned pet animal study has been recently analyzed for evidence of enhanced normal tissue toxicity (DEWHIRST et al. 1984) and the authors concluded that, if the few cases where acute thermal injury occurred were excluded, there was no significant evidence for increased fibrosis or other late normal tissue sequelae.

Normal tissue toxicity has not yet proven to be a problem with regional heating. However, it must not be forgotten that effective clinical heating of critical normal tissues has not yet been performed with sufficient frequency to expect the possible consequences to have become evident. Patients have experienced acute discomforts during the treatment with occasional minor burns or persistence of minor musculoskeletal pain for hours to days after treatment but the only significant complications appear to have been related to consequences of tumor necrosis which has occasionally resulted in ulcers or fistuli (SAPOZINK et al. 1984).

There is one disturbing report of patients developing transverse myelitis of previously irradiated spinal cord after undergoing whole body hyperthermia (DOUGLAS et al. 1981). These incidents were probably caused by heat induced alteration of perfusion in a vascular bed previously damaged by radiation therapy rather than hyperthermic radiosensitization. However, they are the sort of hazards that may become more apparent as clinical studies expand.

7 Conclusions

The clinical results that have been achieved as a result of combined hyperthermia and radiation therapy are exciting. Complete response rates achieved with subcurative radiation doses have been essentially doubled. The maintainence of such responses will probably depend on the accu-

racy with which hyperthermia can be administered, a major point of concern since with presently available techniques accurate control of the thermal dose distributions is severely limited. It is hoped that the use of tolerance dose x-irradiation may lessen the necessity of such stringent control over the minimum tumor thermal dose. There are many details regarding the optimization of the administration of hyperthermia with radiation and chemotherapy that remain to be determined as well as uncertainties regarding the ultimate potential for enhancement of adverse normal tissue effects. Though normal tissue complications have not yet been reported to be a problem in the clinic, normal tissues have generally been spared or inadequately heated with the techniques employed. As attempts to heat more deep seated tumors and adjacent critical tissues progress, toxicity will probably become a greater problem. The biological questions, definition of thermal dose and accurate measurement and prediction of temperature distributions, are significant but soluble. The technical difficulties of heat delivery remain a major problem. If we are to transform hyperthermia from a merely effective clinical modality into a useful one (i.e. develop it into a modality that is good for something more than treating superficial metastases), ongoing efforts to improve our ability to heat selected anatomic regions are urgently needed. Although the interstitial techniques discussed in the adjoining chapter are one potential solution to this problem, it is probable that their ultimate application will be as relatively limited as interstitial irradiation is to the field of radiation therapy. The ultimate potential of hyperthermia will therefore rest with the successful development of non-invasive heating techniques. At the present time, hyperthermia is starting to be used adjunctively in potentially curative settings. The most logical current application for external heating is in the management of unresectable cervical lymph node metastases; it is even conceivable that in a few years it will become standard therapy for this disorder. The developments with regional heating in the pelvis are also encouraging and it will not be long before prospective cooperative trials will be undertaken to evaluate adjunctive regional heating for advanced cervical, rectal, bladder and other pelvic primary carcinomas. If present trends continue it is probable that hyperthermia will gradually establish a foothold in the treatment of specific clinical entities and slowly expand with our knowledge and expertise. There is no longer reasonable doubt that it is effective and it is almost certain that it will be useful to at least a limited extent. How far it will expand is still impossible to say.

References

Arcangelli G, Cividalli A, Nervi C, Creton G (1983) Tumor control and therapeutic gain with different schedules of combined radiotherapy and local external hyperthermia in human cancer. Int J Radiat Oncol Biol Phys 9:1125–1134

Arcangelli G, Nervi C, Cividalli A, Lovisolo GA (1984) Problems of sequence and fractionation in the clinical application of combined heat and radiation. Can Res (Suppl) 44:4857s–4863s

Cetas TC (1984) Will thermometric tomography become practical for hyperthermia treatment monitoring. Can Res (Suppl) 44:4805s–4808s

Dewhirst MW, Sim DA (1984) The utility of thermal dose as a predictor of tumor and normal tissue responses to combined radiation and hyperthermia. Can Res (Suppl) 44:4772s–4780s

Dewhirst MW, Sim DA, Grochowski K (1984) Incidence of thermal injury and radiation induced early and late normal tissue reactions in a phase III trial comparing radiotherapy alone and heat combined with radiation (abstract). Int J Radiat Oncol Biol Phys 10 (supp. 2):110

Douglas MA, Parks LC, Bebin J (1981) Sudden myelopathy secondary to therapeutic total-body hyperthermia after spinal cord irradiation. N Engl J Med 304:583–585

Fessenden P, Lee ER, Anderson TL, Strohbehn JW, Meyer JL, Samulski TV, Marmor JB (1984a) Experience with a multitransducer ultrasound system for localized hyperthermia of deep tissues. IEE Trans Biomed Eng 31:126–135

Fessenden P, Lee ER, Samulski TV (1984b) Direct temperature measurement. Can Res (Suppl) 44:4799s–4804s

Field SB, Morris CC (1983) The relationship between heating time and temperature: its relevance to hyperthermia. Radiother & Oncol 1:179–186

Gibbs FA Jr, Peck JW, Dethlefsen LA (1981) The importance of intratumor temperature uniformity in the study of radiosensitizing effects of hyperthermia in vivo. Rad Res 82:138–145

Gibbs FA Jr (1983) "Thermal mapping" in experimental cancer treatment with hyperthermia: Description and use of a semi-automatic system. Int J Radiat Oncol Biol Phys 9:1057–1063

Gibbs FA Jr. (1984) Regional hyperthermia: A clinical appraisal of noninvasive deep-heating methods. Can Res (Suppl) 44:4765s–4770s

Gibbs FA Jr, Sapozink MD, Stewart JR (1985) Clinical thermal dosimetry – why and how. In: Overgaard J (ed) Hyperthermic Oncology 1984 – Proc. of the 4th Internat. Symp. on Hyperthermic Oncology, Vol. 2. Taylor & Francis, London and Philadelphia, p 155–167

Hiraoka M, Jo S, Takahashi M, Abe M (1984) Thermometry results of RF capacitive heating for human deep-seated tumors. In: Overgaard J (ed) Hyperthermic Oncology 1984 – Proc. of the 4th Internat. Symp. on Hyperthermic Oncology. Vol. 1. Taylor & Francis, London and Philadelphia, p 609

Hume S (1985) Experimental studies of normal tissue response to hyperthermia alone or combined with other modalities. In: Overgaard J (ed) Hyperthermic Oncology 1984 – Proc. of the 4th Internat. Symp. on Hyperthermic Oncology, Vol. 2. Taylor & Francis, London and Philadelphia, p 53–70

Kato H, Hiraoka M, Nakajima T, Ishida T (1985) Depp heating characteristics of an RF heating device. Int J Hyperthermia 1:15–28

Kim JH, Hahn EW, Ahmed SA (1982) Combined hyperthermia and radiation therapy for malignant melanoma. Cancer 50:478–482

Lele PP (1983) Physical aspects and clinical studies with ultrasonic hyperthermia. In: Storm FK (ed) Hyperthermia in cancer therapy. Hall, Boston, 333

Marmor JB, Hahn GM (1980) Combined radiation and hyperthermia in superficial human tumors. Cancer 46:1986–1991

Meyer JL (1984) The clinical efficacy of localized hyperthermia. Can Res (Suppl) 44:4745s–4751s

Oleson JR (1984) A review of magnetic induction methods for hyperthermia treatment of cancer. IEEE Trans Biomed Eng 31:91–97

Overgaard J (1983) Hyperthermic modification of the radiation response in solid tumors. In: Fletcher G, Nervi C, Withers H (eds) Biological bases and clinical implications of tumor radioresistance. Masson Publishing Co., New York, p 337

Paliwal BR, Gibbs FA Jr., Wiley AL (1982) Heating patterns induced by a 13.56 mHz radiofrequency generator in large phantoms and pig abdomen and thorax. Int J Radiat Oncol Biol Phys 8:857–864

Perez CA, Sapareto SA (1984) Thermal dose expression in clinical hyperthermia and correlation with tumor response/control. Can Res (Suppl) 44:4818s–4825s

Roemer RB, Cetas TC (1984) Applications of bioheat transfer simulations in hyperthermia. Can Res (Suppl) 44:4788s–4798s

Ruggera PS, Kantor G (1984) Development of a family of RF helical coil applicators which produce transversely uniform axially distributed heating in cylindrical fat-muscle phantoms. IEEE Trans Biomed Eng 31:98–105

Sapareto SA, Dewey WC (1984) Thermal dose determination in cancer therapy. Int J Rad Oncol Biol Phys 10:787–800

Sapozink MD, Gibbs FA Jr, Gates KS, Stewart JR (1984) Regional hyperthermia in the treatment of clinically advanced deep seated malignancy: Results of a study employing an annular array applicator. Int J Radiat Oncol Biol Phys 10:775–786

Sapozink MD, Gibbs FA Jr, Thomson JW, Eltringham JR, Stewart JR (1985) A comparison of deep regional hyperthermia from an annular phased array and a concentric coil in the same patients. Int J Radiat Oncol Biol Phys 11:179–190

Sapozink MD, Gibbs FA Jr, Egger MJ, Stewart JR (1986a) Regional hyperthermia in the treatment of clinically advanced deep seated pelvic malignancy. Am J Clin Oncol 9:162–169

Sapozink MD, Gibbs FA Jr, Egger MJ, Stewart JR (1986b) Abdominal regional hyperthermia with an annular phased array. J Clin Oncol 4:775–783

Scott R, Johnson R, Story K, Clay L (1984) Local hyperthermia in combination with definitive radiotherapy: Increased tumor clearance, reduced recurrence rate in extended follow-up. Int J Radiat Oncol Biol Phys 10:2119–2123

Stewart JR (1984) Past clinical studies and future directions. Can Res (Suppl) 44:4902s–4904s

Stewart JR, Gibbs FA Jr (1984) Hyperthermia in the treatment of cancer: perspectives on its promise and problems. Cancer 54:2823–2830

Storm FK, Baker HW, Scanlon EF, Plenk HP, Meadows PM, Cohen SC, Olson CE, Thompson J, Khandekar JD, Roe D, Nizze A, Morton DL (1985) Magnetic induction hyperthermia: results of a 5-year multiinstitutional na-

tional cooperative trial in advanced cancer patients. Cancer 55:2677–2687

Strohbehn JW (1984) Calculation of absorbed power in tissues for various hyperthermia devices. Can Res (Suppl) 44:4781s–4787s

Turner PF (1984) Regional hyperthermia with an annular phased array. IEEE Trans Biomed Eng 31:106–114

Vaguine VA, Christensen DA, Lindley JH, Walston TE (1984) Multiple sensor optical thermometry system for application in clinical hyperthermia. IEEE Trans Biomed Eng 31:168–172

9.2 Interstitial Hyperthermia

James R. Oleson

CONTENTS

ABBREVIATIONS

TER   Thermal Enchancement Ratio
TGF   Therapeutic Gain Factor
Rf   Radiofrequency
LCF   Localized Current Field
CR   Complete Response Rate
PR   Partial Response Rate

1 Introduction

A variety of techniques has been investigated for producing elevated temperatures in the whole body, in large body regions or in localized areas. Localized hyperthermia can be produced either with external energy sources in the case of superficial tumors, or with interstitial energy sources in a variety of sites. In this chapter we will only consider the technical and clinical aspects of interstitial approaches.

The rationale for interstitial hyperthermia follows in part from the following brief remarks:

James R. Oleson, M.D., Ph.D., Associate Professor
Duke University Medical Center, Box 3085
Durham, NC 27710, USA

A. Interstitial hyperthermia results in temperature rise localized to the tumor; hence the TER is likely to be greater in tumor than normal tissue regardless of tumor perfusion, intrinsic thermal sensitivity of the malignant cells, or time-sequence between radiation and hyperthermia.
B. Some interstitial hyperthermia techniques are readily combined with conventional brachytherapy techniques that localize radiation dose to the tumor volume.
C. Interstitial hyperthermia techniques allow for a greater degree of sampling of temperatures within the tumor and for a greater degree of control of the temperature distribution than is typically the case with other hyperthermia techniques.

The motivation for improving control of localized bulky disease using interstitial hyperthermia and radiation is particularly strong in sites such as head and neck, breast, brain and pelvis, where disease may be locally advanced, even at initial presentation, and where local control is important in the quality of survival as well as in the possibility of cure.

In the following section, we describe physical aspects of several interstitial techniques that have been proposed. Initial clinical results with some techniques have been reported and are reviewed in the next section. From these results we will formulate an assessment of the status of, and future role for interstitial hyperthermia.

2 Physical Aspects of Interstitial Hyperthermia Techniques

2.1 Sources of Energy

Sources of energy for heat production that are placed directly into tumor volumes include:

A. Metallic needles or wires that conduct radiofrequency currents to produce localized current field (LCF).

B. Microwave antennae.
C. Ferromagnetic seeds that can be heated via eddy current flow in a magnetic induction field.
D. Ferromagnetic fluids and ferrimagnetic glass-ceramic material that can be heated by hysteresis effects in an induction field.

2.2 Localized Current Fields

Most clinical experience has been with the LCF technique. Doss and McCabe (1976) first proposed placing parallel rows of metal needles, such as those used in brachytherapy, into a tumor volume and applying a radiofrequency (RF) voltage across rows of needles to cause RF current flow between the needles. Human tissue has predominantly resistive properties in the frequency range of 0.1 to 1.0 MHZ and this range is usually chosen to minimize capacitive reactance and simplify impedance matching of the source to the implant. These frequencies are high enough to avoid neuronal depolarization and to minimize electrical noise interference with other equipment as well.

Power deposition is proportion to the square of the electrical current density and to the resistivity of the tissue. Since current density is highest near the needles, and diverges between needles, power deposition varies similarly. Also, there can be conductive heat transfer from the high temperature volume immediately surrounding a needle toward intervening regions of lower temperature. The relative contribution of resistive heating and conductive heating at a given point will depend upon the geometry of the implant, tissue/tumor electrical properties, and blood perfusion rates.

Strohbehn (1983) has reported results of theoretical calculations that modelled temperature distributions resulting from rectilinear implants in homogeneously perfused tissue with homogeneous electrical properties. When perfusion rates approached that of resting muscle, the minimum temperature became less than 42° C even though the maximum temperature at the needles exceeded 45° C. As perfusion increased, the likelihood of having a satisfactory temperature distribution (minimum >42° C, maximum <45° C) increased as the spacing between needles decreased.

A number of studies have been performed utilizing conductive needles placed into non-perfused material ("phantom") having electrical properties similar to that of tissue in order to assess power deposition patterns in heterogeneous tissue (Oleson and Cetas 1982; Cetas et al. 1980; Cetas et al. 1982). While these phantom studies have limitations, they do illustrate the marked variations in power deposition that might occur in practice because of heterogeneous tissue properties. These results, together with the theoretical modelling that includes blood perfusion effects, emphasize the need for approximately 1 cm needle spacing in a plane and for ability to vary the power deposition within an implant to compensate for geometrical, electrical, and perfusion effects. Temperatures can be monitored within needles to provide estimates of maximum temperatures and at other sites near the periphery of the implant to estimate minimum temperatures.

Astrahan (1982) has reported on an LCF system that includes computer-controlled switches to sequence power to various combinations of needles with a variable duty cycle.

Cosset et al. (1984a) modified the LCF technique used at the University of Arizona to limit the current field around the metallic electrode to the tumor volume by passing the leads to the needle through electrically-insulating plastic tubes as they traversed the normal tissues. An alternative method of insultating portions of the metallic needle passing through normal tissue was reported earlier by Joseph et al. (1981) and consisted of a plastic coating or angiographic catheter sleeve extending over steel guides within normal tissue.

Brezovich and Young (1981) have published theoretical calculations modelling the electromagnetic fields asociated with an internal electrode and a large area surface electrode, as was suggested by Doss and McCabe (1976).

Phantom and animal testing of this LCF approach (Lilly et al. 1983) confirm that relatively uniform fields and temperature rise can be produced within an internal volume implant of electrodes or Faraday cage together with an external electrode. The radionale of this scheme is that the tumor temperature distribution may not be critically dependent upon the internal electrode geometry, as long as the electrode is near the peripheral portions of the tumor.

Another approach of permanently implanting needle electrodes in intrathoracic lesions has been described by Corry and Barlogie (1982).

2.3 Microwave Antennae

Several investigators have designed microwave antennae that can be inserted into lumens of organs or interstitially into afterloading catheters: absorption of electromagnetic energy radiated into surrounding tissue results in temperature rise.

The antennae developed by Strohbehn and collaborators at Dartmouth (STROHBEHN et al. 1979; KING et al. 1983; STROHBEHN et al. 1982a, b; LYONS et al. 1984; TREMBLY et al. 1982) are made of miniature, flexible coaxial cable, operate at 915 MHZ, and are 1.6 mm or less in diameter. Their size allows placement into 17 gauge plastic or nylon afterloading catheters. The active portion of the antennae is an electromagnetic monopole radiator created by extending the inner conductor beyond the termination of the outer conductor ("junctional region") by a distance equal to one-quarter wavelength (in the dielectric medium). The portion of cable proximal to the termination of the outer conductor also radiates and the resulting power deposition in tissue can depend upon the frequency of operation, dielectric properties of the surrounding catheter and tissue, and the insertion length of the antenna into tissue. At 1 GHZ the power deposition 5 mm from the junction is about 10% of the power deposition at a 1 mm radius. If antennae are inserted into a square array 1.1 cm on a side and excited in phase from a common source, phase reinforcement can result in a significant power deposition at the center of the array. Thus, an array of N antennae can treat more than N times the volume treated by a single antenna.

The power deposition pattern along the direction of the antenna is approximately cigar-shaped shaped, so that non-uniformities in power deposition would call for careful planning of the implant geometry and length of active antenna. By using power splitters and variable attenuators on each antenna feed line, applied power levels can be varied to control the temperature distribution. The active length of the antenna as well as the radius of the half-power point is inversely related to frequency. Small tumors volumes 2 cm or less in diameter could require a 2450 MHZ system, whole lesions larger than 5 cm could be better treated with a 433 MHZ system.

The design of antennae involves many detailed considerations and a variety of designs do appear in the literature. SAMARAS (1984) has described a monopole coaxial slot radiator having greater rigidity than the previously described antenna and has also discussed temperature control problems. MENDECKI et al. (1980) have designed larger diameter, directional antenna for intraluminal applications in the rectum or vagina. TAYLOR (1980) and TAYLOR et al. (1982) have described microwave radiators for both interstitial and intracavitary applications.

LI et al. (1984) have recently reported on the design of a novel intracavitary antenna that can be operated at frequencies of 300 to 915 MHZ. Instead of a quarter-wavelength extension of the inner conductor, the radiating portion has an outer conductor that spirals loosely around the inner conductor. Electric fields that radiate through these loose turns into tissue provide the power deposition.

BICHER et al. (1984) have attempted to reduce the high temperature that can occur adjacent to an antenna by constructing a dipole antenna placed into a jacket through which air is forced to produce cooling of the jacket and adjacent tissue. In animal experiments, more uniform temperatures were produced with than without air flow.

2.4 Induction of Ferromagnetic Seeds

In contrast to the LCF and microwave antennae methods are approaches that require implanting conductive substances or seeds into the tumor that can absorb energy from a magnetic induction field created by current-carrying coils external to the patient. Several physical mechanisms have been used as a basis for this method, including conductive (eddy current) heating of ferromagnetic substances and hysteresis heating of ferromagnetic or ferrimagnetic substances. In each case, heat transfer to surrounding tumor occurs by means of thermal conduction rather than direct electromagnetic power absorption in tissue. In general, establishing a satisfactory temperature distribution with given maxima and minima of temperature requires a greater density of conductive sources than of radiative sources (STROHBEHN et al. 1979).

The implant geometry must be carefully planned in order to achieve desired temperature elevation within the tumor (MATLOUBIEH et al. 1984). Seeds must be or at just outside the target volume for satisfactory solutions using conductive heat transfer. Control of temperature rise with most of these techniques would require adjusting applied power levels to maintain some specified temperature in the implanted volume; the seeds themselves would reach higher temperatures than surrounding tumor. The exception to this situation occurs when ferromagnetic materials are used that have a Curie temperature in the therapeutic range, e.g. 45–50° C. As the Curie temperature is approached, a magnetic phase transition within the substance lower the magnetic moment and hence the absorption of power within the seed. The seed becomes thermally regulating near the predetermined temperature whenever sufficiently intense magnetic fields are applied. This novel idea solves the problem of controlling individual seed temperatures, and invasive thermometry would be needed for dosimetric rather than control purposes. Thermally regulating seeds could be implanted into the unresectable portions of tumor at the time of surgical exploration, for instance, and the actual hyperthermia treatment could be done later.

The ferromagnetic seed concept was originally proposed by BURTON et al. (1971) as a means of producing controlled thermocoagulation in brain tissue, and the application of the concept to hyperthermia treatment of cancer has been investigated at the University of Arizona (STAUFFER et al. 1982; STAUFFER et al. 1984a, b; OLESON and CETAS 1982; FORSYTH et al. 1984) and at the University of Alabama (BREZOVICH et al. 1984a, b; ATKINSON et al. 1984).

Determinants of power absorption in ferromagnetic seeds include the seed geometry and alloy composition, Curie temperature, and frequency and amplitude of the applied magnetic field. These variables have been studied extensively, and nickel-copper and nickel-silicon alloys can be made with Curie temperatures in the desired range of 45–50° C.

Once seeds are implanted, the seed temperature is elevated by placing the patient within a high-power, high-frequency (0.1 to 0.5 MHZ) magnetic induction coil within an electromagnetically shielded room. The technology of coil and power supply design derives from radiofrequency engineering principles and from existing applications of magnetic induction in industry (DAVIES and SIMPSON 1979). Current work with this approach concerns biocompatibility of the seeds, methods of implantation and fixation of seeds, and methods of combining the thermoseeds with interstitial radiation sources.

RAND et al. (1982) described injection of a ferromagnetic fluid into a VX_2 renal carcinoma in rabbits. Exposure of the animal to a 2 KHZ magnetic field resulted in hysteresis heating of the microscopic ferromagnetic particles in the fluid areas to 50–55° C. The mechanism of producing tumor hyperthermia was thermal conduction from the fluid to surrounding tissue, so the considerations of distribution of material required for uniformity of temperature elevation throughout a tumor are similar to those discussed previously for ferromagnetic seeds. The distribution problem would be particularly important in the larger tumors encountered in humans.

Another substance that can be hysteresis-heated after injection into a tumor has been investigated by LUDERER et al. (1983). This is a ferrimagnetic lithium iron phosphate compound that is melted into a glass, then fractured into microscopic spinels that can be combined with a carrier fluid to form an injectable slurry. Experiments have been reported injecting this material around an implanted sarcoma in mice and heating in a 10 KHZ magnetic field. Significant temperature elevations were observed.

3 Clinical Results Using Interstitial Hyperthermia

There has been experience reported in human clinical trials utilizing LCF and microwave antennae, and these results will be emphasized. Most work with other techniques involves feasibility studies with limited numbers of patients or animals. Until further studies are published it will be premature to compare relative advantages of other techniques such as ferroseeds with LCF and microwave techniques.

3.1 University of Arizona Clinical Trials

At the University of Arizona, human clinical trials using LCF in combination with interstitial radiation started in 1977 (MILLER et al. 1977; CETAS et al. 1980, 1982; MANNING et al. 1982a, b; MANNING and GERNER 1983; OLESON and CETAS 1982; OLESON et al. 1984a; OLESON et al. 1984b; ARISTIZABAL and OLESON 1984). The current update of this experience included here includes patients treated from 1977 through 1983.

Patients were eligible who had bulky primary recurrent or metastatic disease for which conventional therapy would offer little chance of palliation or control, who had a survival expected to be greater than 6 months, and who had disease that was accessible for interstitial implantation. Patients with disease recurrent after prior radiotherapy were included.

Fifteen of the 64 total patients were male, 49 were female, with a mean age of 59 years. Tumors histologies included 26 squamous cell carcinomas, 24 adenocarcinomas, 5 melanomas, 5 sarcomas, and 4 other types. Forty-seven patients had pelvic disease; 36 of these were gynecological malignancy and 11 were urological or colorectal in origin. In addition, 9 patients had head and neck malignancy, 3 had breast carcinoma, and 5 had other soft tissue sites involved. Fifty-four patients had received at least one modality of prior treatment.

The first patients treated had radium needle implants done, after which the metallic guide needles were connected to a modified 500 KHZ electrocautery unit that supplied current that flowed through the implanted tissue from one set of needles to another. Subsequently, most patients had 17 gauge hollow needles placed into the tumor according to conventional ^{192}Ir afterloading approaches and dosimetric considerations. Implantation was performed under general or spinal anesthesia and a 30 to 40 minute hyperthermia treatment was performed in the operating room. Temperatures were monitored with thermistors placed into the metallic needle guides as well as into additional plastic catheters within the tumor volume. Periodic translation of the sensors through the catheters mapped temperatures throughout the tumor volume. The temperature distribution was controlled to 42–43° C by adjusting the applied power level as well as by manually varying the particular needles activated as electrodes. Occasionally power was limited because of excessive temperature (greater than 44° C) in normal tissues. Afterloading with ^{192}Ir followed the hyperthermia treatment within 2 to 3 hours.

The average minimum interstitial radiation dose was 2581 ± 290 cGy (mean $\pm$ standard error) with a range of 15 to 45 Gy. The mean tumor volume was 276 ± 118 cm^3, calculated as the product of three orthogonal tumor dimensions. The minimum measured intratumoral temperature (T_{min}), averaged over the treatment period after the initial transient temperature rise, was $41.0 \pm 0.2°$ C in the entire patient series. Similarly, the maximum measured temperature was $44.6 \pm 0.3°$ C. The range of minimum measured temperature was $37.5°$ C to $45.0°$ C, emphasizing that in 50% of cases, minimum temperatures were less than $41.0°$ C.

The complete response rate (CR) observed was 38%, the partial response rate (PR) was 39%, and 23% of tumors showed no response. Multivariate analysis revealed significant correlations only between CR and radiation dose ($p = 0.007$), tumor volume ($p = 0.001$), and T_{min} ($p = 0.005$).

In further analysis of data that included patients treated at the University of Arizona with other techniques as well, there was a stronger correlation between CR and T_{min} for radiation doses less than 24 Gy than for doses 24 Gy or more (SIM et al. 1984a).

Eight of 64 patients had severe toxicity from the treatment that required hospitalization and/or surgical intervention. This toxicity consisted of acute slough of tumor within 10 days of treatment that led to development of pelvic fistulae in patients having had tumor infiltration of hollow organs prior to treatment. We defined this problem as toxicity because the interstitial therapy, especially from the patient's point of view, appeared to have precipitated the problem.

The median survival of these patients was 31 weeks, a survival that reflected presence of disseminated disease in a majority of patients. The short survival precluded estimation of late effects of combined therapy.

The principal conclusions from this study were:
1. Addition of hyperthermia to modest doses of interstitial radiation did yield a greater frequency of complete responses than would be expected with similar doses of radiation alone.
2. The correlation of response rate with minimum intratumoral temperature suggested a thermal dose-response relationship.
3. Even with considerable ability to control the temperature distribution, the presence of subtherapeutic temperatures (less than 41° C) was confirmed in half the patients and constitutes an important reason not to reduce radiation doses from those conventionally established when treating potentially curable lesions.
4. Serious toxicity of treatment did occur and was related in part to predictable sequelae of locally advanced disease and possibly to acute thermal injury of normal tissues.

3.2 City of Hope Medical Center Clinical Trial

Investigators at the City of Hope Medical Center (JOSEPH et al. 1981; ASTRAHAN and GEORGE 1980; ASTRAHAN 1982; VORA et al. 1982) have used a similar LCF technique with a computer controlled switching system on the needle electrodes. Fifteen patients with 16 lesions were treated (VORA et al. 1982). Six patients without prior radiotherapy to the site received 50 to 55 Gy with teletherapy, then 15 to 30 Gy interstitial radiation with hyperthermia. The hyperthermia was given prior to afterloading and consisted of 30 to 40 minutes at 42–43° C. Eight previously irradiated patients were retreated with interstitial radiation plus hyperthermia alone, and one additional patient also received 30 Gy with teletherapy. There was a CR in 6 of 6 lesions in the previously untreated group. In the 10 previously treated sites there were 4 CRs, 1 PR, 3 without response, and 1 patient was inevaluable. One serious complication, a vesicovaginal fistula, was noted.

Although the biology and physiology of tumors recurrent after prior radiotherapy may differ from that of previously untreated tumors, it seems most likely that the difference in radiation dose given between the two groups accounts for the different response rates.

3.3 Institute Gustave-Roussy Clinical Trial

At the Institut Gustave-Roussy, LCF (44° C for 45 min) has been used prior to afterloading with ^{192}Ir (30 Gy) in 14 lesions in 11 patients (COSSET et al. 1984a). Initial response evaluation showed 10/14 CR, 2/14 PR, and 2/14 inevaluable. In an updated report (COSSET et al. 1984b) of treatment of 21 lesions in 18 patients there were 15 CRs in 17 evaluable tumors. However, there were 6 late relapses (median 9 months) amongst the complete responders: 4 were at the margin of the treated volume and 2 were within the volume. There were 4 cases of severe necrosis. These authors planned to extend the volume of treatment as well as the radiation dose to 40 Gy in a subsequent trial.

3.4 Dartmouth Study

In an initial feasibility study, investigators at Dartmouth have utilized combined interstitial hyperthermia with microwave antennae and irradiation (COUGHLIN et al. 1983). Seven patients with locally advanced and unresectable lesions were selected. The catheter spacing was chosen according to radiation dosimetry considerations. The treatment goal was 42° C or more throughout the tumor volume for 60 minutes followed by ^{192}Ir afterloading to give a dose of 25–30 Gy in 2 to 3 days, followed by a second hyperthermia treatment. No normal tissue thermal injuries were noted, and responses were not analyzed in detail in this Phase I study. This group is also applying this combined technique in treatment of brain tumors.

3.5 Washington University School of Medicine Clinical Trial

Emami and collaborators (EMAMI et al. 1984) used LCF (8 patients) or interstitial microwave techniques (21 patients) to treat 31 recurrent or persistent lesions in 29 patients. The average diameter of lesions was 7 to 8 cm. LCF hyperthermia was done once in the operating room and ^{192}Ir afterloading followed in about 4 hours. Interstitial microwave hyperthermia was given in two sessions separated by 72 hours during the course of brachytherapy delivering 40 to 60 Gy in 4 to 7 days. The treatment goal was 42° C minimum temperature for 60 minutes. These authors noted 18/31 CRs and 6/31 PRs. In 5 lesions the hyperthermia treatments were "unsatisfactory" and there were no CRs in this group. Rapid tumor necrosis resulted in slow-healing open wounds in 7 patients. In none of these sites was tumor recurrence noted during follow-up. Response rates did not depend upon the hyperthermia technique.

3.6 University of Maryland School of Medicine Clinical Trial

SALCMAN and SAMARIS (1983) reported on a Phase I trial in which interstitial radiation and hyperthermia were combined in the treatment of six patients with previously treated recurrent or persistent glioblastoma or malignant astrocytoma. These patients had repeat subtotal resection followed by implantation of a single 2450 MHZ microwave antenna into the residual tumor. A temperature of 45° C was maintained adjacent to the antennae for about 20 minutes during surgery, at which time numerous measurements were taken. On the first postoperative day, 45° C was maintained for 60 minutes. This treatment was repeated 48 hours after surgery. No additional treatment was given unless progression was documented. In this study, no permanent complications were encountered and postoperative treatments were well tolerated by the awake patients.

Problems that were identified included the need for a rigid support and fixation system for the antennae as well as CT-guided stereotactic implantation. CSF leaks were found at the dural puncture site that indicated the need for fluid seals at the entry sites.

In general, temperatures ranged from 45 to 47° C near the antenna to 37–39° C at a radius of 2 cm. The authors attributed the relatively large volume of temperature rise in human tumors to reduced blood flow in tumor relative to normal feline brain, in which preclinical studies showed a smaller effective radius of treatment.

4 Discussion of Clinical Results

A variety of clinical experiences have been referenced that have had characterization of equipment, feasibility, and toxicity as primary goals.

In the trial at the University of Arizona the prognostic importance of minimum tumor temperature, tumor volume, and radiation dose was identified. Comparison of results from several institutions also suggests that radiation dose and minimum temperature contribute independently to complete response (ARISTIZABAL and OLESON 1984), although such comparison does not account for the variation of tumor volume that probably existed in different trials.

Since present techniques are unlikely to produce at least 42° C in all gross tumor, especially in tumor peripheries, radiation dose levels must be sufficiently high to sterilize gross underheated disease within the tumor and underheated microscopic deposits within surrounding normal tissue. Insufficient radiation doses may lead to a risk of marginal recurrence that outweighs the hypothesized advantage of radiation plus hyperthermia in sterilizing hypoxic, radioresistant cells within the tumor. The experience of COSSET et al. (1984b) with late marginal recurrences in 4 of 15 patients with an initial CR emphasizes this point.

Thermal necrosis can result in acute tumor slough. In contrast, more gradual regression of disease during conventional courses of radiotherapy alone may allow for normal tissue healing. If combined therapy improves the control of locally advanced disease, reconstructive or reparative surgery may play a major role as well.

There is little information from the human clinical experience regarding the degree of potentiation of late effects of radiation in normal tissue. In part, this reflects short survival of patients in the Phase I trials, and in part it may be a consequence of well-localized enhancement of radiation effect with small volumes of normal tissue exposure to elevated temperatures. This can derive from design (localized power deposition) or good fortune (higher blood perfusion in normal tissue than tumor). More study of late effects is required.

Treatment planning methods and extensive thermometry must still be emphasized to minimize risk to normal tissues. Computerized data acquisition systems are being incorporated into most commercial hyperthermia systems at the present time to facilitate the accumulation of thermometric data. Computer modelling of temperature distributions will be valuable, but routine application of such modelling to clinical treatment of individual patients is not yet available (STROHBEHN and ROEMER 1984; ROEMER and CETAS 1984; CETAS and ROEMER 1984). In addition, blood perfusion will probably need to be measured in order for modelling to be accurate in individual patients.

Although minimum tumor temperature has prognostic significance (DEWHIRST and SIM 1984; OLESON et al. 1984a, 1984b), it is likely that the percentage of tumor volume treated at given thermal dose levels will yield a stronger correlation with response, as FESSENDEN et al. (1984) have hypothesized, and as suggested in further analysis of human and animal clinical data (SIM et al. 1984a, b).

With all the limitations of Phase I/II studies in mind, the range of reported complete response rates (38% to 98%) with combined therapy suggests substantial enhancement of radiation effect by hyperthermia. One may hypothesize that a complementary difference in spatial distribution of thermal and radiation effects within a tumor exists that would make these results difficult to produce with radiation alone by simply increasing radiation doses. Randomized trials comparing radiation alone to combined modalities will be necessary for confirming a therapeutic gain with combined radiation and hyperthermia. This is especially true in sites and with tumor volumes where modern brachytherapy itself yields high response rates, in the range of 70–100% (ARISTIZABAL and OLESON 1984).

More experience using several interstitial techniques in particular sites is necessary to define the most advantageous system for specific situations. The apparent advantages of microwave antennae in an easily implanted site, for instance, could be of less importance in sites difficult to implant such as intrathoracic or intracranial lesions where thermally regulating Curie seeds may be more advantageous.

5 Conclusions

Enhancement of radiation effect by hyperthermia is shown to advantage with interstitial modalities. A variety of techniques are now becoming available commercially. This stage of equipment development should facilitate performing controlled trials of radiation with or without hyperthermia. In such trials, stratification by tumor volume will be important. Thermal isodose distributions must be determined and controlled, raising issues of quality assurance (NUSSBAUM 1984).

Hyperthermia is likely to have its greatest value in treatment of bulky disease. Technical limitations in producing temperature rise greater than 42° C throughout a tumor will persist for the foreseeable future. This implies that radiation doses of proven value should be used in treating potentially curable patients rather than using reduced doses in anticipation of a radiation effect uniformly enhanced by hyperthermia.

References

Aristizabal SA, Oleson JR (1984) Combined interstitial irradiation and localized current field hyperthermia: Results and conclusions from clinical studies. Cancer Res (Suppl) 44:4757s–4760s

Astrahan MA (1982) A localized current field hyperthermia system for use with 192 iridium interstitial implants. Med Phys 9:419–424

Astrahan MA, George III FW (1980) A temperature regulating circuit for experimental localized current field hyperthermia systems. Med Phys 7:362–364

Atkinson WJ, Brezovich IA, Chakraborty DP (1984) Useable frequencies in hyperthermia with termal seeds. IEEE Trans BME 31:70–75

Bicher HI, Moore DW, Wolfstein RW (1984) A method for interstitial thermoradiotherapy. In: Overgaard J (ed) Hyperthermia Oncology 1984, Vol. 1, Taylor & Francis, London, pp 595–598

Brezovich IA, Young JH (1981) Hyperthermia with implanted electrodes. Med Phys 8:79–84

Brezovich IA, Atkinson WJ, Lilly MB (1984a) Local hyperthermia with interstitial techniques. Cancer Res (Suppl) 44:4752s–4756s

Brezovich IA, Atkinson WJ, Chakraborty DP (1984b) Temperature distributions in tumor models heated by self-regulating nickel-copper alloy thermoseeds. Med Phys 11:145–152

Burton C, Hill M, Walker AE (1971) The RF thermoseed – A thermally selfregulating implant for the production of brain lesions. IEEE Trans BME 18:104–109

Cetas TC, Connor WG, Manning MR (1980) Monitoring of tissue temperature during hyperthermia therapy. NY Academy of sciences 335:281–297

Cetas TC, Hevezi JM, Manning MR, Ozimeck EJ (1982) dosimetry of interstitial thermoradiotherapy. Natl Cancer Inst Monogr 61:505–507

Cetas TC, Roemer RB (1984) Status and future developments in the physical aspects of hyperthermia. CA Res (Suppl) 44:4849s–4901s

Corry PM, Barlogie B (1982) Clinical application of high frequency methods for local tumor hyperthermia. In: Nussbaum GH (ed) Physical Aspects of Hyperthermia. Amer Inst of Phys. NY, pp 307–328

Cosset JM, Dutreix J, Dufour J, Janoray P, Damia E, Haie C, Clarke D (1984a) Combined interstitial hyperthermia and brachytherapy: Institute Gustave Roussy technique and preliminary results. Int J Radiat Oncol Biol Phys 10:307–312

Cosset JM, Dutreix J, Gerbaulet A, Damia E (1984b) Combined interstitial hyperthermia and brachytherapy: The Institute Gustave Roussy Experience. In: Overgaard J (ed) Hyperthermic Oncology 1984, Vol. 1, Francis & Taylor, London, pp 587–590

Coughlin CT, Douple EB, Strohbehn JW, Eaton Jr WL, Trembly BS, Wong TZ (1983) Interstitial hyperthermia in combination with brachytherapy. Radiology 148:285–288

Davies J, Simpson P (1979) Induction Heating Handbook. McGraw-Hill Book Co., London

Dewhirst MW, Sim DA (1984) The utility of thermal dose as a predictor of tumor and normal tissue responses to combined radiation and hyperthermia. Ca Res (Suppl) 44:4772s–4780s

Doss JD, McCabe CW (1976) A technique for localized heating in tissue: An adjunct to tumor therapy. Med Instrum 10:16–21

Emami B, Marks J, Perez C, Nussbaum G, Leybovich L (1984) Treatment of human tumors with interstitial irradiation and hyperthermia. In: Overgaard J (ed) Hyperthermic Oncology 1984, Vol. 1. Francis & Taylor, London, pp 583–586

Fessenden D, Lee ER, Samulski TV (1984) Direct temperature measurement. CA Res (Suppl) 44:4799s–4804s

Forsyth K, Deshmukh R, DeYoung DW, Dewhirst MW, Cetas TC (1984) Recent clinical experience in pet animals with hyperthermic therapy in the head and neck region induced with inductively-heated ferromagnetic implants. In: Overgaard J (ed) Hyperthermic Oncology 1984, Vol. 1., Taylor & Francis, London, pp 599–602

Joseph CO, Astrahan M, Lyssett J, Archambeau J, Forell B (1981) Interstitial hyperthermia and interstitial iridium 192 implantation: a technique and preliminary results. Int J Radiat Oncol Biol Phys 7:827–833

King KWP, Trembly BS, Strohbehn JW (1983) The electromagnetic field of an insulated antenna in a conducting or dielectric medium. IEEE Trans MTT 31:574–583

Li DJ, Luk KH, Jiang HB, Chou CK, Hwang GZ (1984) Design and thermometry of an intracavitary microwave applicator suitable for treatment of some vaginal and rectal cancers. Int J Radiat Oncol Biol Phys 10:2155–2162

Lilly MB, Brezovich IA, Atkinson M, Chakraborty D, Durant JR, Ingram J, McElvein RB (1983) Hyperthermia with implanted electrodes: in vitro and in vivo correlations. Int J Radiat Oncol Biol Phys 9:373–382

Luderer AA, Borrelli NF, Panzarino JN, Mansfield GR, Hess DM, Brown JL, Barnett EH (1983) Glass-ceramic-mediated magnetic-field-induced localized hyperthermia: response of a murine mammary carcinoma. Rad Res 94:190–198

Lyons BE, Britt RH, Strohbehn JW (1984) Localized hyperthermia in the treatment of malignant brain tumors using an interstitial microwave array. IEEE Trans BME 31:53–62

Manning MR, Cetas TC, Miller RC, Oleson JR, Conner WG, Gerner EW (1982a) Clinical hyperthermia: Results of a phase I trial employing hyperthermia alone or in combination with external beam or interstitial radiotherapy. Cancer 49:205–216

Manning MR, Cetas TC, Gerner EW (1982b) Interstitial thermoradiotherapy. Natl Cancer Inst Monogr 61:357–360

Manning MR, Gerner EW (1983) Interstitial thermoradiotherapy. In: Storm FK (ed) Hyperthermia in Cancer

Therapy. GK Hall Medical Publishers, Boston, pp 467–477

Matloubieh AY, Roemer RB, Cetas TC (1984) Numerical simulation of magnetic induction heating of tumors with ferromagnetic seed implants. IEEE Trans BME 31:227–234

Mendecki J, Friedenthal E, Botstein C, Paglione R, Sterzer R (1980) Microwave applicators for localized hyperthermia treatment of cancer of the prostate. Int J Radiat Oncol Biol Phys 6:1583–1588

Miller RC, Connor WG, Heusinkveld RS (1977) Prospects for hyperthermia in human cancer therapy and hyperthermic effects in man and spontaneous animal tumors. Radiology 123:489–495

Nussbaum GH (1984) Quality assessment and assurance in clinical hyperthermia: requirements and procedures. CA Res (suppl) 44:4811s–4817s

Oleson JR, Cetas TC (1982) Clinical hyperthermia with rf currents. In: Nussbaum GH (ed) Physical Aspects of Hyperthermia. American Inst of Phys, Inc., NY, pp 280–306

Oleson JR, Manning MR, Sim DA, Heusinkveld RS, Aristizabal SA, Cetas TC, Hevezi JM, Connor WG (1984a) A review of the University of Arizona human clinical hyperthermia experience. Front Radiat Ther Oncol 18:136–143

Oleson JR, Sim DA, Manning MR (1984b) Analysis of prognostic variables in hyperthermia treatment of 161 patients. Int J Radiat Oncol Biol Phys 10:2231–2239

Rand RW, Snow HD, Brown WJ (1982) Thermomagnetic surgery for cancer. J Surg Res 33:177–183

Roemer RB, Cetas TC (1984) Applications of bioheat transfer simulations in hyperthermia. Ca Res (Suppl) 44:4788s–4797s

Salcman M, Samaras GM (1983) Interstitial microwave hyperthermia for brain tumors: Results of a phase-I clinical trial. J Neuro-Oncol 1:225–236

Samaras GM (1984) Intracranial microwave hyperthermia: Heat induction and temperature control. IEEE Trans BME 31:63–69

Sim DA, Oleson JR, Grochowski RJ (1984a) An update of the University of Arizona human clinical hyperthermic experience including estimates of therapeutic advantage. In: Overgaard J (ed) Hyperthermia Oncology, Vol. 1. Francis & Taylor, London, pp 359–362

Sim DA, Dewhirst MW, Oleson JR, Grochowski RJ (1984b) Estimating the therapeutic advantage of adequate heat. In: Overgaard J (ed) Hyperthermic Oncology 1984, Vol. 1. Francis & Taylor, London, pp 359–362

Stauffer PR, Cetas TC, Jones RC (1982) System for producing localized hyperthermia in tumors through magnetic induction heating of ferromagnetic implants. Natl Cancer Inst Monogr 61:483–487

Stauffer PR, Cetas TC, Fletcher AM, DeYoung DW, Dewhirst MW, Oleson JR, Roemer RB (1984a) Observations on the use of ferromagnetic implants for inducing localized hyperthermia. IEEE Trans BME 31:76–90

Stauffer PR, Cetas TC, Jones RC (1984b) Magnetic induction heating of ferromagnetic implants for inducing localized hyperthermia in deep-seated tumors. IEEE Trans BME 31:235–251

Strohbehn JW, Bowers ED, Walsh JE, Douple EB (1979) An invasive microwave antenna for locally induced hyperthermia for cancer therapy. J Microwave Power 14:339–350

Strohbehn JW, Trembly B, Douple EB (1982a) Blood flow effects of the temperature distributions from an invasive microwave antenna array used in cancer therapy. IEEE BME 29:649–661

Strohbehn JW, Trembly BS, Douple EB, De Sieyes DC (1982b) Evaluation of an invasive microwave antenna system for heating deep-seated tumors. Natl Cancer Inst Monogr 61:489–491

Strohbehn JW (1983) Temperature distributions from interstitial RF electrode hyperthermia systems: Theoretical predictions. Int J Radiat Oncol Biol Phys 9:1655–1667

Strohbehn JW, Roemer RB (1984) A survey of computer simulations of hyperthermia treatments. IEEE-Trans BME 31:136–149

Taylor LS (1980) Implantable radiators for cancer therapy by microwave hyperthermia. Proc IEEE 68:142–149

Taylor LS, Samaras GM, Cheung AY, Salcman M, Scott RM (1982) Implantable microwave radiators for clinical hyperthermia. Radio Sci 17:125S–133S

Trembly BS, Strohbehn JW, De Sieyes DC, Douple EB (1982) Hyperthermia induction by an array of invasive microwave antennas. Natl Cancer Inst Monogr 61:497–499

Vora N, Forell B, Joseph C, Lipsett V, Archambeau JO (1982) Interstitial implant with interstitial hyperthermia. Cancer 50:2518–2523

9.3 Internal Fixation and Irradiation for Bone Metastases

Ronald L. Huckstep

CONTENTS

1 Introduction

There are many patients with secondary deposits from carcinoma, particularly carcinoma of the breast, with pathological or potential pathological fractures, who will survive for many months and sometimes years with radiotherapy and systemic therapy after their initial fracture has occurred.

Many, unfortunately, are treated in bed in hospitals and nursing homes by conservative methods instead of by an operation designed to get the patient out of bed, often walking, and usually returned home.

This is despite various references in the literature on the importance of prophylactic and therapeutic stabilization of these fractures to allow mobility for the last few months or years of life (Bennish and Hammond 1955; Devas et al. 1956; Glasko 1974; Huckstep 1969, 1977, 1976, 1983, 1985, 1987; Koskinen and Nieminen 1974; Parish and Murray 1970).

The aims of treatment of these patients should be to relieve pain, to give stable internal fixation wherever possible, to mobilize them early, and to return them to their home environment where their

Ronald L. Huckstep, M.D., Professor
The University of New South Wales
Kensington, Sydney
N.S.W., 2033 Australia

quality of life and that of their relatives will be so much better.

Many patients with pathological fractures of the hip are left untreated in the mistaken view that stability cannot be obtained by the usual pin and plate. Similarly, potential fractures of the femoral shaft or humerus are often not treated by prophylactic blind nailing, which is usually a relatively simple quick operation *before* a fracture has occurred.

Even when no fracture is seen, patients with large secondary deposits of the femur or humerus are often afraid to move the leg or arm. This is probably due to small microscopic stress fractures which are not seen on x-ray, especially if involving the calcar femoris or linea aspera of the femur. The effect of a blade plate or intramedullary nail is to give stability to these areas and often lead to a considerable increase of mobility.

This chapter is based on personal experience gained with 476 documented patients with secondary tumors treated personally from 1973 to June 1985. Two hundred patients with actual or potential pathological fractures required internal stabilization, and 153 bones in these patients were internally fixed.

2 Preoperative Assessment

The risks of operation are obviously greater in patients with multiple secondary deposits and appropriate preoperative investigations are required. These should always include a lateral x-ray of the cervical spine because of the anesthetic risks in patients with secondary deposits. X-rays of both humeri and femora should be performed, as these are common sites of undiagnosed secondary deposits, and also lateral x-ray of the lumbosacral spine and an anterior-posterior view of the pelvis. P.A. and lateral x-ray of the chest should always include the thoracic spine. Lung tomograms may also be indicated. Blood investigations should include a white cell count, erythrocyte sedimentation rate, platelet count, prothrombin index and hemoglobin. They must also include serum calcium and phosphate levels, as postoperative hypercalcemia is a common and lethal complication.

In the case of an unknown primary, serum plasma protein and alkaline and acid phosphate levels may be necessary to confirm a diagnosis of multiple myeloma or secondaries from the prostate while an intravenous pyelogram or a thyroid scan may be necessary to diagnose a suspected renal or thyroid tumor. A bone marrow biopsy may be necessary if other investigations are negative.

It is important to confirm that the bone proposed for stabilization has sufficient strength above and below the destroyed area to hold an implant, especially as bone involvement is often much more extensive than shown on radiological examinations. A bone scan with technetium on a pyro-phosphate carrier will often be invaluable in diagnosing secondaries when x-rays appear normal.

A trephine biopsy with a 2 or 3 mm core is also a simple method of diagnosing secondary deposits where the primary is unknown or the diagnosis in doubt. Most bones such as the femur are easily biopsied. The lumbar spine can also be biopsied safely with a trephine through a posterolateral approach under image intensifier or x-ray control.

Blood loss may be heavy with open operation on secondary deposits from kidney, thyroid, and multiple myeloma and adequate blood should be available, especially for operation on these deposits. Other secondaries are often remarkably avascular and any bleeding may often be stopped by plugging the neoplastic bone with methyl methacrylate bone cement after insertion of the internal fixation.

Consultation with a radiotherapist and medical oncologist is essential before operation is embarked upon by the surgeon, and the closest team work is essential in the management of these patients.

3 Principles of Operative Stabilization

Stabilization should be aimed towards the simplest and quickest available method for a pathological fracture. Methyl methycrylate bone cement is also a very useful additional method of treatment. As previously noted, there is also a definite and important place for prophylactic closed nailing particularly of the neck and shaft of the femur and of the shaft of the humerus if a fracture is imminent.

The anesthetist should be prepared to take a risk with anesthesia in those patients with potential or actual fractures provided the patient and relatives are warned of the increased danger associated with an operation.

In nearly all cases surgery should be followed by radiotherapy, chemotherapy or hormone therapy, which may sometimes be combined. If this is not done there will be local tumor progression, particularly as tumor cells will sometimes be disseminated by reaming of bones at operation. Whenever possible, radiotherapy should follow rather than precede operation as otherwise wound healing may be delayed. Bone grafts should not be inserted as these will often sequestrate following postoperative radiotherapy. Instead methyl methacrylate bone cement, or Huckstep ceramic spacers giving immediate strength, should be used (HUCKSTEP 1983, 1987).

Postoperatively, the patient should be mobilized as soon as possible, usually with full weightbearing. Some risk is justified in this early mobility as the patient's life span is limited. Radiotherapy should be commenced as soon as the wound shows signs of healing without complication. Chemotherapy, if indicated, can often be started 2 or 3 days after operation. The risk of delayed healing is often overestimated provided there is no postoperative infection. Prophylactic antibiotics are recommended in all major internal fixations.

3.1 Humeral Metastases

Secondary deposits in the humerus are common and should be treated, where possible, before a pathological fracture occurs.

In the lower humerus a simple waterproof lightweight skelecast or strut support of thermoplastic will often immobilize a fracture adequately and allow early radiotherapy (HUCKSTEP 1969, 1986).

In the shaft of the humerus, however, internal fixation is the procedure of choice. It is best carried out from above (Fig. 1) but sometimes this can be carried out from below (Fig. 2). In each case this must be followed by radiotherapy, and early union of the fracture will usually occur.

A nail introduced from above should be slightly posterior and well medial. It must also be well impacted into the head of the humerus so as not to interfere with abduction, as it seldom requires removal.

In secondary deposits of the head of the humerus immobilization with a triangular sling and radiotherapy with early active exercises are all that

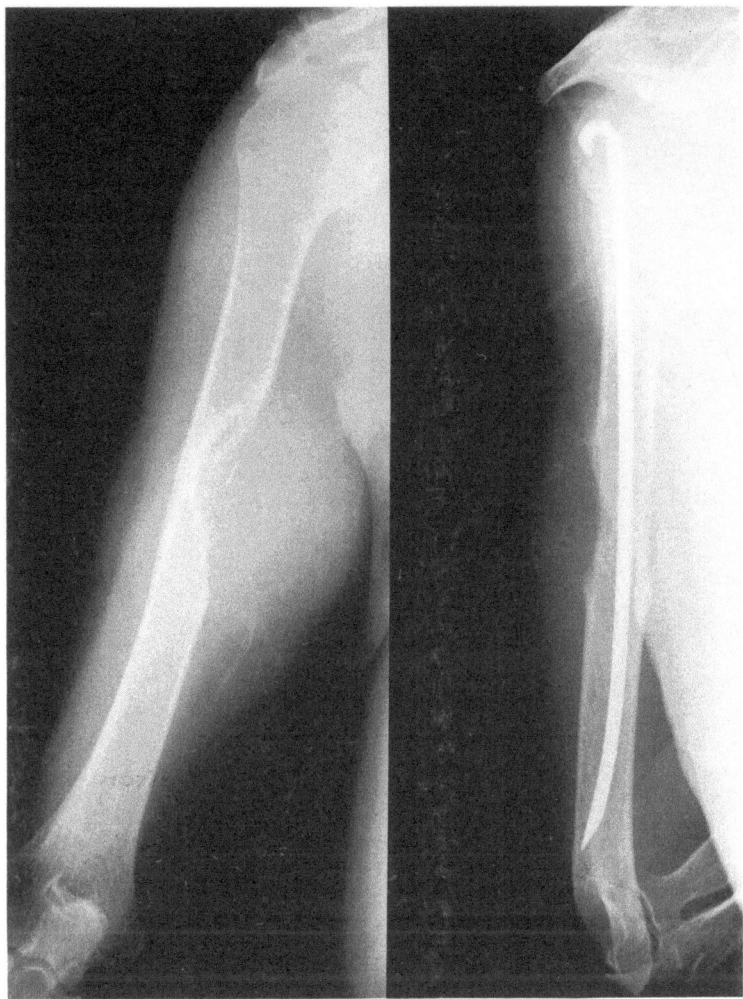

Fig. 1. Secondary deposit from carcinoma of breast in humerus. Prophylactic Rush nailing with consolidation after radiotherapy

is indicated in most cases, but there may be a place for occasional prosthetic replacement.

3.2 Spinal Metastases

Metastases to the cervical spine are common and may be asymptomatic. Prophylactic protection with a neck collar, depending on site or extent, is essential while radiation therapy is given. Operation is seldom indicated for the cervical spine except for emergency decompression for cord pressure. Secondary deposits in the thoracic and lumbar spine are also common and the patient should initially be supported with a Taylor or other type of brace or corset when there are no neurological signs. Where there is neurological involvement, however, early emergency laminectomy is essential. This should be followed by radiotherapy as soon as the wound is healed. Posterior stabilization with Harrington rods or spinal plates and ce-

ment may be indicated at the time of operation if the spine is unstable.

A newer and effective method, especially in the lumbar region, where the patient has neurological involvement, is anterior decompression and stabilization. The tumor can be curretted through a bed of the twelfth rib or by a lateral extraperitoneal approach followed by anterior stabilization with a plate and methyl methacrylate cement (Fig. 3). The discs are left intact to act as shock absorbers for the cement.

3.3 Pelvic and Acetabular Metastases

In secondary deposits in the acetabulum alone the optimal treatment is Russell traction of about 10 lbs with knee flexed over 3 pillows or with a sling and early movement under traction. Radiotherapy should be given, and the patient got up non-weightbearing or partial weightbearing with

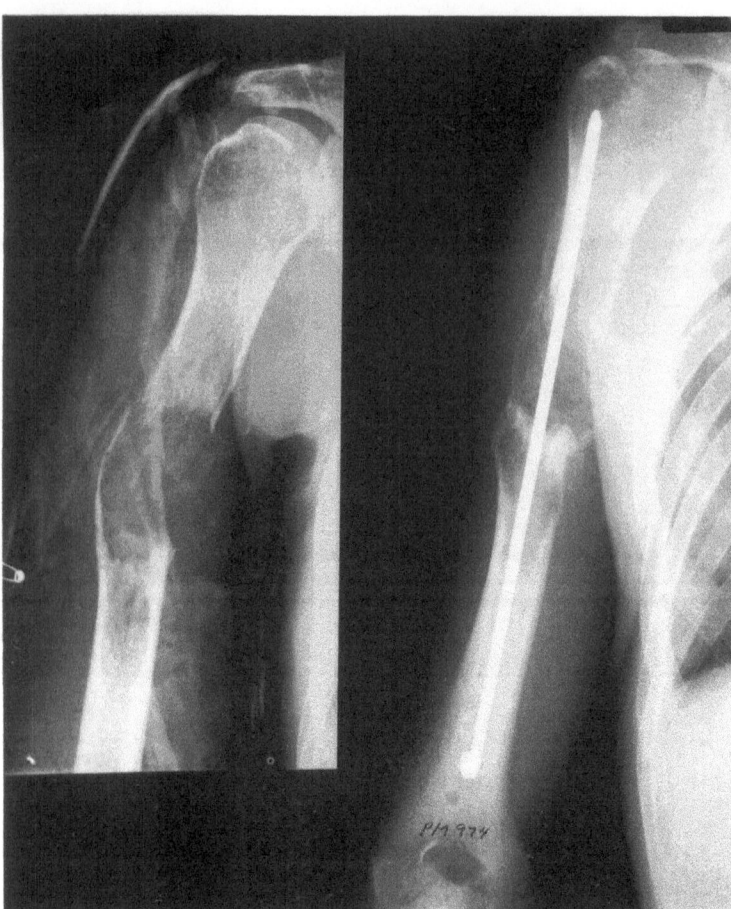

crutches as soon as pain permits. In isolated acetabular fractures, even if there is some protrusion of the head of the femur into the acetabulum, there will seldom be any severe symptoms following radiotherapy.

There is almost *no* place for replacement or reconstruction of the acetabulum except where the head of the femur is involved or fractured. A total hip replacement should then be considered, but only if the patient's condition permits. Total hip replacement is essential rather than a hemiarthroplasty if both the hip and acetabulum are affected (Fig. 4). This may occur due to multiple secondaries, or due to osteonecrosis following radiation therapy for carcinoma of the bladder or uterus. In secondary deposits the replacement should be followed by radiotherapy, but not of course for osteonecrosis alone.

Multiple secondaries in the pelvis should be treated by radiotherapy if symptomatic. The patient meanwhile should be mobilized out of bed and walking if possible with crutches. Many small

secondaries are relatively asymptomatic and surprisingly painless, and may not require treatment.

3.4 Femoral Metastases (Fig. 5)

A secondary in the upper end of the femur may require internal fixation before fracture especially if involving the calcar femoralies. Although small secondaries may not require surgery, bone involvement is always much more extensive than it appears on x-ray, and this area could weaken and fracture with radiotherapy alone. Fig. 6 shows the internal fixation of a hip with a nail, plate and cement.

In the case of involvement of the head, however, a blade plate and cement will not give adequate support. In these cases a Moore prosthesis can be used. A long-stemmed Huckstep hemiarthroplasty is preferable, however, and should be used if possible (HUCKSTER 1987). It should be several in place as there are often other secondary deposits

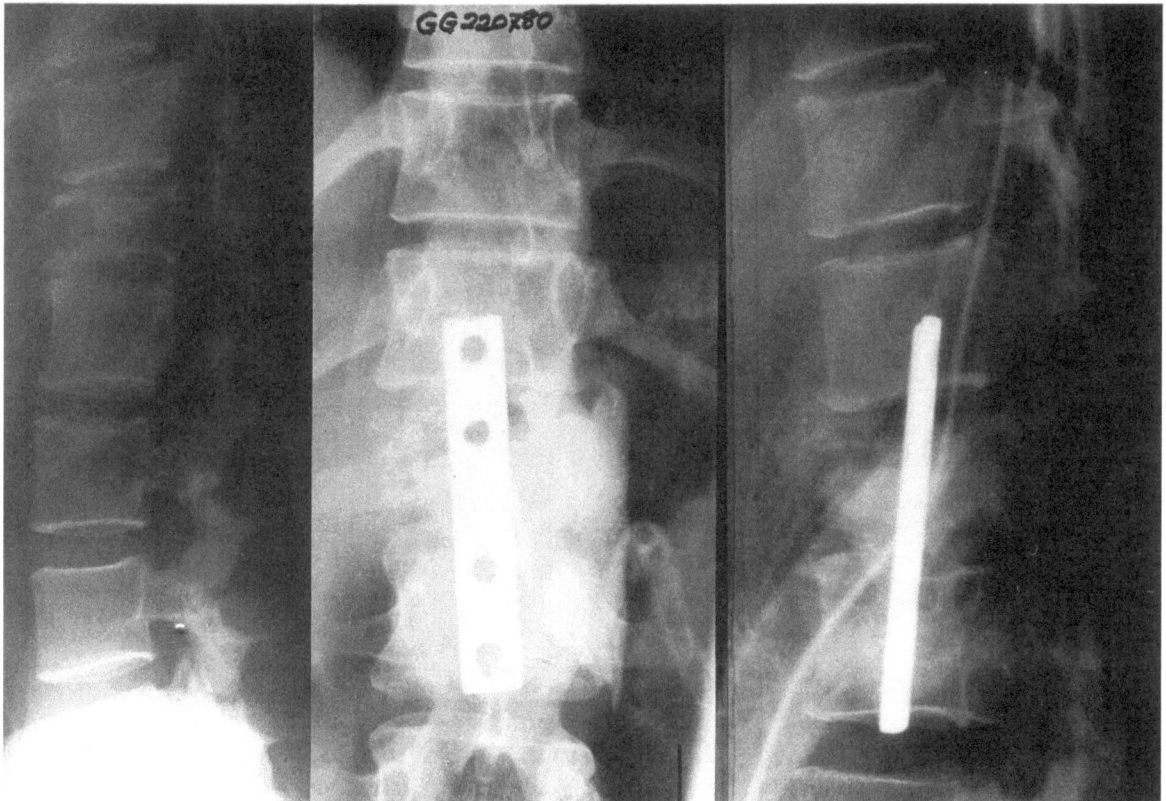

Fig. 3. Secondary deposit from breast in first lumbar verte-brae with paralysis. Anterior decompression plus stabiliza-tion with plate and cement and x-ray therapy. Walking for three years postoperatively without paralysis before recurrence

present in the shaft (Fig. 7). Alternatively a special long-stemmed titanium alloy prosthesis, can be cemented in place. This will stabilize a fracture of the hip associated with multiple areas of weakness due to secondary carcinoma.

In the past six years a ceramic hip has also been developed based on the Huckstep nail to replace the hip and shaft of the femur as a completely modular basis (HUCKSTEP 1983, 1987) (Fig. 8). The stem is coated with 200 μ porous ceramic and held in place with screws while ingrowth of bone occurs. No bone cement is required and the sleeve and spacers are porous to allow for additional bone grafts if necessary. An interchangeable ceramic aluminium oxide hemiarthroplasty or total hip can be used also.

Closed Kuntscher nailing of secondary deposits in shaft of the femur is the treatment of choice where the nail will stabilize the fracture, or before the fracture has occurred.

A special intramedullary nail with screws has, however, been developed for difficult fractures of all types where additional fixation is required. This is also ideal for difficult pathological fractures of the femur (Fig. 9) (HUCKSTEP 1983, 1985, 1987).

In the lower one third of the femur a blade plate and cement may be adequate and should be followed by radiation therapy. If union does not occur, however, the plate may fracture. Figure 10 shows an example of a large secondary deposit in the lower third of the femur which was treated initially with currettage plus a blade plate and cement. The plate and cement broke on two occasions due to non-union of the fracture. They were removed and replaced with a 60 cm Huckstep nail plus four ceramic spacers, with immediate full postoperative weightbearing with one stick.

3.5 Other Skeletal Metastases

Secondary deposits below the knee or below the elbow are uncommon. If possible they should be internally fixed with nails or plates strengthened with methyl methacrylate cement if necessary. The alternative is a simple lightweight waterproof sup-

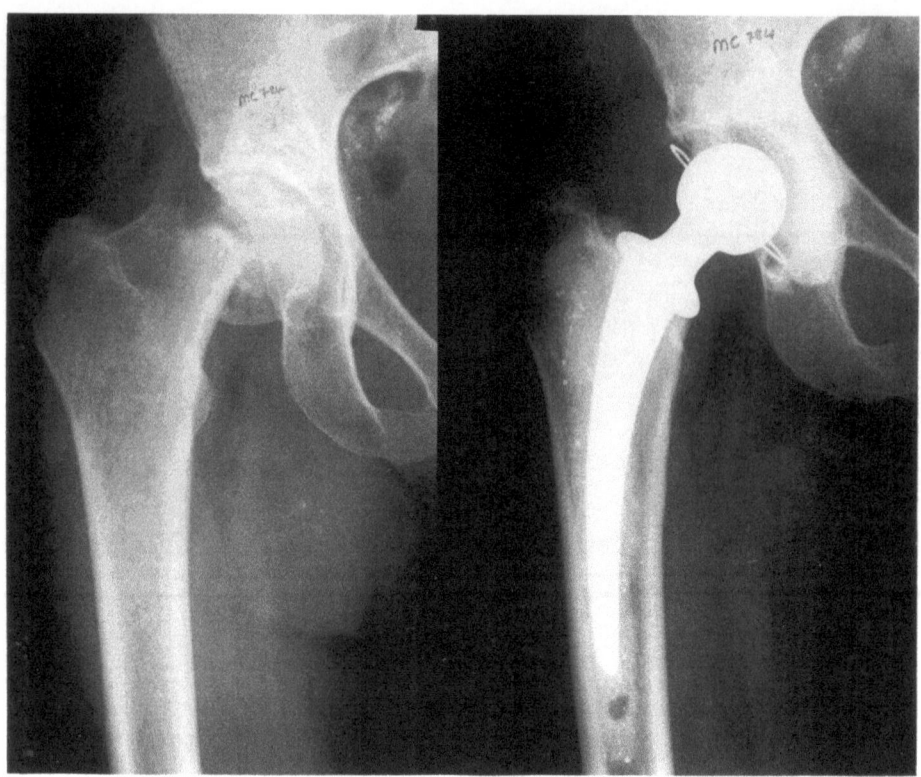

Fig. 4. Pathological fracture of hip and acetabulum following radiotherapy for carcinoma of breast treated with total hip replacement

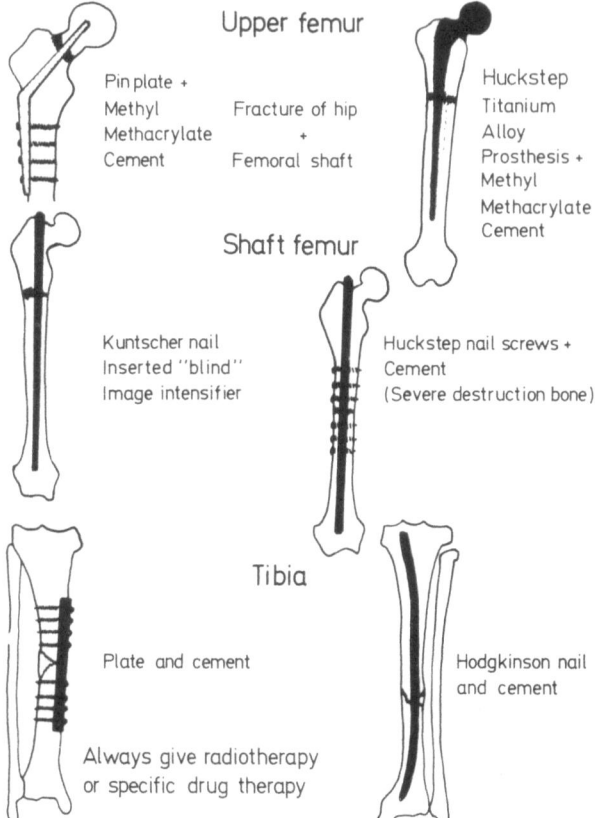

Upper femur

Pin plate +
Methyl   Fracture of hip
Methacrylate   +
Cement   Femoral shaft

Huckstep
Titanium
Alloy
Prosthesis +
Methyl
Methacrylate
Cement

Shaft femur

Kuntscher nail
Inserted "blind"
Image intensifier

Huckstep nail screws +
Cement
(Severe destruction bone)

Tibia

Plate and cement

Hodgkinson nail
and cement

Always give radiotherapy
or specific drug therapy

Fig. 5. (Reproduced with permission from Churchill Livingston, Edinburgh. HUCKSTEP RL (1986) A Simple Guide to Trauma, 4th edition)

Fig. 6. Pathological stress fracture hip. Pin, plate and methyl methacrylate cement followed by x-ray therapy

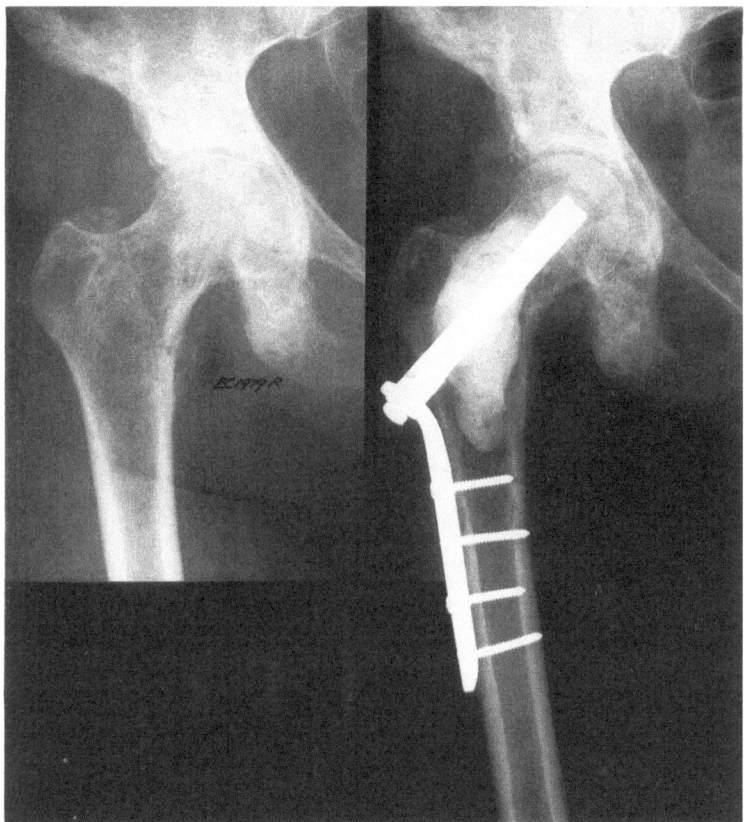

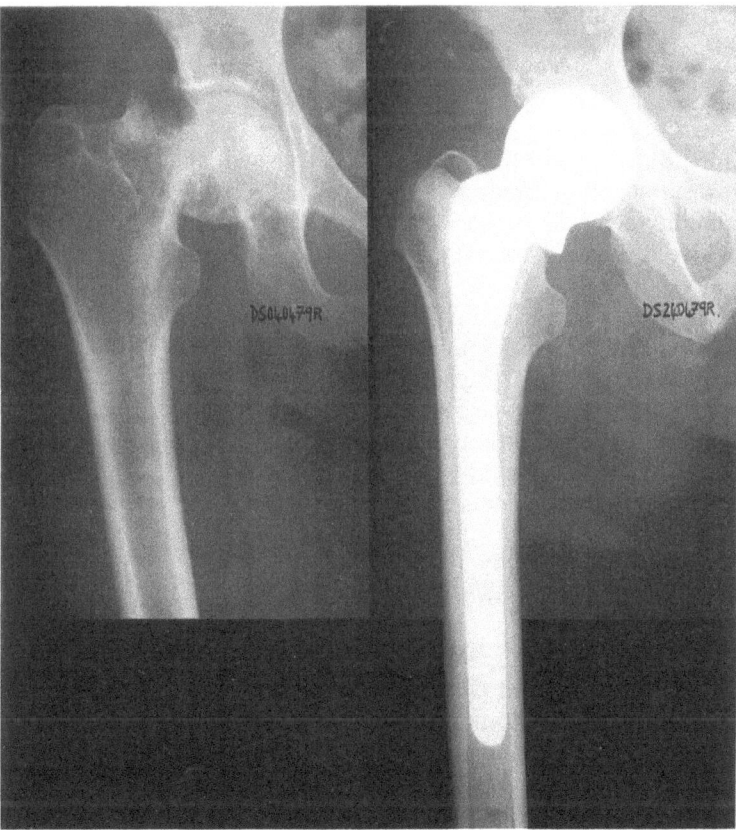

Fig. 7. Pathological fracture treated with Huckstep titanium hip

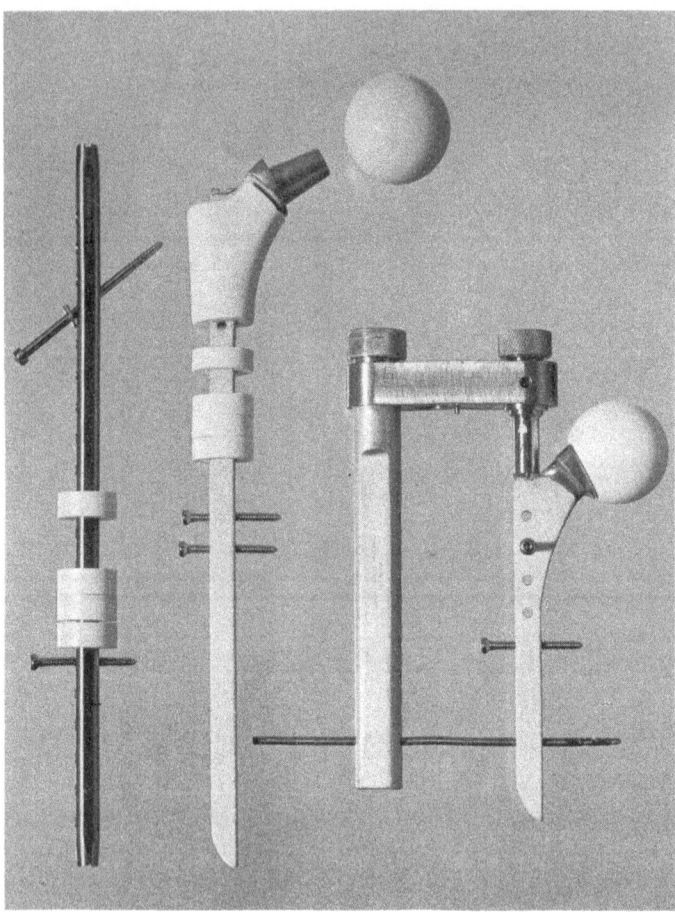

Fig. 8. Huckstep cementless ceramic and titanium alloy hip and femoral replacement. Porous ceramic coating on stem allows bone ingrowth

port (Skelecast) of fibreglass struts which will allow stabilization and deep x-ray therapy. The early mobility achieved is considerably better than that achieved with plaster of Paris and gives good stability.

Secondary deposits in other bones will often only require external splinting. These include the scapula and clavicle which only require a triangular sling and the thoracic and lumbar spine which may need a corset or brace. All, or course, should receive radiation therapy plus chemotherapy or hormone therapy if indicated.

4 Summary of Operative Techniques

Rush nailing of fractures of the shaft of the humerus can be performed closed with the help of an image intensifier. A small longitudinal lateral incision 3 cm or less in length should extend distally from the acromion. It is important to insert the nail medial enough, and just lateral to the articular

cartilage of the head. The hooked end of the nail facing laterally should be impacted into the tuberosity of the humerus so that it is flush with the bone, as it will not require removal. If any difficulty is experienced in reducing the fracture a small anterolateral incision just lateral to the biceps will allow easy manual reduction of the fracture.

Kuntscher nailing of the femur can often be performed "closed" by a small 5 cm longitudinal incision above the trochanter. The largest nail which can be inserted without excessive reaming should be inserted just medial to the trochanter and down to the level of the upper border of the patella. This should aim to stabilize almost the whole length of the shaft, as there may be multiple other involved areas in the lower shaft. Tumor will often be seen coming out of the end of the hollow Kuntscher nail when it is inserted. This tumor should be sent for histology. In the case of secondaries from the breast this tumor should be tested for oestrogen receptors. If any difficulty is experienced in reducing the fracture a small anterolateral

Fig. 9. Huckstep closed nailing for pathological fracture of femur

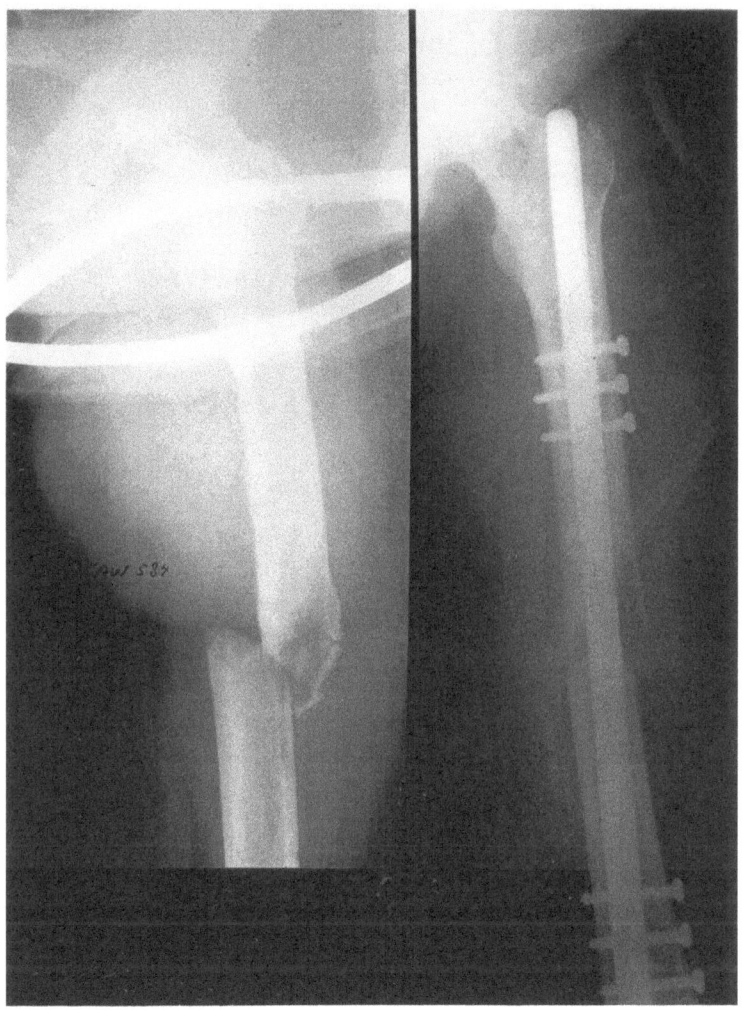

incision between vastus lateralis and rectus will quickly rectify this.

In fractures, or potential fractures, of the head or upper cervical region of the femur, excision of the head and neck should be carried out with replacement with a prosthesis. This can either be a Thompson, Moore or Huckstep titanium alloy long stem prosthesis cemented into the medullary cavity. An improvement on these is a Huckstep modular ceramic hip already discussed which is screwed into the femoral shaft with the help of a special jig to locate the screw holes without the need for x-ray control (HUCKSTEP 1983, 1987). This also has the advantage that the upper femur can be replaced with a sleeve and spacers where the trochanter or upper femur is also involved (Fig. 8).

5 Results of Treatment

A total of 253 internal fixation procedures were performed personally by the author in 200 patients with metastatic cancer from 1973 through June 1985. Table 1 shows the site of the primary tumor in 200 patients. The fixation techniques used are listed in Table 2.

The outcome of treatment by internal fixation was analyzed in detail in the first 100 patients so treated of whom 23 had more than one limb fixed. The distribution of primary sites in this series is listed in Table 3. Nearly half of these patients had primary breast cancer; they were followed for a median of 8.5 months after surgery and had a median survival in excess of 1 year. One patient survived for over 3 years following surgery. The remaining patients with primaries other than breast were followed for a median of 5 months after sur-

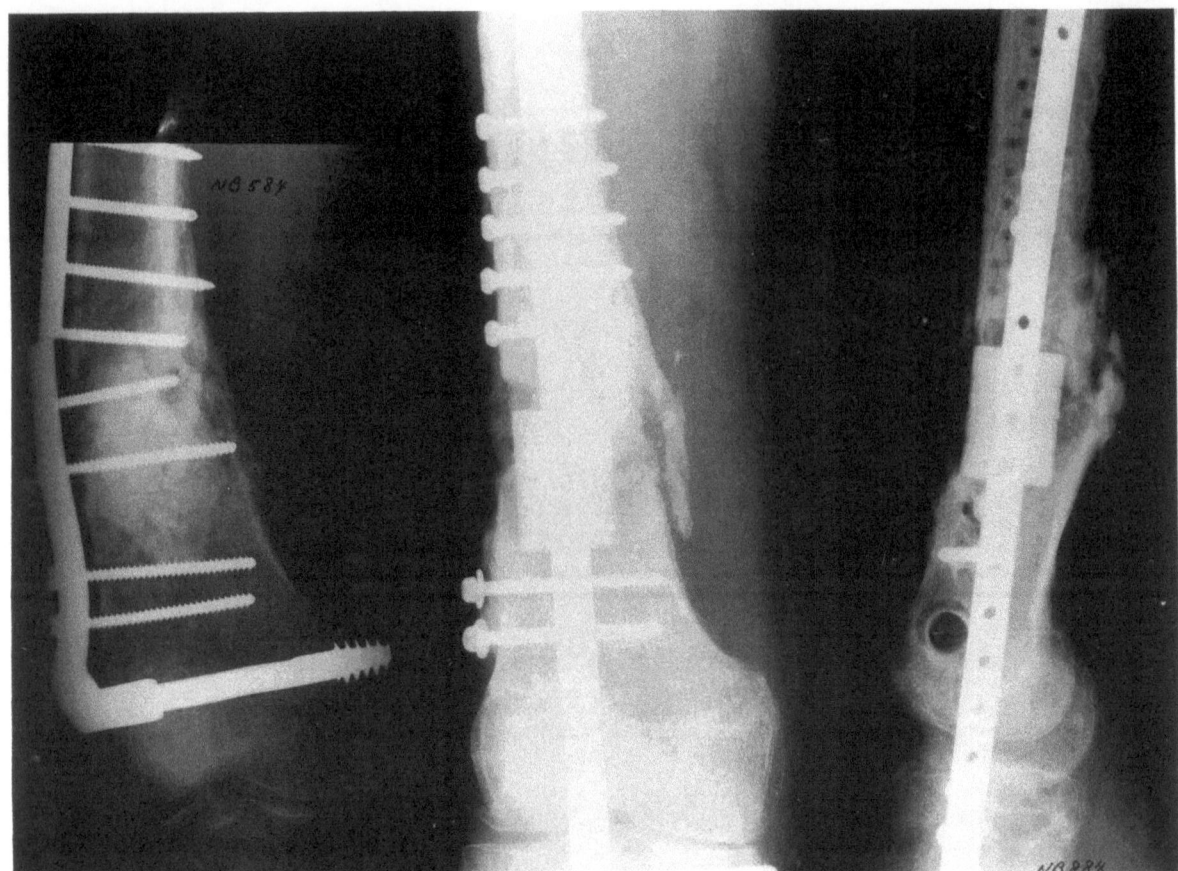

Fig. 10. Huckstep 60 cm nail and four ceramic spacers for failed blade plate and cement for renal secondary deposit of lower femur

Table 1. Primary site patients with internal fixation 1973–1985 (June) R.L.H. patients

Breast	95
Lung	16
Prostate	13
Lymphoma	6
Melanoma	6
Myeloma	8
Kidney	13
Cervix	6
Miscellaneous	25
Unknown	12
Total patients	200

Table 2. Internal fixation secondary tumors 1973–1985 (June) R.L.H. personally operated

Rush Nails to Humerus (3 bilateral)	57
Kuntscher Nail (10 bilateral)	64
Huckstep Nail	19
Huckstep Hips	7
Other Hip Replacements	35
Titanium Nails/Screws	4
Pin Plate Cement/Blade Plate	58
Plate and Cement for spine	3
Hodgkinson Nail for Tibia	1
H-Circlips/Spacers	5
Total fixations	253

Table 3. Primary site first 100 patients (68 female – 32 male) with internal fixation

Breast	47
Lung	9
Lymphoma	9
Kidney	7
Prostate	5
Melanoma	3
Thyroid	2
Myeloma	2
SCC	2
Miscellaneous	7
Unknown	7
	100

Table 4a. Prophylactic internal fixation in first 100 patients

Time to walk (Post-operative)	3 days
Average hospital stay (which includes about 2 weeks of radiotherapy and/or chemotherapy)	30 days

Table 4b. Internal fixation of actual fractures in first 100 patients

Average time to walk (Post-operative)	7 days
Average hospital stay (which includes 3–6 weeks of radiotherapy and/or chemotherapy	40 days

Table 5. Complications in first 100 patients

Hypercalcaemia (All died within 6 weeks)	4
Cardiorespiratory Failure	3
Intraoperative Haemorrhage (Renal Cell Carcinoma)	2
Wound Infection	2
Acute Renal Failure	1
Thrombocytopenia	1
Pulmonary Embolus	1
Obstructive Jaundice	1
	15

gery and had a median survival in excess of 8 months. Details of hospitalization for patients treated prophylactically for impending fractures and for those treated for stabilization of actual pathologic fractures are set out in Table 4. The length of hospitalization was determined primarily by the need for radiation therapy and/or chemotherapy postoperatively. From the surgical point of view, the average requirement for hospitalization was approximately 2 weeks.

6 Complications

The complications occurring in the first 100 patients are set out in Table 5. Fifteen patients sustained operative complications of which 8 were fatal. This included 4 patients who developed postoperative hypercalcemia, emphasizing the importance of preoperative assessment and careful postoperative monitoring. In the second 100 patients, the operative mortality rate was only 4%.

On discharge from the hospital, the great majority of patients were walking and pain free.

7 Conclusions and Summary

In conclusion it is stressed that the treatment of these patients with actual and potential pathological fractures requires a fairly bold approach. The benefit from the treatment of such patients is considerable even if the risks of operation are relatively high.

Ninety two percent of the patients in the first hundred internally fixed returned home or to a nursing home walking, and in the second hundred patients the percentage was 96%.

Early prophylactic fixation of potential and actual pathological fractures is therefore a very worthwhile procedure, despite the risks. It is recommended that the estimated life span be at least 6 weeks before operation. It is also essential that adequate preoperative investigations are carried out, such as serum calcium estimation, and that an analysis of other potential fractures, including the cervical spine, be performed preoperatively.

Acknowledgements. I should like to thank Churchill Livingstone for permission to reproduce Figure 5 from my book, "A Simple Guide to Trauma, 4th edition, 1986".

I should also like to thank Drs. S. QUAIN, B. COURTENAY, A. SARIC, G. FETTKE, G. CAMERON, J. FULLER and various other research workers for correlating the statistics, and Mrs. DAWN DENNIS for secretarial assistance. The Cancer Council of New South Wales for research assistance.

References

Bennish EL, Hammond G (1955) The treatment of actual and imminent pathological fractures of femur by intramedullary nailing. Surg Clin Am 35:865

Devas MB, Dickson JW, Jelliffe AM (1956) Pathological fractures: treatment by internal fixation and indications. Lancet ii:484

Glasko CSB (1974) Pathological fractures secondary to metastatic cancer. Clinical Orthopaedics and Related Research

Huckstep RL (1969) Skelecasts. A concept of lightweight immobilization. East Africa Med J 46:604

Huckstep RL (1976) Early mobilization of patients neoplastic bone diseases. J Bone Jt Surg 56B:262

Huckstep RL (1977) Early mobilization and rehabilitation in orthopaedic surgery and fractures. Australia and New Zealand J of Surg 47:344

Huckstep RL (1983) Huckstep Intramedullary Compression Nail and Ceramic Hip, 3rd edition, Yennora Press, Sydney

Huckstep RL (1985) Intramedullary compression. In: Seligson D (ed), Concepts in Intramedullary Nailing, Grune & Stratton, New York

Huckstep RL (1986) A Simple Guide to Trauma, 4th edition, Churchill Livingstone, Edinburgh

Huckstep RL (1987) Stabilization of prosthetic repleasement in difficult fractures of bone tumours. Clinical Orthopaedics of Related Research

Koskinen EVS, Nieminen RA (1974) Surgical treatment of metastatic pathological fractures of major long bones. *Acta Orthop Scand* 44:34

Parrish FF, Murray JA (1970) Surgical treatment for secondary neoplastic fractures. J Bone Jt Surg 52A:665

Subject Index